The Prevention of Dental Disease

THE PREVENTION OF DENTAL DISEASE

Second Edition

•

Edited by

J. J. MURRAY

Professor of Child Dental Health,
University of Newcastle upon Tyne

Oxford New York Tokyo

OXFORD UNIVERSITY PRESS

Oxford University Press, Walton Street, Oxford OX2 6DP
Oxford New York Toronto
Delhi Bombay Calcutta Madras Karachi
Petaling Jaya Singapore Hong Kong Tokyo
Nairobi Dar es Salaam Cape Town
Melbourne Auckland
and associated companies in
Berlin Ibadan

Oxford is a trade mark of Oxford University Press

Published in the United States
by Oxford University Press, New York

First published 1983
Second edition 1989
Reprinted (with corrections) 1990

British Library Cataloguing in Publication Data
The prevention of dental disease.—2nd ed.
1. Preventive dentistry
I. Title
617.6'01

ISBN 0-19-261807-5
ISBN 0-19-261806-7 Pbk

Library of Congress Cataloging in Publication Data
The prevention of dental disease
(Oxford medical publications)
Includes bibliography and index.
1. Preventive dentistry. I. Murray, John J.
II. Series. [DNLM: 1. Preventive Dentistry.
2. Tooth Diseases—prevention & control.
WU 113 P944151] RK60.7.P7133 1989 617.6'01 88-28902
ISBN 0-19-261807-5
ISBN 0-19-261806-7 (pbk.)

Printed in Great Britain by
Butler & Tanner Ltd, Frome

PREFACE TO THE SECOND EDITION

In the five years since the first edition was prepared the impetus for the prevention of dental disease has increased. Reviews of the book have been generally favourable, but in some cases pointed out areas that might have been included in a text on the prevention of dental disease. Most reviewers appreciated that the aim was not to provide details of clinical techniques but rather to concentrate on documented evidence. This general aim has been maintained; chapters on dental health education, root caries and other problems affecting the dentition in middle and old age, and the difficulties involved in preventing dental disease in handicapped persons have been added. The chapter on fissure sealants has been expanded so that the question of cost-effectiveness of preventive techniques can be considered in greater detail. The downward trend in dental caries in developed countries has been reviewed, together with a consideration of changes in child and adult dental health over the last 20 years, as found by results from national surveys. The implications of providing a preventively orientated service to deal with rapidly changing levels of oral disease are considered against a background of dental services that have developed from a curative base.

I am most grateful to Mr J. R. McCarthy, Chief Dental Adviser, Dental Estimates Board, for providing me with details from the Board's Annual Reports, to Ms Diana Scarrott, Under Secretary, British Dental Association, for information on the General Dental Services, and most especially to Miss Sally Baldwin, who has been responsible for the secretarial work involved in compiling this second edition.

Newcastle upon Tyne J. J. M.
September 1988

PREFACE TO THE FIRST EDITION

THE Survey of Children's Dental Health in England and Wales in 1973 showed that over 90 per cent of our children leave school with untreated dental disease and over 50 per cent have had at least one general anaesthetic for dental treatment. This high level of dental disease seems to have been accepted with equanimity by the public at large, as though it were inevitable. It means that in adult life, at best a large amount of repair is required to maintain teeth in the mouth, at worst, that decayed teeth must be extracted. The extent of the problem can be judged by the fact that 30 per cent of all adults aged 16 years and over in Britain have no natural teeth at all.

And yet, and yet. Are things changing?

Over the last ten years there has been an increasing emphasis on good dental health and a number of encouraging reports, not only from Britain, but also from America, Australia, Scandinavia, and other European Countries that dental caries is decreasing in children. The idea is gaining ground that dental disease is not inevitable, but preventable and that the possibility of keeping one's teeth for life is not just for the lucky few but is possible for almost everyone.

I was delighted to be given the opportunity of trying to draw together some of the main factors involved in the prevention of dental disease and am most grateful to my colleagues for agreeing to contribute the various chapters which make up this book. We do not attempt to cover all dental disease but concentrate on the prevention of dental caries and periodontal disease in order to draw together the available clinical and epidemiological information. In many instances we have referred to previous publications and have reproduced diagrams from other workers: due acknowledgement is made in the text. We would also like to thank our publishers for their help and encouragement. If our present knowledge could be translated into practice the impact on dental health would be immense and the practice of dentistry would change considerably. We hope that this book will help in some small way to encourage the movement towards prevention.

Newcastle upon Tyne J. J. M.
January 1983

To provide the opportunity for everyone to retain a healthy functional dentition for life, by preventing what is preventable and by containing the remaining disease (or deformity) by the efficient use and distribution of treatment resources.

Aim of the Dental Strategy Review Group,
Towards Better Dental Health HMSO 1981

CONTENTS

The plates for Chapter 6 fall between pages 244 and 245
The plates for Chapter 9 fall between pages 308 and 309

CONTRIBUTORS

F. P. ASHLEY
Professor of Periodontology and Preventive Dentistry,
UMDS Guy's Hospital,
London

J. F. BEAL
Department of Community Dental Health,
Leeds Eastern and Western Health Authorities

W. M. EDGAR
Professor of Dental Science,
The University of Liverpool

P. H. GORDON
Department of Child Dental Health,
University of Newcastle upon Tyne

W. M. M. JENKINS
Department of Periodontology,
Glasgow Dental Hospital and School

E. A. M. KIDD
Department of Conservative Dental Surgery,
UMDS Guy's Hospital,
London

J. R. E. MILLS
Emeritus Professor of Orthodontics,
Institute of Dental Surgery,
Eastman Dental Hospital,
London

J. J. MURRAY
Professor of Child Dental Health,
University of Newcastle upon Tyne

M. N. NAYLOR
Professor of Preventive Dentistry,
UMDS Guy's Hospital,
London

J. H. Nunn
Department of Child Dental Health,
University of Newcastle upon Tyne

A. J. Rugg-Gunn
Professor of Preventive Dentistry,
Departments of Oral Biology and Child Dental Health,
University of Newcastle upon Tyne

P. Sutcliffe
Professor of Preventive Dentistry,
University of Edinburgh

A. W. G. Walls
Department of Operative Dentistry,
University of Newcastle upon Tyne

1

Introduction

J. J. MURRAY

THE mouth contains a number of different tissues, some of which, such as mucous membrane, connective tissue, blood vessels, nerves, muscle, and bone, are found throughout the body. Any of these tissues can suffer from infection, trauma, degeneration, or neoplastic change, although fortunately oral cancer is fairly uncommon. Of overwhelming importance to the condition of the mouth are its two specialized tissues—the teeth and the periodontal structures. Indeed dental caries and periodontal disease are so widespread that virtually everybody in the world, certainly every adult, has either one or both of these conditions.

The cost of dental treatment in the General Dental Services in England and Wales in 1980 was over £410 million (figures from Dental Estimates Board, England and Wales—Annual Report 1980 (by kind permission of Mr N. R. Elwis)). Half of this was spent on restoring teeth that had been attacked by dental caries, and nearly £70 million on the provision of dentures to replace teeth extracted because of dental caries or periodontal disease. Six years later the cost of treatment for General Dental Services had increased to £753 million (Table 1.1), but the pattern of expenditure on various items had hardly changed at all. Table 1.1 also shows that the cost of restoring teeth had dropped by 3 per

Table 1.1. Cost of various items of dental treatment in the General Dental Services of the National Health Service in England and Wales. (Source—The Dental Estimates Board 1985)

	1980		1985		1987	
	£m	per cent	£m	per cent	£m	per cent
Examination and X-rays	65	16	101	15	125	17
Restoration of teeth	199	49	307	46	356	47
Dentures, bridges etc.	69	17	122	18	136	18
Periodontal treatment	46	11	90	14	81	11
Extractions, other surgical treatment (except periodontal) and general anaesthetics	14	3	19	3	23	3
Orthodontic treatment	14	3	22	3	23	3
Other items	3	1	7	1	9	1
Total	410	100	668	100	753	100

cent and the cost of treatment of periodontal disease had increased by 3 per cent over a 5-year period.

In addition the cost of treatment carried out by dental practitioners, the cost of the Community Dental Services and the Hospital Dental Services, and to a much smaller extent the cost of dentistry in the Armed Forces and in industry, all of which are difficult to quantify, must be considered in any estimate of the total cost of dental disease in Britain, which must have reached £1 billion in 1987.

It has been reported that in terms of a single specific illness or disease the cost of dentistry is second only to the cost of mental illness and is greater than direct National Health Service expenditure on conditions such as pregnancy or the treatment of heart disease, bronchitis, or tuberculosis (Office of Health Economics 1969).

A considerable amount is known already about how to prevent both dental caries and periodontal disease. If put into practice this would affect dramatically their prevalence or at least would slow down the rate at which they progress, so that the vast majority of people would be able to keep their teeth, in reasonable condition, for the whole of their lives. At present, in Britain, only one adult in every thousand is caries free, and 25 per cent of adults aged 16 years and over have no natural teeth at all—they have to rely on plastic dentures for the rest of their lives. This is, in part, due to attitudes of the general public to the importance of good dental health, and also to the attitudes of dentists in their management of dental disease.

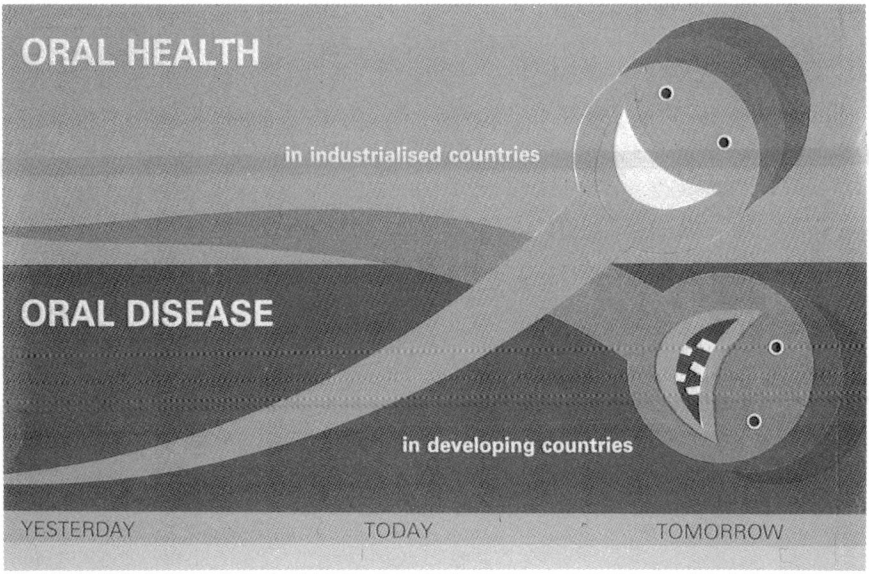

Fig. 1.1. 'Healthy mouths for all by the year 2000'—part of a World Health Education poster. (World Health Organization 1984).

Although the prevalence of dental diseases and the provision of dental services varies in different countries, the same underlying general principles of prevention must apply throughout the world. The World Health Organization has pointed out the potentially disastrous consequences of the rise in dental caries in developing countries (Fig. 1.1). The provision of dental treatment consumes economic resources and requires highly trained personnel. The only possible way forward in improving dental health for all is to reduce the prevalence of dental disease.

The aim of this book is to draw together the available epidemiological and clinical knowledge on the prevention of dental caries and periodontal disease in order to highlight the tremendous improvement in oral health which could be achieved if preventive measures were put into practice.

Reference

Office of Health Economics (1969). *The Dental Services*, No. 29.

2

Diet and dental caries

A. J. Rugg-Gunn

Introduction

Diet can affect the teeth in two ways, first, while the tooth is forming before eruption and, second, a local oral effect after the tooth has erupted into the mouth. On present evidence the post-eruptive local effect would seem to be very much more important and sugar the most important dietary factor in this local effect. But although there is overwhelming evidence incriminating sugar in the aetiology of dental caries, it is impractical to eliminate sugar completely from our diet. It is therefore important to discover in what way sugar is harmful—whether there is a threshold of sugar intake, below which caries is minimal, and whether there are any particular sugary food or drinks, or any particular eating habits which are especially harmful, so that our advice may be as practical and effective as possible. Much of this chapter will be devoted to a review of the evidence relating sugar to dental caries. It should be pointed out that clinical studies relating diet and caries in human subjects are much more difficult to conduct than fluoride studies for example. It would be impossible, if not ethically unacceptable, to ask groups of people to consume strictly controlled diets, perhaps with high amounts of sugar, for a 2-year period, which is the shortest time that caries increments can be reasonably measured. Our evidence therefore comes from a number of sources—human observational sources, human interventional studies, animal experiments, plaque pH studies, and laboratory experiments, and these will be discussed in turn.

Various food items, other than sugar, have received attention such as the cariogenicity of starch, the effect of detersive (cleansing) foods, and the existence of various 'protective factors' in our diet. Since sugar, particularly sucrose, is so heavily incriminated as the major cause of caries (and other diseases as well), the search for alternative sweeteners has been active and evidence is now accumulating on their effect on caries and general health. This evidence will also be briefly reviewed.

Pre-eruptive effect

For many years dental health advice recommended that, in order to aid the satisfactory development of their children's teeth and their subsequent resistance to caries, mothers should during pregnancy eat a diet rich in calcium; phosphate; and vitamins A, C, and D, and continue feeding such a diet to the child during the time their teeth were developing. Despite the fact that much of the evidence on which this advice is based is now some 40 to 60 years old, it is still unclear whether pre-natal and infant diets have any appreciable influence on a child's future susceptibility to dental caries. The following example helps to illustrate the problem of determining the relative importance of nutritional items.

Sognnaes and White (1940) obtained detailed medical and dietary histories from a group of American children aged 4 to 13 years (mean 9 years) and their parents. Fourteen children were caries free (CF) and 18 caries susceptible (CS). The family per capita income was similar in the two groups. The mothers' condition during pregnancy was poorer in the CS group, breast-feeding was less prevalent and of shorter duration in the CS group, the child's physical condition on medical examination was poorer in the CS group, although there was no difference in the number of episodes of illness. Dental hypoplasia was more prevalent and severe in the CS group (especially in two children born prematurely), the diets at the time of the survey were lower in 'protective factors' in the CS children and higher in 'adhesive foods', vitamin D intake was lower in the CS group and between-meal eating of carbohydrates was higher in the CS group. The difficulty of separating the relative importance of these many factors in human subjects is obvious. Hence much of the evidence on pre-eruptive nutrition and caries susceptibility comes from animal experiments.

Because of its intimate involvement in calcification, the effect of vitamin D upon a tooth's structure and resistance to decay was studied fairly extensively in the 1920s and 30s. Mellanby (1923, 1937) observed that vitamin D deficiency in puppies resulted in hypoplastic teeth. She also observed that many children had hypoplastic teeth and that these tended to be more carious than teeth with sound enamel. It therefore seemed probable that vitamin D deficiency was responsible for the hypoplastic enamel which in turn resulted in decreased resistance to caries. After preliminary positive observations (Mellanby and Pattison 1928) a three-year experiment was undertaken (Mellanby 1937; Young 1937) in which three groups of Birmingham children, initially aged $9\frac{1}{2}$ years, were given dietary supplements of either cod-liver oil (rich in vitamin D), olive oil (low in vitamin D), or treacle. The children receiving cod-liver oil had statistically significantly less caries in their newly erupted teeth than those in the olive oil or treacle groups. There was also a non-significant trend towards less caries in the teeth already erupted before the experiment began. In support of her theories, Mellanby (1937) pointed out that Africans (whose skin is exposed to plenty of sun) and Eskimos (who ate an animal fat diet rich in vitamin D) had very low caries prevalence. Other experiments showed that children receiving high cereal diets developed more caries, and she suggested that this was because the cereals reduced the absorption of calcium. Mellanby's experiments suggesting that vitamin A also had a protective effect were probably invalid because vitamin D was also present in the vitamin A supplement. Recently, Harris and Navia (1980) have shown that a deficiency of vitamin A during tooth formation resulted in defective tooth structure and increased caries susceptibility, although variations in vitamin A intake after eruption are likely to be ineffective (Shaw 1949).

Not all dental workers in the 1930s and 40s agreed with Mellanby's conclusions. Bunting (1935) and Jay (1940) both working in America, stated quite clearly that they could not accept that caries could be controlled by the addition of Ca, P, vitamins, or by altering the acid/base balance of the diet, and they considered dietary sugar was very much more important. In England, Weaver (1935) also found Mellanby's evidence unconvincing. An epidemiological investigation into the caries-preventive effect of vitamin D was reported in Hungary (Bruszt *et al.* 1977). The dental health of 1017 3-6 year-old children, who had received regular vitamin D prophylaxis, was measured in 1975 and compared with the dental health of 620 children of the same age examined in 1955 and who had not received vitamin D prophylaxis. Caries experience rose from 3.8 dmft in 1955 to 5.3 dmft in 1975. However, sugar consumption in Hungary increased from 24 kg/person/year in 1955 to 38 kg/person/year in 1975, leading the authors to conclude 'that vitamin D either does not possess a protective effect against caries or that the employed vitamin D doses are not sufficient to counteract the deleterious effect of the high carbohydrate consumption.'

Experiments of Howe *et al.* (1933) suggested that vitamin C might be protective, while Hawkins (1932) advised a diet high in vegetables to increase the alkalinity of the diet; these were however considered post-eruptive effects. The effect of protein deficiency on caries susceptibility has been investigated mainly by Navia and co-workers in America: they remark that these studies 'may help to explain the increase in dental caries incidence in technologically emerging societies' who may experience increasing sugar availability against a background of protein deficiency. In their earlier investigations, increased caries susceptibility was observed in rats whose mothers received low protein diets during pregnancy and lactation (Navia *et al.* 1970; Navia 1972). As it was possible, under these conditions, that milk production was low in quantity as well as changed in quality, further experiments were conducted which separated the effects of protein and caloric malnutrition (Menaker and Navia 1973). Specific protein malnutrition was shown to be responsible for increased caries susceptibility; the addition of protein alone was able to restore the low incidence of caries observed in well-fed rats. It is not known whether this effect is mediated directly through a deficient and more susceptible tooth structure, or indirectly through reduced salivary function.

The ratio of Ca/P in the diet has been considered by some workers. Sobel and Hanok (1948, 1958) and Sobel *et al.* (1958) showed, in rats, that a massive decrease in the ratio of dietary P to Ca results in an increase in enamel carbonate and, some ten years later, Stanton (1969) published remarkable data suggesting that the optimum dietary Ca/P ratio (by weight) is 0.57 in man. As the subjects of Stanton's study were mainly adults, it is clear that he was principally interested in a post-eruptive effect. The mean Ca/P ratio in the diet of 80 caries-free and 103 caries-susceptible patients was very similar, but the caries-susceptible subjects clearly separated into 58 patients with a low Ca/P ratio (mean 0.39) and 45 with a high Ca/P ratio (mean 0.79), while the caries-free patients had a mean ratio of 0.57. Stanton's hypothesis was tested by Rugg-Gunn *et al.* (1984) using data from a study of diet and dental caries in 405 12–14 year-old English children. The range of Ca/P ratio in this study was 0.56 to 1.04, much narrower than the range reported by Stanton (0.24 to 1.05). Nevertheless, within this range, Rugg-Gunn *et al.* found no relationship between Ca/P ratio in the diets of adolescents and their caries prevalence or two-year increment.

During and after the two World Wars, it has been reported in many countries that caries experience decreased (see p. 21). Toverud (1956, 1957), Toverud *et al.* (1961), and Sognnaes (1948) observed that there was several years delay between the use of the wartime diet and the decrease in caries prevalence and severity, and a similar delay in caries increase when the diet returned to the pre-war level. They therefore concluded that the alteration in diet (particularly sugar) was having an important pre-eruptive effect resulting in a change in the caries susceptibility of the teeth. Animal experiments in America appeared to support this view (Sognnaes 1947). Animals born from mothers fed high-sugar diets developed more caries than animals whose mothers were fed diets containing less sugar, but further experiments showed that when the ash of the low-sugar diet was added to the high-sugar diet the caries susceptibility of the offspring was much reduced (Sognnaes and Shaw 1954). The ash contained trace elements, including fluoride, and it was likely therefore that these trace elements were responsible for the difference in caries in the offspring, rather than the mothers' high-sugar diet. However, Hartles (1951) reported that a high-sugar diet in young rats resulted in higher carbonate levels and lower enamel Ca/P ratios. Luoma (1961) later confirmed that increases in blood-sugar concentration decreased phosphate and increased carbonate levels in bone and enamel.

A very large number of studies have shown that fluoride has a substantial pre-eruptive caries preventive effect (see Chapter 3). On present evidence, fluoride is by far the most important trace element, dwarfing the observed effects of molybdenum, strontium, boron, and lithium. These minerals have been associated, individually or in combination, with low caries prevalence in the United Kingdom (Anderson *et al.* 1976), New Zealand (Cadell 1964), the United States (Curzon and Losee 1978), and in New Guinea (Barmes 1969; Barmes *et al.* 1970). In contrast, selenium has been associated with higher caries prevalence. Foods (e.g. vegetables) are the main source of trace elements, and fluoride and strontium are alone in that water is the main dietary source. The evidence relating trace elements to caries prevalence has been reviewed in a book by Curzon and Cutress (1983). Most of the evidence is confined to epidemiology and animal experiments, and is very much less extensive than evidence relating fluoride to caries.

The possible influence of hardness and calcium content of water upon caries

Table 2.1. Correlations between mean caries experience (DMFT) and water fluoride concentration, water hardness, and water calcium concentration in 21 cities in America. (Data from Dean *et al.* (1942))

Bivariate correlations	
DMFT v. fluoride	−0.86*
DMFT v. hardness	−0.30
Fluoride v. hardness	+0.14
Calcium v. hardness**	+0.99*
Partial correlations	
DMFT v. fluoride (controlling for hardness)	−0.86*
DMFT v. hardness (controlling for fluoride)	−0.36

* $p < 0.01$
** for 14 cities only.

prevalence has been suggested by many but investigated by only a few, mainly in America and South Africa. In America, Mills (1937) and East (1941) reported moderate inverse relationships between water hardness and caries experience of children, but the findings of Dean *et al.* (1942) were less impressive. Waters with appreciable levels of natural fluoride tend to be hard, leading most people to conclude that water hardness is of negligible importance compared with the fluoride content of the water. This conclusion seems justified when the data presented by Dean *et al.* (1942) are subjected to partial correlation analysis (Table 2.1). It can be seen that the correlation between caries experience and fluoride level is negative and high (only linear correlations have been attempted), and is not altered when the level of water hardness is controlled. The negative correlation between caries experience and hardness is weaker (and not statistically significant), and little altered when the fluoride content of water is controlled.

However, a South African study by Ockerse (1944) contradicts this conclusion. He correlated the caries experience of 78 563 children in 109 towns and 86 districts with water hardness, pH, and fluoride content. Not only did he find high negative correlations between caries and water fluoride levels (−0.6 to −0.7), and between caries and water hardness (−0.7 to −0.8) but, by partial correlation analysis, he showed that the relation between caries and fluoride was not influenced by differences in water hardness, and that the relation between caries and hardness was not influenced by fluoride level. The extent to which Ockerse's findings are relevant to modern industrialized countries (with fairly adequate levels of dietary calcium) is unclear. The very high correlation between water hardness and calcium content can be seen in Table 2.1. Some of the South African districts have very high calcium levels in their water supplies (400 p.p.m.) capable of providing daily calcium intakes of 1 g, which is about the daily calcium requirement. Whether these dental effects of differing water hardness levels are principally pre-eruptive or post-eruptive is also unclear.

Because human milk is a better source of vitamin D than cows' milk, Mellanby (1937) recommended breast-feeding. Some reports from America suggested that 'on demand' breast-feeding may result in caries development because erupted teeth may be frequently exposed to lactose—this will be discussed further on p. 85. From the dental viewpoint, there is no evidence to go against present medical preference for breast-feeding, with the exception that since milk is very low in fluoride, fluoride supplementation might be considered if breast-feeding is the only source of nutrient and is very prolonged.

In conclusion, on present evidence it would seem clear that fluoride is the most important dietary item influencing the caries resistance of the developing tooth. Other trace elements have a smaller effect. The pre-eruptive influence of Ca, P, Ca/P ratio, of vitamins, and sugar is uncertain even after many years research, but their effect is unlikely to be great. These conclusions are supported by a recent report by Navia *et al.* (1980) of an extensive dietary survey in many Guatemalan villages. Although malnourished children had higher caries experience than moderately nourished children, the difference in caries experience between these two groups of children was less than the effect of differing levels of fluoride in the villages' water supplies.

Human observational studies

Epidemiology is concerned with observing the relationship between disease and social, environmental, and other factors. This information might then indicate possible causes and possible ways of preventing disease. Epidemiological surveys are basically observational and should be distinguished from interventional studies in which factors are purposely altered and the effect on the pattern of disease observed. Interventional studies will be considered on page 34.

World-wide epidemiology

At its crudest level, sugar intake and caries can be compared on a country basis. Marthaler (1978) compared the caries experience of 11–12-year-old children in 19 countries with annual sugar consumption data from those same countries and showed a close correlation between the two. The same type of comparison was undertaken by Sreebny (1982), who correlated the caries experience in the primary dentition (dmft) of 5–6-year-olds with sugar availability in 23 countries, and the caries experience of 12-year-olds (DMFT) with sugar availability in 47 countries. The data on sugar supplies were obtained from the Food and Agriculture Organization of the United Nations, and the caries data from the WHO Global Oral Epidemiology Bank. For both the primary and permanent teeth the correlation coefficients were positive—+0.31 for the primary dentition and +0.72 for the permanent dentition. Sreebny's data for the 47 countries are shown graphically in Fig. 2.1. On a linear regression, for each rise in sugar supply of 20 g/person/day, caries increased by 1 DMFT. For the 21 nations with a sugar supply less than 50 g/person/day, caries experience was consistently below 3 DMFT. For the 7 nations with sugar supplies greater than 120 g/person/day, in 6 nations caries experience was over 5 DMFT and in 1 nation between 3 and 5 DMFT. For the 19 nations with sugar supplies between 50 and

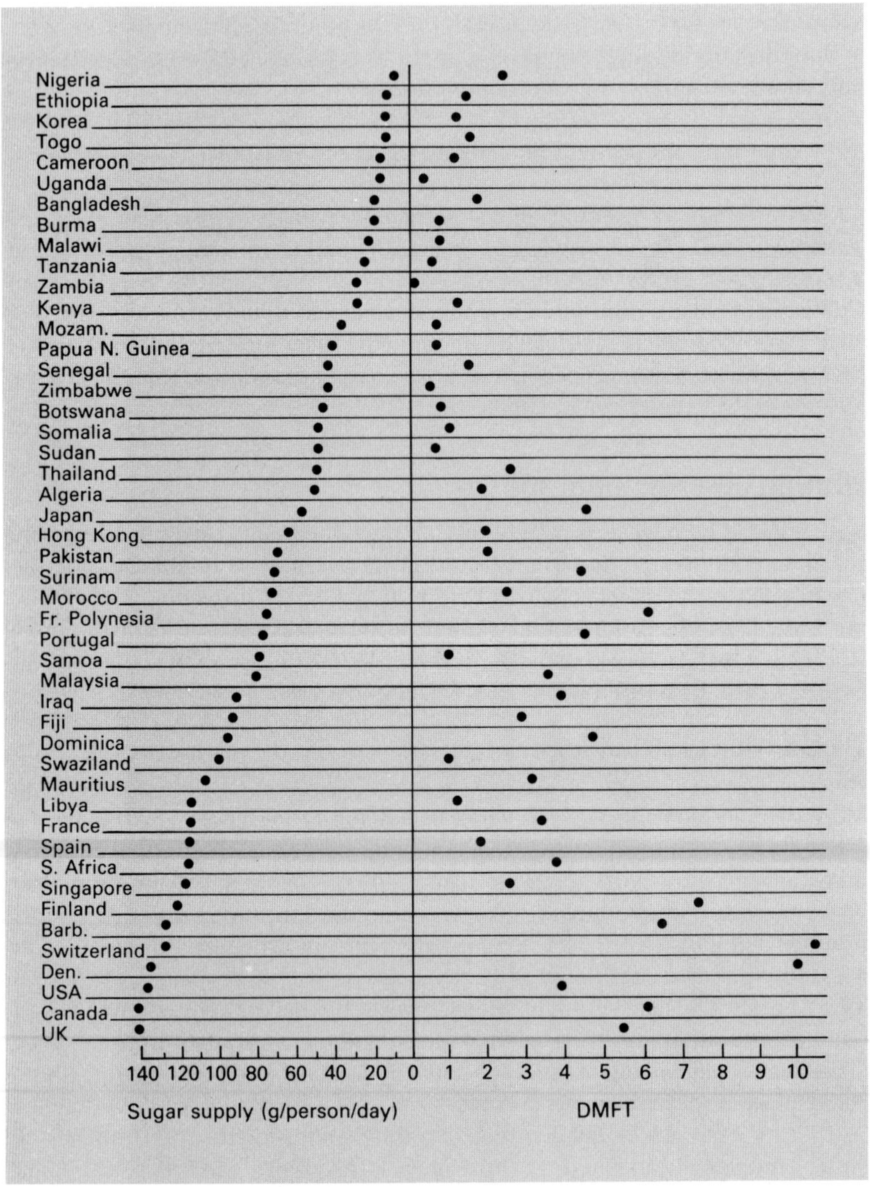

Fig. 2.1. Caries experience (DMFT) of 12-year-old children and sugar supply (g/person/day) in 47 countries. (Data from Sreebny (1982).)

120 g/person/day, caries experience was below 3 DMFT in 9 nations, between 3 and 5 DMFT in 9 nations, and above 5 DMFT in 1 nation. It should be appreciated that this type of epidemiological comparison is imperfect as sugar availability figures do no refer specifically to 5- or 12-year-olds, and both caries levels and sugar consumption will vary widely within each country. Sreebny (1983) published similar data comparing cereal availability and caries, and these results will be discussed on page 75.

Caries experience in groups of people before and after increase in sugar consumption

The consumption of sugar is a fairly recent phenomenon in many areas of the world. For one reason or another, isolated communities have become exposed to increased trade with 'westernized' countries and have subsequently adopted their high-sugar diet. In some of these communities, it is fortunate that the caries status of the population was recorded before as well as after the increase in the availability of sugar.

Eskimos

Numerous reports have stated that Eskimos living on their natural diet have low caries experience (Zitzow 1979), but that their dental health declined rapidly after exposure to a westernized lifestyle including a high-sugar western diet (Price 1936; Moller *et al.* 1972; Mayhall 1975, 1977; Curzon and Curzon 1970, 1979). Results of one such survey will be given to illustrate this point.

Between 1955 and 1957, Bang (1964) observed the dental health and diet of Alaskan Eskimos in three communities. The inhabitants of two of these (Point Ley and Point Hope) had traded with 'white' people for many years and weekly mail-planes brought in food supplies including flour, sugar, and candy. In the third community (Anaktuvuk), although a small trading store was opened in 1953, the import of foodstuffs was very much less, and it was observed that the young children tended to eat the imported food. The inhabitants of Anaktuvuk were examined again 8 years later (Bang and Kristoffersen 1972). In the intervening period three more stores had opened and a weekly mail-plane service had been established so that by 1965 only 20 per cent of the food was native. The caries experience of inhabitants of these communities is given in Table 2.2. All examinations were by the same examiner. A low caries experience, particularly in the adults, was observed in Anaktuvuk in 1955/57, compared with Point Ley and Point Hope. However, by 1965, caries experience in the deciduous dentition had increased to the very high levels previously observed in Point Ley and Point Hope. Caries experience in permanent teeth had also increased but had not reached levels seen in Point Ley and Point Hope. The change in the proportion of carbohydrate, fat, and protein consumed by the Anaktuvuk inhabitants between 1955/57 and 1965 can be seen in the lower part of Table 2.2: carbohydrate had replaced half the protein previously consumed in 1955/57.

Greenland has the largest group of people of Eskimo descent. Dental caries

Table 2.2. Caries experience in three Alaskan Eskimo communities

	Point Ley	Point Hope	Anaktuvuk	
Age group	(1955/56)	(1956/57)	(1955/57)	(1965)
1½–5 years (dmft)	7.2	9.8	4.1	10.3
6–12 years (DMFT)	2.4	4.2	0.7	2.4
13–19 years (DMFT)	9.1	9.4	1.3	1.9
20–29 years (DMFT)	10.6	12.3	1.6	4.9
30–39 years (DMFT)	15.4	11.5	0.0	6.3
Number examined	49	148	75	75
Per cent contribution to calories	Protein		33	15
	Fat		41	40
	Carbohydrate		26	45
			100	100

Stores (replenished weekly) had been established in Point Ley and Point Hope many years before 1955. Although a small, infrequently replenished store opened in Anaktuvuk in 1953, three new stores (replenished weekly) were opened there between 1957 and 1963.

used to be virtually unknown (Pedersen 1938). However, by 1977, the mean dmfs of 7-year-olds was 20 and the mean DMFS of 14-year-olds was 19. These figures are amongst the highest in the world (Jakobsen 1979).

Bantu

Osborn and Noriskin (1937) dentally examined 609 Bantu from the Transkei area of South Africa, who had had little previous contact with Europeans. Details of their usual diet were obtained by questioning. The caries experience of the Bantu eating diets containing various types of food were compared. According to the authors, machine-ground mealie meal, European bread, sugar, nuts, green tea, and coffee were associated with higher caries experience. The greater number of types of sugar-containing foods eaten, the greater the caries experience. In addition, the authors concluded that sugar-cane and unprocessed wheat contained a 'protective agent' that is lost in the refinement of these foods.

Nearly 40 years later, Retief *et al.* (1975) reported that Africans living near Johannesburg had very much lower caries experience than the white, coloured, or Indian inhabitants of Johannesburg despite a very similar sugar intake in all four racial groups. This general finding of differences in caries levels between races in South Africa being unrelated to any difference in sugar consumption or eating habits has been the theme of a number of articles by this group of workers. Their study populations have been infants (Richardson *et al.* 1981*a*), pre-school children (Richardson *et al.* 1978, 1981*b*; Cleaton-Jones *et al.* 1981, 1984), and older schoolchildren (Walker *et al.* 1981). Richardson *et al.* (1984) point out that changes in caries levels in different racial groups living in the Johannesburg area between 1976 and 1981 were unrelated to changes in sugar consumption. They suggest that dietary factors other than sugar (possibly fibre) and racial differences should be considered as reasons for the observed differences in caries experience. However, surveys in the United States and United

Kingdom have revealed that when negroids are exposed to the same dietary environment as Caucasians, the caries experiences of the two races are similar. Also, Enwonwu (1974) reported that privileged Nigerians had as high caries experience as Europeans. The reasons, therefore, for the different caries experience in the different racial groups in South Africa remains obscure.

Sudan and Ethiopia

Emslie (1966) examined 995 persons, 645 of whom were between 16 and 19 years of age, in many areas of the Sudan. Caries experience was generally low, but higher in Khartoum and Omdurman, where sugar consumption was also high (Fig. 2.2).

Olsson (1978, 1979) examined 1700 persons in Arussi province, Ethiopia, and 200 children in private schools in Addis Ababa. Caries experience of persons under 40 years of age was low (1.61 DMFT) in Arussi in 1974 but higher than that observed 16 years previously by Littleton (1963) (0.3 DMFT). This increase in caries experience paralleled the increase in sugar consumption in Ethiopia, which rose from 1.2 kg/person per year in 1958 to 4.2 kg/person per year in 1974. Olsson also reported that caries experience was statistically significantly higher in persons using sugar in tea and coffee (2.2 DMFT) compared with those who did not (1.7 DMFT). Caries experience in Addis Ababa children was about twice as high as similarly aged children in the less developed Arussi province. The use of sugar in tea or coffee and the eating of candy was reported to be much more prevalent in the previleged Addis Ababa children.

Ghana and Nigeria

MacGregor (1963) examined 468 six-year-olds, 516 12-year-olds, and 592 adults in nine areas of Ghana and found caries prevalence was highest in the 12-year-olds, indicating a rapid rise in caries prevalence in that country. Between 1950 and 1960 the import of sugar into Ghana increased over fourfold and the import of sugar confectionery increased by over sixfold but, despite their wider availability, sugar and confectionery remained luxury foods enjoyed by the more affluent. Caries prevalence was highest (59 per cent) in people with a good living standard, 46 per cent in people with fair living standard, and lowest (28 per cent) in those with a poor living standard; according to MacGregor, correlating well with their ability to buy sugar products. Of those children and adults who said they regularly ate sweets, 62 per cent had caries and 42 per cent severe caries, while only 24 per cent of those not eating sweets had caries. MacGregor concluded that it is difficult to see what other factors, other than the increased use of refined carbohydrates, could explain the increased prevalence and the pattern of caries in Ghana.

Sheiham (1967), in a survey of 4888 children and adults in 1964, observed that caries prevalence was very low in Southern Nigeria—98 per cent were caries-free. However, between 1966 and 1975 sugar consumption in Nigeria increased 27-fold, from 0.06 to 1.64 kg/person per year, and Enwonwu (1974)

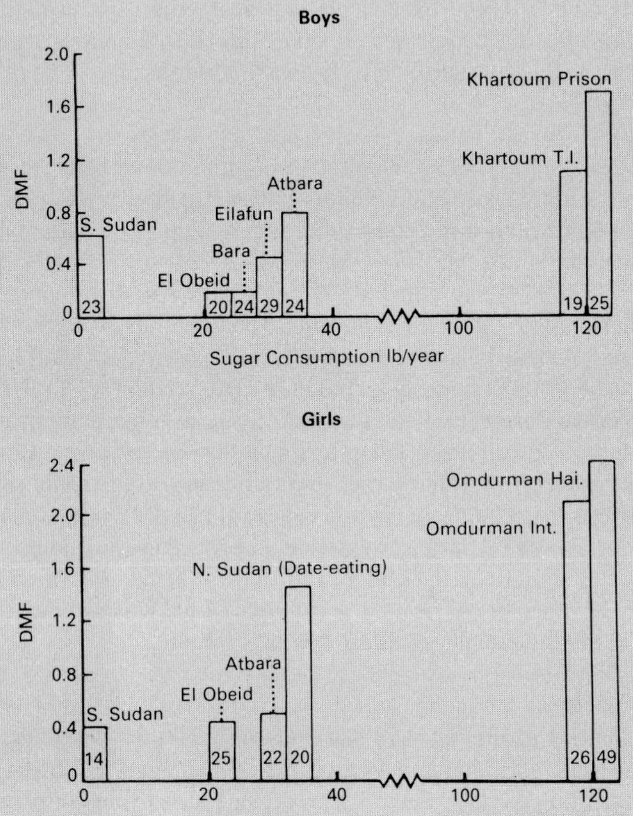

Fig. 2.2. Caries experience (DMFT) for adolescent boys and girls from regions of Sudan with different sugar consumption. (Emslie (1966), with permission of the editor *British Dental Journal.*)

recorded that privileged urban Nigerians had a similar sugar consumption and similar caries experience to western Europeans, although sugar consumption and caries were still very much lower in rural Nigeria. Henshaw and Adenubi (1975), in a survey of 1396 people of all ages in North Nigeria, observed caries prevalence to be highest in the 20- to 29-year age-group, indicating a rapid rise in caries in this population, and the consumption of confectionery between meals to be widespread. Akpata (1979) found that the caries experience of a sample of 820 Lagos secondary-school children was higher (about 1.3 DMFT) than that recorded by Sheiham (about 0.3 DMFT) 12 years earlier, although the

Table 2.3. Consumption (g/person per day) of sugar- and flour-containing foods in Tristan da Cunha. (Fisher (1968))

	1938	1966
Sugar	1.8	150
Cakes and Biscuits	0.5	24
Jam and condensed milk	0.2	20
Bread	1.7	
White flour		110
Sweets and chocolates	0	50

figure was still low by Western European standards. This low level of caries did not last long. A well-conducted study in Ondo State, Nigeria, found that between the years 1977 and 1983, the mean dmft of 5-year-olds rose from 0.8 to 2.0, and the mean DMFT of 12-year-olds rose from 0.1 to 2.2. In both age-groups the higher social-class children had substantially more caries than children from lower social classes (Olojugba and Lennon 1987).

Ojofeitimi *et al.* (1984) reported that the caries prevalence of 60 10-13-year-old children attending fee-paying schools was significantly higher than that of 120 children attending non-fee-paying schools in Ile-Ife, Nigeria. The frequency of consumption of sweets, biscuits and cakes was much higher in the children attending the fee-paying schools.

Island races

Baume (1969) reviewed data on the caries and nutritional status of the inhabitants of many of the Pacific islands and reported on the examination of 12 344 4- to 19-year-olds in French Polynesia. He observed that the variation in caries experience between islands coincided with their nutritional status. Caries experience was highest in those islands who had abandoned their traditional low-sugar diet for high-sugar imported foodstuffs.

Hankin *et al.* (1973) found a high caries experience in 910 13-year-old children in Hawaii. In all three racial groups (Hawaiian, Japanese, and Caucasian) caries experience increased with increasing frequency of eating candy and gum.

The island of Tristan da Cunha

Tristan da Cunha is a remote, rocky island in the south Atlantic, 1500 miles west-south-west of Cape Town. The inhabitants, approximately 200, are of mostly European origin and have only occasional contact with the outside world. Because of a volcanic eruption, the islanders were evacuated to England between 1961 and 1963. Prior to 1940 their diet was very low in sugar, but since 1940 the island store has sold sugar and sugar-containing foods. The dramatic increase in consumption of imported sugary foods can be seen in Table 2.3. The dental health of the islanders has been recorded many times before and after the opening of the trading store in 1940. The results of the surveys (Fig. 2.3) show a very low caries experience in 1937 but a steady deterioration in

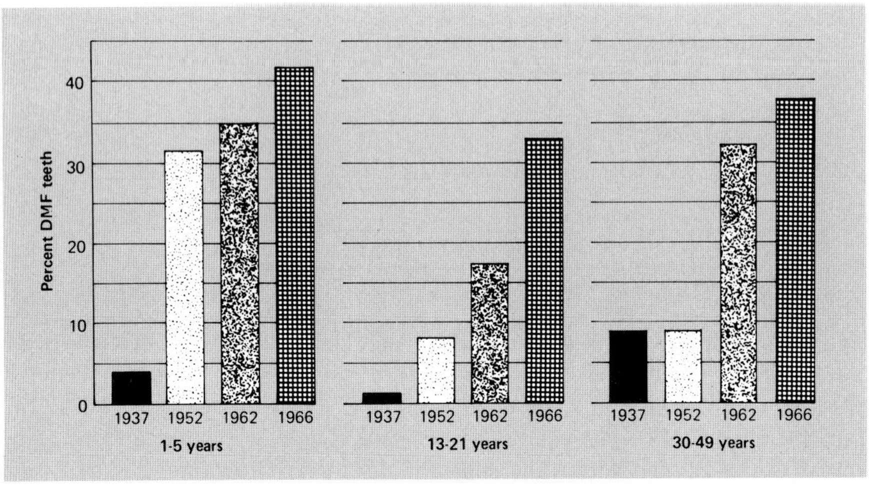

Fig. 2.3. Caries severity (per cent DMFT) in three age-groups of islanders of Tristan da Cunha at four examinations between 1937 and 1966.

their dental health since then; faster in the children than in the adults. The study is valuable in that it shows an increase in caries experience paralleling an increase in sugar consumption in the same population. In their isolated community, the major change in their lifestyle was dietary and the increase in sugar consumption was the major part of this.

England

There is probably no disease whose pattern is known so accurately throughout the ages as dental caries, as teeth are the most resistant of our tissues after death. Hardwick (1960), in a thorough review of caries prevalence in England since prehistoric times, concluded that there was a striking correlation between the consumption of refined sugars and caries incidence. He pointed out, however, that this increase in sugar consumption was accompanied by (i) a decrease in bread consumption; (ii) a rise in the extraction rate of flour; (iii) the preparation of flours, bread, and other cereal foods of finer texture; and (iv) removal of factors in the flour which might protect against caries. Figure 2.4 is taken from Moore and Corbett (1978) and shows the parallel rise in sugar consumption and caries in England over many centuries. A major reason for the rapid rise in sugar consumption during the last half of the nineteenth century (from 19 lb/person per year in 1850 to 90 lb/person per year in 1900) was the removal of duty on sugar between 1845 and 1875. The authors infer that starch may also be important in caries aetiology since they point out that repeal of the Corn Laws and improvements in milling led to substantially increased consumption of finely ground imported flour during this same period.

In conclusion, although many of the above dental epidemiological surveys

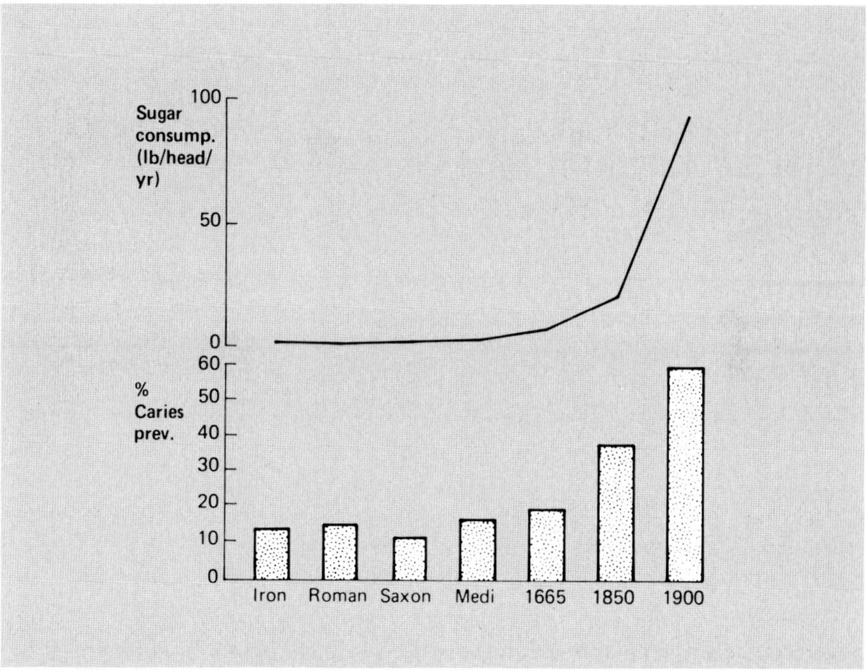

Fig. 2.4. Per cent caries prevalence related to mean sugar consumption in British populations from the Iron Age to modern times. (After Moore and Corbett (1978), with permission of Professor W. J. Moore.)

can be criticized because of poor response rates, different non-standardized examiners recording their findings over the years, and other technical reasons, it would be obdurate not to be impressed by the close parallel between the increase in consumption of sugar in many communities throughout the world and the increase in caries prevalence and severity. Some caries occurs in man in the absence of cane or beet sugar, but this is very small compared with the caries experience which occurs in populations consuming the usual high-sugar, modern European diet.

Studies on groups of people eating low amounts of sugar

Hopewood House

Hopewood House is a home in rural New South Wales, Australia, housing about 80 children of low socio-economic background. Children enter the home soon after birth and remain under close supervision until about 12 years of age when they can move to other accommodation but remain associated with the House. Dental examinations were conducted annually between 1947 and 1962, and thorough dietary surveys made (Harris 1963). The diet could be classed as lacto-

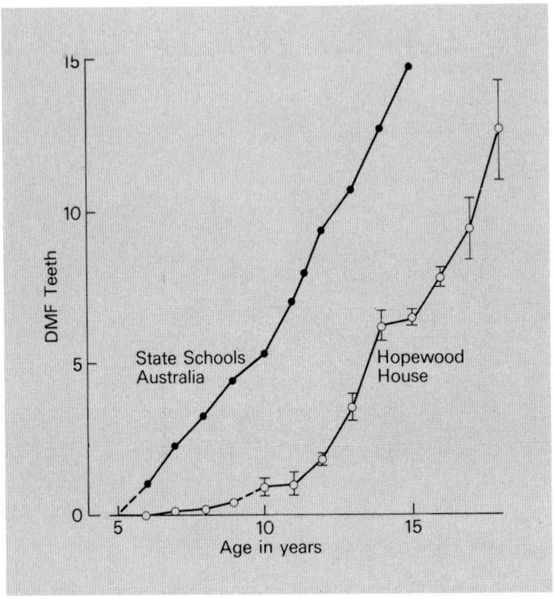

Fig. 2.5. Caries experience (DMFT) in children in Hopewood House (with SE of means) and children in state schools of South Australia. (Marthaler (1967), with permission of the editor *Caries Research*.)

vegetarian. Only wholemeal flour was used to bake bread, biscuits and make porridge, and many of the vegetables were taken raw. Protein and vitamin levels exceeded the minimum recommended level. Sugar and white-flour products were virtually absent from the diet. On the other hand, their fluoride intake was estimated to be low and oral hygiene measures were virtually absent.

The dental surveys revealed a very low prevalence and severity of dental caries, much lower than children of the same age and socio-economic background attending state schools in New South Wales, who were examined using the same methods (Fig. 2.5). Up to the age of 12 years caries prevalence was very low: 46 per cent of Hopewood House 12-year-olds being caries-free compared with only 1 per cent in the state schools. However, the rate of caries development increased in the Hopewood House children after 12 years of age (when their close supervision ended) to become virtually the same rate as observed in children in the state schools. This indicates that the diet received up until 12 years did not confer any protection from caries development in subsequent years.

Synonon Ranch community

Children in this community in California live in a boarding school environment where, 5 years before a dental survey was conducted, refined sugar was eliminated from the diet (Silverstein *et al.* 1983). It was found that 53 per cent of the 73 children aged 5 to 17 years were caries-free. The mean DMFS for 5–10-year-olds was 0.5 compared with 1.3 DMFS for the USA in general. For the age group 11–17 years, the mean DMFS was 3.3 compared with 7.0 for the USA. It should

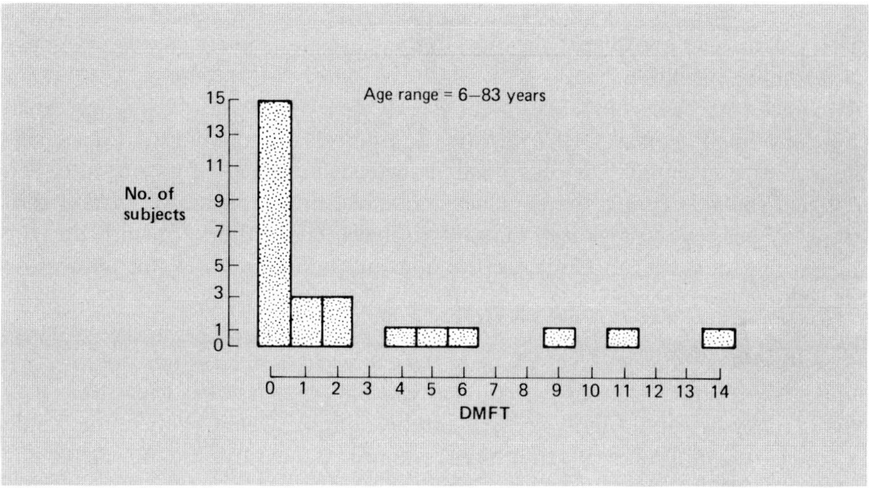

Fig. 2.6. Frequency distribution of the caries experience (DMFT) for 27 people with hereditary fructose intolerance. (Data from Newbrun (1978).)

be noted, however, that in addition to receiving a low-sugar diet, the children also received dietary fluoride supplements.

Patients with hereditary fructose intolerence

This is a rare hereditary disease caused by an inborn error of metabolism, first recognized in 1956 (Marthaler 1967). These patients do not possess a liver enzyme (fructose 1-phosphate-splitting aldolase) and ingestion of foods containing fructose or sucrose (which contains fructose) causes severe nausea. On the other hand, starchy foods (not containing fructose) are well tolerated. Marthaler (1967) and Newbrun (1978) have reviewed the dental state of 27 patients of age range 6 to 82 years (Fig. 2.6). Their caries experience was very low—15 of the patients were caries-free. Those extreme cases having DMFT of 9, 11, and 14 were aged 14, 20, and 34 years, respectively. The third patient had been made to eat sugar up to the age of 12 years. There is a need for further information on the oral status of this group of people, now that their disease is well recognized.

Diabetes

Diabetes mellitus is usually treated by insulin and dietary restriction. Although some authors have reported high caries incidence in diabetics (Wegner 1971), explained by slightly increased salivary glucose levels and reduced salivary flow, most surveys show a lower caries experience in diabetics (Starkey *et al.* 1971; Bernich *et al.* 1975). Matsson and Koch (1975) compared the caries experience of 33 dietary- and insulin-controlled diabetics aged 9 to 16 years with a group of 33 age- and sex-matched social twins. While the control children had a mean of 20.5 DFS, the diabetic children had a mean of only 13.4 DFS ($p < 0.01$); the differences being predominantly in approxial surfaces. The severe restriction of dietary sugar was considered the most likely cause of the lower caries experience in the diabetic children.

However, no such difference in caries experience was found by Sarnat *et al.* (1985). While the mean DMFT and mean carbohydrate consumption were both similar in a group of 24 controlled diabetics, aged 11–14 years, and two matched control groups, the diabetics consumed half as much sugar and consumed 17 per cent more starch than the controls. The authors conclude that the substitution of starch for sugar in the diabetics apparently did not reduce the cariogenicity of their diet.

Seventh Day Adventists

Adventists' Dietary Councils, written a century ago, advised that the use of sugar, sticky desserts, highly refined starches, and between-meal eating should be restricted. All the surveys that have compared the caries state of Seventh Day Adventist (SDA) children with other children have found lower caries experience in the SDA (see Glass and Hayden 1966). The differences are, however, small. For example, in their study, Glass and Hayden found 5.0 per cent DF surfaces in the 132 SDA children aged 9 to 11 years, compared with 6.0 per cent DF surfaces in the 158 control children.

Children of dentists

Bradford and Crabb (1961, 1963) asked British dentists to record the number of carious deciduous teeth in their own children and complete a dietary questionnaire. The caries experience of the children who were subject to full parental control of sugar consumption was less (half in the five-year-olds) than for the children who had only partial parental sugar restriction (Fig. 2.7). Low caries experience in children of dentists has also been reported in New Zealand (Ludwig *et al.* 1960) and Finland (Ainamo and Holmberg 1974) although dietary information was not recorded in these two studies. McDonald *et al.* (1981) attempted to analyse the reasons for the lower caries experience of dentists' children and concluded that dietary restriction of sugar was the most effective single method of prevention when compared with fissure sealing, topical fluoride, and toothbrushing. Although dietary habits and caries experience were strongly correlated, sugar-eating habits cannot be assumed to explain all this difference, as it is very likely that these parents took other steps to prevent caries occurring in their children.

Restrictions of sale of sweets in Australian schools

There have been two studies into the effect of selling sweets in school canteens on the caries increment of schoolchildren. Both studies were conducted in Australia and both showed that children had a lower caries increment in schools not selling sweets.

Fanning *et al.* (1969) recorded a 2-year increment of 10.9 DMFS in 981 chil-

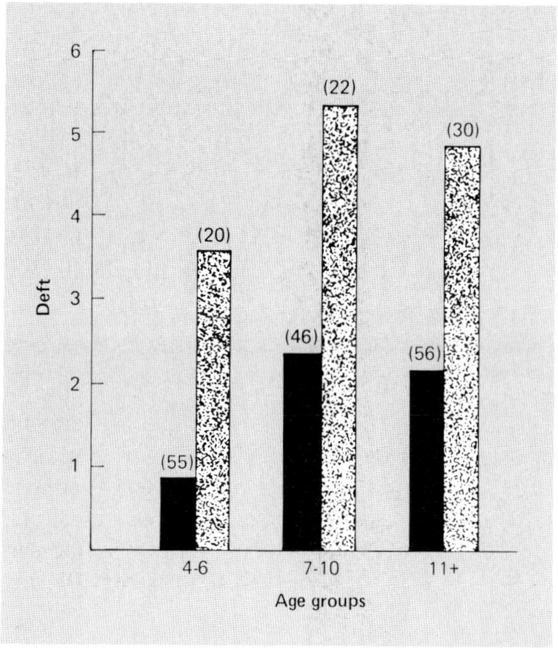

Fig. 2.7. Caries experience (deft) of children in three age groups who (a) had restriction of sweet and biscuit consumption both between meals and at bedtime (black columns); and (b) had restriction of sweet and biscuit consumption at bedtime only (stippled columns). (Bradford and Crabb (1961), with permission of the editor *British Dental Journal*.)

dren attending Adelaide secondary schools where sweets were sold, and 9.3 DMFS in 285 children attending schools not selling sweets; a difference of 1.57 surfaces or 14 per cent ($p < 0.05$). A few years later, in a further study in South Australia, Roder (1973) also recorded 2-year caries increments in children attending government or private schools. In half the schools of each type, sweets were not on sale. The 337 5- to 9-year-old children attending the government schools which did not sell sweets developed 0.9 DMFS, 16 per cent less caries ($p < 0.01$), than the same number of matched children in the schools which sold sweets. Similarly in the private schools, 314 7- to 13-year-old children in schools not selling sweets had 2.6 DMFS, 30 per cent less caries ($p < 0.01$) than matched children in the private schools selling sweets. Furthermore, the frequency with which the children attended the canteens was recorded and the frequent users of the canteens selling sweets had the highest caries increments. The profitability of the canteens not selling sweets was unchanged after removal of sweets.

War-time diets

A country at war usually experiences a reduction in availability of sugar. This was severe in Japan, for example, where sugar consumption fell from 15 kg/person per year before the Second World War to 0.2 kg/person per year in 1946. In many countries attempts have been made to relate the level of sugar consumption before, during, and after war years to the caries prevalence in children

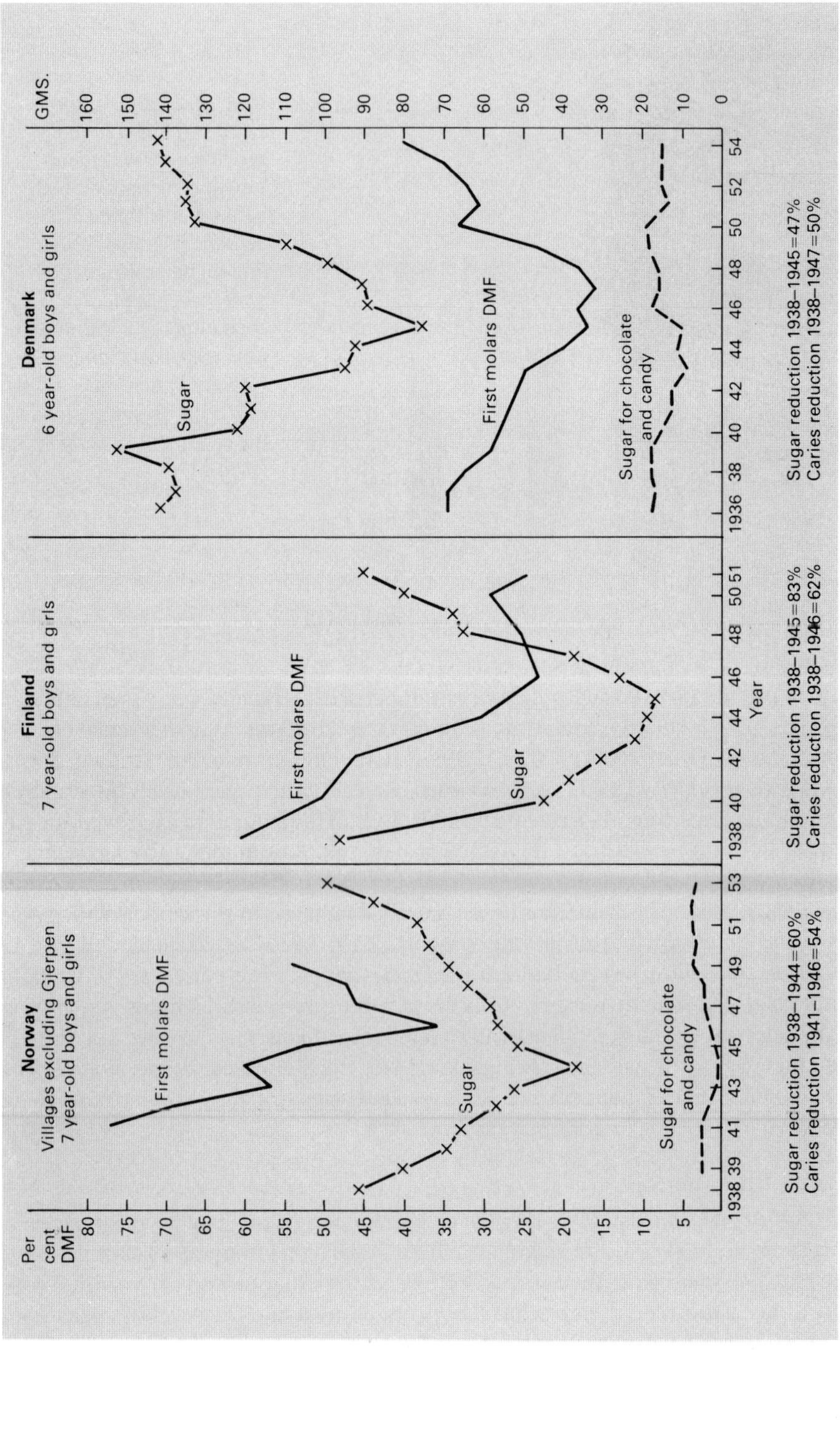
Norway
Villages excluding Gjerpen
7 year-old boys and girls
First molars DMF
Sugar
Sugar for chocolate
and candy
Sugar recuction 1938–1944=60%
Caries reduction 1941–1946=54%
Finland
7 year-old boys and g rls
First molars DMF
Sugar
Sugar reduction 1938–1945=83%
Caries reduction 1938–1946=62%
Denmark
6 year-old boys and girls
Sugar
First molars DMF
Sugar for chocolate
and candy
Sugar reduction 1938–1945=47%
Caries reduction 1938–1947=50%
Per
cent
DMF
GMS.
Year

over that period. The relation between sugar consumption and caries development in first permanent molars in children in Norway, Finland, and Denmark is shown clearly in Fig. 2.8.

One of the most thorough literature surveys was made by Sognnaes (1948), who reviewed 27 wartime studies from 11 European countries covering 750 000 children. Table 2.4 gives data from Sognnaes (1948) but only where the caries figures were given over the war years. Reductions in caries prevalence and severity were observed in all these studies. Because of the high prevalence of caries in Europeans, reductions in severity were usually greater than reductions in caries prevalence. Sognnaes (1948) observed that in many of the studies there appeared to be a delay of about 3 years between the reduction (or increase) in sugar consumption and a reduction (or increase) in caries severity. Although he accepted that sugar restriction after a tooth had erupted was a cause of the lower caries experience by a reduced intra-oral effect, he supported the views of Mellanby and Toverud (see pp. 6–7) that a reduction in sugar also influenced the forming tooth, making it less susceptible to caries after it had erupted. This viewpoint did not have much support subsequently, and Parfitt (1954), Takeuchi (1960, 1961) and Marthaler (1967) have published data in support of the view that the pre-eruptive effect of sugar restriction was unimportant.

Weaver (1950) observed a reduction in caries between 1943 and 1949 in both high- and low-fluoride areas in the north of England. Unlike many of the other surveys where there were many examiners, he examined all the children in both 1943 and 1949 (Table 2.5). Jackson (1979) has suggested that the increase in caries experience in British children after the Second World War has been negligible. However, his data show a rise in caries experience in 5-year-olds from about 4.3 dmft in 1948 to 5.1 dmft in 1963, during which time sweet consumption rose from 5.1 to 11.0 kg/person per year, and sugar consumption from 37 to 49 kg/person per yar. In common with many studies of this type, sweet and sugar consumption data are not available for the age-groups of children being studied, but only for the whole population. Knowles (1946) reported that Jersey (Channel Islands) children who had stayed on the island during the German occupation, and who consumed one-third the amount of sugar during this time than Guernsey children who were evacuated to the United Kingdom for the war years, had much better teeth than the evacuees.

Both Parfitt (1954), who re-examined Toverud's Norwegian data, and Takeuchi (1960) in Japan, pointed out that while there was a delay in the fall in caries experience per person after sugar restriction, there was no delay in the reduction in the rate at which teeth became carious; the difference being in the way the data were expressed. The Takeuchi study is very thorough and shows this point

---

Fig. 2.8. Sugar consumption (g/person/day) in pre-war, war and post-war years, and the per cent of first permanent molars decayed, missing, or filled in 7- or 6-year-old children in Norway, Finland, and Denmark. (Reproduced from Toverud (1957).)

Table 2.4. Reductions in dental caries observed in European countries following wars. (Data from Sognnaes (1948))

Country		Approx. number examined per year	Age (years)	Time period	Caries reductions (%) over time period in	
					Prevalence	Severity
England		50 000	5	1910–20	40	
Sweden		9000	7–12	1914–19	50	
Germany	(a)	30 000	6–7	1914–18	3	
	(b)	1442	6–9	1914–22	36	
France		500	4–18	1942–45	37	
England	(a)	700–1800	5	1943–45	20	
	(b)	3000	5–14	1938–45	23	
Scotland		?	5–18	1939–45	30	
Denmark	(a)	400	pre-school	1941–45	7	14
	(b)	7000	6–7	1939–45	7	40
	(c)	800	6–7	1938–45	6	
Finland		200	6	1938–45		60
		200	8	1938–45		80
Norway	(a)	300	6–7	1938–45	8	78
	(b)	10 000	8–9	1940–44	15	83
	(c)	2500	6–7	1940–44		50
	(d)	300	5–6	1939–45		35
	(d)	200–400	4–5	1939–45	22	59
	(d)	200–500	3–4	1939–45	44	76
	(e)	148	6–7	1939–46	4	48
	(e)	208	4–5	1939–46	30	63
	(e)	113	2–3	1939–46	80	87
	(f)	150	14	1939–45		35
	(f)	150	7	1939–45		73
	(g)	70–172	14	1939–46		83
	(g)	130–150	7	1939–46		61
Sweden	(a)	8000	7–12	1938–45		20
	(b)	8000	7–12	1938–45		30
	(c)	10 000	7	1941–45		17

Table 2.5. Caries experience of 5- and 12-year-old children in North Shields (fluoride-low area) and South Shields (1.4 p.p.m. F) in 1943 and 1949; 500 children in each group, all examined by the same examiner. (Data from Weaver (1950))

	5-year-olds (dmft)		12-year-olds (DMFT)	
	1943	1949	1943	1949
N. Shields	6.6	4.4	4.3	2.4
S. Shields	3.9	3.5	2.4	1.3

very clearly in data from dental charts of 7894 children born between 1929 and 1951. These were analysed using both Sognnaes (1948) method, where changes were expressed in terms of whole-mouth caries experience, and Takeuchi's own method, where the annual caries incidence rate of a tooth was measured and compared with sugar consumption. He observed no delay when

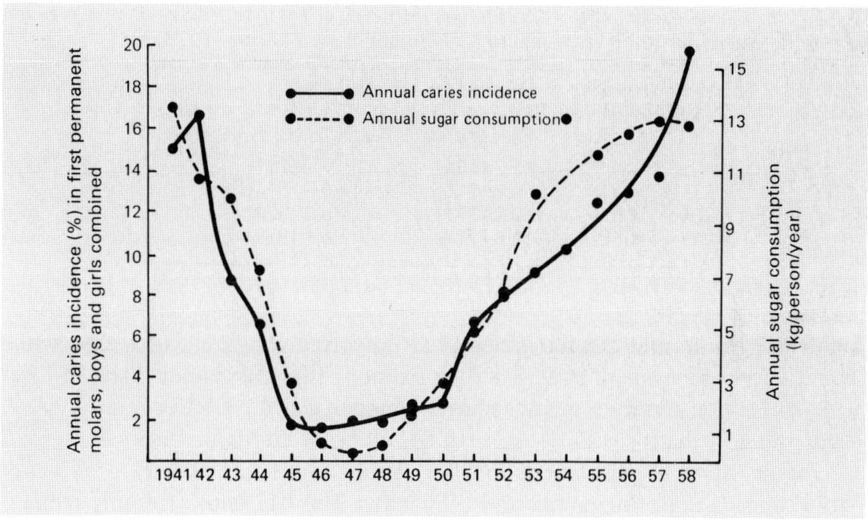

Fig. 2.9. The relation between the annual caries incidence in first molars in 7894 Japanese school children and the annual sugar consumption in Japan between 1941 and 1958. (Data from Takahashi (1961); graph drawn by J. J. Murray and reproduced with permission.)

using his own method of analysis and dismissed the idea of a pre-eruptive influence of sugar on a tooth's future caries experience. Figure 2.9 is compiled from Takeuchi's data as presented by Takahashi (1961): the close correlation between the annual caries incidence in first molars and annual sugar consumption between 1941 and 1958 can be seen clearly. This view is supported by Marthaler (1967), who provided new evidence from Switzerland as well as reanalysing Norwegian and New Zealand wartime data.

Recently, Alanen *et al.* (1985), using data collected in the 1979 Finnish National Dental Survey, suggested that the level of sugar consumption in the first few years after tooth eruption had a lasting effect upon caries experience. Sugar consumption reached a minimum in Finland in 1945. Caries experience of premolars and second permanent molars in people born in 1931–33 was significantly less than that in people born before or after these years, even after 40 years.

Groups of people with high sugar consumption

Sugar-cane chewers

There appear to have been five surveys of caries experience of people who habitually chew sugar-cane. An habitual chewer might chew 4 to 5 kg of cane per day, which could contain about 500 g of sugar. The reslts are equivocal. The two studies on Bantu workers in South African plantations (Osborn and Noris-

Table 2.6. Caries experience of adult Israelis working either in four sweet factories or five textile factories, according to their length of employment. (Anaise (1978))

No. of years employed	DFMT (no. of subjects)	
	Sweets industry	Textile industry
Up to 3	12.7 (150)	7.7 (171)
3–10	14.7 (210)	9.8 (314)
Over 10	17.3 (371)	9.3 (324)
All workers	15.6 (722)	9.1 (812)

$p < 0.001$.

kin 1937; Harris and Cleaton-Jones 1978) reported very low caries experience. Thirty-seven per cent of the 98 adults examined by Harris and Cleaton-Jones were caries-free and their mean caries experience was 3.2 DMFT.

In contrast, the three Caribbean studies all reported higher caries experience in workers in sugar plantations in Cuba (Driesen and Spies 1952; Künzel *et al.* 1973) and Jamaica (Steggerda and Hill 1936). The 147 adults (mainly white of Spanish background) in the study of Driesen and Spies had a mean DMFT of 15.1, which was similar to that reported by Künzel (16.5 DMFT) for adult white workers in Cuba.

It is unclear whether the low caries experience reported in South Africa is due to protective factors supposed to be present in raw cane sugar (see p. 81), or due to racial factors.

Workers in confectionery industry

There have been two studies comparing the caries experience of confectionery industry employees with similar groups of other workers. Anaise (1978) found the caries experience of 722 Israeli confectionery workers to be 71 per cent higher than the caries experience of 812 workers from textile factories (Table 2.6). This table also shows the increase in caries experience with increasing length of time spent in the industry was greater in confectionery workers. However, it is surprising that such a large difference in caries experience was found in those who had worked for less than 3 years, indicating that either the employees had entered the confectionery industry with abnormally high caries experience or else caries developed very rapidly after they had entered the confectionery factories. Although no consumption figures are given, it could be that confectionery consumption was at its highest level very soon after a worker joined the factory. A further study (Anaise 1980) confirmed previous results and, in addition, reported higher caries experience in production-line workers compared with non-production-line workers in the confectionery industry. The possibility that caries was caused by airborne sugar particles rather than by actual consumption should be borne in mind.

In Japan, Katayama *et al.* (1979) also found a higher caries experience in confectionery workers (17.2 DMFT) compared with age-matched workers in other industries (11.4 DMFT).

Phenylketonuria

This is a rare inherited metabolic defect in which there is a deficiency of the liver enzyme, phenylalanine hydroxylase. Unless a diagnosis is made within the first few weeks of life, and treated with special, high-carbohydrate diets which are low in phenylalanine, severe mental deficiency can occur. However, despite the fact that their diets from birth to 8 years contain about twice as much sucrose as is consumed by normal children, Winter *et al.* (1974) found that the caries experience of 105 phenylketonuric children in London and Liverpool was of the same order as that found in normal, similarly aged, London children. The reason for this lack of interest in caries experience following high sucrose ingestion is unclear.

Children taking syrup medicines long-term

Paediatric medicines are conveniently given in syrup form; almost always sucrose based. One of the first reports of syrup medicines causing damage to teeth was by James and Parfitt (1953). Roberts and Roberts (1979) compared the caries experience of 44 children, aged 9 months to 6 years (mean 47 months), who had been receiving syrup medicines for at least 6 months, with the caries experience of 47 similarly aged (mean 41 months) children who attended the same out-patient clinic but either did not take medicines or took tablets. Children receiving carbohydrate-controlled diets were excluded. There was no difference between the groups in the type of milk feeding they had received, use of dummies or other feeders, sweet or snack consumption, and the use of fluoride as tablets or toothpaste. The children taking the syrup medicines had much higher caries experience (5.6 defs) than the control children (1.3 defs).

Cross-sectional observational studies relating caries experience to the level of consumption of sugar and confectionery

There have been many cross-sectional observational studies in several countries—they are listed in Tables 2.7 to 2.9 with an attempt to indicate whether a statistically significant relationship was observed between the two parameters, sugar (or confectionery) consumption and caries.

Tables 2.7 to 2.9 were not easy to compile. Dietary information had been collected in a variety of ways; some reports subdivided confectionery into type of sweets only some of which were significantly related to caries experience. Definitions of a 'sugary food' were seldom given, which frequently made interpretation of the correlation between caries and frequency of sugar intake difficult. Some studies only looked at one aspect of sugar consumption, such as bedtime eating habits (Palmer 1971). In most of the studies, children were not selected for inclusion via their level of caries experience but, in some studies (see footnotes to tables), the eating habits of children at the two extremities of the caries experience distribution only were compared. Absolute sizes of figures for caries experience are not given as many articles only give correlation coefficients; and it should be emphasized that in some studies, although significant correlations

Table 2.7. Cross-sectional observational studies relating dental caries prevalence or experience to sugar and confectionery consumption. NS = not statistically significant and Sig = significant relation observed. Subjects aged 0–5 years

Reference	Country	Subjects No.	Age (years)	Caries Index	Dietary parameters and their relation to caries: Sugar		Confectionery		How Obtained
					Total weight	Frequency	Total weight	Frequency	
James *et al.* (1957)	UK	245	1–4	% prev. inc. car.	—	Sig¶	—	—	Int
Savara and Suher (1955)	USA	279	1–6	deft	—	NS	—	NS	Q
Weiss and Trithart (1960)	USA	783	5	deft	—	Sig*	—	—	24R
Bradford and Crabb (1961)	UK	75	4–6	deft	—	Sig†	—	—	Q
Tank and Storvick (1965)	USA	134	1–6	dmft	—	—	—	Sig‡	7 day R
Winter *et al.* (1966)	UK	200	1–5	deft§	—	Sig‖	—	NS‖	Int
Goose (1967)	UK	304	1–2	% prev. (inc. only)	—	Sig¶	NS	—	Q
Goose and Gittus (1968)	UK	6837	1–2	% prev. (inc. only)	—	Sig¶	NS	—	Q
Kato *et al.* (1969)	Japan	155	2–3	% prevalence	—	Sig	—	—	?
Winter *et al.* (1971)	UK	602	1–5	prevalence	—	Sig	—	—	Int
Holm *et al.* (1975)	Sweden	187	4	defs	—	—	—	Sig	24R
Iizuka *et al.* (1977)	Japan	247	4	dft	—	Sig	—	—	Q
Granath *et al.* (1978)	Sweden	515	4	BL and AP**	—	Sig	—	—	Int
Roberts and Roberts (1979)	UK	91	1–6	deft	—	Sig	—	—	Int
Kleemola-Kujala (1979)	Finland	167	5	dmfs§	Sig	—	Sig	NS	24R and Int
Messer *et al.* (1980)	USA	305	3–5	defs	—	—	—	NS	Q
Silver *et al.* (1987)	UK	161	3	dmft	—	Sig¶	—	—	Int

* No statistical analysis given, but strong relationship and large sample indicates significant differences very likely.
† Restriction of sweet and biscuit consumption between meals.
‡ Significant for children in fluoride-low areas only.
§ Comparison of groups with high or low caries experience.
‖ Caries highly significantly related to use of sweetened comforters but not to other sugary sweets.
¶ For sugared comforters.
** BL = buccal and lingual surfaces; AP = approximal caries; Q = questionnaire; 24R = 24-hour recall; Int = interview; 7 day R = 7 day record.

Table 2.8. Cross-sectional observational studies relating dental caries prevalence or experience to sugar and confectionery consumption. NS = not statistically significant and Sig = significant relation observed. Subjects aged 6–10 years

Reference	Country	Subjects No.	Age (years)	Caries Index	Dietary parameters and their relation to caries: Sugar		Confectionery		How Obtained
					Total weight	Frequency	Total weight	Frequency	
Sognnaes and White (1940)	USA	32	4–13	% carious t*	Sig†	Sig†	NS	—	Int
Zita *et al.* (1959)	USA	200	5–13	DMFS	NS‡	NS‡	—	—	Diary
Bradford and Crabb (1961)	UK	68	7–10	deft	—	Sig§	—	—	Q
Palmer (1971)	UK	731	7–11	dmf and DMF	—	Sig‖	—	—	Q
Bagramian *et al.* (1974)	USA	749	9	DMFS	NS	NS	—	NS	Int
Bagramian *et al.* (1974)	USA	749	9	defs	Sig¶	NS	—	Sig¶	Int
Ranke *et al.* (1974)	W. Germany	187	7–14	DFT	—	—	Sig	—	?
Granath *et al.* (1976)	Sweden	85	6	BL and AP**	—	NS	—	—	Int
Richardson *et al.* (1977)	Canada	234	6	DMFS	NS	NS	—	—	Diary
Kleemola-Kujala (1979)	Finland	186	9	DMFS*	NS	—	NS	NS	24R and Int
Hargreaves *et al.* (1980)	USA	360	5–17	DMF	NS	Sig	—	—	Diary
Silver (1987)	UK	161	8–10	dmft and DMFT	—	—	NS	—	Int

* Comparison of groups with high or low caries experience.
† Data for between-meals only given.
‡ But high correlations found between caries and weight of between-meal sugar.
§ Restriction of sweet and biscuit consumption between meals.
‖ Food or drink within 15 min of bed—majority sugar-containing.
¶ Significant when eaten as snacks, not significant when eaten at meals.
** BL = buccal and lingual surfaces; AP = approximal caries; Q = questionnaire; 24R = 24-hour recall; Int = interview.

Table 2.9. Cross-sectional observational studies relating dental caries prevalence or experience to sugar and confectionery consumption. NS = not statistically significant and Sig = significant relation observed. Subjects aged over 10 years.

Reference	Country	Subjects No.	Age (years)	Caries Index	Dietary parameters and their relation to caries: Sugar		Confectionery		How Obtained
					Total weight	Frequency	Total weight	Frequency	
Mansbridge (1960)	UK	426	12–14	DMFT	—	—	Sig	—	Int
Macgregor (1963)	Ghana	974	6–68	% prev.	—	—	—	Sig	Int
McHugh *et al.* (1964)	UK	2905	13	DMFT	—	—	NS	—	Int
Martinsson (1972)	Sweden	307	14	DFS*	Sig†	—	—	Sig‡	24R
Duany *et al.* (1972)	USA	86	12–14	DT*	—	Sig§	—	—	Int
Bagramian and Russell (1973)	USA	1486	14–17	DMFT	—	NS	—	—	Q
Hankin *et al.* (1973)	Hawaii	910	13	DMFT	—	—	—	Sig	24R × 3
Retief *et al.* (1975)	S.Africa	478	16–17	DMFT	NS	—	—	—	Q
Clancy *et al.* (1977)	USA	143	12	DMFT	—	—	—	Sig‖	Int
Richardson *et al.* (1977)	Canada	223	12	DMFS	NS	NS	—	—	Diary
Clancy *et al.* (1978)	USA	92	12	DMFT	—	—	—	Sig¶	Q
Kleemola-Kujala (1979)	Finland	181	13	DMFS*	Sig	—	Sig	NS	24R and Int
Shaw and Murray (1980)	UK	81	13–15	DMFS*	—	—	Sig	—	Int
Garn *et al.* (1980)	USA	2514	10–16	DMFT	Sig	—	—	—	24R
Hausen *et al.* (1981)	Finland	2024	7–16	DMFT	—	Sig	—	—	Q
Lachapelle-Harvey (1985)	Canada	159	12–16	DMFT	—	—	Sig	—	Diary + Q
Kristoffersson *et al.* (1986)	Sweden	388	13	DFS	—	NS	—	—	Int
Steyn *et al.* (1987)	S. Africa	100	12 W♂	DMFS	NS	NS	Sig	—	24R
Steyn *et al.* (1987)	S. Africa	97	12 W♀	DMFS	NS	NS	NS	—	24R
Steyn *et al.* (1987)	S. Africa	122	12 C♂	DMFS	NS	NS	NS	—	24R
Steyn *et al.* (1987)	S. Africa	133	12 C♀	DMFS	Sig	NS	NS	—	24R
Steyn *et al.* (1987)	S. Africa	68	12 B♂	DMFS	Sig	Sig	NS	—	24R
Steyn *et al.* (1987)	S. Africa	128	12 B♀	DMFS	NS	NS	NS	—	24R
Steyn *et al.* (1987)	S. Africa	98	12 I♂	DMFS	Sig	Sig	NS	—	24R
Steyn *et al.* (1987)	S. Africa	97	12 I♀	DMFS	NS	NS	NS	—	24R

* Comparison of groups with high or low caries experience.
† Boys only.
‡ For the majority of sugary snacks.
§ Special index used.
‖ Only significant for chocolate candy.
¶ Only for chewy candy, not for hard candy or chocolate.
Q = questionnaire; 24R = 24-hour recall; Int = Interview; W = White; C = Coloured; B = Black I = Indian.

Table 2.10. The percentage of DMF tooth surfaces for three types of teeth in 402 12–14-year old Ayrshire children according to their sweet consumption. (After Mansbridge (1960))

Teeth	Sweet consumption		
	<8 oz/week (n = 177)	>8 oz/week (n = 225)	Difference
First molars	35.8	36.5	2% more
Premolars	8.0	10.5	31% more
Second molars	13.8	16.7	21% more
Mean DMFT (all teeth)	9.60	10.83	13% more

were found, the absolute differences in caries experience were small (e.g. Mansbridge 1960, Tables 2.9 and 2.10). In other cases (e.g. Read and Knowles 1938) large differences in sugar-eating habits were observed but insufficient data given to allow their inclusion. Nevertheless, Tables 2.7–2.9 are useful as they list the studies, giving some information of their findings.

Several studies have investigated the effect of sugar in various methods of infant feeding on caries, particularly 'rampant caries' (or labial incisor caries) in the very young. Five British studies (James *et al.* 1957; Winter *et al.* 1966; Goose 1967; Goose and Gittus 1968; Winter *et al.* 1971) have all shown a strong relationship between labial incisor caries and sugared infant comforters, especially reservoir feeders. One study which did not show such a relationship was reported by Richardson *et al.* (1981*a*) in South Africa. The worldwide use of comforters and their effect on oral health has been reviewed by Winter (1980).

The two studies of Granath *et al.* (1976, 1978) are of particular interest because not only was the level of consumption of sugary foods compared with caries severity, but two other important confounding factors, fluoride supplementation and oral hygiene practices, were also considered. In both studies, diet was the most important of these factors in its relationship to dental caries and analysis showed that differences in caries experience between children with the highest and lowest between-meal sugar intake could not be explained by differences in fluoride supplementation or oral hygiene practices. The first study, on 6-year-olds (Granath *et al.* 1976), was small (179 children) and the higher levels of caries found in the children consuming more sugary foods between meals was not statistically significant. However, the second study, on 4-year-olds (Granath *et al.* 1978), was larger (515 children) and differences between the dietary groups were highly significant. When the effect of oral hygiene and fluoride were kept constant, the children with 'low between-meal sugar intakes' had 86 per cent less buccal and lingual caries and 68 per cent less approximal caries than children with a 'high between-meal sugar intake'.

The sensible approach, first used by Granath and co-workers, of attempting to quantify the importance of the three widely available methods of caries control (diet, tooth-cleaning and fluoride) has been followed by other workers, almost all Scandinavian. Advanced statistical techniques have been used to identify clinically important aetiological factors, but one important criticism of all these studies is their cross-sectional nature: this aspect of study design will be discussed later.

Hausen *et al.* (1981), in a study involving over 2000 Finnish children, aged 7–16 years, reported that water fluoride level, tooth-brushing frequency and sugar exposure were all important determinants of caries experience, although sugar exposure was the least important. Similarly, in another study in Finland, involving 543 children of three age-groups (5, 9, and 13 years), Kleemola-Kujala and Rasanen (1982) found the relation between poor oral hygiene and caries to be stronger than the relation between high sugar consumption and caries, although both were important. Again, very similar results were reported by Lachapelle-Harvey and Sevigny (1985) in a study of 159 12–16-year-old French Canadians.

Holund *et al.* (1985) found that caries-active 14-year-old Danes consumed liquid sugar drinks more frequently than caries-inactive children.

Continuing the work begun by Granath in the 1970s, Schroder and Granath (1983) found that poor dietary habits and poor oral hygiene were both good predictors of high caries in 3-year-old Swedish children. A few years later, Schroder and Edwardsson (1987) reported that the predictive ability of diet and oral hygiene could be increased by additional tests involving counts of Lactobacilli and *Streptococcus mutans*. Another Swedish group (Kristofferson *et al.* 1986) also found *Strep. mutans* counts good predictors of caries experience in 13-year-old Karlstad children. They found no difference in caries between those who ate high, medium or low levels of sugar.

Stecksen-Blicks *et al.* (1985) conducted a large survey of diet, tooth-brushing and caries experience in children of three age groups (4, 8 and 13 years) living in two northern and one southern community in Sweden. Children from the south had considerably more caries than children in the north in both deciduous and permanent teeth. The authors concluded that this difference was best explained by differences in tooth-brushing frequency and the age at which dental care started, and that the lack of observed differences in diet between north and south indicated that diet was an unimportant factor (Persson *et al.* 1984).

A large cross-sectional study in America looked specifically at the relation between the consumption of soft drinks and caries experience (Ismail *et al.* 1984). Analyses of data from 3194 Americans aged 9–29 years revealed significant positive associations between frequency of between-meal consumption of soft drinks and high DMFT scores. These associations remained even after accounting for the reported concurrent consumption of other sugary foods and other confounding variables.

Some studies have correlated caries experience with the dietary habits of the same person some years previously. Persson *et al.* (1985) found, in 275 Swedish children, that the consumption of sucrose-rich foods as 12 months of age was positively related to the presence of caries at 3 years of age. Both consumption of sugary foods and caries experience were linked to the educational status of the mother. The importance of social factors as determinants of eating habits and caries experience of young children has been highlighted in a number of studies, such as that of Blinkhorn (1982), who found caries and sugar-eating to be much higher in children from socially-deprived backgrounds in Edinburgh, Scotland.

Another study concerning past dietary experience was conducted in Hertford, England, by Silver (1987). He collected data on infant feeding and caries status at the age of 3 years, and dietary habits and caries status at the age of 8–10 years, in 161 children. There was a positive relation between 'poor infant feeding' (including the use of sugared foods and drinks) and caries experience at 3 years and at 8–10 years. Children given sweetened drinks in bottles in infancy were more likely to be consuming sugar-containing snacks at the age of 8–10 years, supporting the idea that the development of a sweet tooth in infancy persists into later childhood.

While a few of the studies (e.g. those investigating sugar intake in infant feeding) attempted to assess life-long habits of sugar consumption, nearly all the studies tried to relate caries experience at one point in time to sugar or confectionery consumption at the same point in time or, at the most, over the previous 3 to 7 days. While this approach may be acceptable for young children whose teeth have only erupted and become carious over the preceding few years and whose sugar-eating habits may not have changed appreciably since the time dentition erupted, it may not be acceptable in older age groups. For a child aged 12 years much of the caries experience will reside in the first permanent molars which erupted six years previously and may have become carious fairly soon after that. It is impossible to say that the child's sugar-eating habits had not changed between aged 6 and 12 years and it would seem unfair, therefore, to compare sugar-eating habits at one point in time (e.g. at 12 years) with caries experience over a very much longer period (e.g. 6 to 12 years). But many studies have attempted to do this. A good example of the possible effect of comparing sweet-eating habits at one point in time with lifelong caries experience can be found in the study of Mansbridge (1960). The 225 12- to 14-year-old Ayrshire children who said they consumed more than 8 oz (227 g) of sweets per week had a mean DMFT of 10.83, 13 per cent more caries experience than the 177 children who said they consumed less than 8 oz of sweets per week. The difference, although statistically significant, is of modest size. But in Table 2.10 it can be seen that there was virtually no difference in first-molar caries experience but a more substantial difference in premolar and second-molar caries experience. The first molars had erupted about 6 to 8 years before the sweet-eating habits were assessed, but the premolars and second molars had erupted less than 4 years before.

It would seem, therefore, that there is a need for studies which assess sugar-eating habits over a defined period of time and relate this to caries which develop over the same period. Only three studies appear to have done this. In two of these only 1-year caries increments were recorded and related to diet recorded at one point in time (Clancy *et al.* 1977; Stecksen-Blicks and Gustafsson 1986); the third study lasted for two years and related the 2-year caries increment to dietary intake assessed on five occasions during the same two years (Rugg-Gunn *et al.* 1984*b*). All three studies showed statistically significant positive correlations between sugar intake and caries increment.

The data collected in the study of Rugg-Gunn *et al.* (1984*b*) has been analysed fairly fully. The 405 children, initially aged 11–12 years, living in south Northumberland, England, received annual dental examinations including bitewing radiographs. Diet was recorded by each child in a 3-day diet diary, followed by an interview with a nutritionist on the fourth day. This was repeated on five occasions during the two years. The data were analysed in three ways: first, by correlating caries increment with dietary habits for all 405 subjects; second, by comparing the caries increments of children with the highest and lowest sugar intakes; and third, by comparing the diets in children who developed the highest or lowest caries increments. Correlations between diet and caries increments were generally low. The highest correlation was between fissure caries and weight of daily sugar intake (+0.146, $p < 0.01$). Multivariate analyses revealed that this relationship could not be explained by differences in sex, social class, tooth-brushing habits, or level of plaque as measured by gingival inflammation. Weight of sugar intake appeared to be more strongly related to caries than frequency of intake. The 31 children who consumed the most sugar developed 56 per cent (0.9 DMFS/person/year) more caries than the 31 children who had the lowest sugar intake. When the diets of the children who developed no caries during the two years were compared with the diets of children with the highest caries increment, the former had lower intakes of confectionery ($p = 0.05$), sugared coffee and drinking chocolate ($p = 0.05$), and higher intakes of unsugared tea ($p = 0.06$) and cheese ($p = 0.07$). Some 69 per cent of all sugar consumed came from three sources—confectionery, table sugar, and soft drinks (Rugg-Gunn *et al.* 1986).

Human interventional studies

The number of planned, interventional studies on human subjects in the field of diet and dental caries is few. This is because of the difficulties of placing groups of people on rigid dietary regimes for long periods of time. Many of the studies have involved providing daily sugar supplements to subjects—a practice which would now be considered ethically unacceptable. Nevertheless, these studies form an important contribution to our knowledge and so are discussed in some detail.

The Vipeholm studies

The Vipeholm study (Gustaffson *et al.* 1954) is probably the biggest single study in the field of dental caries ever undertaken; it lasted from 1945 to 1953 and cost SwK 596 000 up until 1951. The study was planned because it was appreciated in 1938 that the costs of the proposed Swedish Public Dental Service

Table 2.11. The Vipeholm study: Distribution of the 436 patients who completed the main study (1946–51) into the control and eight test groups. (Gustaffson *et al.* (1954))

Group	No. of subjects Male	Female	Age in 1946 (years)	Sound tooth surfaces in 1946	DMFT in 1946
Control	60		34.9	85.3	15.3
Sucrose	57		34.7	81.8	16.4
Bread—male	41		30.4	85.0	17.1
Bread—female		42	28.0	88.4	14.5
Chocolate	47		29.1	79.0	17.7
Caramel	62		35.6	87.3	15.5
Eight-toffee	40		26.3	96.9	11.7
24-toffee—male	48		31.0	88.1	15.1
24-toffee—female		39	31.1	89.1	14.1
Total	436		31.9	86.4	15.6

would be heavy. In 1939 the Government requested the Swedish Medical Board to undertake 'a general investigation concerning what means should be taken to decrease the frequency of the most common dental diseases in Sweden', since previous studies had not provided an answer to whether caries was a deficiency disease or whether it was due to the local oral effect of diet.

The Vipeholm Hospital is situated near Lund in the south of Sweden and in 1951 containing 964 mentally-deficient patients from all parts of Sweden, supervised by about 700 staff. The drinking water contained 0.4 p.p.m. F. To be accepted into the investigation a patient had to (i) be amenable to dental examinations, (ii) have no illness requiring special dietary measures, and (iii) have at least 10 natural teeth. The patients were housed in 12 wards which were largely independent; about 80 per cent of the patients were male.

The main purpose of the study was to investigate how caries activity is influenced (i) by the ingestion *at meals* of refined sugar with only a slight tendency to be retained in the mouth (non-sticky form), (ii) by ingestion *at meals* of sugar with a *strong tendency to be retained* in the mouth (sticky form, e.g. sugar-rich bread), and (iii) by the ingestion *between meals* of sugar with a *strong tendency to be retained* in the mouth (sticky form, e.g. toffees, etc.). There was one control group and six main test groups, although the 'bread' and '24-toffee' groups were both divided into separate male and female groups (Table 2.11). The groups lived in separate wards eliminating the possibility of exchange of diet between groups. Of the 633 patients examined in 1946, 436 completed the main study in 1951 (Table 2.11). In general, their caries experience was low—15.6 DMFT at the age of 32 years, compared with 18.4 DMFT found in 20-year-old Swedish army conscripts (Westin and Wold 1943).

The dental examination system was developed during the preparatory period (1945–46) and examinations were conducted each year by the same two examiners, although it is not clear which subjects were examined by which examiners. Five bitewing films were taken annually, together with models and photographs. The teeth were cleaned and dried with compressed air prior to examination. Caries was diagnosed at two severity levels, including and excluding precavitation carious lesions. Caries activity was the sum of all new primary and secondary carious lesions and new filled surfaces.

It should be appreciated that individual patients wre not randomly allocated to the different groups but rather that all suitable patients in a ward belonged to a group. This ensured minimum exchange of diet between groups (an important factor) but meant that the groups were likely to be imbalanced in certain factors which might influence caries susceptibility (e.g. age, number of sound tooth surfaces, initial caries experience). These imbalances can be seen in Table 2.11.

The study was in five parts: preparatory period (1945–46), vitamin period (1946–47), the first (1947–49) and second (1949–51) carbohydrate periods, and a post-study period (1951–53). The purpose of the vitamin trial was to find out whether differences in the amounts of vitamins ingested were capable of producing changes in caries activity. During this period all groups received an 'all-round diet', which contained half the average level of sugar in Sweden (which was 37 kg/person per year in 1946), and the diet of different groups was supplemented with vitamins, calcium fluoride, calcium lactate, or bone meal. The caries activity in all groups was very low and unaffected by the additions, although the test period was too short for adequate evaluation (less than one year).

The basal diets during the two carbohydrate periods differed from each other. In the first period it was low in sugar and contained only 1800 kcal, but this was raised to 3000 kcal by sugar supplements in the test groups, and by 150 g margarine (on bread) in the control group. However, during the second carbohydrate period the basal diet was made as similar as possible to that of an ordinary Swedish household, but because the sugar supplements (40 g margarine for the control group) continued during this second period the subjects gained weight.

The changes in dental caries experience (DMFT) in each of the groups can be seen in Fig. 2.10, which is taken straight from the report (Gustafsson *et al.* 1954, Fig. 6), and Fig. 2.11, which is compiled from their data on tooth surface caries increments including precavitation lesions. The DMFT data (Fig. 2.10) include teeth which were lost through causes other than primary caries (overall about 51 per cent of score), while only primary caries increment is included in Fig. 2.11. The dietary regime and results for each groups are given below and are shown graphically in Fig. 2.12.

Control group

These 60 males received a carbohydrate-poor, high-fat diet, practically free from sugar. Caries increment was almost nil. The increase in sugar in the second carbohydrate period was accompanied by a small but statistically significant increase in caries. Nothing was eaten between meals in any of the study periods.

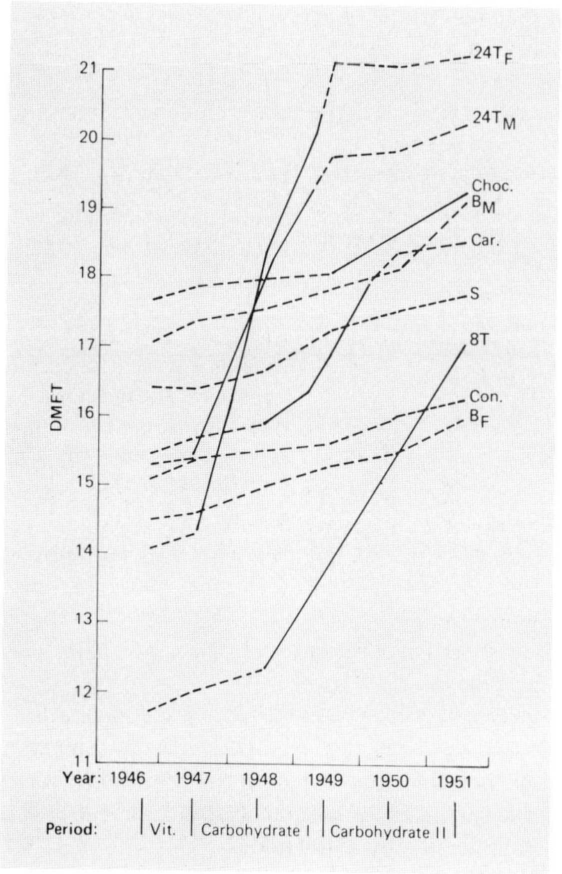

Fig. 2.10. Caries experience (DMFT) for the control group and eight test groups as recorded at the seven or eight examinations between 1946 and 1951. Solid line indicates that the subjects ate sugar both at and between meals; interrupted line indicates that subjects received sugar only at meals. (Gustaffson *et al.* (1954), with permission of the editor *Acta odontologica scandinavica*.)

Sucrose group

During the first carbohydrate period, these 57 males consumed about twice the national average level of sugar, but only at meals in solution (300 g). Sugar consumption was reduced in the second carbohydrate period to just over the national average and again only in solution in meals. Nothing was consumed between meals in any of the periods. Caries increment was slightly higher in both carbohydrate periods compared to the vitamin period but the changes were not statistically significant.

Bread groups

During the carbohydrate periods, the 41 males and 42 females consumed 345 g of especially sweetened bread (containing 50 g sugar) per day. Since the bread was fresh it had a sticky consistency. During the first period it was eaten at afternoon coffee-time only, while during the second period it was eaten at all four meals. Nothing was consumed between meals. All the males ate all their ration,

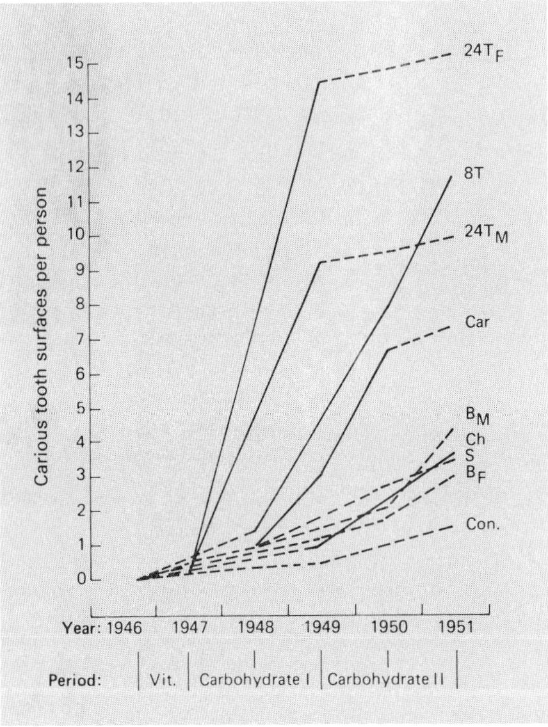

Fig. 2.11. The cumulative number of tooth surfaces attacked by primary caries only (including pre-cavitation lesions) in the control group and eight test groups, between 1946 and 1951. Solid line indicates that the subjects ate sugar both at and between meals; interrupted line indicates that subjects received sugar only at meals. (Data from Gustaffson *et al.* (1954), Table 12.)

but one-third of the females did not. This may account for the higher caries activity in the last year of the study in the males compared with the females. This moderate rise was statistically significant only in the males.

Chocolate group

During the first carbohydrate period, the 47 males consumed the same diet as the sucrose group (300 g in solution at meals). In the second period, the sugar in solution was reduced to 110 g but supplemented by 64 g milk chocolate (30 g sugar) in four portions eaten between meals. Caries increment was low in the first carbohydrate period but increased, statistically significantly, in the second period. Further analysis of the data revealed that in the patients under 30 years of age, the consumption of chocolate was accompanied by a threefold increase in caries activity, but the effect was less in the older patients.

Caramel group

The 62 males received 345 g stale sugar-rich bread during the first year of the first carbohydrate period. Caries increment was unchanged from that observed in the vitamin period. During the second year of the first period and most of the first year of the second period, they received 22 caramels (155 g containing 70 g sugar) per day; the caramels being issued between meals twice a day in the former year and four times a day in the latter. Only three of the 62 patients were reported to consume less than all their ration. The consumption of caramels was accompanied by a statistically significant increase in caries increment. This increase was so great that the caramels were withdrawn before the last year of the second carbohydrate period and replaced with an isocaloric quantity (40 g) of margarine. This withdrawal of the caramel ration without any reduction in other carbohydrates was accompanied by a fall in caries increment to its previous level.

Eight-toffee group

During the first year of the first carbohydrate period, the 40 male patients received a low-carbohydrate, high-fat diet: caries activity was low. During the second year of the first carbohydrate period and the two years of the second carbohydrate period the diet was supplemented with eight toffees (60 g containing 40 g sugar) per day. During the first carbohydrate period the toffees were issued at breakfast and after lunch and were often eaten straight away; during the next two years the toffees were issued only between meals. To bring the sugar intake to the same level as the other test groups, 250 g sucrose were taken in solution at meals in the first carbohydrate period and 25 g taken similarly in the second period. A statistically significant, marked rise in caries increment was observed in all the three years during which toffee was consumed. This was greatest in the third year, when the data were calculated for cavities only.

24-toffee groups

During the first carbohydrate period, the 48 males and 39 females received 24 toffees (120 g sugar) per day, which were available throughout the day. This was accompanied by a very marked rise in caries increment, which was 70 per cent greater in females than males. In both sexes the increment, when all carious lesions were included, was approximately equal in the first and second years, but the increment of carious cavities was twice as high in the second year as in the first. Many of the patients did not eat their full ration of 24 toffees per day, although consumption was higher in the females than the males. Twenty-two of the 39 females ate all their daily ration: only two did not eat any toffee at all and 15 ate less than their ration. Thirty-one out of the 48 males ate all their ration, 12 did not consume any toffee, two ate more than their ration, and the remaining three less than their ration.

Because of the very great increase in caries in these groups, issue of toffee was stopped just before the end of the first carbohydrate period and replaced by an isocaloric amount of fat. Also, consumption between meals was not allowed. This was accompanied by a dramatic fall in caries increment in both sexes to near the pre-carbohydrate period level. The lower level of consumption of toffee in the males might be an explanation for their smaller increase in caries. This view is strengthened by the observation that of the 10 males who showed no increase in caries during the toffee-eating period, seven of these had consumed no

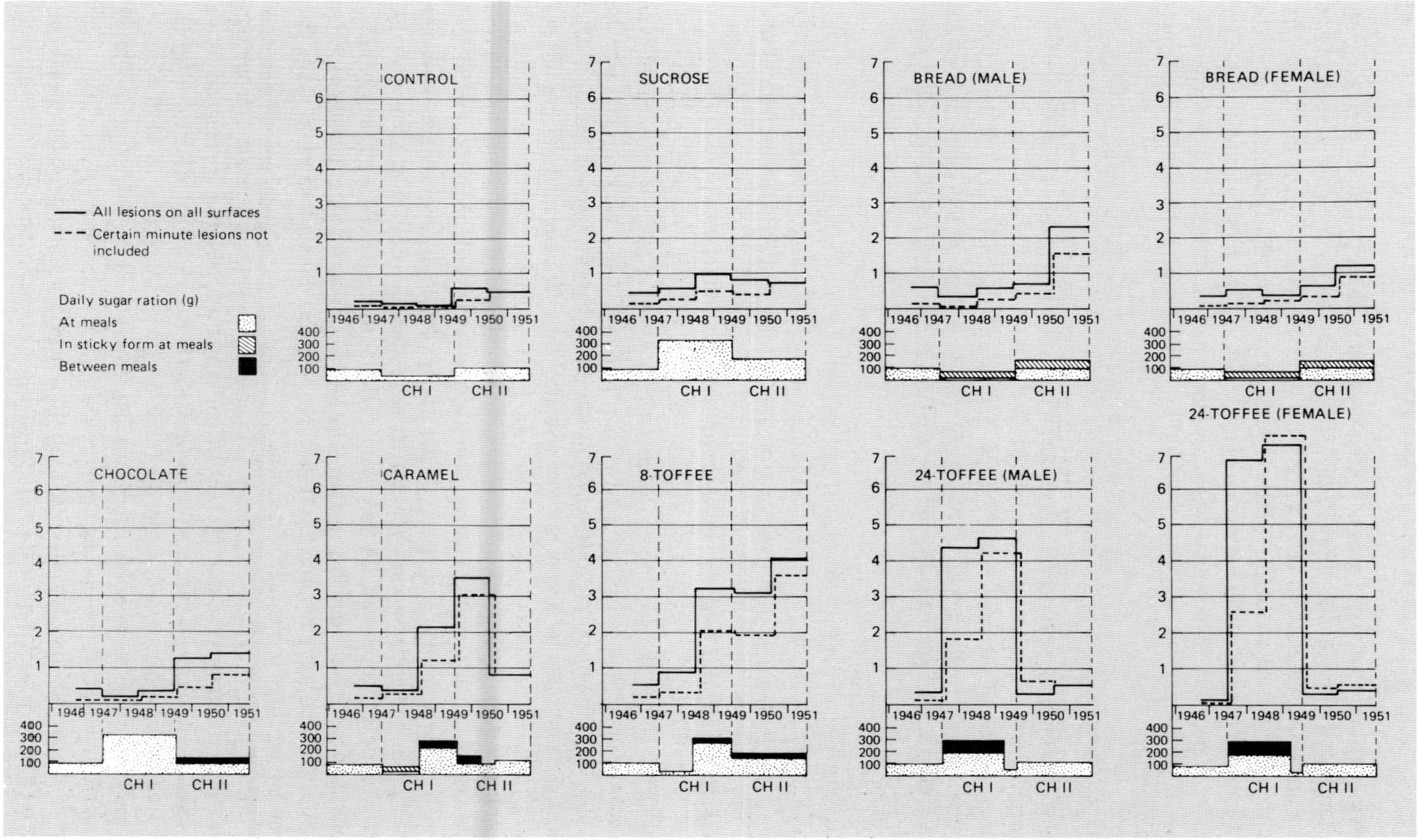

All lesions on all surfaces
Certain minute lesions not included
Daily sugar ration (g)
At meals
In sticky form at meals
Between meals
CONTROL
SUCROSE
BREAD (MALE)
BREAD (FEMALE)
CHOCOLATE
CARAMEL
8-TOFFEE
24-TOFFEE (MALE)
24-TOFFEE (FEMALE)
1946 1947 1948 1949 1950 1951
CH I
CH II

toffee. In addition, the male 24-toffee group was the only group to receive bone-meal (containing 1 mg F) during the vitamin period: the bone-meal was spread on bread and thus could have had a topical anticaries effect. As in the caramel group, caries activity was highest in lower anterior teeth, although 25 per cent of lesions occurred in cementum.

Comment

The main conclusions of the Vipeholm study are:

1. Consumption of sugar, even at high levels, is associated with only a small increase in caries increment if the sugar is taken up to four times a day at meals and none between meals.
2. Consumption of sugar both between meals and at meals is associated with a marked increase in caries increment.

Other conclusions were:

(i) the increase in caries activity, under uniform experimental conditions, varies widely from person to person;
(ii) the increase in caries activity disappears on the withdrawal of the sugar-rich foods;
(iii) carious lesions occurred despite avoidance of sugar.

Both the study itself and the use of the findings of the study in dental health education have been criticized by a few authors (The Cocoa, Chocolate and Confectionery Alliance 1974, 1979; Jackson 1978). Their criticisms are based largely on the fact that the subjects were mentally-deficient patients kept in unique conditions and fed abnormally high levels of sugary foods. The authors of the Vipeholm report point out that because the study was planned to be long-term and involved a large number of subjects, adults had to be used. The authors suggest that the subjects seemed to be more caries-resistant than the general population and that the greater caries resistance was found in the more mentally ill patient; therefore increases in caries in the Vipeholm patients might be even greater in normal subjects. In both the caramel and 24-toffee groups the increase in caries was so great that the between-meal sweet-eating was stopped before the end of the project.

One factor which complicated the Vipeholm study is the vitamin period before the two carbohydrate periods. Although this lasted for $1\frac{1}{2}$ years, the dental examinations were less than one year apart—too short a period to compare increments adequately. Nevertheless, no dramatic differences in increment were observed. While most of the groups received vitamins A, C, D, or calcium supple-

---

Fig. 2.12. Number of new carious surfaces per year (both including and excluding pre-cavitation lesions) together with the daily sugar ration for the control and eight test groups, during each period of the study. (Compiled from Gustaffson *et al.* (1954).)

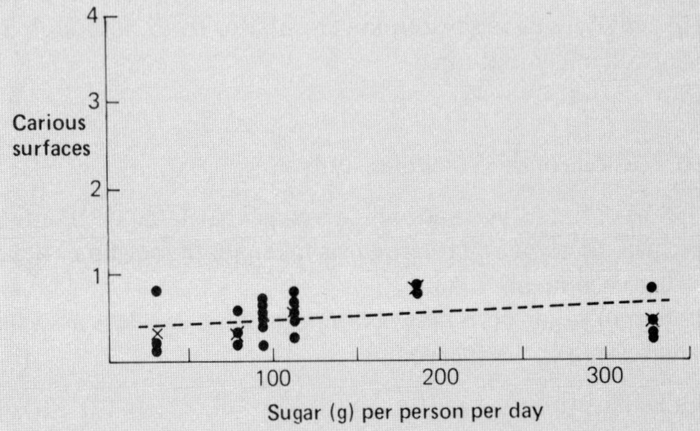

Fig. 2.13. Relationship between quantity of sugar taken at meals only and the number of new carious lesions per person per year (caries activity). (Gustaffson *et al.* (1954), with permission of the editor *Acta odontologica scandinavica.*)

ments, the future sucrose and male 24-toffee groups received 1 mg F per day. On present knowledge, these two groups would seem to be the only ones likely to benefit from the vitamin period, but what influence the $1\frac{1}{2}$ years of fluoride supplementation had upon the caries increment of these two groups remains conjectural.

Studies relating diet and dental caries are very difficult to conduct as caries is a chronic disease, and diet is infinitely variable and very prone to strongly held personal preferences. It is very difficult to keep a large group of people on the same diet for a year or more, and this is only likely to be achieved in institutions. Mental institutions have a high staff:patient ratio (almost 1:1 at Vipeholm) and supervision of diet is likely to be more thorough. It would seem unreasonable, therefore, not to obtain as much information as possible from the Vipeholm study; despite its complicated nature and the abnormality of the subjects, the main conclusions appear to be valid. Figures 2.13 and 2.14 show the difference in caries increment in groups that received sugar at meal times only, with groups that received between-meal and meal-time sugar. The effect can clearly be seen.

Of the groups receiving between-meal sugar, the chocolate group developed the lowest number of new lesions. The authors point out that this could be due to (i) the lower sugar concentration in chocolate compared with caramels and toffees; (ii) the higher fat concentration in chocolate; and (iii) possible anti-enzymatic properties of chocolate. These findings agree with other reports sug-

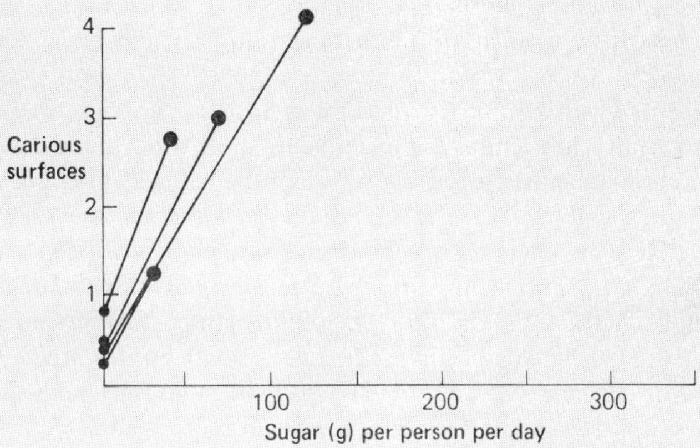

Fig. 2.14. Relationship between quantity of sugar taken both at and between meals, and the number of new carious lesions per person per year (caries activity). (Gustaffson *et al.* (1954), with permission of the editor *Acta odontologica scandinavica.*)

gesting that chocolate is likely to be less cariogenic than other confections (see p. 85).

The authors suggest that the stickiness of the sugary foods was an important factor responsible for the high caries increments in the sweet-eating groups. However, this stickiness does not seem to have been of importance if the food was eaten only at meals, since the caries increment of the bread and sucrose groups appear to be similar. In retrospect, it is regrettable that a group receiving a non-sticky sugary snack between meals (such as cups of sugared coffee) was not included, as more recent evidence suggests that the ability of toffees and sugared coffee to depress plaque pH is similar (Rugg-Gunn *et al.* 1978).

It can be seen from Table 2.11 and Fig. 2.10 that the groups were rather imbalanced in past caries experience at the beginning of the study. Caries increments during the vitamin period were low and therefore rather similar for all groups (Fig. 2.12), but because the groups received different dietary supplements during the vitamin period it is impossible to be certain that imbalance in baseline caries experience was unimportant. However, although many studies have shown that baseline caries experience and subsequent caries increment are correlated, this is very unlikely to account for the large differences in caries experience observed in the Vipeholm study.

The Turku sugar studies

By 1970, there was considerable evidence of variation in the rate of acid production from different sugars by plaque micro-organisms: for example, the sweet polyalcohols produced virtually no acid. Animal experiments had also demonstrated that sugars differed in their cariogenicity (p. 62). In order to test whether the cariogenicity of sugars was also different in human subjects, a clinical study was conducted in Turku, Finland between October 1972 and October 1974 (Scheinin and Mäkinen 1975). The object was to study the effect on dental caries increment of nearly total substitution of sucrose in a normal diet with either fructose or xylitol. Because full co-operation of the subjects in adhering to their diet was essential, and because it was planned that the subjects would undergo a wide range of biochemical and microbiological tests, it was decided to restrict the study largely to adults, most of whom were connected with the Turku dental or medical schools. Of the 125 adults who began the study, 115 remained after two years. Two-thirds of the subjects were female. The mean initial age of the subjects completing the study was 27.7 years, and although the age range was wide (12–53 years), 65 per cent of the subjects were initially aged 20–29 years.

The 125 subjects were allocated to three groups—sucrose (S), fructose (F), and xylitol (X). Because full co-operation was essential, the subjects could choose which group they wished to be in. Slight taste and texture differences between foods made with fructose, xylitol, or sucrose, made it impossible for the trial to be double-blind and the subjects knew their group allocation. Slightly more subjects were allocated to the X group as it was anticipated that some of them would drop out of this group because of persistent diarrhoea: in the event, only one of the 52 X-group subjects withdrew for this reason. Nine others did not complete the two years, mainly due to failure to adhere to the strict dietary regime and other personal reasons, although three subjects were withdrawn (two in the S group and one in the F group) because of high caries increment in the first year.

The caries examination was conducted blind by one person throughout the study; it was thorough, taking about 60 min per subject. In addition, two standardized bitewing radiographs were taken of each side of the mouth. Both precavitation and cavitation lesions were recorded, for both primary and secondary caries. Because of the short duration of the trial (24 months), and because it was conducted in a largely adult population in whom low caries increment could be expected, the majority of caries results were expressed including the precavitation caries grade. Secondary caries (caries in previously filled surfaces) is rare in adolescent children and usually not included in the analyses of caries increment studies in chidren, but because adults were used in the Turku studies, a seemingly more complicated method of caries data analysis had to be used whereby secondary caries was included in the analyses.

The organization of the dietary regimes for the subjects in the three groups was very considerable. Virtually all foods which normally contained sucrose had to be manufactured with fructose or xylitol substituting for the sucrose. Altogether about 100 dietary items were especially manufactured by 12 food firms in Finland in order to ensure that as wide a variety of foods were available to sub-

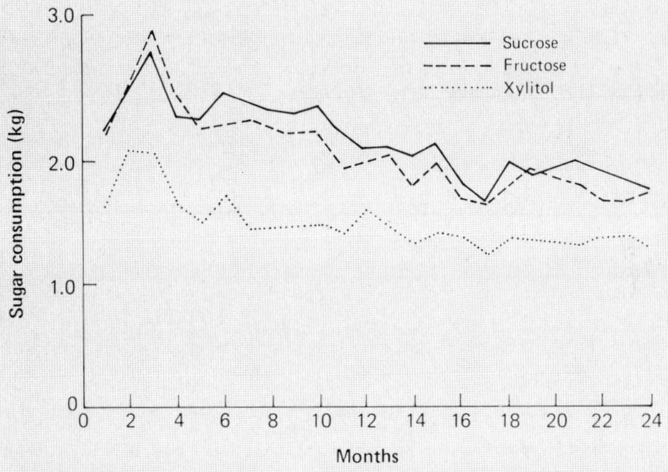

Fig. 2.15. The mean monthly sugar consumption by subjects in the three groups. This does not include sugar in manufactured items. (Scheinin and Makinen (1975), with permission of the editor *Acta odontologica scandinavica.*)

jects in the F and X groups as for the S group or normal subjects. Sugar and sugar-containing foods were provided free during the 2-year study. All subjects were asked to avoid sweet fruits such as dried figs, raisins, and dates, because the sugars in these foods could not be substituted. The fructose products presented no manufacturing problems, but some foods were more difficult to manufacture with xylitol, partly owing to its lower solubility and partly because it is not metabolized by yeast cells used in making dough. Some products, though, were considered better tasting than their sucrose-containing counterparts. Participants kept a dietary diary for all 745 days of the study. From these, the consumption of sugars in the three groups during the 2-year study was obtained (Fig. 2.15): consumption by the S and F groups was very similar but consistently higher than consumption by the X group. The advent of free food and initial curiosity resulted in higher consumption for the first few months. Overall, average sugar consumption in all groups was slightly lower than in the general Finnish population (about 45 kg/person per year).

In addition to a difference in the mean daily weight of xylitol consumed and the mean daily weight of sucrose of fructose consumed (Fig. 2.15), there was a difference in the frequency of consumption of sugars. It has been possible to determine these data from the very full information provided in the survey report. The mean frequencies of sugar intake per day for each group were: F 4.3, S 4.8,

Table 2.12. The base-line conditions of the 115 subjects who completed the 2-year Turku sugar study

	Group		
	F	S	X
Total clinical and radiographic carious surfaces	13.9	11.0	13.4
Filled surfaces	29.4	27.3	29.8
DMFS	48.0	42.1	50.7
Number of subjects	35	33	47
Mean age (years)	26.2	27.2	29.1

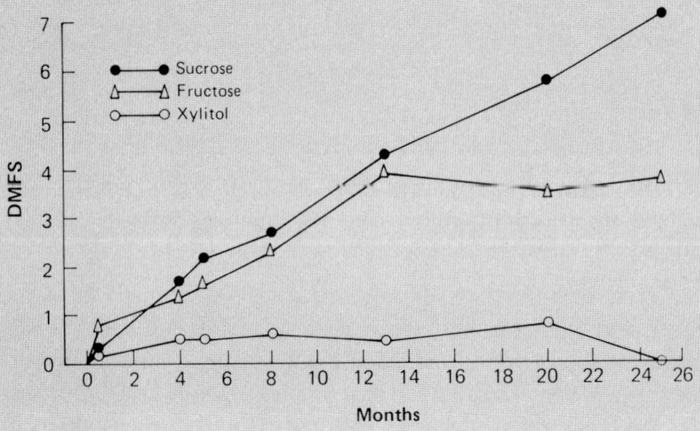

Fig. 2.16. The cumulative development of decayed, missing, or filled surfaces including cavitation and pre-cavitation carious lesions, diagnosed both clinically and radiographically, but not including secondary caries. At 24 months, differences between all groups were statisically significant ($p<0.01$). (Scheinin and Makinen (1975), with permission of the editor *Acta odontologica scandinavica*.)

and X 3.4. The difference between the xylitol group and the other two groups is statistically significant ($p<0.05$).

Data analyses revealed that there were no substantial differences in baseline caries scores between the three groups (Table 2.12). The cumulative development of caries (DMFS), diagnosed both clinically and radiographically, is given in Fig. 2.16. These results include both precavitational (C1) and cavitation (C2) lesions. The 24-month DMFS increments were 7.2 in the S group, 3.8 in the F group, and 0.0 in the X group. Although data given in Fig. 2.16 include pre-

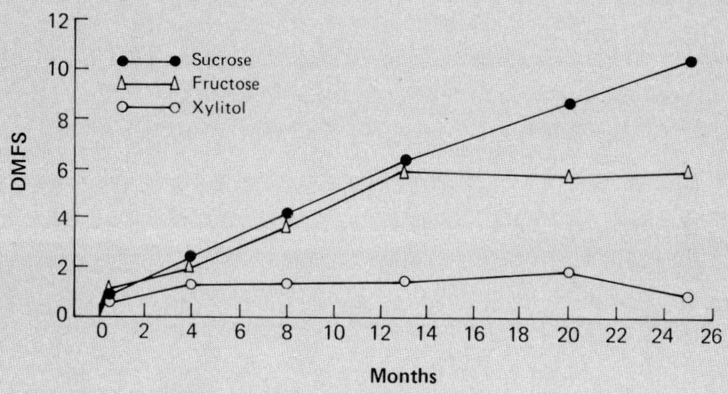

Fig. 2.17. The cumulative DMFS (as in Fig. 2.16) but including the development of secondary caries. At 24 months, differences between all groups were statistically significant ($p < 0.05$). (Scheinin and Makinen (1975), with permission of the editor *Acta odontologica scandinavica*.)

cavitation carious lesions, they do not include the development of secondary caries. Figure 2.17, though, includes both the DMFS data given in Fig. 2.16 and the development of secondary caries. The size of the increments is considerably increased (10.5, 6.1, and 0.9 DMFS in the S, F, and X groups respectively after 24 months), indicating the importance of secondary caries in adults. The relative sizes of the increments for the group are, however, unaltered: the increments in the F and S groups were approximately equal at the end of the first year but during the second year the development of the S-group caries increment continued at the same rate while virtually no increase was observed in the F group. Little caries occurred in the X group and that which developed was cancelled out by the 'healing' (reverting to the appearance of a sound surface) of precavitation lesions by the 24th month, resulting in a zero (excluding secondary lesions) or near zero (including secondary lesions) 2-year increment. The differences in 2-year caries DMFS increments calculated either way were statistically significant between all three groups ($p < 0.05$). Differences between the X group and the other two groups were also significant after one year ($p < 0.005$).

It was previously noted that the above DMFS scores included precavitation lesions. Subsequently, Scheinin (1979) published DMFS increments for the three groups, excluding precavitation lesions. The 2-year mean DMFS increments for

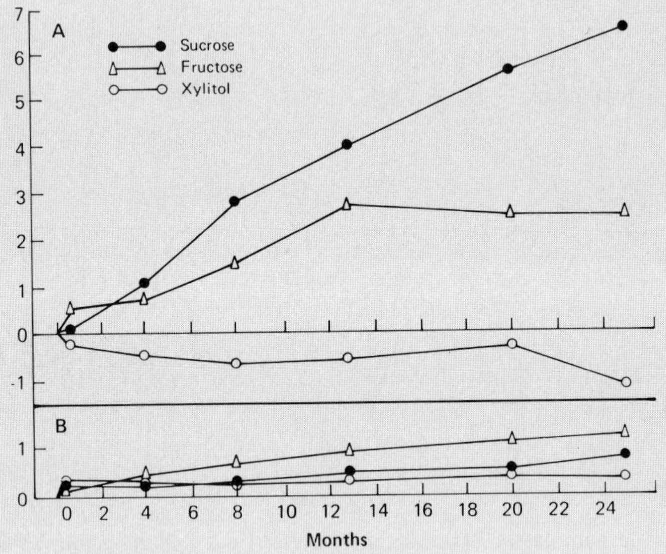

Fig. 2.18. Cumulative primary caries increments. A: for precavitation carious lesions. At 24 months, differences between all groups were statistically significant ($p<0.01$). B: for carious cavities. At 24 months, the difference between X and F groups only statistically significant ($p<0.01$). (Scheinin and Makinen (1975), with permission of the editor *Acta odontologica scandinavica.*)

each group were: S group 3.33, X group 1.47, and F group 3.57. The 56 per cent reduction in the X group compared with the S group was statistically significant ($p<0.01$). However, no difference between the S and F groups was observed, in fact the F group increment was slightly larger than the S group increment. An explanation of the unusual occurrence in the X group of a higher increment recorded when precavitation lesions were excluded than when they were included, can be seen in Figs. 2.18 and 2.19, which give cumulative increments for both primary and secondary caries respectively, for both precavitation (A) and cavitation (B) lesions. Figure 2.18A shows the healing effect of xylitol on primary precavitation lesions, although a net healing effect of xylitol is not seen for secondary precavitation lesions (Fig. 2.19A). Statistically significantly fewer precavitation lesions were observed in the X and F groups compared with the S group after two years for both primary (Fig. 2.18A) and secondary (Fig. 2.19A) lesions. However, for precavitation carious lesions only, more primary and secondary lesions occurred in the F group: the difference between the S and X

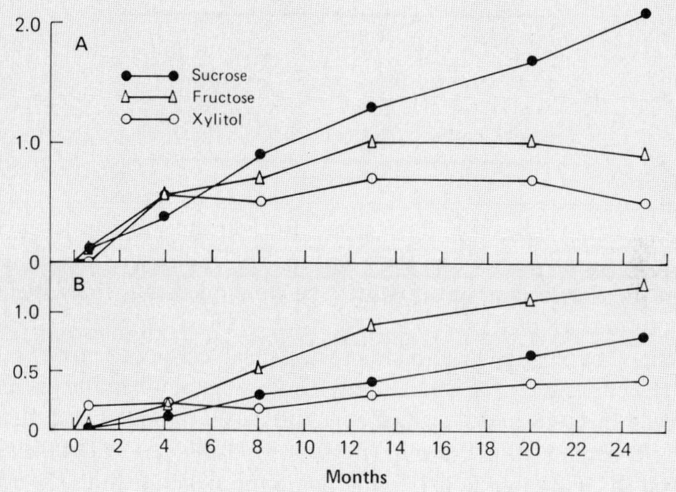

Fig. 2.19. Cumulative secondary caries increments. A: for pre-cavitation carious lesions. At 24 months, differences between S and X groups, and between S and F groups were statistically significant ($p<0.05$). B: for carious cavities. At 24 months, the difference between X and F groups only was statistically significant ($p<0.01$). (Scheinin and Makinen (1975), with permission of the editor *Acta odontologica scandinavica*.)

groups was statistically significant ($p<0.01$), but no significant difference was observed between the F and S groups. Figures 2.16 to 2.17 show that, in this experiment, the total DMFS increment for all caries grades and types of cavity is dominated by the number of primary precavitation carious lesions (6.6 out of 10.5 DMFS in the S group).

Recently, Rekola (1987) has re-examined the radiographs from the Turku study in order to quantify changes in the size of approximal carious lesions. Using a planometric method, Rekola showed there was no difference in the mean size of the lesions in the X and S groups at baseline but at the end of the 2-year study the mean size was significantly smaller in the X group than in the S group ($p<0.01$). The size of the carious lesions increased almost linearly at 0.12 mm^2/year in the S group, but remaïned virtually unchanged (-0.01 mm^2/year) in the X group.

In summary, analyses of the caries data over the 2-year study period indicated that substitution of xylitol for sucrose in a normal Finnish (high-sucrose) diet resulted in a very much lower caries increment of both carious cavities and precavitation lesions. While subjects in the S group developed more precavitation

Table 2.13. Mean plaque wet weight (mg) at the beginning and end of the Turku study in the three groups. At 24 months, differences between the X and the other two groups were statistically significant ($p<0.005$)

	Group		
	F	S	X
At base-line	23.5	23.4	25.1
At 24 months	21.1	20.6	11.9

carious lesions than subjects in the F group, the F group subjects developed more carious cavities than subjects in the S group, The X diet was clearly less cariogenic than the S or F diet, but it cannot be concluded that the F diet was less cariogenic than the S diet.

Comprehensive biochemical and microbiological tests were carried out in parallel with the caries assessments. Although a very slight fall in the plaque weight was observed in the S and F groups over the 2-year study period, the fall was very much greater in the X group ($p<0.005$) (Table 2.13) Detailed analyses showed that the few subjects with a high amount of plaque in the X group were habitually high consumers of starch-containing foods. Despite the lower plaque levels in the X group, there was no difference in gingival inflammation (GI) between the groups at the end of the study. The X group had a lower level of salivary amylase, which was in agreement with and enhances previous work suggesting that dietary starch influences amylase secretion. The finding that salivary lactoperoxidase activity was higher in the X group is of interest, because of its role in the lactoperoxidase-thiocyanate anti-caries system (Hoogendoorn 1974). However, salivary thiocyanate levels were not raised in the X group and the clinical significance of these findings remains uncertain.

Replacement of dietary sucrose with xylitol did not affect the proportion of major bacterial groups in dental plaque but did reduce the number of most organisms, especially the acidogenic and aciduric flora, including *Strep. mutans*. Plaque from X group subjects showed a reduced rate of sucrose hydrolysis. No adaptation by plaque organisms to produce acid from xylitol was observed during the 2-year study.

Results of serum analyses and liver-function tests indictated that neither dietary xylitol nor fructose altered metabolic parameters of liver function as compared with a normal sucrose diet. The only adverse side-effect of xylitol consumption appeared to be a raised incidence of osmotic diarrhoea. This was, however, less than had been expected and only one subject withdrew from the study for this reason. Over the two years, the incidence of diarrhoea or flatulence was 1.2 occurrences per subject per month in the X group, although symptoms decreased in these subjects during the study (Table 2.14). The occurrence of diarrhoea did not correlate well with the quantity of xylitol consumed as it was noted that 200 g of xylitol per day caused diarrhoea on some days, whereas the same or much higher doses led to no symptoms on other days.

Table 2.14. The occurrence of diarrhoea-like conditions and flatulence per subject per month

	Group		
Mean for period	F	S	X
First 8 months	0.38	0.38	2.25
Second 8 months	0.38	0.25	0.88
Final 8 months	0.38	0.38	0.50
Total 24 months	0.38	0.34	1.21

In summary, the Turku sugar study required a considerable amount of careful planning and organization. Almost total substitution of sucrose by xylitol resulted in a substantial reduction in caries incidence. Although slight differences in amounts of sugars eaten and in frequency of intake, changes in salivary enzymes, the amount of plaque, and incidence of some micro-organisms may have contributed to the observed results, the persistent inability of plaque organisms to metabolize xylitol to acids is likely to be the main explanation for its caries-preventive effect. The lack of any undesirable general metabolic processes, and the fairly low incidence of osmotic diarrhoea, indicates that xylitol is likely to be a suitable substitute for sucrose from the dental point of view. On the other hand, substitution of dietary sucrose by fructose did not lead to a clear-cut reduction in caries increment, and it cannot be concluded that substitution by fructose is a worthwhile caries-preventive measure. This lack of difference between sucrose and fructose in caries development and in plaque weight, casts doubt on the importance of plaque dextrans in caries aetiology.

Turku 1-year xylitol chewing-gum study

Because of the considerable success of near total substitution of sucrose by xylitol in reducing caries increment, a subsidiary study was conducted on 102 young adults over one year (Scheinin *et al.* 1975). The subjects were mainly medical and dental students and were randomly divided into two groups (S and X groups). At the end of the one year, each group contained 50 subjects. The subjects were asked to maintain their normal dietary habits and oral hygiene procedures. In addition, they were given an ample supply of chewing-gum and asked to consume between three and seven sticks per day. Each stick weighed 3 g and contained 1.5 g of either sucrose (S) or xylitol (X). The mean daily consumption was 4.0 sticks per day in the S group and 4.5 per day in the X group. From the dietary diaries completed by the subjects, it was observed that the mean daily frequency of sucrose intake was 4.2 in the S group and 4.9 in the X group.

Caries incidence was much lower in the X group subjects compared with the subjects in the S group ($p < 0.001$) (Figs. 2.20 and 2.21): precavitation carious lesions are included in both Figs. 2.20 and 2.21 while data in Fig. 2.21 includes the development of secondary caries. Data analyses excluding precavitation carious lesions have been presented by Scheinin (1979): the 50 S-group subjects

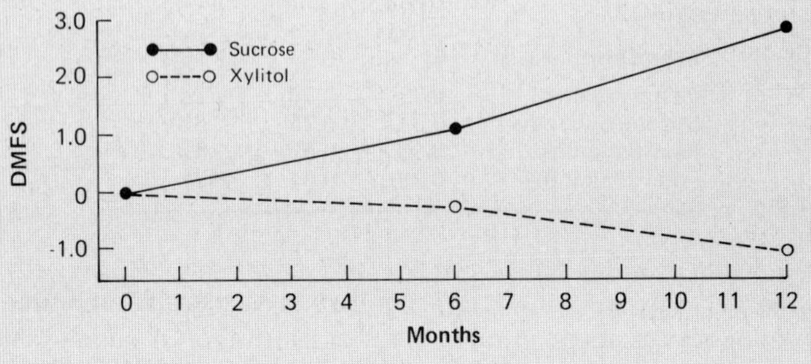

Fig. 2.20. The cumulative development of DMFS, including cavitation and pre-cavitation carious lesions, diagnosed both clinically and radiographically. At 12 months, the difference between groups was statistically significant ($p < 0.001$). (Scheinin *et al.* (1975), with permission of the editor *Acta odontologica scandinavica*.)

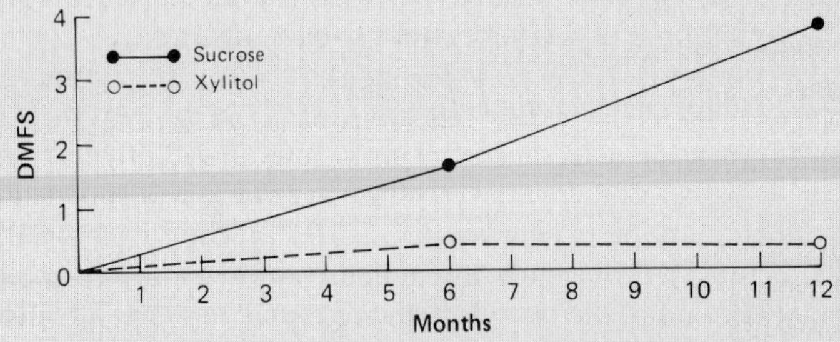

Fig. 2.21. The cumulative DMFS (Fig. 2.20) but including the development of secondary carious lesions. At 12 months, the difference between groups was statistically significant ($p < 0.001$). (Scheinin *et al.* (1975), with permission of the editor *Acta odontologica scandinavica*.)

developed 2.12 DMFS, while the 50 X-group subects developed 0.84 DMFS, a difference of 60 per cent ($p < 0.001$). In agreement with the previous 2-year study of replacement of sucrose by xylitol, significantly less plaque was found in the X group subjects at the end of the 1-year study period. However, the changes in salivary enzyme activity observed in the main study were not observed in the subjects using xylitol chewing-gum.

The favourable results observed in the chewing-gum study would appear to be due to the non-acidogenicity of the xylitol chewing-gum rather than any anti-acidogenic action of xylitol, although this action has been claimed (Makinen 1985). However, it is now well recognized that remineralization as well as demineralization of enamel occurs, and that caries is a result of greater demineralization than remineralization. Fast-flowing saliva is alkaline and possesses adequate concentration of minerals for enamel remineralization (see Fig. 2.25, p. 66, for effect of sugarless gum on plaque pH). Chewing a non-acidogenic gum is therefore very likely to favour enamel remineralization.

Other xylitol substitution studies

Two other trials have investigated the partial substitution of dietary sucrose by xylitol. The foods have included other forms of confectionery as well as chewing-gum. Both studies were supported by the WHO—one in Hungary and one in French Polynesia.

In Hungary (Scheinin *et al.* 1985*a*), a 3-year study was undertaken in 11 children's homes, involving children who were aged 6–11 years at the start of the study. Children in five institutions were allocated to the xylitol (X) group and received xylitol confectionery (giving about 14 to 20 g xylitol/day/person). Children from three institutions did not receive xylitol confectionery but consumed fluoridated milk or fluoridated water (F group), while children from the three remaining institutions constituted the control (C) group and received restorative treatment only. The X and F groups, but not the C group, received fluoride toothpaste. It was concluded that the dietary partial substitution of xylitol for sucrose resulted in a pronounced caries reduction—43 per cent when compared with the C group, and 26 per cent when compared with the F group. Results of a 2-year trial were also published (Scheinin *et al.* 1985b) and supported the findings of the 3-year trial.

The investigations in French Polynesia took place between 1981 and 1984, and also involved partial substitution of sucrose by xylitol (Kandelman *et al.* 1988). Seven varieties of confectionery especially made with xylitol were provided, giving a daily xylitol intake of about 20 g/person. The children on one island were assigned to the control group while children on two other islands formed the xylitol group. Out of 746 6–12-year-olds who began the trial, 468 completed the 32-month study. The mean caries increment in the control group was 7.1 DMFS compared with 4.5 DMFS in the xylitol group—a reduction of 37 per cent.

Sorbitol chewing-gum trials

In a 2-year trial of the use of sorbitol-containing chewing-gum upon caries in 8–12-year-old Danish children, 174 children in one school were given three sticks of gum per day to be chewed after breakfast, lunch, and supper; 166 children, at another school, acted as control and were given no gum or other supplements (Möller and Poulsen 1973). The difference of about 10 per cent in the 2-year caries increment was statistically significant. As no group of children chewed a comparable amount of sucrose-containing chewing-gum, the results do not necessarily indicate the effect of substitution of sucrose dietary items by sorbitol gum. Banoczy *et al.* (1981) reported that the substitution of sorbitol in sweets eaten between meals by children in a Hungarian closed children's home resulted in a 41–45 per cent reduction in 3-year caries increment.

The effect of giving a group of 9–11-year-old American children sucrose-containing gum, to be chewed twice daily, was reported by Glass (1981). These children developed a 36 per cent ($p < 0.01$) larger 2-year caries increment than a control group who were given no gum. This result was not expected at the time Glass planned his study, because Slack *et al.* (1972) had reported no increased caries increment in Greek children who chewed five sticks of sucrose gum over a 3-year period.

United Kingdom Medical Research Council (MRC) 2-year sugar supplement study

Between 1949 and 1951 a study was conducted of the effect on caries increment of supplementing the diet of children living in children's homes with additional sugar (King *et al.* 1955). Because previous work had suggested that raw brown sugar contained factors which might protect enamel against caries, it was planned that some children should receive brown sugar.

It had been hoped that many centres throughout England would participate, but only three (London, Liverpool, and Sheffield) finally took part. Separate investigators were involved in the three centres. The study was planned to consist of one control and two study groups: the control group consuming wartime (1939–45) levels of sugar, while the two test groups consumed pre-war sugar levels of either white or raw brown sugar. However, it was not possible to include a raw sugar group in Liverpool or Sheffield, which thus became two group studies. The investigation was planned to last 2 years, but in Sheffield it was terminated after 18 months because the subjects were unable to accept the sugar supplement any longer.

Because strict dietary control was necessary, the study was conducted in children's homes. In the London area the 678 children, aged 2–5 years, starting the study were housed in 23 homes throughout Greater London. Two of these homes withdrew, leaving 21 homes to complete the study. Only 82 of the 678 London children completed the 2 years (88 per cent loss of subjects) due to them leaving the homes.

In the Liverpool area one suitable home was found. After 2 years, 161 children, aged 4–14 years, remained out of nearly 300 children examined at baseline. The age range was the same (4–14 years) in Sheffield where 199 children from 16 children's cottages began the study, 93 of whom were still available at the end of the 18-month study period.

Table 2.15. Medical Research Council sugar supplement study. Results expressed as per cent of teeth which were decayed, extracted, or filled (% deft) and the change over the study period. Data for older children (i.e. 7–10 years for deciduous molars and 11–14 years for first permanent molars) are not given because teeth would have been erupted for many years before trial period

A. London

2–4-years old (all deciduous teeth)

	Control	White	Brown
N	30	32	20
At base-line	0.3	2.5	1.3
After 2 years	9.1	6.8	9.3
% sound teeth developing caries	8.8	4.4*	8.1

*Stat. sig. smaller than other groups.

B. Liverpool

4–6-years old (deciduous molars only)

	Control	Sugar
N	21	21
At base-line	12.3	13.7
After 2 years	20.2	31.5
% sound teeth developing caries	9.1	20.7*

*Stat. sig. larger.

7–10-years old (first permanent molars only)

	Control	Sugar
N	39	32
At base-line	32.5	39.4
After 2 years	66.2	73.2
% sound teeth developing caries	50.0	55.8

C. Sheffield

4–6-years old (deciduous molars only)

	Control	Sugar
N	10	10
At base-line	24.4	8.8
After 18 months	29.5	16.3
% sound teeth developing caries	5.4	8.1

7–10-years old (first permanent molars only)

	Control	Sugar
N	16	23
At base-line	26.6	19.3
After 18 months	40.6	43.2
% sound teeth developing caries	19.1	29.6

In London, each child's sugar supplement was 11 oz (312 g) per week, which doubled their total sugar intake. But in Liverpool and Sheffield, 22 oz (624 g) sugar per week were given to each child in addition to their basic dietary sugar level of about 15–25 oz (425–710 g) per week. In all three areas the issue of sugar was carefully supervised and confined to 2–4 meals per day. Owing to a misunderstanding, Demerara (semi-refined) sugar was given in place of some of the raw sugar, and some of the sugar supplement was white in the raw brown-sugar group.

The results of the main analyses are shown in Table 2.15. The caries data were expressed as the per cent of teeth that were carious (or extracted or filled), rather than the more usual deft/DMFT indices (which give a caries score per child). In London, the groups were very unbalanced in caries experience at base-line. However, the 32 children receiving the white sugar supplement developed significantly less caries than the control (sugar-low) children and the children receiving the brown sugar. On the other hand the children receiving the sugar supplement in both older age groups in Liverpool and Sheffield developed more caries than the control (sugar-low) group children. This difference reached statistical significance in the 4–6-year-old Liverpool children in whom the groups were well balanced at base-line. On the whole, though, the equivocal findings, the small number of subjects in some of the groups, and the inbalance of some of the base-line scores, precludes firm conclusions being drawn from this study. A tentative conclusion might be that approximately doubling daily intake in children did not result in a clear increase in caries incidence over a $1\frac{1}{2}$–2-year period. However, it can now be appreciated that one very important point was that the sugar supplements were given only at meal times (i.e. 2–4 times per day), so that the frequency of sugar intake was unlikely to have been different in the control and sugar supplement groups. It was shown in the Vipeholm study that the amount of sugar taken at meal times only could be increased considerably with only slightly increased caries increment, so that the results of the MRC study, to some extent, are in agreement with those of the Vipeholm study. It is not possible to draw any conclusions about the cariogenicity of raw brown sugar.

United Kingdom bedtime carbohydrate supplements study

King (1946) reported a study which investigated the effect on caries increment of giving pre-school children sweets and/or biscuits at bedtime, for periods up to 2 years. The children, who lived in two children's homes in the south of England, were aged 3–4 years. The number of children studied was small and their caries experience was extremely low.

In the first children's home, 22 children received one boiled sweet the last thing at night for 6 months. Twenty-one out of the 22 children were caries-free before the study (one child having two carious teeth) and no change in caries experience was observed at the end of the 6-month period.

The 46 children in the second home were divided into three groups: a control group (no supplement), a biscuit-only group (one chocolate biscuit at night), and a sweet and a biscuit group (one chocolate biscuit plus one to two boiled sweets at night). All these children were studied over a 24-month period. All 16 control group children were caries-free before the study, 12 remained at the end of the 24-month period, one of whom had developed one carious tooth. All 13 children in the biscuit group were caries-free before the study, and all 10 still present at the end of the period were still caries-free. In the sweets and biscuit group, 14 children were still present at the end of the 24-month period out of 17 present before the study. The one child who had any caries (six carious teeth) at base-line, developed one further carious tooth during the study.

In conclusion, although the number of subjects was very small (an average of 12 per group after 24 months), there was no indication that sugar supplements last thing at night led to increased caries development in these pre-school children who were, initially, caries-free.

Other studies

The Roslagen study

Frostell *et al.* (1974) reported a study designed to investigate the effect upon dental caries increment of substituting sucrose in candies by Lycasin. Lycasin is a hydrogenated starch hydrolysate and was at that time made by the Lyckeby Co., Sweden. Since then an improved product has been made in France (see p. 91). Initially, 225 children, aged $2\frac{1}{2}$–4 years, took part in the study. They were allocated to a Lycasin and a control group. but it is uncertain whether this was random. Some 77 per cent of the children remained in the study after 1 year and 50 per cent after 2 years. Dental examinations were conducted 'blind'. Substitution of Lycasin for sucrose in candies was only partial but, from examination of thc data, the authors seen justified in their conclusion that the reduction in caries increment in the Lycasin group was about 25 per cent.

The Gustavsberg study

The results of the Turku study (see p. 43) have been interpreted by some as showing that fructose is less cariogenic than sucrose, and led Frostell *et al.* (1981) to undertake the Gustavsberg study. A number of families who had 3-year-old children, living in the Gustavsberg suburb of Stockholm, were invited to participate in a 2-year clinical study designed to investigate the effect of substituting invert sugar (a mixture of glucose and fructose) for dietary surcose. The study was complicated, the subjects were not allocated to groups at random, and the examinations were not 'blind'. Because of these shortcomings, the results, which suggested that 2-year caries increments, and plaque and gingivitis scores were lower in the invert sugar group compared with the 'contrast' (control) groups, should be treated cautiously.

Effect of pre-sweetened cereals on caries increment

The sugar content of breakfast cereals can be very high. The 78 cereals analysed by Shannon (1974) varied from 1 to 70 per cent in their sucrose + glucose content. The mean figure for the 78 cereals was 25 per cent sucrose and 2 per cent glucose, 58 containing over 10 per cent sucrose + glucose. There has therefore been concern at their possible cariogenic potential.

Two studies, both in the United States, have reported caries increments in adolescent children who did or did not consume pre-sweetened cereals over a defined period of time. The study of Glass and Fleisch (1974) lasted 2 years and that of Rowe *et al.* (1974) for 3 years. The cereals were provided to the families *ad libitum*. In both studies no difference was found between the two groups of children. But, as Glass and Fleisch pointed out, these findings should not be construed to dilute in any way the evidence associating dental caries with sucrose in general. Some 94 per cent of the cereals were taken with milk, which will reduce acidogenicity, and cereals are usually eaten at meal times. It is also exceptionally difficult to test the importance of just one dietary item per day on caries because its effect is likely to go undetected amongst the many other sugar-containing foods and drinks.

Effect of acidulated carbonated beverages on caries increment

Steinberg *et al.* (1972) conducted a study in which 119 institutionalized mentally subnormal patients, aged 8–21 years, consumed 6 oz of sugar-containing acidulated carbonated beverage at mid-morning and at bedtime each day for 3 years. At the same times, an age-matched control group (132 patients) in the same institution consumed 6 oz of water. The 3-year caries increment in the group receiving the sugared beverage (12.2 DMFS) was slightly higher than that for the control group (10.3 DMFS) but the difference was not statistically significant. However, the experimental group had significantly more caries than the control group in the buccal surfaces of maxillary anterior teeth and the buccolingual surfaces of mandibular teeth. It is possible that these surfaces had greater contact with the acid sugared beverage.

The consumption of soft drinks is increasing in many countries. Dental caries, caused by the presence of sugar, is not the only threat these pose to teeth. These drinks almost invariably have a low pH due to the presence of citric or phosphoric acid, which is considered to be an important cause of dental erosion (Eccles 1982; Smith and Shaw 1987; Asher and Read 1987).

Von de Fehr short-term caries experiments

Von der Fehr *et al.* (1970) reported on the development of an experimental caries system in which optical changes in enamel (similar to early carious lesions) were produced and subsequently reversed. It was hoped that this system could be used to test the cariogenicity of different sugars and diets, and the efficacy of various dietary additives or enamel pre-treatments in preventing lesion formation. In the experimental caries system, 12 dental students ceased oral hygiene for 23 days, and six of the 12 also rinsed nine times per day with 10 ml of 50 per cent sucrose solution. At the end of this test period, an increased 'caries index' score was observed in both groups, but the increase was more marked in the sucrose-rinse group (Fig. 2.22). As the authors pointed out, the control group did not refrain from sucrose intake, so the comparison is not between no sucrose and frequent intakes, but rather between different levels of sucrose intake.

Geddes *et al.* (1978), using the same experimental system but with only 14 days of no oral hygiene and sucrose rinsing, also reported a greater increase in 'caries index' in the sucrose-rinsing group compared with a control group. In both experiments, the caries-like lesions were reversed by scrupulous oral hygiene in combination with fluoride rinsing.

Although this experimental caries model looked promising, because of the fairly high inter-subject variation in caries-index increments, the minimum sample size per treatment group has to be large, and it is unlikely that further studies will be undertaken using this method (Edgar *et al.* 1978).

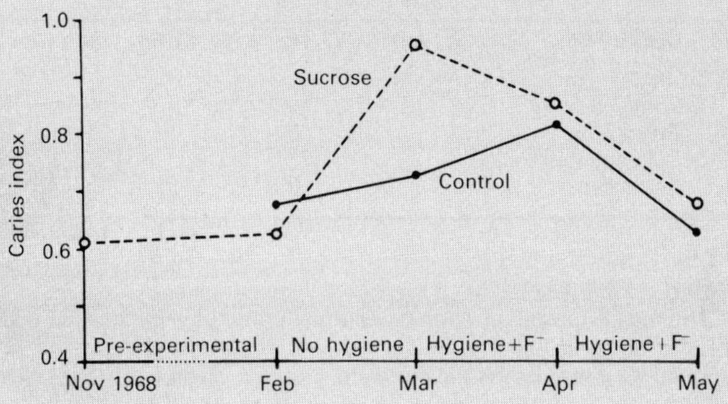

Fig. 2.22. Mean 'caries index' scores for buccal surfaces of canine, premolar, and maxillary incisor teeth in Danish dental students during the experimental caries study. (von der Fehr *et al.* (1970), with permission of the editor *Caries Research*.)

Two other short-term experiments

Koehne *et al.* (1934) and Koehne and Bunting (1934) supplemented the diets of caries-low children in orphanages with candy. In the first, the supplement was 3 lb of candy per week: at the end of the 5 months, 22 of the 31 orphans had developed active caries. In the second study, 100 g of candy/day was given for 5 to 18 months: caries developed in nine of the 13 girls.

In an even shorter trial, Hewat *et al.* (1950) observed that caries increment was lower in a group of 38 student dental nurses in New Zealand who consumed a low-carbohydrate diet (particularly a reduction in sugar) for 6 weeks, than 40 nurses in the control group who did not alter their diet.

The time periods were too short to draw definite conclusions in either of these studies.

Animal experiments

This section will only include discussion of animal experiments concerned with sugar and dental caries. Experiments concerned with pre-eruptive dietary effects have already been discussed (p. 4), the effect of adding phosphates to diets will be found on p. 81, the cariogenicity of starch on p. 74, and alternative sweeteners and caries development on p. 89. The rat is the most commonly used animal, but hamsters, mice, and monkeys have also been used.

Table 2.16. Caries development in rats fed a cariogenic diet and living in either conventional conditions (mixed microbial flora) or under germ-free conditions. (Orland *et al.* (1954))

Experiments	Conditions	No. of animals	No. with caries	Mean no. of carious molars
Series I	Conventional	16	16	4.8
	Germ-free	13	0	0
Series II	Conventional	23	23	3.2
	Germ-free	9	0	0

Table 2.17. The mean number of carious lesions in rats fed a cariogenic diet either conventionally or by stomach tube. The salivary glands of some of the animals in each group had been removed. Number of animals in each group is given in parentheses. (Kite *et al.* (1950))

	Conventional	Tube fed
Intact	6.7 (13)	0 (13)
Desalivated	28.8 (4)	0 (3)

The importance of micro-organisms and the importance of the local effect of diet

Two animal experiments are milestones in our knowledge of dental caries. Orland *et al.* (1954) developed a system for rearing rats under germ-free conditions. When these rats were fed a cariogenic diet, caries did not develop, in contrast to similar rats fed on the same diet but not reared under germ-free conditions and allowed to acquire their usual mixed microbial flora (Table 2.16). Although the weight gain was slightly lower for the germ-free animals, this was within acceptable limits. Both the liquid and solid phases of the diet were low in fluoride. These experiments clearly show that micro-organisms are essential for caries development.

The importance of the local effect of diet in the mouth was demonstrated by Kite *et al.* (1950). Rats were allocated to four groups (Table 2.17) and all were fed a cariogenic diet. When intact or desalivated animals were fed adequate amounts of the cariogenic diet by stomach tube (therefore avoiding the diet contacting the plaque-covered teeth) caries did not develop. In contrast, caries occurred in the normally fed rats; the severity being much higher in the desalivated animals. Although the number of animals was small and the technique of tube feeding imperfect, resulting in the loss of animals, it clearly demonstrated that diet has to be present in the mouth for caries to occur. A second important finding was the significance of saliva in the control of dental caries.

Frequency of feeding

The careful control of the frequency with which an animal could feed on a cario-

Table 2.18. The mean caries severity, daily food intake, and weight gain in five groups of rats fed at different frequencies per day; six animals per group. (König *et al.* (1968))

Group	Eating frequency per day	No. of fissure lesions	Daily food intake (g)	Weight gain during experiment (g)
1	12	0.7	6.0	23
2	18	2.2	6.0	34
3	24	4.0	6.0	28
4	30	4.7	6.0	29
5	*ad libitum*	4.2	11.7	64

genic diet became available when the Zurich Dental Institute developed an automatic feeding machine (König *et al.* 1968). Food could then be presented to animals at precisely controlled times and under-feeding ensured the animals ate all of the known quantity of foods. The results of the study by König *et al.* (1968) clearly showed a positive correlation between frequency with which animals ate a cariogenic diet and caries severity (Table 2.18). The group of rats feeding *ad libitum* consumed 11.7 g of food per day, nearly twice the 6 g consumed by the other groups. The level of caries severity in the groups indicates that frequency of eating a cariogenic diet is likely to be more important than the total amount of diet consumed.

More recently, Firestone *et al.* (1984) have shown that another relevant factor is the length of the time interval between meals. They devised an experiment in which all animals ate a cariogenic diet (56 per cent sucrose) 18 times a day: half the animals received their diet in three groups of 6 meals with no interval between the 6 meals in each group, but all the 18 meals consumed by the second group of animals were separated by intervals of 30 minutes. In both groups, each meal lasted 10 minutes. Caries development was greater in the latter group whose meals were spread out during the day, compared with the former group whose meals were bunched close together.

Concentration of sugar

Although a large number of experiments have shown that diets containing some sugar (e.g. about 10 per cent of the total diet) produce more caries in rats than diets with no sugar, further increases in caries have not always been observed when the sugar content is raised above 10 per cent. It would seem that differences in results have been due to, first, the type of diet used and, second, whether or not the rats were superinfected with cariogenic organisms. The composition of the non-carbohydrate part of the diet is also very important in determining how cariogenic a given amount of sugar will be. In gnotobiotic rats mono-infected with *Strep. mutans*, Michalek *et al.* (1977) found that a sucrose concentration of 1 per cent produced marked caries development, and maximum caries development occurred at 5 per cent concentration. As little as 2.5 per cent sugar causes much caries in the presence of 50–70 per cent starch, while five times as much sugar is necessary in a high-fat diet (Shaw 1979).

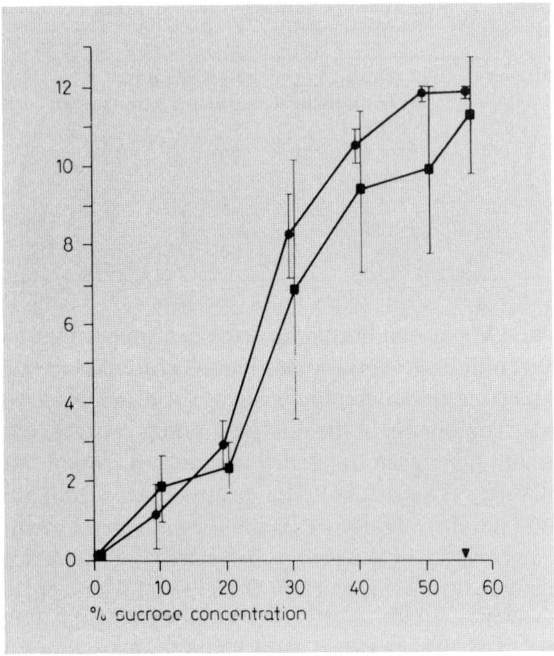

Fig. 2.23. Incidence of carious lesions (± SE) in fissures (●) and smooth surfaces (■) in rats fed '*ad libitum*', diets containing 0, 10, 20, 30, 40, 50, and 56 per cent sucrose. (Hefti and Schmid (1979), with permission of the editor *Caries Research*.)

In a comprehensive study, Huxley (1977) investigated two strains of rat, two basic diets (diet '2000' or 'DD') with up to five levels of sugar concentration, fed either *ad libitum* or fed 17 times/day by programmed feeding. He found that in all cases caries was higher in animals receiving the 15 per cent compared with 0 per cent sugar. While caries increased linearly with dietary sugar concentration (0, 15, 30, and 56 per cent sugar) in Sprague–Dawley rats receiving the '2000' basic biet, those receiving the 'DD' basic diet showed no linear increase in caries for sugar concentrations above 15 per cent. The linear response between dietary sugar concentrations and caries severity observed with the 2000 diet supported previous results (Huxley 1971), while the non-linear response with the DD diet agreed with Green and Hartles (1970) and Kreitzman and Klein (1976). Unlike Huxley (1977), Hefti and Schmid (1979) heavily superinfected their Osborne–Mendel rats with cariogenic *Strep. mutans* and *Actinomyces viscosus*. Their results (Fig. 2.23) showed that caries severity increased with increasing sugar concentration although the increase in severity fell with sugar concentrations above 40 per cent.

Types of sugar

Most animal experiments have used a basic starch diet and any added sugar has almost always been sucrose (usually as icing sugar). Dietary studies using rats (Guggenheim *et al.* 1966) suggested that the addition of 25 per cent glucose, fructose, lactose, or maltose did not produce significantly more caries than starch, while sucrose was much more cariogenic. However, all these animals were inoculated with a dextran-producing streptococcus. Grenby *et al.* (1973) also found that sucrose was more cariogenic than glucose in gnotobiotic rats mono-infected with *Strep. mutans*. Some strains of streptococci utilize sucrose preferentially and do not thrive in its absence. Experiments, therefore, where the animals are superinfected with such organisms are likely to exaggerate differences between the cariogenicity of sucrose and other sugars. Grenby and Hutchinson (1969) also observed, in three out of four experiments, that in rats sucrose was more cariogenic than glucose or fructose but the differences were small. There was no difference in the cariogenicity of glucose and fructose. Grenby and Leer (1974) found that 20 per cent glucose syrup was less cariogenic than 20 per cent sucrose syrup when taken by rats in drinking water, the difference being particularly marked in smooth surface caries. These findings agree with those of Green and Hartles (1969), who found sucrose diets slightly more cariogenic than diets containing glucose, fructose, galactose, lactose, or maltose, although the authors emphasized that all the sugars were highly cariogenic.

Colman *et al.* (1977) studied the development of caries in monkeys fed diets containing either sucrose, glucose + fructose, or fructose alone. The sucrose and glucose + fructose diets were of almost equal cariogenicity, while fructose appeared to be slightly less cariogenic than sucrose. Their former finding does not support the view that sucrose is the most cariogenic of sugars, except that it is so widely present in our diet, but their latter finding supports the 24-month results of the Turku human studies where the analyses included precavitation carious lesions (see p. 46). These findings cast doubt on the theory that sucrose is uniquely cariogenic because it increases dextran formation in plaque. Schemmel *et al.* (1982) also observed that dextran production was an unimportant determinant of caries because rats fed maltose formed little plaque but developed a considerable amount of caries. However, a different result was reported by Birkhed *et al.* (1981). They found that glucose + fructose (invert sugar) was less cariogenic than sucrose, but the significance of this is uncertain as the rats who received the sucrose diet were superinfected with *Strep. mutans* but the rats who received the invert sugar were not.

Cariogenicity testing of foods in animals

While the introduction of the Zurich programmed feeder was a major advance in experimental design, two further improvements have been suggested recently. Bowen *et al.* (1980) advocated that test products should be fed to rats by mouth in the usual way using a programmed feeder, while essential nutrients should be given twice a day by stomach tube, so by-passing the mouth. Because this method is technically difficult and results in loss of animals, Navia and Lopez (1983) suggested that essential nutrients should be given by mouth but in a gel form which ensures minimal contact time with the teeth. These methods were compared in a collaborative study in the USA (Shaw 1986) and, as similar results were found using either method, the nutrient supplement gel method was considered preferable. It must be appreciated, however, that these methods move further away from usual methods of human food consumption so that, while their results may be more clear-cut and reproducible, extrapolating such results to the human situation is more difficult.

Plaque pH studies

If the acidogenic theory of caries aetiology is accepted, measurement of plaque pH before, during, and after a food is eaten should be a guide to the cariogenic potential of that food. If measurements of plaque pH are made, under standardized conditions, the acidogenicity of various foods, drinks, and meal patterns can be compared and the results used as a basis for advising on their potential cariogenicity. It is emphasized that it is acidogenicity not cariogenicity which is being measured but these might be expected to be strongly correlated, and only the possible presence of 'protective factors', which may protect the enamel against dissolution even at low pH, or 'chelators', which might cause loss of Ca at neutral pH, may confuse their close relationship (see p. 81).

Methods of measuring plaque pH

There are four main methods of measuring plaque pH. Firstly, metal probes (antimony, iridium, or palladium), which can be inserted *in situ* into plaque. The antimony probe micro-electrode was used by Stephan (1940, 1943, 1944) in his original 'Stephan curve' experiments, and by many workers since then (e.g. Forscher and Hess 1954; Kleinberg 1958; Kleinberg *et al.* 1982; Mörch 1961; Neff 1967; Bowen 1969). Yankell *et al.* (1983) used iridium oxide probes fitted into upper removable intra-oral appliances; Harper *et al.* (1985) used a palladium–palladium oxide miniature probe.

Secondly, glass probes have been used (Charlton 1956). Thirdly, a more complicated, but potentially more useful system employs a miniature glass electrode built into a partial denture that stays in the mouth for several days while plaque forms over the teeth and electrode. Recordings of pH are made either via wires coming from the mouth or by radio-telemetry, which avoids the possibility of wires interfering with eating (Imfeld 1977). This system, which was developed in Zurich and has given consistent results for many years (Firestone *et al.* 1987), has also been used by Clarke and Fanning (1971), and Clarke and Dowdell (1976) in Australia, and by Newman *et al.* (1979) in Glasgow.

The fourth method involves the removal of small samples of plaque from representative teeth and the measurement of the pH of this plaque on a small saucer-shaped glass ('one-drop') electrode outside the mouth. This method was developed by Fosdick *et al.* (1941), and Forscher and Hess (1954), and used subsequently by workers in Sweden (Frostell 1969), America (Edgar *et al.* 1975), and the United Kingdom (Rugg-Gunn *et al.* 1975, 1978). Each method has its advantages and disadvantages. The metal–metal oxide probes can be made with very fine points well suited to reaching the deep layers of interproximal plaque. They react faster than glass electrodes, but are very prone to poisoning. The indwelling glass electrode permits continuous recording of pH at the deepest part of plaque, but concern has been expressed that plaque does not adhere to glass (Winter and Ridge 1982), and that plaque contacts an unreactive glass surface rather than a reactive enamel surface. The method records plaque pH at a single, highly cariogenic site in only a few subjects whose plaque is known to exhibit a large pH drop, thus maximizing the pH response (Edgar and Geddes 1986). The plaque 'harvesting' method involves removal of rather superficial plaque and disrupts the plaque structure, but it has the advantages of sampling plaque from many sites per mouth, and of simplicity, which enables large numbers of subjects to be studied. However, regardless of methods used, there is reasonable agreement in the order in which foods and drinks are ranked according to their acidogenicity, although the methods differ in the absolute pH values recorded (Harper *et al.* 1985; Edgar and Geddes, 1986).

Snack foods and plaque pH

The largest survey of snack foods was carried out by Edgar *et al.* (1975) in America. They ranked 54 snack foods and drinks according to the value of the minimum pH reached by the plaque. This varies from pH 6.8 (virtually no pH depression) for 'sugarless' chewing-gum to pH 5.2 for a 'cherry sucker' (a hard fruit-flavoured sucrose sweet). Rugg-Gunn *et al.* (1978) ranked 22 British snacks and again found a boiled sweet gave the lowest pH minimum value. Sugared coffee and tea also gave low pH minimum values. Figure 2.24 shows curves for four of the 22 snack foods tested. Peanuts tended to raise plaque pH, while the curves for apple and chocolate were similar. The importance of sugar in causing plaque pH to fall is shown in Fig. 2.25: sugared (containing sucrose) gum caused a depression of plaque pH, while the pH rose to the high level of pH 7.5 when 'sugarless' (called 'sugarless' although sweetened with non-metabolizable sorbitol and mannitol) gum was chewed. Similar results were shown by Graf (1970) using the indwelling electrode technique. It should be appreciated that the rise in plaque pH is principally caused by salivary flow: as the flow increases so the alkalinity of the saliva increases. The availability of non-sucrose flavoured snacks and drinks has increased in recent years and Figs. 2.26 and 2.27 further illustrate the difference in the acidogenicity of sucrose and non-sucrose containing snacks. Diabetic chocolate and 'Diet Pepsi' are sweetened with sorbitol and saccharin, respectively. In addition to sorbitol and mannitol, a third sugar alcohol, xylitol has been shown to be non-acidogenic (Mühlemann and Boever 1970; Imfeld 1977). Similarly, sorbose (a ketohexose, like fructose) does not depress plaque pH (Mühlemann and Schneider 1975). Another artificial sweetener, Lycasin, a starch hydrolysate, has also been shown to produce only a moderate Stephan curve (Frostell 1973, Imfeld 1977). Because of the much higher acidogenicity of confectionery made with sucrose and glucose

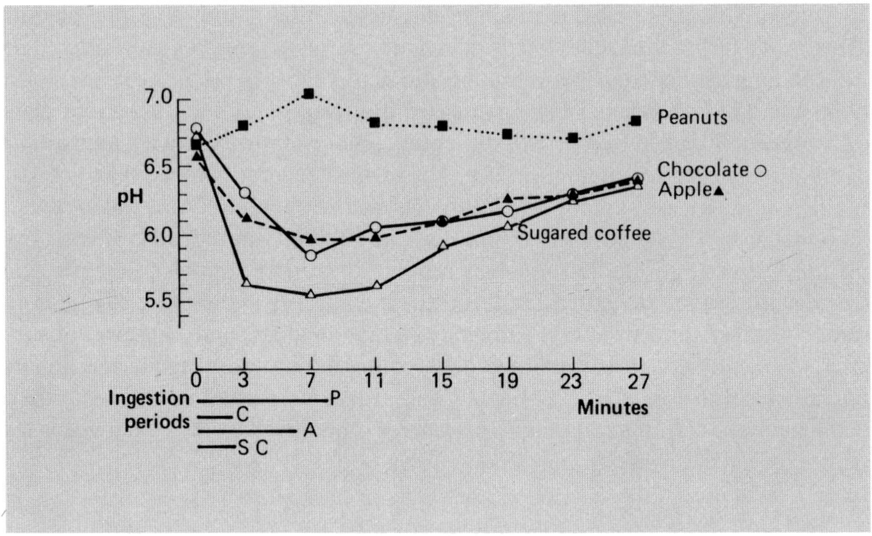

Fig. 2.24. Stephan curves produced by chocolate, apple, salted peanuts, and sugared coffee. (Rugg-Gunn *et al.* (1978), with permission of the editor *British Dental Journal.*)

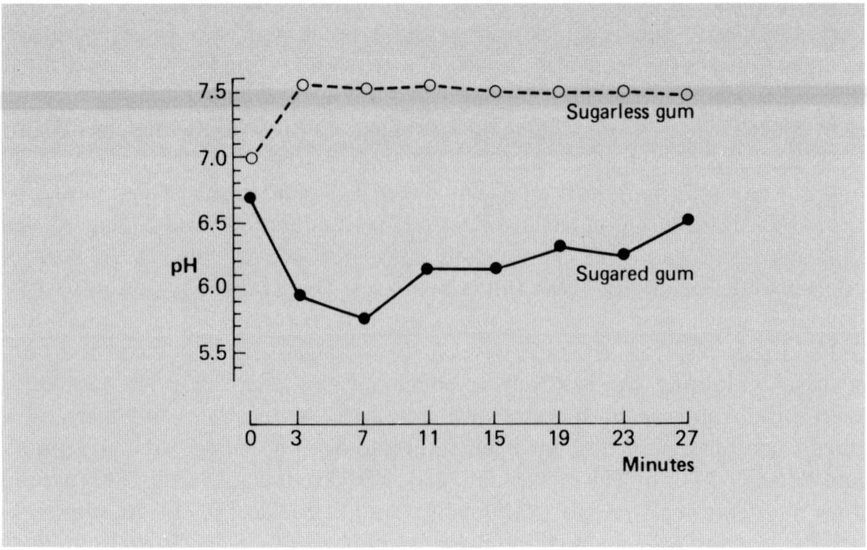

Fig. 2.25. Stephan curves produced by sugared and sugarless chewing-gum. (Rugg-Gunn *et al.* (1978), with permision of the editor *British Dental Journal.*)

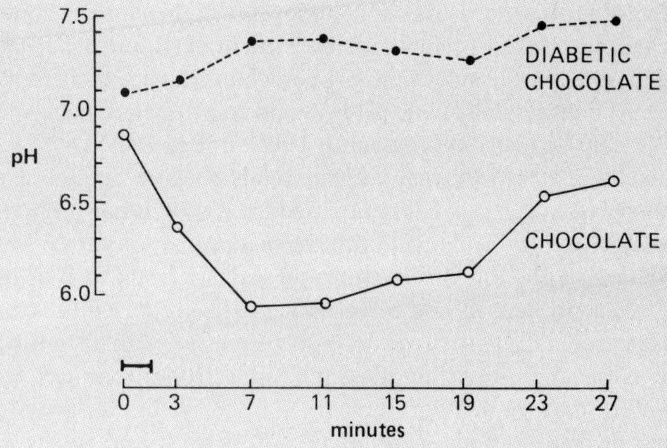

Fig. 2.26. Stephan curves produced by dark ('plain') chocolate (containing sugar) and 'diabetic' chocolate (containing sorbitol).

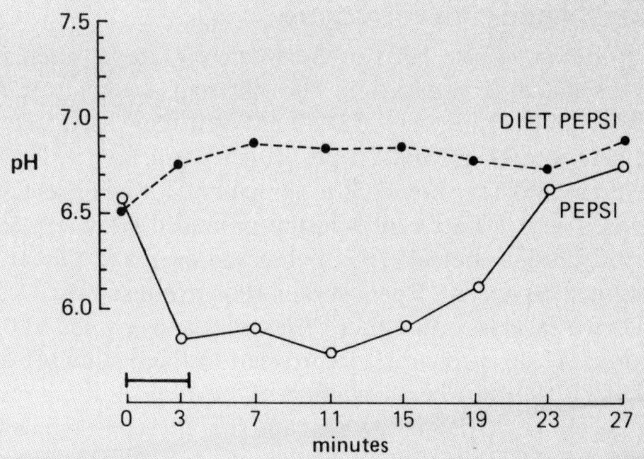

Fig. 2.27. Stephan curves produced by Pepsi Cola (sugar-containing) and Diet Pepsi (sugarless).

compared with that of sorbitol, mannitol, xylitol, sorbose, and Lycasin, preventive dentistry advanced one step further in Switzerland in 1969, when the Swiss Office of Health pronounced that non-acidogenic confectionery could be classed as 'safe for teeth'. The test involves an assessment of plaque pH using the Zurich indwelling glass electrode system; many confectionery products have passed the test (plaque pH does not fall below pH 5.7) and can therefore be advertised under Swiss law as 'safe for teeth' (Mühlemann 1969; Imfeld 1977).

The indwelling glass electrode system tends to give an 'all-or-nothing response to foods' (Edgar 1985; Edgar and Geddes 1986). It has been very useful in demonstrating the non-acidogenic nature of non-carbohydrate foods but less useful at indicating the low acidogenicity of starchy foods such as bread (Edgar 1985). For example, Jensen and Schachtele (1983) reported that starchy foods (wheat-flakes and bread) produced deep pH responses, similar to those produced by sucrose, using the indwelling glass micro-electrode technique (see p. 79 for discussion of the cariogenicity of starch).

The effect of fruit cordials, carbonated soft drinks, and sports drinks upon plaque pH has been studied by Birkhed (1984) and Grobler *et al.* (1985). They found that well-buffered acid drinks produced the greatest adverse effect on plaque pH and were also more likely to cause tooth erosion. Drinking through a straw seemed to be the least harmful method of imbibing sugar-containing drinks.

The beneficial effect upon plaque pH of substituting sucrose or glucose by non-fermentable sweeteners, such as sorbitol or Lycasin, in syrup medicines has been reported by Lokken *et al.* (1975), Feigal and Jensen (1982), and Rugg-Gunn (1988).

Different sugars and concentrations

Plaque pH studies have also been used to differentiate between the potential cariogenicity of different sugars and the different concentrations of sugar. Sucrose solutions in the range of 0.05–50 per cent have been tested by Frostell (1969), and between 0.025 and 15 per cent by Imfeld (1977). Their results (using different methods) are not in close agreement, for whereas Frostell (1969) found that rinses with 50 per cent solution produced a lower plaque pH than with 5 per cent solution, Imfeld (1977) observed deep and similar curves after rinses containing 2.5 per cent, 5 per cent, or 10 per cent sucrose. A fall in plaque pH of 1.5 units was also recorded after rinses with a very weak (0.025 per cent) sucrose solution, yet no comparable depression in the plaque pH was observed by Frostell (1969). This may be an example of the all-or-nothing response of the indwelling glass electrode (Edgar, 1985), and it is therefore impossible to state, at present, a theshold concentration below which a sucrose solution may be considered safe. Using an antimony micro-electrode, Abelson and Pergola (1984) observed that a 10 per cent solution of sucrose was more acidogenic than a 40 or 70 per cent solution when rinsed for 1 minute.

Frostell (1973) showed that lactose (in both 10 per cent and 50 per cent solu-

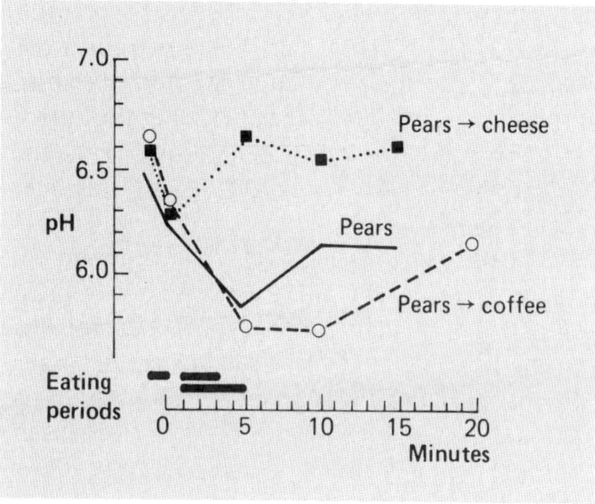

Fig. 2.28. Stephan curves produced by eating either cheese or sugared coffee after tinned pears in syrup. (Rugg-Gunn *et al.* (1975), with permission of the editor *British Dental Journal*.)

tion) produced less severe falls in plaque pH than sucrose, glucose, or fructose. These results were confirmed by Imfeld (1977) who also showed that galactose was of similar acidogenicity to lactose, and maltose of similar acidogenicity to sucrose, glucose, and fructose. Cows' milk contains 5 per cent lactose. Although milk (Frostell 1970) and milk-containing unsugared tea (Rugg-Gunn *et al.* 1978) causes a slight fall in plaque pH, and milk chocolate produces a slightly greater fall in plaque pH than dark (plain) chocolate, milk must be considered to be of very weak cariogenic potential, especially in view of its other favourable properties such as high Ca, P, protein, and fat content (Jenkins and Ferguson 1966; Rugg-Gunn *et al.* 1985).

Meals and plaque pH

Although the effect of individual snacks has been investigated by many people, the acidogenicity of meals has not received much attention. Rugg-Gunn *et al.* (1975) showed that eating cheese after a sugary food (e.g. tinned pears in syrup) prevented the depression of plaque pH which otherwise would have been caused by the sugary food (Fig. 2.28). Sugared coffee instead of the cheese further depressed plaque pH. The favourable action of cheese is likely to be due to (i) the high salivary flow rate induced by the strongly flavoured food; (ii) absence of fermentable carbohydrates. Peanuts and sugarless chewing-gum also have similar actions in raising the pH of plaque after it has been depressed by a sugary food (Geddes *et al.* 1977; Jensen 1986*a*, *b*). On the other hand, eating an apple was found to have little beneficial effect compared with peanuts (Geddes *et al.* 1977).

Rugg-Gunn *et al.* (1981) investigated the effect of a three-course 'breakfast' upon plaque pH. The breakfast consisted of one sugary course (sugared coffee) and two non-sugary courses (a boiled egg, and crispbread and butter). The Stephan curve produced when the sugared coffee was taken first, second, or last can be seen in Fig. 2.29. When sugared coffee was taken last (curve C) the

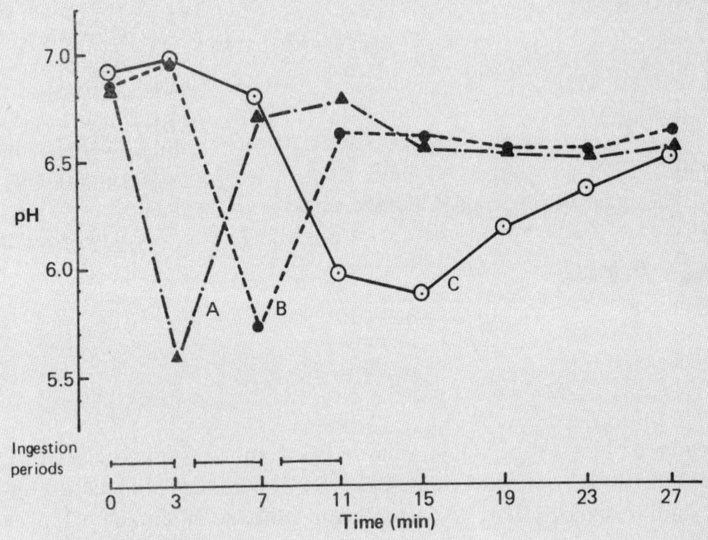

Fig. 2.29. Stephan curves produced when sugared coffee was the first (A), second (B), or last (C) food in a three course meal. The other two courses were non-acidogenic. (Rugg-Gunn *et al.* (1981), with the permission of the editor *Journal of Dental Research.*)

Stephan curve is longer but shallower than when it was first (A) or second (B). The most favourable curve was produced when all three foods were taken together (curve F in Fig. 2.30); the fall in plaque pH being much less than when sugared coffee was taken alone (curve E). The potential harmful effect of having a gap after the sugary course can be seen in Fig. 2.31 (curve D): plaque pH staying at a low level until a non-acidogenic food was eaten. These experiments clearly show that one food can influence the acidogenicity of another.

Plaque pH studies have the advantage of being quick and, for the 'harvesting' or one-drop glass electrode method at least, relatively easy to do. They have been useful at ranking snacks and meals according to their acidogenicity which in turn indicates their potential cariogenicity.

Other methods of assessing cariogenicity

Incubation experiments

These are simple tests and examine the ability of plaque micro-organisms to metabolize a test food to acid. They are done outside the mouth and can be classed as 'test-tube experiments'. Saliva, which contains oral micro-organisms,

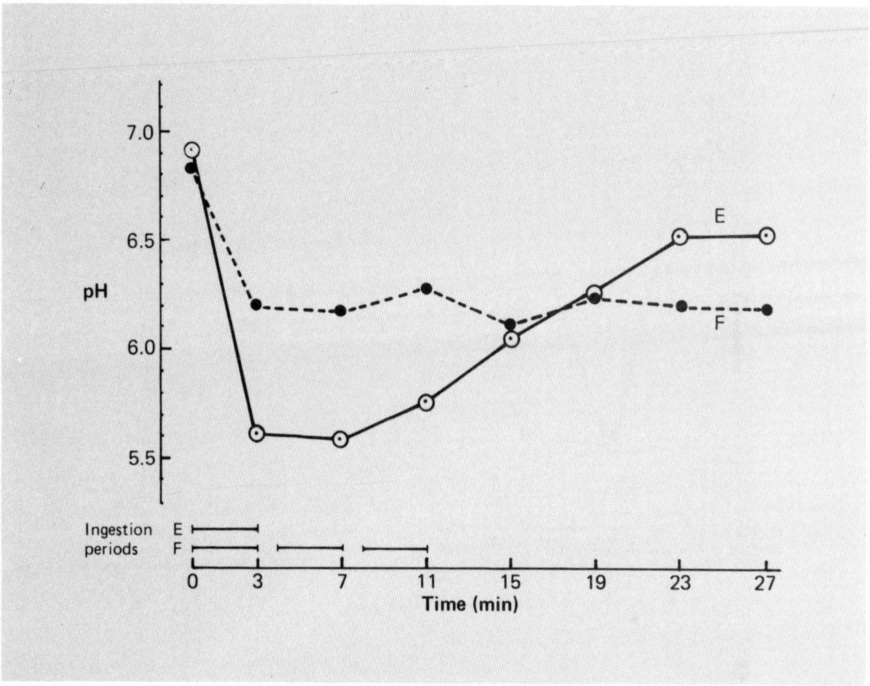

Fig. 2.30. Stephan curves produced when sugared coffee was taken alone (E) or taken together with the other two non-acidogenic foods (F). (Rugg-Gunn *et al.* (1981), with permission of the editor *Journal of Dental Research.*)

or pure cultures of oral micro-organisms, have substituted for plaque (Bibby *et al.* 1951; Grobler 1982). This is a very stringent test, as some acid may be formed from some foods but as such a slow rate that it has to be of little clinical relevance. Conversely, rapid acid production indicates that the food under test is potentially cariogenic.

In some of these experiments, teeth, or parts of teeth, have been incubated with the bacteria and substrate, and the degree of dissolution of the enamel quantified. This has led to the construction of 'artificial mouths' (Huang *et al.* 1981). However, the conditions in the mouths of living people are constantly changing and it is impossible to reproduce all of these, many of which may be protective. Because of these limitations it is unlikely that artificial mouths will become a wholly reliable guide to the cariogenicity of foods.

Changes in plaque flora

A number of studies have suggested that micro-organisms of the *Strep. mutans* group are more capable of causing caries than other organisms. In fact, caries has been labelled a 'specific plaque' disease (Emilson and Krasse 1985). It has been suggested that any potential caries-preventive effect of foods can be

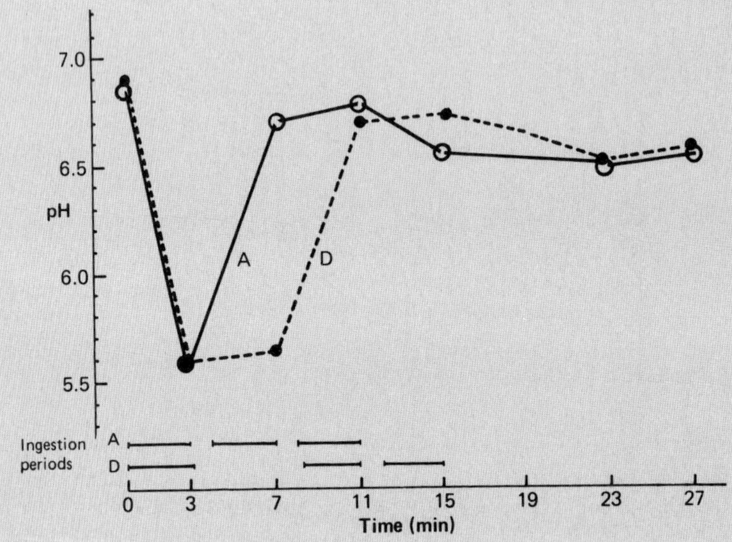

Fig. 2.31. Stephan curves produced when there was no gap (A), or a 5-minute gap (D) after drinking sugared coffee and before eating two non-acidogenic foods. (Rugg-Gunn *et al.* (1981), with permission of the editor *Journal of Dental Research.*)

assessed by their ability to alter plaque flora in one direction or another (Loesche 1985). However, the unique relationship between oral levels of *Strep. mutans* and the development of dental caries is not universally accepted and, at the present time, it must be considered a weak method of measuring cariogenicity.

Food clearance from the mouth

A number of factors influence the rate at which foods are removed from the mouth by swallowing. These are (a) physical properties, such as adhesiveness; (b) the resting salivary flow rate; and (c) the degree of salivary flow induced by food in the mouth. The main food ingredients studied have been total carbohydrate and sugars. Bibby *et al.* (1951) determined the 'decalcification potential' as the product of the intra-oral retention of carbohydrate and the quantity of acid produced after incubation of food and saliva, but found no simple relation between carbohydrate content and food retention. This same group has shown recently (Bibby *et al.* 1986) that starchy foods remain in the mouth longer than sugary foods, and they have suggested that starch enhances the cariogenicity of dietary sugars. On the other hand, foods such as toffee, caramel, and chocolate have high intra-oral adhesion and long clearance times (Lundqvist 1952).

Theoretical and practical aspects of sugar clearance have been studied extensively by Dawes (1983) and co-workers. Britse and Lagerlof (1987) have shown that intra-oral sugar clearance is quickest in the lower incisor region and slowest in the upper incisor region, with little difference in the clearance rates in the upper and lower molar regions. As the greater the salivary concentration of sugars, the greater the fall in plaque pH (Lindfors and Lagerlof 1988), rapid clearance of cariogenic food is important in caries prevention.

Enamel slab experiments

In order to overcome some of the drawbacks of the artificial mouth, intra-oral appliances have been made that can hold slabs of enamel. Plaque forms on the surface of the slabs, which remain in the mouth for 1 to 6 weeks. The experimental system is extremely flexible so that by using either sound or partially demineralized enamel, the cariogenic effect or the remineralizing effect of diets can be assessed.

Because of this flexibility of design, a variety of methods have been used. Some workers have used slabs made from bovine enamel (Koulourides *et al.* 1976); others have used human enamel (Pearce and Gallagher 1979). In some experiments the slabs have been covered with Dacron (Koulourides *et al.* 1976) or terylene (Pearce and Gallagher 1979) gauze to encourage plaque formation, but in others no gauze was used (van Herpen and Arends 1986). The gauze is, in some experiments, infected with suspensions of *Strep. mutans* to encourage caries formation (Tehrani *et al.* 1983). Slabs have been held in full dentures (van Herpen and Arends 1986), partial dentures (Koulourides *et al.* 1976), or orthodontic retainers (Pearce and Gallagher 1979; Tehrani *et al.* 1983). In most experiments, the appliances have been removed from the mouth several times a day so that the slabs can be inserted into solutions of test foods (Koulourides *et al.* 1976), but in some (van Herpen and Arends 1986) the foods are eaten with the appliance in place. While the former methods allows different slabs on the one appliance to be placed in different test solutions, the latter design takes into account the effect of eating the food and the stimulating effect on salivary flow that may be induced. From the work of van Strijp *et al.* (1988) it would seem important that the temperature of the test solutions into which the slabs are placed out of the mouth is 37°C rather than room temperature. Lesion formation has been measured by micro-hardness tests (Koulourides *et al.* 1976), microradiography (Pearce and Gallagher 1979), and iodine dye permeability (Brudevold *et al.* 1984).

An example of an appliance made to fit over mandibular teeth is shown in Fig. 2.32. There seems to be reasonably good agreement between results obtained by different methods of measuring lesion formation, as can be seen in Fig. 2.33, in which demineralization has been quantified in three ways. In this experiment, it can be seen that eating two extra 'filled chocolate products' (FCPs) per day led to an increase in lesion formation (van Herpen and Arends 1986). Other workers have shown that sugars cause demineralization while non-fermentable alternat-

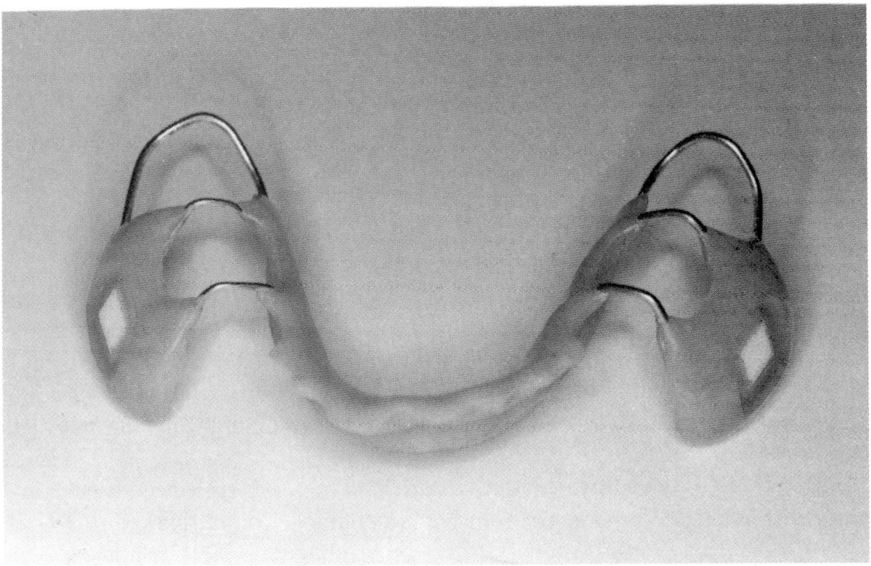

Fig. 2.32. An example of an acrylic resin appliance showing two buccal flanges each containing a terylene mesh-covered slab of enamel. (Illustration kindly supplied by E.I.F. Pearce; reproduced with permission of the editor *New Zealand Dental Journal*.)

ive sweeteners (see p. 88) aid remineralization (Koulourides *et al.* 1976; Pearce and Gallagher 1979). Tehrani *et al.* (1983) showed that increasing the concentration of sugars and the frequency of exposure to sugars increased demineralization.

Enamel slab experiments seem to have a number of advantages over *in vitro* incubation and demineralization experiments and *in vivo* plaque pH experiments, especially if the test foods are eaten with the appliance in place.

Starchy foods and dental caries

It has been suggested that all carbohydrate foods should be considered cariogenic (Biscuit, Cake, Chocolate, and Confectionery Alliance 1987). The term fermentable carbohydrate has been widely used as the dietary cause of dental caries; indeed, Miller (1890) launched the acidogenic theory of caries with his experiments on the incubation of starchy foods, saliva, and enamel. In Britain, as in many countries, current advice for healthy eating is to decrease consumption of fat, sugar, salt, and alcohol, and to increase consumption of starchy foods, fresh fruit, and vegetables. Because of this, it is sensible to consider the relative cariogenicity of starch compared with sugars as a separate issue. As with all aspects of cariogenicity, it is important to look at evidence from all sources and these will be discussed in turn. A fuller review of this subject has been published by the Health Education Authority (Rugg-Gunn 1988).

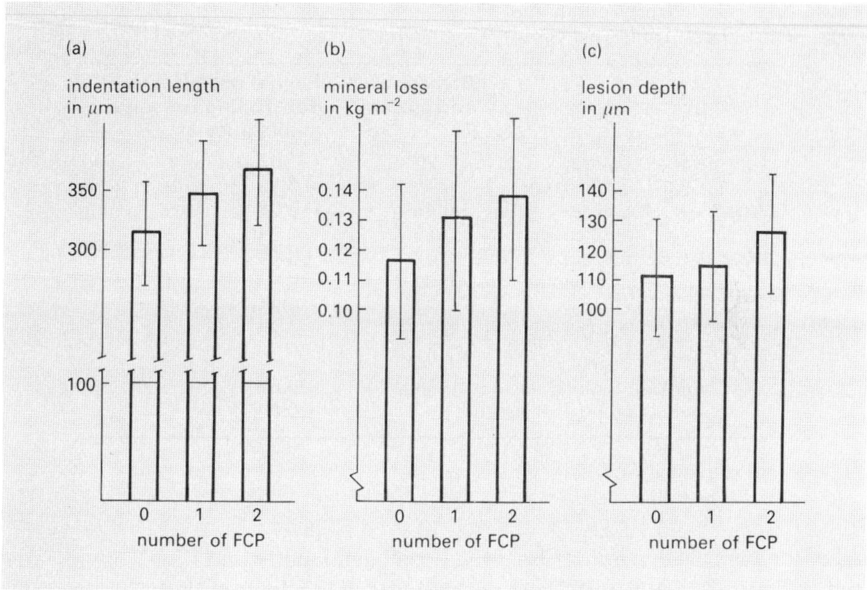

Fig. 2.33. Demineralization of enamel slabs used in intra-oral cariogenicity testing of foods. Filled chocolate products (FCP) were consumed by the subjects at frequencies of 0, 1, or 2 per day, over and above normal food consumption. Demineralization is expressed in three ways: (a) length of indentation made with a Knoop diamond; (b) mineral loss calculated from microradiographs scans; and (c) lesion depth, also calculated from microradiograph scans. Sound enamel gave an indentation length of 100 μm (a). (van Herpen and Arends (1986), with permission of the editor of *Caries Research*.)

Human observational studies

In two publications, Sreebny (1982, 1983) listed and correlated the caries status of 47 countries with the availability of sugar and cereals in those countries. The caries status was measured by the DMFT index for 12-year-old children, obtained primarily from the WHO Global Epidemiology Bank; data on sugar and grain availability were obtained from the food balance sheets compiled by the Food and Agricultural Organization of the UN. Cereal availability was quantified in two ways: (a) as the number of calories provided by the cereal per day; and (b) as the proportion of total energy intake provided by that cereal. Sreebny gave only bivariate correlations and showed that, while the correlation between sugar availability and DMFT was +0.72, the correlation between total cereals availability and DMFT was −0.25 (calculated as cal/day) and −0.45 (calculated as per cent of total energy). However, for wheat, positive correlations with DMFT were found (+0.45 and +0.30). Sreebny's data have been examined further, using partial correlation analyses (Table 2.19); this allows an examination of the caries versus cereal relationship, when the effect of differences in sugar availability is removed. It can be seen (in the right-hand column of Table 2.19) that

Table 2.19. Correlations and partial correlations between DMFT (for 12-year-olds) and sugar or cereal availability in 47 countries. Raw data taken from Sreebny (1982; 1983)

		Bivariate correlation	Partial correlation, controlling for sugar availability
Total cereals	cal/day	−0.25	−0.03
	% of energy	−0.45***	−0.13
Wheat	cal/day	+0.45***	+0.05
	% of energy	+0.29	−0.03
Rice	cal/day	−0.07	+0.10
	% of energy	−0.09	+0.10
Maize	cal/day	−0.37*	−0.24
	% of energy	−0.40**	−0.26
Sugar	(g/day)	+0.70***	
controlling for total cereal (cal/day)			+0.67***
controlling for wheat (cal/day)			+0.60***

*** $p<0.005$
** $p<0.01$
* $p<0.05$

all of the partial correlations between cereal availability and DMFT are low and not statistically significant. On the other hand, it can be seen in the lower part of Table 2.19 that when the correlation between DMFT and sugar availability (r = +0.70, using Sreebny's data) was controlled for cereal availability, the correlation fell only slightly to +0.67 ($p<0.001$) and +0.60 ($p<0.001$) when controlling for the two measures of wheat availability. These findings suggest a much closer positive relation between DMFT and sugar availability than between DMFT and cereal availability.

Many countries have or have had staple diets which are high in starch and low in sugar. Afonsky (1951) described the very low caries experience in Chinese eating crude polished rice. Russell *et al.* (1960) commented upon the exceptionally low caries rates in Vietnamese, Ethiopians, and Middle- and South-American Indians.

One of the best surveys of an increase in caries prevalence coinciding with a change of diet took place in the island of Tristan da Cunha (Fisher 1968). However, both sugar and refined flour were introduced in 1942, so that is not possible to blame the deterioration of the islanders' teeth solely on the introduction of sugar. It can be noted, though, that prior to 1942 the staple food was potatoes, which would have been cooked before eating.

Newbrun *et al.* (1980) compared diets and the dental status of 17 subjects with the rare disorder—hereditary fructose intolerance (HFI)—with 14 control subjects who were unaffected and mostly blood-relations. The mean ages were 29 years for the HFI subjects and 27 years for the control subjects. The respective mean DMFT scores were 2.1 and 14.3, and DMFS 3.3 and 36.1. The respective daily sucrose consumption was 3 g and 48 g, and the respective mean daily starch consumption was 160 g and 140 g. The nutrient, vitamin, and mineral contents of the diets of the two groups were similar. The finding that the HFI subjects consumed high levels of starch (higher than the control subjects) and yet developed minimal caries levels must indicate that starch is not particularly caries-inducive. Newbrun also concludes that while a diet with a high content and a high frequency of sucrose is cariogenic, a diet with an extremely low content of sucrose is non-cariogenic.

Although over 30 cross-sectional studies have correlated sugar-eating habits with dental caries experience, only a few of these have considered starch intake. In a comprehensive cross-sectional study of Swedish 14-year-old children, Martinsson (1972) compared the diet of children with high (H) caries experience (mean DFS = 37) with the diet of children with low (L) caries experience (DFS = 8). The H-group had a higher intake of sucrose, but this difference was statistically significant in the boys only. The intake of potatoes and bread was similar in the two groups, but the consumption of groats and flakes was higher in the caries-low children. The author states that 'only the carbohydrate intake in the form of sucrose, especially between meals, was found to be significantly higher in the H-group than in the L-group'. Hankin, Chung, and Kau (1973) reported the relationship between the dietary patterns and caries prevalence in Hawaiian schoolchildren. They found that the consumption of sugared gum and candy was strongly positively associated with DMFT ($p<0.001$), but the consumption of breads and cereals was negatively associated with DMFT ($p<0.05$). Kleemola-Kujala and Rasanen (1979) reported the dietary intake of low-caries and high-caries children of three different age groups (5, 9, and 13 years). While the total carbohydrate was similar in each pair of high- and low-caries groups, the intake of sugar was higher in each of the three high-caries groups, although the differences were statistically significant for the 5- and 13-year-old groups only. Calculated by subtraction, the intake of starch would have been higher in the low-caries groups.

When examining the relationship between diet and dental caries, a longitudinal design is better than a cross-sectional design because diet and the occurrence of dental caries can be measured over the same time period. A longitudinal observational study was conducted between 1979 and 1981 in northern England (Rugg-Gunn *et al.* 1984*b*): 405 children initially aged 11.5 years completed the 2-year study. Sugars intake was positively correlated with DMFS increment ($p<0.05$), but starch intake was not. When the starch versus caries correlations were controlled for sugars intake, they became negative, although not statistically significantly so. The children who had a high sugar/low starch diet developed 4.1 DMFS compared with 2.8 DMFS in the children who had a low sugar/high starch diet, although this difference of 1.3 tooth surfaces was not statistically significant (Rugg-Gunn *et al.* 1987).

Human interventional studies

The main purpose of the Turku sugar studies (Scheinin and Mäkinen 1975; see p. 43 for detail) was to investigate the effect on dental caries of total substitution of dietary sugars with either fructose or xylitol. About 100 dietary items were especially manufactured by 12 food firms in Finland, in order to ensure that as wide a variety of foods as possible was available. Fructose or xylitol was substituted for sucrose but the starch content of the foods was not altered. The mean 2-year DMFS increments for the sugar, fructose, and xylitol groups were 7.2, 3.8, and 0.0 respectively when precavitation carious lesions were included. When such lesions were excluded from the analyses and only cavities recorded, the 2-year increments were 3.33, 3.57, and 1.47 for the sugar, fructose, and xylitol groups respectively. The trial showed that substitution of sucrose by xylitol resulted in a substantial reduction in caries incidence. Although changes in salivary enzymes, the amount of plaque, and the incidence of some microorganisms may have contributed to the results, the persistent inability of plaque organisms to metabolize xylitol to acids is likely to be the main explanation for the caries-preventive effect. As the starch intake was unaltered, dietary starch cannot have contributed significantly to caries development in these human subjects.

Animal experiments

Animal experiments which have assessed the cariogenicity of starch have given variable results. Raw starches would appear to have very low cariogenicity, regardless of the method of feeding. In experiments where the animals were fed *ad libitum*, cooked starch caused caries, but the amount was less than that caused by sucrose: for example, in the study by Frostell and Baer (1971) pregelatinized starch caused half as much caries as sucrose. Mixtures of starch and sucrose caused more caries than starch alone (Green and Hartles 1967), and the amount of caries developing was positively related to the amount of sugar in the starch/sugar food (Hefti and Schmid 1979). Baking of starch/sugar mixtures increases their cariogenicity markedly (Grenby and Paterson 1972). The oral flora of rats (or the amylase levels in the rat's salivary glands) did not adapt to metabolize starch more rapidly when several generations of rats were fed a starch diet (Shaw and Ivimey 1972).

In animal experiments where frequency of feeding was standardized, cooked starch or starchy foods (e.g. bread) were shown to be capable of causing caries but were less cariogenic than sucrose (König 1969). Caries development increased as frequency of feeding starchy foods increased. When only the test foods were taken orally by the rats and the rest of the diet fed by stomach tube, a similar picture emerged with some caries developing when starchy foods were eaten but less than that caused by sucrose (Bowen *et al.* 1980). The relevance of this type of feeding can be questioned as it is not the way foods are eaten in man, and there is no opportunity for foods to interact to influence caries development. Krasse (1985) has pointed out that foods in animal experiments have to be given in a powdered form and not in the physical form in which they are consumed by humans. A further problem in extrapolation of findings on starch cariogenicity in the rat to its effect in man was highlighted by Beighton and Hayday (1984), who pointed out that the buffering capacity of rat saliva is less than that of primates such as monkeys or humans. They suggested that this 'difference in buffering capacity of rodent and macaque (monkey) saliva is a major obstacle to the extrapolation of caries results obtained in rodents to man.' Clearly, animal experiments are useful in giving an indication of the cariogenicity of foods in man, but caution in their interpretation is necessary.

Plaque pH studies

Plaque pH experiments investigate acidogenicity, not cariogenicity. Any 'protective factors' present in starchy foods would not affect the measurement of acidogenicity but would decrease cariogenicity. Almost all of the plaque pH experiments with starch have been carried out using either the sampling method or the indwelling glass electrode method. The sampling method, used by Frostell (1972), Edgar *et al.* (1975), and Rugg-Gunn *et al.* (1978), has tended to indicate that cooked starch or starchy foods are less acidogenic than sugar or high sugar foods. Frostell (1972) showed that uncooked starch was virtually non-acidogenic. On the other hand, indwelling glass electrode experiments (Imfeld 1983; Schachtele and Jensen 1981; Jensen and Schachtele 1983) have shown that starch is capable of depressing plaque pH to below what is commonly called the 'critical pH' (pH 5.5) to a similar extent as sugar and, by these criteria, starch cannot be labelled 'safe for teeth'. These findings have led Bibby *et al.* (1986) to conclude 'that the starch in foods may be a more important contributor to the acidogenicity of sugar-containing foods than generally is believed'. Whether this adequately reflects what occurs naturally in man has been questioned by some workers. Newbrun (1984) remarked that 'the pH response seen with the glass electrodes might be hyper-responsive'. Similarly, Edgar (1985) suggested that the indwelling glass electrode (see p. 64) 'tends to give an all-or-nothing response to foods—any carbohydrate-containing food leading to a maximum drop in pH. This feature makes the application of the method to evaluating relative cariogenicity of normal snack foods difficult, as foods such as bread, judged to be of low relative cariogenicity by other methods, appear highly cariogenic, and the technique has mainly found favour in verifying the low cariogenicity of some sugar substitutes.'

Enamel slab experiments

There have been two reports of the effect of starchy foods upon the demineralization of enamel slabs worn in the mouth of volunteers; both indicated that starch is about one-quarter as 'cariogenic' as sugar. Thompson and Pearce (1982) compared the effect of a biscuit made from wheat, oats, butter, honey, and mollasses, and a sugar-free biscuit (78 per cent flour), with that of 5 per cent sucrose. While sucrose gave a demineralization score of 38, the sweetened biscuit gave a score of 6, and the sugar-free biscuit a score of 10. The authors suggest that the difference in the demineralization caused by the two biscuits may be due to 'protective factors', particularly present in the sweetened biscuit.

A second intra-oral demineralization test using enamel slabs was described by Brudevold *et al.* (1985). They compared the effect of rinsing with solutions of either raw starch or cooked starch, with no rinsing at all. The degree of demineralization was assessed by measuring the change in the iodine permeability of the enamel slab. Cooked starch caused a slight increase in the enamel permeability (+3.6 units) while the raw starch produced a significant decrease in the permeability (−6.7 units). In comparison with these results, rinsing with a 10 per cent sucrose rinse solution increased enamel permeability by 15.6 units, indicating that sucrose had a considerably greater demineralization effect than either starch.

Incubation experiments

Miller (1890) established, nearly a century ago, that when carbohydrate foods (such as bread) were incubated with oral organisms, acid was produced and this acidic incubate was capable of demineralizing tooth enamel. Since then many experiments have been conducted to elucidate the cariogenicity of foods, and these experiments have used a variety of methods.

Despite this diversity of methods, incubation experiments, as a whole, do not appear to provide very much useful information concerning the cariogenicity of starch, other than showing that acids can be produced from starchy foods. Some of the results appear to bear little relation to other evidence of the cariogenicity of foods: e.g. Bibby and Mundorff (1975) reported that sorbitol sweets produced eight times as much enamel dissolution as 2 per cent sucrose, while lemon-flavoured sugar candies produced only one-fifth as much enamel dissolution as sucrose. The artificial mouth is an attempt to overcome some of these drawbacks of food/saliva/enamel incubation experiments but this is still too far removed from what happens in man to be of much assistance.

Unlike sugars, starch is not transported across the cell membrane of plaque micro-organisms (Birkhed and Skude 1978) and must be split into sugars before it can be used by the cell and acid produced. This is achieved by amylase in saliva and plaque, but the rate at which it happens will vary, depending on salivary amylase levels and the nature of the starchy food. Mormann and Mühlemann (1981) showed that solutions of starch are quickly degraded to sugars, but this is not the form in which starch is commonly eaten.

Conclusions

1. Cooked staple starchy foods, such a rice, potatoes and bread would appear to be of very low cariogenicity in man.
2. If finely ground, heat-treated and eaten frequently, starch can cause caries but the amount is much less than that caused by sucrose.
3. The addition of sugar increases the cariogenicity of cooked starchy foods. Foods containing baked starch and substantial amounts of sucrose appear to be as cariogenic as a similar amount of sucrose.

Phosphates and other dietary items protective against caries

The observations of Osborn an his colleagues (Osborn and Noriskin 1937; Osborn *et al.* 1937*a*, *b*) that South African Bantu have very low caries prevalence, despite a high-carbohydrate diet, began the search for factors in human diets which may protect teeth against dental caries. As they also observed that less enamel dissolved from teeth incubated with 'unrefined' than with 'refined' foods, they suspected that these 'protective factors' act locally in the mouth rather than systematically via the developing tooth. However, it must be noted that the observed high-carbohydrate diets were low in sugar. Since then many possible 'protective factors', not necessarily normal constituents of food, have been studied, and their relevance in caries prevention will be briefly discussed. Some of the most widely studied of these 'protective factors' are inorganic phosphates and the cation is frequently calcium. This would seem logical because the caries process involves dissolution of enamel, which is very largely calcium and phosphate, and therefore any rise in the concentration of these two ions in plaque or saliva surrounding the tooth would, by the law of mass action, result in less enamel dissolving. The availability of calcium and phosphate during remineralization phases would also be increased aiding repair of the lesions. Phosphates have the additional advantage of being good buffers and their presence in plaque would therefore resist depression of plaque pH towards the 'critical pH'. Some organic phosphates have also been tested but, unlike inorganic phosphates, act mainly by binding to the tooth surface and reducing its solubility. The evidence concerning the effectiveness of protective factors comes principally from three sources, all important: animal experiments; laboratory experiments (largely enamel dissolution experiments in acid buffer or saliva incubates); and human clinical trials. A useful review of phosphates and dental caries has been made by Lilienthal (1977).

Inorganic phosphates

From a thorough review of over a hundred animal experiments, Nizel and Harris (1964) concluded that there was almost unanimous agreement that addition of inorganic phosphates to cariogenic diets reduced caries experience in rodents. The degree of protection varied with type of anion and cation tested. The cations H, Na, and K were more effective than Ca or Mg, probably owing to the lower solubility of Ca- and Mg-containing compounds. They concluded that addition of phosphates to water was very much less effective than the addition to food, and that the mode of action was principally local on erupted teeth, although the observed rise in salivary phosphate levels might also account for some of the effect. They also concluded that the amounts of added phosphate (e.g. 2 per cent Na_2HPO_4) were not considered excessive from the general health point of view, as this only doubled the daily intake of phosphorus. Shaw (1979, 1980) does not entirely agree with their view on the safety of phosphates and this is discussed further on p. 83.

There have been several clinical trials of the addition of inorganic phosphates to diets in human subjects, but the results are equivocal. Stralfors (1964) investigated the effect of adding dibasic calcium phosphate at 2 per cent concentration to bread, wheat flour, and sugar used in school lunches for about 1000 9-year-old Malmo schoolchildren. Caries was assessed only by radiological examination of four approximal surfaces in two upper incisor teeth. At the end of the 2-year study period about 44 per cent less caries was observed in the children in the six test schools compared with children in the seven control schools. The authors point out, though, that the phosphate additive also contained an appreciable amount of fluoride during the first year, and that this could account for some, or all, of the effect. Two other studies reported at the same conference were negative (Ship and Mickelsen 1964; Averill and Bibby 1964) on testing 2 per cent $CaHPO_4$ and dicalcium phosphate respectively.

Further trials have investigated the caries-preventive effect of dietary phosphate supplements in man. Averill *et al.* (1966) studied the effect of 2 per cent dicalcium phosphate on the teeth of 6–13-year old children in Brazil who had previously received diets very low in calcium. They observed a reduced caries incidence over 20 months, and increased serum and saliva calcium levels.

Finn and Jamison (1967) and Richardson *et al.* (1972) reported that the addition of dicalcium phosphate to chewing-gum counteracted the effect of sugar in the gum but did not confer any additional benefit. In a 3-year clinical trial on London schoolchildren aged 11–15 years, Ashley *et al.* (1974) reported no reduction in caries in children consuming sweets supplemented with 3 per cent dicalcium phosphate, compared with control children consuming unfortified sweets.

Sodium salts have been investigated with marginally more success. Stookey *et al.* (1967) recorded a 20 to 40 per cent reduction in 5–16-year-old children consuming cereals fortified with 1 per cent NaH_2PO_4, over 2 years. On the other hand, Rowe *et al.* (1975) observed only a very small and non-significant reduction in 13-year-old children who consumed cereal fortified with sodium phosphates for three years, and Wilson (1979) found no effect.

Although not a phosphate, calcium lactate has been investigated as a possible anti-caries food additive. It is already commonly used in a number of food products. Shrestha *et al.* (1982) found that 5 per cent calcium lactate reduced enamel dissolution by half in three types of experiment—incubation studies, artificial mouth, and rat experiments. Van der Hoeven (1985) confirmed this finding in rats.

Trimetaphosphates

As a result of earlier work, Harris *et al.* (1967*a*) concluded that trimetaphosphates (TMP) were likely to be the most effective polyphosphate in preventing dental caries. The addition of sodium trimetaphosphate to chewing-gum was tested by Finn *et al.* (1978) with positive results. The children (in a deaf and blind school) were asked to chew three sticks of gum each day for 3 years. This frequency and length of time that the teeth were exposed to the extra phosphates per day would be greater than that likely to occur with fortified cereals and may explain the positive result with gum.

Subsequently, Shaw (1979; 1980) has expressed concern at the use of sodium TMP. Although NaTMP is an accepted food additive in the United States, the relatively high levels which may be required to prevent caries in man may be undesirable—first because of the high sodium intake and, second, because of the reduced dietary Ca:P ratio. CaTMP has not yet been tested in man.

Calcium sucrose phosphate and calcium glycerophosphate

The caries preventive effect of these two organic compounds has been investigated in many parts of the world over the last 20 years. As with the inorganic phosphate compounds, their principal modes of action were thought to be raising plaque calcium and phosphate levels, and increasing plaque buffering power. However, as with phytate, their mode of action is now thought to be mainly a tooth surface adsorption effect preventing the dissolution of enamel. The saga of calcium sucrose phosphate (marketed for many years in Australia as 'Anticay') has been reviewed by Craig (1975). Rat studies (Lilienthal *et al.* 1966; Grenby 1973) have shown a protective effect, and Harris *et al.* (1967*b*) have confirmed this in a 3-year trial on Australian children. Unfortunately, due to considerable loss of subjects, the groups were unbalanced making interpretation of Harris's trial difficult (Craig 1975).

No clinical trial testing the effectiveness of calcium glycerophosphate as a dietary additive on caries in human subjects appears to have been reported, although its effectiveness in a toothpaste has been assessed (Naylor and Glass 1979). Nevertheless, Grenby (1973) reported that it was more effective than calcium sucrose phosphate or sodium phytate in rat experiments, and also in laboratory enamel incubation experiments (Grenby and Bull 1980). Calcium glycerophosphate was more effective than sodium glycerophosphate, in rats, although the effectiveness of the sodium salt was increased by adding calcium nitrate. These were effective when added to the rats' food and were ineffective in drinking-water (Grenby and Bull 1975). When icing sugar fortified with 1 per cent calcium glycerophosphate was fed to monkeys five times a day, caries experience was reduced compared with monkeys eating unfortified icing sugar (Bowen 1972). Plaque calcium levels were raised in the test animals, but Bowen considered the increased buffering power of plaque the more important reason for its effectiveness. A mouthrinse containing 1 per cent calcium glycerophosphate appeared to be ineffective at preventing the occurrence of caries-like lesions in human teeth in a short term study (Edgar *et al.* 1978).

In summary, despite promising results from animal experiments, the superiority of these organic to inorganic sodium or calcium phosphate compounds has not been established in human clinical trials.

Phytate

Jenkins *et al.* (1959) confirmed earlier observations by Osborn and others (loc. cit.) that 'unrefined' carbohydrate foods contain protective factors. Jenkins *et al.* (1959) went on to confirm Osborn's earlier speculation that the principal active substance was phytate. Comprehensive reviews have since been published (Jenkins 1965, 1966, 1968). Unlike the previous inorganic and organic phosphate compounds, the effectiveness of phytate appears to be due to its ability to adsorb readily and firmly to enamel surfaces and so prevent the dissolution of enamel by acid (Magrill 1973). Grenby (1967*a*) showed that the active ingredient was present in wheat-bran and not in wheat-germ, and that the protective action disappeared on exposure to phytase (Grenby 1967*b*). The sodium salt appears to be the most effective. It would be thought, therefore, that rats fed on a cariogenic diet containing brown bread would develop less caries than rats fed white bread. However, the reverse has been observed (König 1967) due, probably, to the limited release of phytate during the few seconds it is in the mouth (Jenkins and Smales 1966), and due to the superior vitamin and mineral content of brown bread favouring the growth and acid production by plaque bacteria.

However, when added to a diet, as opposed to being inside branny particles, phytate has been shown to be an effective dietary additive. Cole *et al.* (1980) observed a marked reduction in caries in monkeys fed on cariogenic diets in which sugar was supplemented with 1 per cent sodium phytate. No difference in amount of plaque was observed, suggesting that the possibility that phytate acts by preventing the deposition of proteins on enamel surface was unimportant. They failed to observe a rise in the plaque phosphate, and supported the view of Jenkins *et al.* (1959) that phytates act by preventing dissolution through surface actions on enamel.

In a rat experiment, Grenby (1973) found sodium phytate less effective than calcium glycerophosphate as a dietary additive. The reason for this finding is unclear as other rodent experiments have shown phytate to be an effective additive. It has been suggested that it could be due to a species difference between rodents and primates: a mode of action of calcium glycerophosphate may be to raise plaque P level, an action which may be less important in primates (Ericsson 1962; Tatevossian *et al.* 1975).

The presence of antibacterial factors in 'unrefined' foods are considered unimportant because those that have been identified are only extractable in alcohol and not in water (Jenkins and Smales 1966). Phytates reduce the absorption of dietary Ca, Mg, Fe, and Zn from the gut (Jenkins 1978), and although humans can adapt to an increased level of phytate and restore their level of absorption, for Ca at least, it is probable that this side-effect may make it difficult for phytate to gain wide acceptance as a food additive.

Honey and partially refined crystallized sugar

It is unlikely that honey is any less cariogenic than refined sugar—although the sugar content of honey varies, approximate values are: fructose 45 per cent, glucose 35 per cent, and sucrose 5 per cent (Shannon *et al.* 1979). Edgar and Jenkins (1974) have shown that honey contains esters which may reduce dissolution of enamel, but their effectiveness is likely be be at least equalled by the presence of nutrients which would encourage the metabolism of plaque microorganisms and thus increase acid production. Findings of rat experiments support their conclusions (Nizel 1973). König (1967) observed that the cariogenicity of sucrose, jam, or honey when spread on bread was approximately equal, while Shannon *et al.* (1979) reported that honey was as cariogenic, in rats, as (i) sucrose and (ii) a mixture of fructose, glucose, and sucrose in the same proportion as occurred in the honey.

Edgar and Jenkins (1974) also showed that 'raw' (Barbados or Demerara) sugar contains cations (probably Ca^{2+}, Fe^{3+} and Cu^{2+}) which reduced enamel solubility in buffer solutions, but their effect is unlikely to negate the cariogenic potential of the sugar *in vivo*.

Cocoa factor and liquorice

In the Vipeholm study (p. 34) the patients in the chocolate group developed less caries than other groups receiving similar sugar levels and frequency of eating. This led to speculation that chocolate might contain 'protective factors'. A subsidiary experiment to test this was, for various reasons, indecisive (Gustaffson *et al.* 1954). Animal experiments also suggested that cocoa may have a caries-protective effect (Stralfors 1966). 's-Gravenmade and Jenkins (1986) described a method for extracting the active ingredient and showed that it was most effective between pH 4 and 5. They considered that, as extraction was expensive, application of cocoa factor as a method of caries prevention would be less efficient than the use of fluoride. The findings, though, could explain the favourable results of the Vipeholm study and Stralfors' rat experiments. Dunning and Hodge (1971) conducted a clinical trial of the caries-preventive effect of cocoa in milk, but the trial was unsatisfactory and the results inconclusive.

Likewise, the major constituent of liquorice—glycyrrhizinic acid—has potentially caries-preventive properties (Edgar 1978). He showed that glycyrrhizinic acid acted in three ways: it reduced enamel dissolution in acid buffer/enamel systems, inhibited glycolysis, and increased plaque buffering power. However, it does have the undesirable properties of strong taste, dark staining, and, more importantly, it disturbs the body electrolyte balance. Its usefulness as a dietary additive may therefore be limited.

Fats and protein

Fat in diet has been thought to help reduce the cariogenicity of dietary sugar, probably by the physical action of accelerating its clearance from the mouth (Frostell 1969). Proteins are known to adsorb onto enamel surfaces (Pearce and Bibby 1966) but the degree to which they protect against caries is unknown. Milk contains both fat and protein. The fall in plaque pH after drinking milk is minimal (Jenkins and Ferguson 1966; Frostell 1970), and the high protein content, with its possible enamel-surface protective effect, and the high levels of calcium and phosphate make it unlikely that milk is cariogenic (Jenkins and Ferguson 1966). Bibby *et al.* (1980), using an artificial mouth test system (Orofax), found that the inclusion of milk solids reduced the cariogenicity of sugar-containing foods; similar results were obtained by Thompson *et al.* (1984) using an enamel slab system. Reynolds and Johnson (1981) observed that rats who were provided with milk to drink had less caries than rats given water, when both groups were fed the same cariogenic diet. The difficulty in extrapolating results of animal experiments to man was emphasized by Harper *et al.* (1987) who, nevertheless, considered that the caries-preventive effect of Ca and P in milk was greater than that of casein.

However, other reports (Kroll and Stone 1967; Kotlow 1977; Gardner *et al.* 1977; Ripa 1978) have suggested that prolonged bottle-feeding of human infants with bovine or formula milk, and 'on demand' breast-feeding, may be responsible for caries development. Although some of these reports can be criticized because of lack of information on the rest of the infants' diet, it has to be noted that human milk contains higher levels of lactose than cows' milk (7.0 g/100 ml compared with 4.8 g/100 ml), lower calcium (33 mg/100 ml compared with 125 mg/100 ml), lower phosphorus (15 mg/100 ml compared with 96 mg/100 ml), and lower protein (1.2 g/100 ml compared with 3.3 g/100 ml) levels. All these factors would increase the cariogenic potential and lessen the caries protective effect of human milk compared with cows' milk. The fat levels are similar (3.8 g/100 ml and 3.7 g/100 ml, respectively) (Darke 1976).

Using plaque pH and 'in vitro' demineralization experiments, Rugg-Gunn *et al.* (1985) found that both human and bovine milk had considerably less cariogenic potential than solutions of lactose or sucrose, but that human milk was a little less protective than bovine milk. Because of the popularity of 'on-demand' breast-feeding and the very few associated cases of infant caries, it would be wise not to discourage breast-feeding (Abbey 1979; Hackett *et al.* 1984).

The caries-preventive effect of cheese is now well established from plaque pH studies (Rugg-Gunn *et al.* 1975), enamel slab experiments (de A. Silva *et al.* 1986), and rat experiments (Edgar *et al.* 1982) although, to date, no clinical trial in man has been reported.

Detersive foods and dental caries

Philip of Macedon decreed that all his royal household should end a meal with an apple 'to cleanse the mouth and aid digestion'. This advice has been propagated by the dental profession for many years. Apples have commonly featured in dental health programmes (Finlayson and Wilson 1961) and have become, to some extent, a symbol of dental health. They have been advocated mainly as a cleansing food at the end of a meal, but evidence concerning the effectiveness of detersive foods in preventing caries and gingivitis is equivocal.

There have been two clinical trials investigating apple-eating and caries and one investigating carrots and caries. Slack and Martin (1958) observed children living in National children homes or family group homes who were offered half-inch slices of firm crisp apple at the end of each meal and after any between-meal snacks. Unfortunately 53 per cent of these subjects left during the study and the size of the groups was small (90 in the apple group and 81 in the control group), especially as the children were in three age groups—under 6 years, 6–10 years, and 11–15 years at the start of the 2-year study period. Caries development was less in the apple-group children in all three age groups. This was statistically significant in the two younger age groups although there was some inbalance in caries experience at base-line. Gingival health was also statistically significantly better in the apple-group children at the end of the 2-year study. The method of allocating children to groups was unfortunately not given and random allocation cannot be assumed, but the findings give some indication of a positive effect. The second trial was a little less thorough: Averill and Averill (1968) studied caries, debris, and other health parameters in 17–25-year-olds over a 21-month period. The 46 subjects in the apple group were provided with apples to eat after the last meal every day and were compared with 56 control subjects. No differences in caries experience or debris scores were observed.

Reece and Swallow (1970) provided 155 4–9-year-old children with pieces of raw carrot after their midday meal in school for 2 years. No differences were observed in caries or gingival disease compared with 191 control children.

Only one animal experiment appears to have investigated the effect of apple eating on dental caries (Karle and Gehring 1976). One of the four groups of animals were fed pieces of apple between all the nine meals of a cariogenic diet per day. The remaining three groups ate sweets, a sucrose-containing diet, or bananas, between meals. The banana group had the highest caries score. The sweets and apple groups had the next highest, and the control group eating the sucrose-containing diet only, the lowest experience.

Some studies have indicated that apples can cause a fall in plaque pH (Graf 1970; Rugg-Gunn *et al.* 1978). Others have shown that following a sugar lump with an apple does not significantly raise plaque pH, compared with salted peanuts, which are effective at raising plaque pH that has been previously lowered by sugar (Geddes *et al.* 1977). These findings are not surprising because apples contain 10 per cent sugar and are acid. It would seem that their favourable action in stimulating a powerful salivary flow is not sufficient to overcome the harmful properties of containing sugar and acid.

Despite the observations of Slack and Martin (1958) that gingival health was better in the apple group, six other articles have reported no effect on gingival health or plaque scores after eating fibrous foods (*British Medical Journal* 1977). The evidence concerning detersive foods and caries is confused. While there appear to be no reports of apples actually causing caries, there is likewise little

Table 2.20. Some sweet-tasting compounds

		Approx. sweetness relative to sucrose
Sugars	Glucose	0.7
	Fructose	1.2
	Sorbose	0.9
	Sucrose	**1.0**
	Lactose	0.3
	Maltose	0.4
Sugar compounds	Glucosylsucrose*	—
	Maltosylsucrose*	—
	Trichlorosucrose*	2000
	Sucralose	600
Sugar alcohols	Xylitol	1.0
	Sorbitol	0.5
	Mannitol	0.7
	Maltitol	0.75
	Lactitol	0.35
Complex	Hydrogenated glucose syrup*	0.75
	Isomalt*	0.5
Dipeptide	Aspartame*	180
Polypeptides	Monellin	3000
	Thaumatin	4000
Miscellaneous	Saccharin*	500
	Cyclamate*	50
	Stevioside	200
	Acesulfame potassium*	130
	Glycyrrhizin	50

* Not naturally occurring.

evidence that they improve dental health. Although other foods might be preferable snacks, from the dental viewpoint, apples are a convenient snack and are probably preferable to many more highly sugared items (Rugg-Gunn 1988*b*).

Relative cariogenicity of sweetening agents

Sweetness

The sweet taste is one of man's basic taste sensations (see Jenkins 1978). The sweet taste sensation is thought to be due to the 'AH-B' system (Shallenberger and Acree 1967), where A and B are a pair of electronegative atoms 25–40 nm apart with a hydrogen atom (H) attached to one of them at a distance of 30 nm. This configuration in a sweet substance is then presumed to bind to the appropriate receptor in the oral mucosa causing stimulation of an afferent nerve ending. Many diverse substances have the ability to produce a sweet sensation.

Types of sweeteners

Table 2.20 lists the more commonly discussed of the many sweet-tasting compounds. The number which are synthesized, rather than being naturally occurring compounds, has been steadily growing since the last century. Fluctuations in the price of natural sweeteners (e.g. sucrose) and their incrimination in the cause of disease such as caries, has accelerated the search for alternative sweeteners and, although many are at present expensive to manufacture, new technology and increased production will, no doubt, make them financially competitive. Not all the compounds give the same sweet taste. The slightly bitter after taste of saccharin is well known, although a combination of cyclamate and saccharin has a pleasant sweet taste. Glycyrrhizin has a liquorice taste. Xylitol has a negative heat of dissolution resulting in a cool taste when xylitol-containing sweets are eaten. Many other sugar alcohols also possess this property. Polypeptides are known for their prolonged sweet taste. Sweetness relative to sucrose varies widely (Table 2.20); some of the compounds are not thermostable and are destroyed in food manufacture.

Although a very large number of sweet compounds are known, relatively few are permitted to be used in foods; those that are permitted will vary from country to country. In the United Kingdom, the list of permitted sweeteners was revised in 1982 (Ministry of Agriculture, Fisheries and Food 1982). This report of the Food Additives and Contaminants committee of the MAFF recommended an increase in the number of sweeteners that might be included in foods and drinks in the United Kingdom, although restrictions were placed on the use of some of them. Permitted sugars (which were outside their report) were unchanged and are glucose, fructose, sucrose, lactose, and maltose. Previously, only sorbitol and mannitol were permitted as 'bulk sweeteners', but the 1982 report recommended that three more—hydrogenated glucose syrup, isomalt, and xylitol—be permitted, in addition to sorbitol and mannitol. The report also recommended that three 'intense sweeteners' be permitted: acesulfame potassium, aspartame, and saccharin (as sodium and calcium salts), where previously only saccharin was allowed. The intense sweetener thaumatin was permitted subsequently. Glycerol is permitted under the Solvents in Foods Regulations (Ministry of Agriculture, Fisheries and Food 1967). It is hoped that this expansion of the list of permitted sweeteners will allow manufacturers, particularly of confectionery and soft drinks, to increase their range of 'sugarless' foods and drinks. Although the Committee on Toxicity of Chemicals in Food, Consumer Products and the Environment (COT) recommended that cyclamates be restored to the permitted list, this recommendation was not accepted by the Food Additives and Contaminants Committee, and cyclamates are thus not permitted for use in foods and drinks in the United Kingdom.

Relative cariogenicity of sugars

Sucrose has been termed the 'arch criminal of dental caries' (Newbrun 1967). It is certainly the most common sugar in our diet and for this reason alone it is a major cause of dental caries. When all types of cariogenicity test are considered, no other sugar has been shown to be more acidogenic or cariogenic than sucrose. A property of sucrose which makes it more likely than other sugars to cause caries is its unique ability to enhance production of extracellular polysaccharides or glucans, such as dextran, in dental plaque. Dextran is not easily metabolized in plaque and increases the bulk of plaque. It is also sticky and increases adherence of plaque to enamel. The practical importance of this unfavourable property of sucrose is difficult to determine. While some studies (mainly rat experiments where the animals have been inoculated with *Strep. mutans*) have shown sucrose to be more cariogenic than glucose, fructose, or maltose, other studies have suggested that all these sugars cause similar levels of caries, plaque pH depression, or enamel softening. The Turku sugar study was inconclusive in indicating whether fructose was less cariogenic than sucrose in man. From the practical viewpoint, it would seem that there is little to be gained by substituting glucose, fructose, or maltose for sucrose for the prevention of dental caries. Lactose and galactose are significantly less cariogenic than other dietary sugars.

Relative cariogenicity of alternative sweeteners

A review of some of the general and dental properties of these sweeteners has been published (Rugg-Gunn and Edgar 1985). In general, the bulk sweeteners are isocaloric and approximately as sweet as sugars, whereas the intense sweeteners provide virtually no calories.

Sorbitol and mannitol

Sorbitol and mannitol occur naturally in small quantities in a number of plants. Sorbitol is used extensively in foods manufactured for diabetics as the metabolism of sorbitol is insulin-independent. Sorbitol is commonly used as the sweetener in sugarless syrup medicines. Mannitol is used mainly in chewing-gum and the amount consumed is very small compared with sorbitol.

The cariogenicity of sorbitol has been reviewed by Birkhed *et al.* (1984). Mannitol has been studied less extensively than sorbitol but the results have been similar. Sorbitol and mannitol are fermented slowly by plaque organisms (Hayes and Roberts 1978) but the rate is very much slower than that of glucose or sucrose. Sorbitol and mannitol depress plaque pH only slightly (Imfeld 1977; Rugg-Gunn 1988) (Figs. 2.34; 2.35). When diets containing sorbitol were fed to rats (Shaw and Griffiths 1960) or monkeys (Cornick and Bowen 1972) little caries developed in comparison with glucose or sucrose diets. *Strep. mutans* can adapt to metabolize sorbitol *in vivo* but only when sorbitol is the sole energy source and this is very unlikely to occur in man. In enamel slab experiments, sorbitol and mannitol gave rise to 45 per cent of the demineralization of enamel attributable to sucrose. Clinical trials of sorbitol have been limited to use in chewing-gum (see page 53) providing partial substitution of dietary sugars. The conclusions from these trials is that sorbitol is 'non-cariogenic' and 'does not promote tooth decay'.

Xylitol

Xylitol also occurs naturally in foods in small quantities. Its use at present is confined to confectionery and toothpaste.

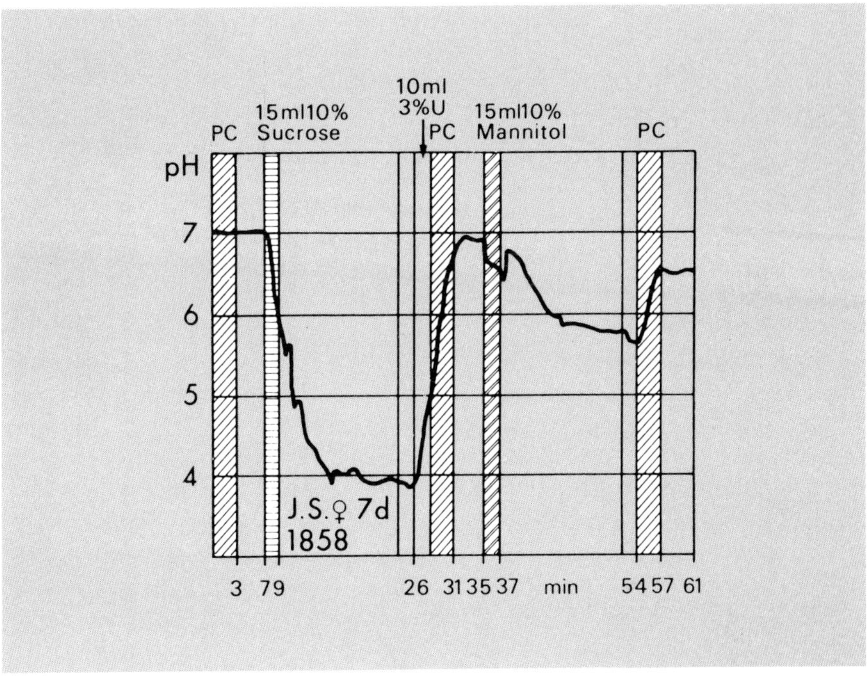

Fig. 2.34. Telemetrically recorded plaque pH after rinsing with (a) 15 ml of 10 per cent sucrose solution, (b) 15 ml of 10 per cent mannitol solution. (From Imfeld (1977), with permission of the editor *Helvetica odontologica acta*.)

In all tests of cariogenicity it would appear to be non-cariogenic. Numerous incubation experiments have demonstrated that xylitol is fermented to acid very slowly (if at all) in comparison with glucose or even sorbitol (Hayes and Roberts 1978). Plaque pH studies confirm the non-acidogenicity of xylitol (Imfeld 1977), and rat experiments have shown xylitol to be non-cariogenic. The Turku sugar study (see page 43) showed that total substitution of dietary sugar by xylitol resulted in very low caries incidence; the use of xylitol chewing-gum reduced caries increments in clinical trials conducted in Hungary and French Polynesia (see page 53).

Hydrogenated glucose syrup

The hydrogenated glucose syrup approved for use in foods is manufactured by Roquette (France) and sold under the trade name Lycasin^{R}. It contains less than 0.3 per cent free sugars, and is used in the manufacture of a variety of foods, drinks, and liquid medicines.

Lycasin is fermented slowly compared with sucrose (Havenaar *et al.* 1979) and causes minimal depression of plaque pH when taken as a syrup or as a boiled sweet (Imfeld 1983; Rugg-Gunn 1988) (Figs. 2.35; 2.36). It is much less

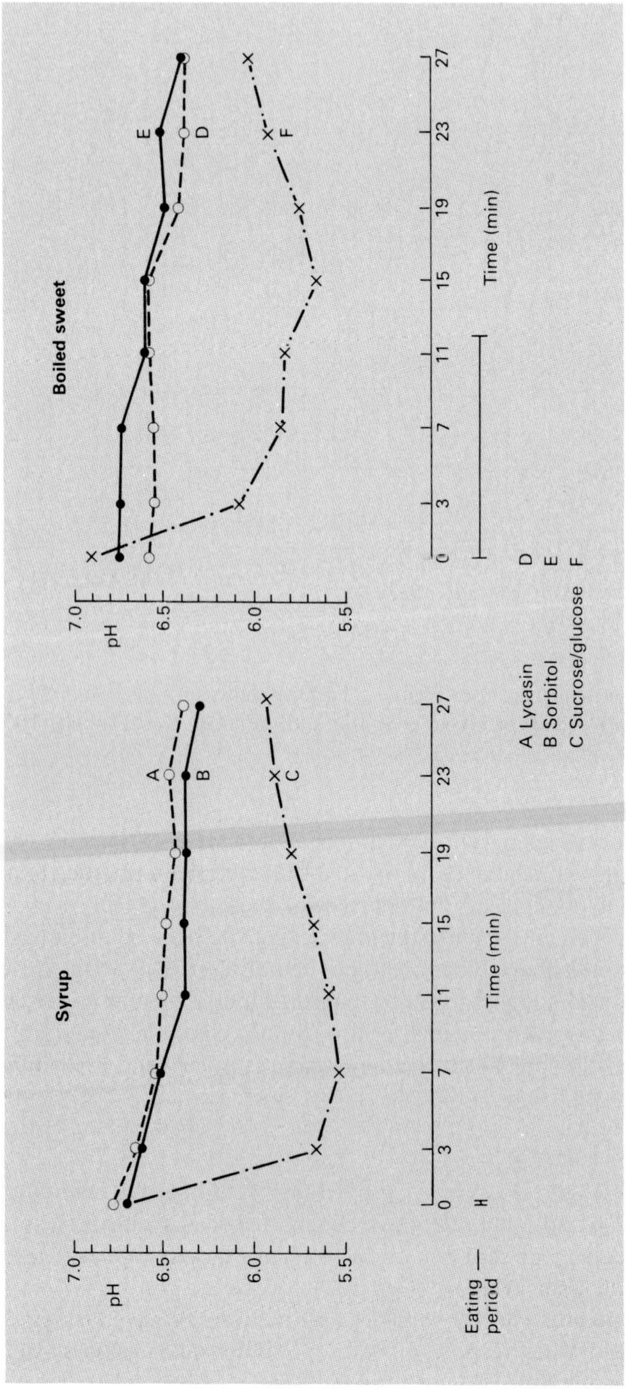

Fig. 2.35. Stephan curves for Lycasin, sorbitol, and sucrose/glucose when taken as a 70 per cent syrup or as a boiled sweet. (From Rugg-Gunn (1988*a*), with permission of the editor *Caries Research*.)

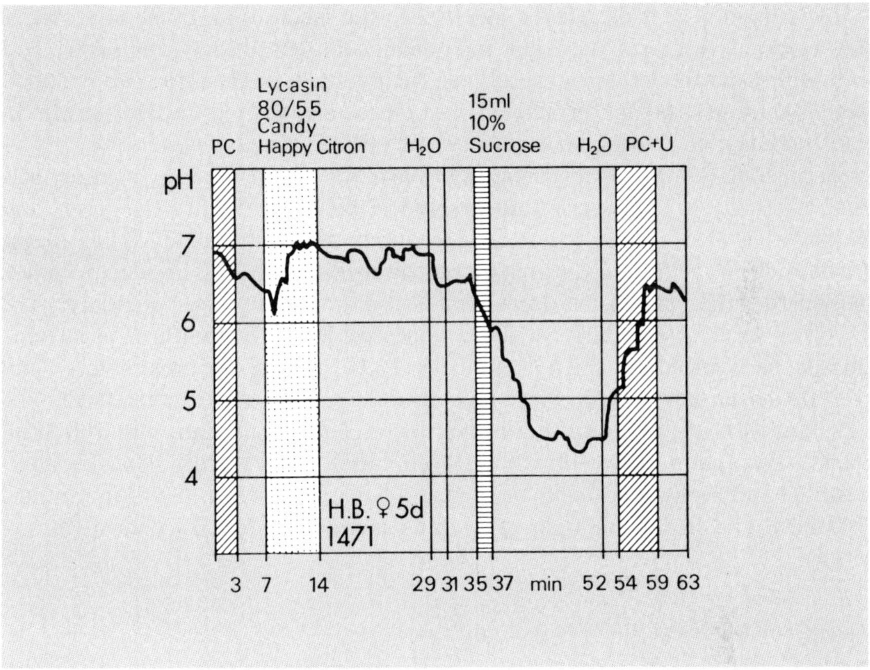

Fig. 2.36. Telemetrically recorded plaque pH after (a) eating a hard sweet containing Lycasin, (b) rinsing with 15 ml of 10 per cent sucrose solution. (From Imfeld (1977), with permission of the editor *Helvetica odontologica acta*.)

cariogenic than sucrose when fed to rats (Grenby and Saldanha 1983) and did not contribute the softening of enamel in intra-oral enamel slab experiments (Rundegren *et al.* 1980).

Isomalt

Isomalt is, basically, a mixture of two polyols. It is manufactured in FGR and marketed under the trade name Palatinit^R. It can be used in the manufacture of a number of foods and drinks. Isomalt causes little acid production when incubated with oral streptococci, and plaque pH is virtually unaffected after exposure to a 10 per cent solution (Imfeld 1983). Isomalt's cariogenicity in rats is low (van der Hoeven 1980).

Intense sweeteners

Saccharin was discovered in 1879 and has been used widely as a food additive for more than 80 years. It has a bitter taste in concentrations over 0.1 per cent although the degree of appreciation of bitterness varies considerably between people. It is used as a 'table-top' sweetener and extensively in soft drinks, especially those marketed as 'calorie-low'.

Acesulfame K was discovered in 1967 in the laboratories of Hoescht AG. It has a clean, sweet taste. It is stable in aqueous solutions of wide-ranging pH, and can withstand moderately severe heat treatment. It is thought to have good potential as a sweetener, principally in 'reduced energy' soft drinks, but also in confectionery, chewing-gum, preserves and other foods.

Aspartame is a dipeptide, consisting of aspartic acid and phenylalanine. It is manufactured by G D Searle and Co under the trades names Canderel^{R} and NutraSweet^{R}. It is moderately stable in solution although prolonged heat treatment and storage hastens its breakdown with subsequent loss of sweetness. It is now used extensively in soft drinks, but is also thought to have potential for use in other foods, particularly in dried or frozen foods. Ingestion of aspartame should be avoided by phenylketonuric (PKU) persons (approximately 1 in 10 000 live births) who have a genetic defect of phenylalanine metabolism.

Thaumatin is a sweet-tasting protein extracted from a plant found in West Africa. Perception of sweetness is delayed and it has a slightly liquorice after-taste. Thaumatin is reported to be used as a flavour enhancer in pharmaceutical products, and in combination with other sweeteners (e.g. saccharin) in soft drinks.

Cariogenicity of the intense sweeteners

Little is known of the effects of the intense sweeteners on caries development. Because of their composition, they are very unlikely to promote caries and research has been directed at investigation the caries-inhibitory properties of these substances. Saccharin has been reported to inhibit bacterial growth and metabolism (Linke 1977), although its inhibitory effect on rat caries development was small (Grenby 1984). Thaumatin has been shown to favour remineralization of early caries in rats when added to starch to give a sweetness equivalent to sucrose (Leach *et al.* 1983). Because the intense sweeteners are used at low concentrations, possible direct effects (inhibitory or otherwise) on bacterial metabolism are likely to be less important than indirect effects on caries through salivary stimulation.

Adverse effects of sweet-tasting compounds

Drucker (1979) has drawn attention to some of the adverse effects of sweeteners, and no compound would appear to be completely clear of undesirable side-effects. He points out that sorbose has been associated with haemolytic anaemia, xylitol and sorbitol with diarrhoea, glycyrrhizin with hypertension, cyclamate and saccharin metabolites with bladder tumours, and sucrose with caries, obesity, diabetes, and coronary heart disease. Although thorough toxicity testing of sweeteners is essential, many people consider that the banning of cyclamate and saccharin in America and Europe was premature and prompted Cowan (see Drucker 1979) to remark that a 'diet drink' (containing saccharin) reduced life expectancy by nine seconds in contrast to the alternative sucrose which would decrease life expectancy by a hundred times more than the cancer risk thereby avoided.

The side effect of using alternative sweeteners most likely to cause concern is the tendency of polyols to cause osmotic diarrhoea. This is unlikely to be a problem in adults, but they should be recommended for young children with caution.

Summary

It would seem that sucrose, glucose, maltose and fructose are the most cariogenic sugars, while lactose would seem to be less cariogenic. The bulk sweeteners sorbitol, mannitol, hydrogenated glucose syrup, and isomalt are non-cariogenic or virtually so. Xylitol, saccharin, aspartame, and thaumatin are non-cariogenic. Effective caries prevention by sugar control includes (i) deciding which types of food or eating habits are the most harmful: substitution of sugar in these foods by less cariogenic sweeteners might then be cost-effective; (ii) development of new technology to reduce the cost difference between sucrose, glucose, and fructose and other less cariogenic sweeteners; (iii) development of sweeteners free from adverse effects.

Summary

At the beginning of this chapter it was emphasized that our knowledge concerning the relation between diet and dental caries comes from many sources, largely because human dietary clinical studies are so difficult to carry out. Taking all these sources of evidence into account the following conclusions and comments can be made:

1. In the development of dental caries, the influence of diet is much more important after a tooth has erupted into the mouth than any dietary influence on the forming tooth before its eruption. Sugar would appear to be the most important dietary item in caries aetiology and its presence around plaque-covered tooth surfaces essential for more than very limited caries development. Starch-containing foods, especially if finely-ground, cooked and eaten frequently, can cause some caries.

2. Some sugars would appear to be more cariogenic than others. Sucrose is likely to be the most cariogenic sugar, although glucose, fructose, and maltose are virtually as cariogenic as sucrose. Lactose is less cariogenic than other dietary sugars. The alternative sweeteners (bulk and intense) are non-cariogenic or virtually so.

3. Dietary sugars come from two sources—those naturally present in foods and those added by manufacturer, cook, or consumer. By far the majority of natural sugars come from milk and fruit. Milk can be considered non-cariogenic or virtually so. Fresh fruits, as eaten by man, are of low cariogenicity. Therefore, sugars naturally present in foods are of negligible importance as a cause of dental caries in man compared with added sugars.

4. Cooked staple starchy foods, such as rice, potatoes, and bread, are of low

cariogenicity in man. Refined, finely ground and heat-treated starch can cause caries but the addition of sugar increases the cariogenicity of cooked starchy foods.

5. The frequency of sugar intake would appear to be a more important dietary variable than the total quantity of sugar eaten. However, frequency of eating sugar and total quantity of sugar consumed are closely correlated in many epidemiological surveys, so that as sugar becomes available to a population both total quantity of sugar eaten increases as well as the frequency with which it is eaten. Hence in many countries there is a correlation between total amount of sugar consumed and caries experience. The aim should be to decrease both the amount eaten and the frequency of intake.

6. The acidogenicity of a sugar-containing food can be modified by other items in that food, and the acidogenicity of a sugar-containing meal can be modified by other foods in that meal.

7. Dietary factors that protect tooth enamel from caries development during acid attack have been isolated. Phytate appears to be the most effective *in vitro* although inorganic and other organic phosphates also have an effect. Organic phosphates act primarily by forming a tightly bound protective layer on the enamel surface, whereas inorganic phosphates act mainly by a common ion effect. However, clinical studies have shown these compounds less effective at caries prevention than might have been expected from animal and laboratory experiments.

8. Although a large number of dietary compounds have been thought to influence a developing tooth's future caries susceptibility, only fluoride has been established to have any appreciable influence (see Chapter 3). Other trace elements may have a smaller effect, and the influence of calcium, phosphates, and vitamins A and D remains uncertain.

9. If our eating habits (with a high number of snack meals) are accepted, in order to modify our 'high-sugar' diet so that it becomes less cariogenic there seems to be three alternatives: (i) to remove sugar from foods (or selected foods) altogether. In many foods this leads to little change in taste (Okholm 1980). (ii) To substitute non-cariogenic sweeteners for sucrose/glucose in foods. It may be necessary for only a limited type of food (e.g. common snack foods) to be altered to have a significant effect on a community's caries experience (Scheinin *et al.* 1975). (iii) To modify sugar-containing foods so that they are less cariogenic. Co-operation between nutritionists, physicians, dentists, economists, and food manufacturers is required to achieve these aims.

References

Abbey, L.M. (1979). Is breast feeding a likely cause of dental caries in young children? *J Am. dent. Ass.* **98**, 21–3.

Abelson, D.C. and Pergola, G. (1984). The effect of sucrose concentration on plaque pH in vivo. *Clin. Prev. Dent.* **6**, 23–6.

Afonsky, D. (1951). Some observations on dental caries in central China. *J. dent. Res.* **30**, 53–61.

Ainamo, J. and Holmberg, S.M. (1974). The oral health of children of dentists. *Scand. J. dent. Res.* **82**, 547–51.

Akpata, E.S. (1979). Patterns of dental caries in urban Nigerians. *Caries Res.* **13**, 241–9.

Alanen, P., Tiekso, J., and Paunio, I. (1985). Effect of wartime dietary changes on dental health of Finns 40 years later. *Commun. Dent. oral Epidemiol.* **13**, 281–4.

Anaise, J.Z. (1978). Prevalence of dental caries among workers in the sweets industry in Israel. *Commun. Dent. oral Epidemiol.* **6**, 286–9.

Anaise, J.Z. (1980). Prevalence of dental caries among workers in the sweets industry in Israel. *Commun. Dent. oral Epidemiol.* **8**, 142–5.

Anderson, R.J., Davies, B.E., and James, P.M.C. (1976). Dental caries prevalence in a heavy metal contaminated area of the West of England. *Br. dent. J.* **141**, 311–14.

Asher, C. and Read, M.J.F. (1987). Early enamel erosion in children associated with the excessive consumption of citric acid. *Br. dent. J.* **162**, 384–7.

Ashley, F.P., Naylor, M.N., and Emslie, R.D. (1974). Clinical testing of dicalcium phosphate supplemented sweets. *Br. dent. J.* **136**, 361–6; 418–23.

Averill, H.M. and Averill, J.E. (1968). The effect of daily apple consumption on dental caries experience, oral hygiene status and upper respiratory infection. *NY St. dent J.* **34**, 403–9.

Averill, H.M. and Bibby, B.G. (1964). A clinical test of additions of phosphate to the diet of children. *J. dent. Res.* **43**, 1150–5.

Averill, H.M., Freire, P.S., and Bibby, B.G. (1966). The effect of dietary phosphate supplements on dental caries incidence in tropical Brazil. *Archs. oral Biol.* **11**, 315–22.

Bagramian, R.A. and Russell, A.L. (1973). Epidemiologic study of dental caries experience and between-meal eating patterns. *J. dent. Res.* **52**, 342–7.

Bagramian, R.A., Jenny, J., Frazier, J., and Proshek, J.M. (1974). Diet patterns and dental caries in third grade U.S. children. *Commun. Dent. oral Epidemiol.* **2**, 208–13.

Bang, G. (1964). A comparison between the incidence of dental caries in typical coastal populations and inland populations with particular regard to the possible effect of a high intake of salt water fish. *Odont. Tidskr.* **72**, 12–43.

Bang, G. and Kristoffersen, T. (1972). Dental caries and diet in an Alaskan Eskimo population. *Scand. J. dent. Res.* **80**, 440–4.

Banoczy, J., Hadas, E., Esztary, I., Marosi, I., and Nemes, J. (1981). Three year results of sorbitol in clinical longitudinal experiments. *J. Int. Ass. Dent. Child.* **12**, 59–63.

Barmes, D.E. (1969). Caries etiology in Sepik villages—trace element, micronutrient and macronutrient content of soil and food. *Caries Res.* **3**, 44–59.

Barmes, D.E., Adkins, B.L., and Schamschula, R.G. (1970). Etiology of caries in Papua-New Guinea. Associations in soil, food and water. *Bull. Wld. Hlth. Org.* **43**, 769–84.

Baume, L.J. (1969). Caries prevalence and caries intensity among 12,344 schoolchildren of French Polynesia. *Archs. oral Biol.* **14**, 181–205.

Beighton, D. and Hayday, H. (1984). The establishment of the bacterium *Streptococcus mutans* in dental plaque and the induction of caries in macaque monkeys (*Macaca fascicularis*) fed a diet containing cooked wheat flour. *Archs. oral Biol.* **29**, 369–72.

Bernick, S.M., Cohen, D.W., Baker, L., and Laser, L. (1975). Dental disease in children with diabetes mellitus. *J. Perio.* **46**, 241–5.

Bibby, B.G. and Mundorff, S.A. (1975). Enamel demineralization by snack foods. *J. dent. Res.* **54**, 461–70.

Bibby, B.G., Goldberg, H.J.V., and Chen, E. (1951). Evaluation of caries-producing potentialities of various foods. *J. Am. dent. Ass.* **42**, 491–509.

Bibby, B.G., Huang, C.T., Zero, D., Mundorff, S.A., and Little, M.F. (1980). Protective effect of milk against 'in vitro' caries. *J. dent. Res.* **59**, 1565–70.

Bibby, B.G., Mundorff, S.A., Zero, D.T., and Almekinder, K.J. (1986). Oral food clearance and the pH of plaque and saliva. *J. Am. dent. Ass.* **112**, 333–7.

Birkhed, D. (1984). Sugar content, acidity and effect on plaque pH of fruit juices, fruit drinks, carbonated beverages and sports drinks. *Caries Res.* **18**, 120–7.

Birkhed, D. and Skude, G. (1978). Relation of amylase to starch and Lycasin metabolism in human dental plaque '*in vitro*'. *Scand. J. dent. Res.* **86**, 248–58.

Birkhed, D., Topitsaglou, V., Edwardsson, S., and Frostell, G. (1981). Cariogenicity of invert sugar in long-term rat experiments. *Caries Res.* **15**, 302–7.

Birkhed, D., Edwardsson, S., Kalfas, S., and Svensater, G. (1984). Cariogenicity of sorbitol. *Swed. dent. J.* **8**, 147–54.

Biscuit, Cake, Chocolate and Confectionery Alliance (1987). *Submission to the COMA panel on sugars.* London.

Blinkhorn, A.S. (1982). The caries experience and dietary habits of Edinburgh nursery school children. *Br. dent. J.* **152**, 227–30.

Bowen, W.H. (1969). The monitoring of acid production in dental plaque in monkeys. *Br. dent. J.* **126** 506–8.

Bowen, W.H. (1972). The cariostatic effect of calcium glycerophosphate in monkeys. *Caries Res.* **6**, 43–51.

Bowen, W.H., Amsbaugh, S.M., Monell-Torrens, S., Brunelle, J., Kuzmiak-Jones, H., and Cole, M.F. (1980). A method to assess cariogenic potential of foodstuffs. *J. Am. dent. Ass.* **100**, 677–81.

Bradford, E.W. and Crabb, H.S.M. (1961). Carbohydrate restriction and caries incidence: a pilot study. *Br. dent. J.* **111**, 273–9.

Bradford, E.W. and Crabb, H.S.M. (1963). Carbohydrates and the incidence of caries in the deciduous dentition. In *Advances in Fluoride Research and Dental Caries Prevention*, (ed. Hardwick, Dustin and Held), pp. 319–23, Pergamon, London.

British Medical Journal (1977). Apples and the teeth—'Natures toothbrush' reappraised. Editorial. *Br. med. J.* **i**, 1116.

Britse, A. and Lagerlof, F. (1987). The diluting effect of saliva on the sucrose concentration in different parts of the human mouth after a mouth-rinse with sucrose. *Archs. oral Biol.* **32**, 755–6.

Brudevold, F., Attarzadeh, F., Terani, A., van Houte, J., and Russo, J. (1984). Development of a new intraoral demineralization test. *Caries Res.* **18**, 421–9.

Brudevold, F., Goulet, D., Tehrani, A., Attarzadeh, F., and van Houte, J. (1985). Intraoral demineralization and maltose clearance from wheat starch. *Caries Res.* **19**, 136–44.

Bruszt, P., Banoczy, J., Esztary, I., Hadas, E., Marosi, I., Nemes, J., and Albrecht, M. (1977). Caries prevalence of preschoolchildren in Baja, Hungary in 1955 and 1975. *Commun. Dent. oral Epidemiol.* **5**, 136–9.

Bunting, R.W. (1935). Diet and dental caries. *J. Am. dent. Ass.* **22**, 114–20.

Cadell, P.B. (1964). Geographic distribution of dental caries in relation to New Zealand soils. *Australia dent. J.* **9**, 32–8.

Charlton, G. (1956). Determination of hydrogen ion concentration in the mouth—comparison of the glass, antimony and quinhydrone microelectrodes. *Australia dent. J.* **2**, 228–32.

Clancy, K.L., Bibby, B.G., Goldberg, H.J.V., Ripa, L.W., and Barenie, J. (1977). Snack food intake of adolescents and caries development. *J. dent. Res.* **56**, 568–73.

Clancy, K.L., Goldberg, H.J.V., and Ritz, A. (1978). Snack consumption of 12-year-old inner-city children and its relationship to oral health. *J. publ. Hlth. Dent.* **38**, 227–34.

Clarke, N.G. and Dowdell, L.R. (1976). Capacity of buffers to inhibit acid production within dental plaque. *J. dent. Res.* **55**, 868–74.

Clarke, N.G. and Fanning, E.A. (1971). Plaque pH and calcium sucrose phosphate: a telemetric study. *Australia dent. J.* **16**, 13–16.

Cleaton-Jones, P., Richardson, B.D., and McInnes, P.M. (1981). Dental caries in coloured and Indian children aged 1–5 years. *J. dent. Ass. S. Afr.* **36**, 61–3.

Cleaton-Jones, P., Richardson, B.D., Winter, G.B., Sinwell, R.E., Rantsho, J.M., and Jodaikin, A. (1984). Dental caries and sucrose intake in five South African preschool groups. *Commun. Dent. oral Epidemiol.* **12**, 381–5.

Cocoa, Chocolate and Confectionery Alliance (1974). *Confectionery and the statistics of dental caries*. London.

Cocoa, Chocolate and Confectionery Alliance (1979). *Confectionery in perspective*. London.

Cole, M.F., Eastoe, J.E., Curtis, M.A., Korts, D.C., and Bowen, W.H. (1980). Effect of pyridoxine, phytate and invert sugar on plaque composition and caries activity in the monkey. *Caries Res.* **14**, 1–15.

Colman, G., Bowen, W.H., and Cole, M.F. (1977). Effects of glucose, fructose and mixtures of glucose and fructose on the incidence of dental caries in Monkeys. *Br. dent. J.* **142**, 217–23.

Cornick, D.E.R. and Bowen, W.H. (1972). The effect of sorbitol on the microbiology of the dental plaque in monkeys. (*Macaca irus*). *Archs. oral Biol.* **17**, 1637–48.

Craig, G.C. (1975). The use of a calcium sucrose phosphates-calcium orthophosphate complex as a cariostatic agent. *Br. dent. J.* **138**, 25–8.

Curzon, M.E.J. and Curzon, J.A. (1970). Dental caries in Eskimo children of the Keewatin district in the northwest territories. *J. Can. dent. Ass.* **36**, 342–5.

Curzon, M.E.J. and Curzon, J.A. (1979). Dental caries prevalence in the Baffin Island eskimo. *Pediatr. Dent.* **1**, 169–3.

Curzon, M.E.J. and Cutress, T.W. (1983). *Trace elements and dental disease*. Wright; PSG, Boston.

Curzon, M.E.J. and Losee, F.L. (1978). Dental caries and trace element composition of whole human enamel: Western United States. *J. Am. dent. Ass.* **96**, 819–22.

Darke, S.J. (1976). Human milk versus cow's milk. *J. hum. Nutr.* **30**, 233–8.

Dawes, C. (1983). A mathematical model of salivary clearance of sugar from the oral cavity. *Caries Res.* **17**, 321–34.

de A. Silva, M.F., Jenkins, G.N., Burgess, R.C., and Sandham, H.J. (1986). Effects of cheese on experimental caries in human subjects. *Caries Res.* **20**, 263–9.

Dean, H.T., Jay, P., Arnold, F.A., and Elvolve, E. (1941). Domestic water and dental caries II. *Publ. Hlth. Rep.* **56**, 761–92.

Dean, H.T., Arnold, F.A., and Elvolve, E. (1942). Domestic water and dental caries V. *Publ. Hlth. Rep.* **57**, 1155–79.

Dreisen, S. and Spies, T.D. (1952). The incidence of dental caries in habitual sugar cane chewers. *J. Am. dent. Ass.* **45**, 193–200.

Drucker, D.B. (1979). Sweetening agents in food, drinks and medicine; cariogenic potential and adverse effects. *J. hum. Nutr.* **33**, 114–24.

Duany, L.F., Zinner, D.D., and Jablon, J.M. (1972). Epidemiologic studies of caries-free and caries-active students. II Diet, dental plaque and oral hygiene. *J. dent. Res.* **51**, 727–33.

Dunning, J.M. and Hodge, A.T. (1971). Influence of cocoa and sugar in milk on dental caries incidence. *J. dent. Res.* **50**, 854–9.

East, B.R. (1941). Association of dental caries in schoolchildren with hardness of communal water supplies. *J. dent. Res.* **20**, 323–6.

Eccles, J.D. (1982). Erosion affecting the palatal surfaces of upper anterior teeth in young people. *Br. dent. J.* **152**, 375–8.

Edgar, W.M. (1978). Reduction in enamel dissolution by liquorice and glycyrrhizinic acid. *J. dent. Res.* **57**, 59–64.

Edgar, W.M. (1985). Prediction of the cariogenicity of various foods. *Int. dent. J.* **35**, 190–4.

Edgar, W.M. and Geddes, D.A.M. (1986). Plaque acidity models for cariogenicity testing; some theoretical and practical observations. *J. dent. Res.* **65**, 1498–502.

Edgar, W.M. and Jenkins, G.N. (1974). Solubility-reducing agents in honey and partially-refined crystalline sugar. *Br. dent. J.* **136**, 7–14.

Edgar, W.M., Bibby, B.G., Mundorff, S., and Rowley, J. (1975). Acid production in plaques after eating snacks: modifying factors in foods. *J. Am. dent. Ass.* **90**, 418–25.

Edgar, W.M., Geddes, D.A.M., Jenkins, G.N., Rugg-Gunn, A.J., and Howell, R. (1978). The effect of calcium glycerophosphate and sodium fluoride on the induction 'in vivo' of caries-like changes in human dental enamel. *Archs. oral Biol.* **23**, 655–61.

Edgar, W.M., Bowen, W.H., Amsbaugh, S., Monnell-Torrens, S., and Brunelle, J. (1982). Effects of different eating patterns on dental caries in the rat. *Caries Res.* **16**, 384–9.

Emilson, C.G. and Krasse, B. (1985). Support for and implications of the specific plaque hypothesis. *Scand. J. dent. Res.* **93**, 96–104.

Emslie, R.D. (1966). A dental health survey in the Republic of the Sudan. *Br. dent. J.* **120**, 167–78.

Enwonwu, C.O. (1974). Socio-economic factors in dental caries prevalence and frequency in Nigerians. *Caries Res.* **8**, 155–71.

Ericsson, Y. (1962). Some differences between human and rodent saliva of probable importance for the different specie reactions to cariogenic and cariostatic agents. *Archs. oral Biol.* Suppl. 327–36.

Fanning, E.A., Gotjamanos, T., and Vowles, N.J. (1969). Dental caries in children related to availability of sweets at school canteens. *Med. J. Austral.* **i**, 1131–2.

Feigal, R.J. and Jensen, M.E. (1982). The cariogenic potential of liquid medications; a concern for the handicapped patient. *Special Care in Dentistry*. **2**, 20–4.

Finlayson, D.A. and Wilson, W.A. (1961). Dental health education: results of Dundee's campaign. *Br. dent. J.* **111**, 103–6.

Finn, S.B. and Jamison, H.C. (1967). The effect of a calcium phosphate chewing-gum on caries incidence in children: 30 month result. *J. Am. dent. Ass.* **74**, 987–95.

Finn, S.B., Frew, R.A., Leibowitz, R., Morse, W., Manson-Hing, L., and Brunelle, J. (1978). The effect of sodium trimetaphosphate (TMP) as a chewing gum additive on caries increments in children. *J. Am. dent. Ass.* **96**, 651–5.

Firestone, A.R., Schmid, R., and Muhlemann, H.R. (1984). Effect of the length and number of intervals between meals on caries in rats. *Caries Res.* **18**, 128–33.

Firestone, A.R., Imfeld, T., Schiffer, S., and Lutz, F. (1987). Measurement of interdental plaque in humans with an indwelling glass pH electrode following a sucrose rinse; a long-term reptrospective study. *Caries Res.* **21**, 555–8.

Fisher, F.J. (1968). A field study of dental caries, periodontal disease and enamel defects in Tristan da Cunha. *Br. dent. J.* **125**, 447–53.

Forscher, B.K. and Hess, W.C. (1954). The validity of plaque pH measurements as a method of evaluating therapeutic agents. *J. Am. dent. Ass.* **48**, 134–9.

Fosdick, L.S., Campaigne, E.E., and Fancher, O.E. (1941). Rate of acid formation in carious areas: the etiology of dental caries. *Ill. dent. J.* **10**, 85–95.

Frostell, G. (1969). Dental plaque pH in relation to intake of carbohydrate products. *Acta odont Scand.* **27**, 3–29.

Frostell, G. (1970). Effects of milk, fruit juices and sweetened beverages on the pH of dental plaques. *Acta odont. Scand.* **28**, 609–22.

Frostell, G. (1972). Effect of a cooked starch solution on the pH of dental plaque. *Swed. dent. J.* **65**, 161–5.

Frostell, G. (1973). Effects of mouthrinses with sucrose, glucose, fructose, lactose, sorbitol and Lycasin on the pH of dental plaque. *Odont. Revy.* **24**, 217–26.

Frostell, G. and Baer, P.K. (1971). Effects of sucrose, starch and a hydrogenated starch derivative on dental caries in the rat. *Acta odont. Scand.* **29**, 253–9.

Frostell, G., Blomlöf, L., Blomqvist, T., Dahl, G.M., Edward, S., Fjellstrom, A., Henrikson, C.O., Larje, O., Nord, C.E., and Nordenvall, N.J. (1974). Substitution of sucrose by Lycasin in candy: the Roslagen study. *Acta odont. Scand.* **32**, 235–54.

Frostell, G., *et al.* (1981). Reduction of caries in preschool children by sucrose restriction and substitution with invert sugar; the Gustavsberg study. *Acta odont. Scand.* **39**, 333–47.

Gardner, D.E., Norwood, J.R., and Eisenson, J.E. (1977). At will breast feeding and dental caries: four case reports. *J. Dent. Child.* **44**, 186–91.

Garn, S.M., Cole, P.E., Solomon, M.A., and Schaefer, A.E. (1980). Relationships between sugar-foods and DMFT in 1968-1970. *Ecol. Food Nutr.* **9**, 135–8.

Geddes, D.A.M., Edgar, W.M., Jenkins, G.N., and Rugg-Gunn, A.J. (1977). Apples, salted peanuts and plaque pH. *Br. dent. J.* **142**, 317–19.

Geddes, D.A.M., Cooke, J.A., Edgar, W.M., and Jenkins, G.N. (1978). The effect of frequent sucrose mouthrinsing on the induction 'in vivo' of caries-like changes in human dental enamel. *Archs. oral Biol.* **23**, 663–5.

Glass, R.L. (1981). Effects on dental caries incidence of frequent ingestion of small amounts of sugars and stannous EDTA in chewing gum. *Caries Res.* **15**, 256–62.

Glass, R.L. and Fleisch, S. (1974). Diet and caries: dental caries incidence and the consumption of ready-to-eat cereals. *J. Am. dent. Ass.* **88**, 807–13.

Glass, R.L. and Hayden, J. (1966). Dental caries in Seventh-Day Adventist children. *J. Dent. Child.* **33**, 22–3.

Goose, D.H. (1967). Infant feeding and caries of the incisors: an epidemiological approach. *Caries Res.* **1**, 167–73.

Goose, D.H. and Gittus, E. (1968). Infant feeding methods and dental caries. *Publ. Hlth. Lond.* **82**, 72–6.

Graf, H. (1970). The glycolytic activity of plaque and its relation to hard tissues pathology; recent findings from intraoral pH telemetry research. *Int. dent. J.* **20**, 426–35.

Granath, L.-E., Rootzen, H., Liljegren, E., and Holst, K. (1976). Variation in caries prevalence related to combinations of dietary and oral hygiene habits in 6-year-old children. *Caries Res.* **10**, 308–17.

Granath, L.-E., Rootzen, H., Liljegren, E., Holst, K., and Köhler, L. (1978). Variation in caries prevalence related to combinations of dietary and oral hygiene habits and chewing fluoride tablets in 4-year-old children. *Caries Res.* **12**, 83–92.

Green, R.M. and Hartles, R.L. (1967). The effect of uncooked and roll dried wheat starch alone and mixed in equal quantities with sucrose on dental caries in the albino rat. *Br. J. Nutr.* **21**, 225–30; 921–4.

Green, R.M. and Hartles, R.L. (1969). The effect of diets containing different mono- and disaccharides on the incidence of dental caries in the albino rat. *Archs. oral Biol.* **14**, 235–41.

Green, R.M. and Hartles, R.L. (1970). The effects of diets containing varying percentages of sucrose and maize on caries in the albino rat. *Caries Res.* **4**, 188–92.

Grenby, T.H. (1967*a*). Wheat bran factors in decalcification tests. *Archs. Oral Biol.* **12**, 523–9.

Grenby, T.H. (1967*b*). Flour, bread and wheat grain fractions in decalcification tests. *Archs. Oral Biol.* **12**, 513–21.

Grenby, T.H. (1967*c*). Investigations in experimental animals on the cariogenicity of diets containing sucrose and/or starch. *Caries Res.* **1**, 208–21.

Grenby, T.H. (1972). The effect of glucose syrup on dental caries in the rat. *Caries Res.* **6**, 52–9.

Grenby, T.H. (1973). Trials of three organic phosphorus-containing compounds as protective agents against dental caries in rats. *J. dent. Res.* **52**, 454–61.

Grenby, T.H. (1984). Can saccharin suppress dental caries in laboratory rats? *Caries Res.* **18**, 178.

Grenby, T.H. and Bull, J.M. (1975). Protection against dental caries in rats by glycerophosphates or calcium salts or mixtures of both. *Archs. oral Biol.* **20**, 717–24.

Grenby, T.H. and Bull, J.M. (1980). Chemical studies of the protective action of phosphate compounds against the demineralization of human dental enamel 'in vitro'. *Caries Res.* **14**, 210–20.

Grenby, T.H. and Hutchinson, J.B. (1969). The effects of diets containing sucrose, glucose or fructose on experimental dental caries in two strains of rats. *Archs. oral Biol.* **14**, 373–80.

Grenby, T.H. and Leer, C.J. (1974). Reduction in 'smooth-surface' caries and fat accumulation in rats when sucrose in drinking-water is replaced by glucose syrup. *Caries Res.* **8**, 368–72.

Grenby, T.H. and Paterson, F.M. (1972). Effect of sweet biscuits on the incidence of dental caries in rats. *Br. J. Nutr.* **27**, 195–9.

Grenby, T.H. and Saldanha, M.G. (1983). Trials of Lycasins in the diet of caries-active laboratory animals. *Proc. nutr. Soc.* **42**, 78A.

Grenby, T.H., Paterson, F.M., and Cawson, R.A. (1973). Dental caries and plaque formation from diets containing sucrose or glucose in gnotobiotics rats infected with *Streptococcus* strain IB-1600. *Br. J. Nutr.* **29**, 221–8.

Grobler, S.R. (1982). Carbohydrate fermentation by human dental plaque. *J. dent. Ass. S. Afr.* **37**, 13–17.

Grobler, S.R., Jenkins, G.N., and Kotże, D. (1985). The effects of the composition and method of drinking soft drinks on plaque pH. *Br. dent. J.* **158**, 293–6.

Guggenheim, B., König, K.G., Herzog, E., and Mühlemann, H.R. (1966). The cariogenicity of different dietary carbohydrates tested on rats in relative gnotobiosis with a Streptococcus producing extracellular polysaccharide. *Helv. odont. Acta.* **10**, 101–13.

Gustaffson, B.E., Quensel, C.E., Lanke, L.S., Lundquist, C., Grahnen, H., Bonow, B.E., and

Krasse, B. (1954). The Vipeholm dental caries study. The effect of different levels of carbohydrate intake on caries activity in 436 individuals observed for five years. *Acta odont Scand.* **11**, 232–364.

Hackett, A.F., Rugg-Gunn, A.J., Murray, J.J., and Roberts, G.J. (1984). Can breast feeding cause dental caries? *Hum. Nutr. appl. Nutr.* **38A**, 23–8.

Hankin, J.H., Chung, C.S., and Kau, M.C.W. (1973). Genetic and epidemiologic studies of oral characteristics in Hawaii's schoolchildren: diet patterns and caries prevalence. *J. dent. Res.* **52**, 1079–86.

Hardwick, J.L. (1960). The incidence and distribution of caries throughout the ages in relation to the Englishman's diet. *Br. dent. J.* **108**, 9–17.

Hargreaves, J.A., Thompson, G.W., Anderson, G.H., and Peterson, R.D. (1980). Dental caries in Canadian children related to between meal sugar consumption. *J. dent. Res.* **59** (spec. iss. B), 968. (Abstr. 325).

Harper, D.S., Gray, R., Lenke, J.W., and Hefferen, J.J. (1985). Measurement of human plaque acidity; comparison of interdental touch and indwelling electrodes. *Caries Res.* **19**, 536–46.

Harper, D.S., Osborn, J.C., Clayton, R., and Hefferen, J.J. (1987). Modification of food cariogenicity in rats by mineral-rich concentrates in milk. *J. dent. Res.* **66**, 42–5.

Harris, R. (1963). Biology of the children of Hopewood House, Bowral, Australia, 4. Observations on dental caries experience extending over 5 years (1957–61). *J. dent. Res.* **42**, 1387–99.

Harris, R.S., Nizel, A.E., and Walsh, N.B. (1967*a*). The effect of phosphate structure on dental caries development in rats. *J. dent. Res.* **46**, 290–4.

Harris, R.S., Schamschula, R.G., Gregory, G., Roots, M., and Beveridge, J. (1967*b*). Observations on the cariostatic effect of calcium sucrose phosphate in a group of children aged 5–17 yrs. Preliminary report. *Australia dent. J.* **12**, 105–13.

Harris, S. and Cleaton-Jones, P. (1978). Oral health in a group of sugarcane chewers. *J. dent. Ass. S. Afr.* **33**, 255–8.

Harris, S.S. and Navia, J.M. (1980). Vitamin A deficiency and caries susceptibility of rat molars. *Archs. oral Biol.* **25**, 415–21.

Hartles, R.L. (1951). The effect of high sucrose diet on the calcium and phosphorus content of the enamel and dentine in rat incisors. *Biochem. J.* **48**, 245–9.

Hausen, H., Heinomen, O.P., and Paunio, I. (1981). Modification of occurrence of caries in children by toothbrushing and sugar exposure in fluoridated and non-fluoridated area. *Commun. Dent. oral Epidemiol.* **9**, 103–7.

Havenaar, R., Huis in't Veld, J.H.J., Backer Dirks, O., and de Stoppelaar, J.D. (1979). Some bacteriological aspects of sugar substitutes. In *Health and sugar substitutes*' (ed. B. Guggenheim), pp 192–8. Karger, Basel.

Hawkins, H. (1932). Manipulation of food in the control of dental caries and systemic pyorrhea. *J. Am. dent. Ass.* **19**, 963–6.

Hayes, M.L. and Roberts, K.R. (1978). The breakdown of glucose, xylitol and other sugar alcohols by human dental plaque bacteria. *Archs. oral Biol.* **23**, 445–51.

Hefti, A. and Schmid, R. (1979). Effect on caries incidence in rats of increasing dietary sucrose levels. *Caries Res.* **13**, 298–300.

Henshaw, N.E. and Adenubi, J.O. (1975). The increase in dental diseasc in the Northern States of Nigeria and its manpower implications. *J. Dent.* **3**, 243–50

Hewat, R.E.T., Abraham, M., and Rice, F.B. (1930). An experimental study on the control of dental caries. *NZ dent. J.* **46**, 78–85.

Hoeven, J.S. van der (1980). Cariogenicity of disaccharide alcohols in rats. *Caries Res.* **14**, 61–6.

Holm, A. -K., Blomquist, K., Crossner, C. -G., Grahnen, H., and Samuelson, G. (1975): A comparative study of oral health as related to general health food habits and socio-economic conditions of 4-year-old Swedish children. *Commun. Dent. oral Epidemiol.* **3**, 34–9.

Holund, U., Theilade, E., and Poulsen, S. (1985). Validity of a dietary interviewing method for use in caries prevention. *Commun. Dent. oral Epidemiol.* **13**, 219–21.

Hoogendoorn, H. (1974). The effect of lactoperoxidase-thiocyanate-hydrogen peroxide on the metabolism of cariogenic micro-organisms *in vitro* and in the oral cavity. Thesis, Mouton, Den Haag.

Howe, P.R., White, R.L., and Rubine, M. (1933). Retardation of dental caries in out-patients of a dental infirmary. *Am. J. Dis. Child.* **46**, 1045–9.

Huang, C.T., Little, M.F., and Johnson, R. (1981). Influence of carbohydrates on 'in vivo' lesion production. *Caries Res.* **15**, 54–9.

Huxley, H.G. (1971). The cariogenicity of various percentages of dietary sucrose and glucose in experimental animals. *NZ dent. J.* **67**, 85–98.

Huxley, H.G. (1977). The cariogenicity of dietary sucrose at various levels in two strains of rat under unrestricted and controlled frequency feeding condition. *Caries Res.* **11**, 237–42.

Iizuka, Y., Yashaki, T., Ahiko, R., Koike, T., and Matsuzawa, A. (1977). The relation of dietary and/or oral hygiene habits to dental caries experience of four-year-old children. *Bull, Kanagawa dent. Coll.* **5**, 61–73.

Imfeld, T. (1977). Evaluation of the cariogenicity of confectionery by intraoral wire telemetry. *Helv. odont. Acta* **21**, 1–28.

Imfeld, T.N. (1983). *Identification of low caries risk dietary components.* Karger, Basel.

Ismail, A.I., Burt, B.A., and Eklund, S.A. (1984). The cariogenicity of soft drinks in the United States. *J. Am. dent. Ass.* **109**, 241–5.

Jackson, D. (1978). Sugar and dental caries: myth and fact. *Probe* **20**, 7–30.

Jackson, D. (1979). Caries experience in deciduous teeth of 5-year-old English children 1947–1977. *Probe* **20**, 404–6.

Jakobsen, J. (1979). Recent reorganisation of the public dental health service in Greenland in favour of caries prevention. *Commun. Dent. oral Epidemiol.* **7**, 75–81.

James, P.M.C. and Parfitt, G.J. (1953). Local effects of certain medicaments on the teeth. *Br. Med. J.* **ii**, 1252–3.

James, P.M.C., Parfitt, G.J., and Falkner, F. (1957). A study of the aetiology of labial caries of the deciduous incisor teeth in small children. *Br. dent. J.* **103**, 37–40.

Jay, P. (1940). The role of sugar in the etiology of dental caries. *J. Am. dent. Ass.* **27**, 393–6.

Jenkins, G.N. (1965). Natural protective factors of foods. In *Nutrition and caries prevention*, (ed. G. Blix), pp. 67–73. Almqvist and Wiksells, Upsalla.

Jenkins, G.N. (1966). The refinement of foods in relation to dental caries. *Adv. oral Biol.* **2**, 67–100.

Jenkins, G.N. (1968). Diet and caries: protective factors. *Alabama J. med. Sci.* **5**, 276–83.

Jenkins, G.N. (1978). *The physiology and biochemistry of the mouth*, 4th edn. Blackwell, Oxford.

Jenkins, G.N. and Ferguson, D.B. (1966). Milk and dental caries. *Br. dent. J.* **120**, 472–7.

Jenkins, G.N. and Smales, F.C. (1966). The potential importance in caries prevention of solubility-reducing and anti-bacterial factors in unrefined plant products. *Archs. oral Biol.* **11**, 599–608.

Jenkins, G.N., Forster, M.G., Spiers, R.L., and Kleinberg, I. (1959). The influence of the refinement of carbohydrates on their cariogenicity. *Br. dent. J.* **106**, 195–208.

Jensen, M.E. (1986*a*). Effects of chewing sorbitol gum and paraffin on human interproximal plaque pH. *Caries Res.* **20**, 503–9.

Jensen, M.E. (1986*b*). Responses of interproximal plaque pH to snack foods and effect of chewing sorbitol-containing gum. *J. Am. dent. Ass.* **113**, 262–6.

Jensen, M.E. and Schachtele, C.F. (1983). The acidogenic potential of reference foods and snacks at interproximal sites in the human dentition. *J. dent Res.* **62**, 889–92.

Kandelman, D., Bar, A., and Hefti, A. (1988). Collaborative WHO xylitol field study in French Polynesia, I; Baseline prevalence and 32-month caries increment. *Caries Res.* **22**, 55–62.

Karle, E.J. and Gehring, F. (1976). About the cariogenicity of fruit and special sweets. *J. dent. Res.* **5** (suppl. D), 155. (Abstr. 20).

Katayama, T., Nagagawa, E., Honda, O., Tani, H., Okado, S., and Suzuki, S. (1979). Incidence and distribution of *Strep. mutans* in plaque from confectionery workers. *J. dent. Res.* **58** (spec. iss. D) 2251. (Abstr. 11).

Kato, T., Sakai, S., Okuyama, T., Nagahama, M., Akiyoshi, T., Sasaki, F., Kuriyama, S., and Motomura, S. (1969). Research on between-meal eatings in 2 and 3 year-old infants, especially their relationship with susceptibility to dental caries. *Jap. J. dent. Hlth.* **19**, 1–8.

King, J.D. (1946). Dental caries: effect of carbohydrate supplements on susceptibility of infants. *Lancet* **250**, 646–9.

King, J.D., Mellanby, M., Stones, H.H., and Green, H.N. (1955). *The effect of sugar supplement on dental caries.* MRC Report 288. HMSO, London.

Kite, O.W., Shaw, J.H., and Sognnaes, R.F. (1950). The prevention of experimental tooth decay by tube-feeding. *J. Nutrit.* **42**, 89–103.

Kleemola-Kujala, E. and Rasanen, L. (1979). Dietary pattern of Finnish children with low and high caries experience. *Commun. Dent. oral Epidemiol.* **7**, 199–205.

Kleemola-Kujala, E., and Rasanen, L. (1982). Relationship of oral hygiene and sugar consumption to risk of caries in children. *Commun. Dent. oral Epidemiol.* **10**, 224–33.

Kleinberg, I. (1958). The construction and evaluation of modified types of antimony microelectrodes for intra-oral use. *Br. dent. J.* **104**, 197–204.

Kleinberg, I., Jenkins, G.N., Chatterjee, R., and Wijeyeweera, L. (1982). The antimony pH electrode and its role in the assessment and interpretation of dental plaque pH. *J. dent. Res.* **61**, 1139–47.

Knowles, E.M. (1946). The effects of enemy occupation on the dental condition of children in the Channel Islands. *Month. Bull. Min. Hlth.* August, 162–72.

Koehne, M. and Bunting, R.W. (1934). Studies in the control of dental caries II. *J. Nutr.* **7**, 657–78.

Koehne, M. and Morrell, E. (1934). Control of dental caries in children. *Am. J. Dis. Child.* **48**, 6–29.

König, K.G. (1967). Caries induced in laboratory rats. Post eruptive effect of sucrose and of bread of different degrees of refinement. *Br. dent. J.* **123**, 583–9.

König, K.G. (1969). Caries activity induced by frequency controlled feeding of diets containing sucrose or bread to Osborne-Mendel rats. *Archs. oral Biol.* **14**, 991–3.

König, K.G., Schmid, P., and Schmid, R. (1968). An apparatus for frequency-controlled feeding of small rodents and its use in dental caries experiments. *Archs. oral Biol.* **13**, 13–26.

Kotlow, L.A. (1977). Breast feeding: a cause of dental caries in children. *J. Dent. Child.* **44**, 192–3.

Koulourides, T., Bodden, R., Keller, S., Manson-Hing, L., Lastra, J., and Housch, T. (1976). Cariogenicity of nine sugars tested with an intraoral device in man. *Caries Res.* **10**, 427–41.

Krasse, B. (1985). The cariogenic potential of foods; a critical review of current methods. *Int. dent. J.* **35**, 36–42.

Kreitzman, S.N. and Klein, R.M. (1976). Non-linear relationship between dietary sucrose and dental caries. *I ADR 54th Gen. Meet. Miami Beach*, p. B. 175.

Kristofferson, K., Axelsson, P., Birkhed, D., and Bratthall, D. (1986). Caries prevalence, salivary *Streptococcus mutans* and dietary scores in 13-year-old Swedish schoolchildren. *Commun. Dent. oral Epidemiol.* **14**, 202–5.

Kroll, R.G. and Stone, J.H. (1967). Nocturnal bottle-feeding as a contributory cause of rampant dental caries in the infant and young child. *J. Dent. Child.* **34**, 454–9.

Künzel, W., Borroto, R.C., Lanier, S., and Soto, F. (1973). Auswirkungen habitnellen Zuckerrohrkanens auf Kariesbefall und Parodontalzustand kubanischer Zuckerrohrarbeiter. *Dt. Stomatol.* **23**, 554–61.

Lachapelle-Harvey, D. and Sevigny, J. (1985). Multiple regression analysis of dental status and related food behaviour of French Canadian adolescents. *Commun. Dent. oral Epidemiol.* **13**, 226–9.

Leach, S.A., Agalamanyi, E.A., and Green, R.M. (1983). Remineralisation of teeth by diet ary means. In *Demineralisation and remineralisation of the teeth*, (Ed. S.A. Leach and W.M. Edgar), pp 51–73. IRL Press, Oxford.

Lilienthal, B. (1977). *Phosphates and dental caries*. Karger, Basel.

Lilienthal, B. *et al.* (1966). The cariostatic effect of carbohydrate phosphates in the diet. *Australia dent. J.* **11**, 388–95.

Lindfors, B. and Lagerlof, F. (1988). Effect of sucrose concentration in saliva after a sucrose rinse on the hydronium ion concentration in dental plaque. *Caries Res.* **22**, 7–10.

Linke, H.A.B. (1977). Growth-inhibition of glucose-grown cariogenic and other streptococci by saccharin in vitro. *Z. Naturforsch.* **32**, 839–43.

Littleton, N.W. (1963). Dental caries and periodontal disease among Ethiopian civilians. *Publ. Hlth. Rep., Wash.* **78**, 631–40.

Loesche, W.J. (1985). The rationale for caries prevention through the use of sugar substitutes. *Int. dent. J.* **35**, 1–8.

Lokken, P., Birkeland, J.M., and Sannes, E. (1975). pH changes in dental plaque caused by sweetened, iron-containing liquid medicine. *Scand. J. dent. Res.* **83**, 279–83.

Ludwig, T.G., Denby, G.C., and Struthers, W.H. (1960). Dental health: 1. Caries prevalence amongst dentists children. *NZ dent. J.* **56**, 174–7.

Lundqvist, C. (1952). Oral sugar clearance. *Odont. Revy.* **3** (suppl. 1) 1–123.

Luoma, H. (1961). The effect of injecting monosaccharides upon the mineralization of rat molars. *Archs. oral Biol.* **3**, 271–7.

McDonald, S.P., Cowell, C.R., and Sheiham, A. (1981). Methods of preventing dental caries used by dentists for their own children. *Br. dent. J.* **151**, 118–21.

MacGregor, A.B. (1963). Increasing caries incidence and changing diet in Ghana. *Int. dent. J.* **13**, 516–22.

McHugh, W.D., McEwen, J.D., and Hitchen, A.D. (1964). Dental disease and related factors in 13-year-old children in Dundee. *Br. dent. J.* **117**, 246–53.

Magrill, D.S. (1973). The reduction of the solubility of hydroxyapatite in acid by adsorption of phytate from solution. *Archs. oral Biol.* **18**, 591–600.

Makinen, K.K. (1985). New biochemical aspects of sweeteners. *Int. dent. J.* **35**, 23–35.

Mansbridge, J.N. (1960). The effects of oral hygiene and sweet consumption on the prevalence of dental caries. *Br. dent. J.* **109**, 343–8.

Marthaler, T.M. (1967). Epidemiological and clinical dental findings in relation to intake of carbohydrates. *Caries Res.* **1**, 222–38.

Marthaler, T.M. (1978). Sugar and oral health: epidemiology in humans. In *Health and sugar substitutes*, (ed. B. Guggenheim), pp. 27–34. Karger, Basel.

Martinsson, T. (1972). Socio-economic investigation of schoolchildren with high and low caries frequency, III. A dietary study based on information given by the children. *Odont. Revy.* **23**, 93–114.

Matsson, L. and Koch, G. (1975). Caries frequency in children with controlled diabetes. *Scand. J. dent. Res.* **83**, 327–32.

Mayhall, J.T. (1975). Canadian Inuit caries experience 1969–1973. *J. dent. Res.* **54**, 1245.

Mayhall, J.T. (1977). The oral health of a Canadian Inuit Community, an anthropological approach. *J. dent. Res.* **56**, C55–61.

Mellanby, M. (1923). The relation of caries to the structure of teeth. *Br. dent. J.* **44**, 1–13.

Mellanby, M. (1937). The role of nutrition as a factor in resistance to dental caries. *Br. dent. J.* **62**, 241–52.

Mellanby, M. and Pattison, C.L. (1928). The action of vitamin D in preventing the spread and promoting the arrest of caries in children. *Br. med. J.* **ii**, 1079–82.

Menaker, L., Navia, J.M. (1973). Effect of undernutrition during the perinatal period on caries development in the rat: II. Caries susceptibility in underfed rats supplemented with protein or caloric additions during the suckling period. *J. dent. Res.* **52**, 680–7.

Messer, L.B., Messer, H.H., and Best, J. (1980). Refined carbohydrate consumption by caries-free and caries-active children. *J. dent. Res.* **59** (spec. iss. B), 968. (Abstr. 324.)

Michalek, S.M., McGhee, J.E., Shiota, T., and Devenyns, D. (1977). Low sucrose levels promote extensive *Streptococcus mutans*-induced dental caries. *Infec. Immun.* **16**, 712–14.

Miller, W.D. (1890). *The micro-organisms of the human mouth*, (ed. K. Konig). Karger, Basel.

Mills, C.A. (1937). Factors affecting the incidence of dental caries in population groups. *J. dent. Res.* **16**, 417–30.

Ministry of Agriculture, Fisheries and Food (1967). Solvents in foods regulations. S1 1967 No. 1582. HMSO, London.

Ministry of Agriculture, Fisheries and Food (1982). Food additives and contaminants committee report on the review of sweeteners in food. FAC/REP/34. HMSO, London.

Möller, I.J. and Poulsen, S. (1973). The effect of sorbitol-containing chewing gum on the incidence of dental caries; plaque and gingivitis in Danish schoolchildren. *Commun. Dent. oral Epidemiol.* **1**, 58–67.

Möller, I.J., Poulson, S., and Orholm Nielsen, V. (1972). The prevalence of dental caries in Godhavn and Scoresbysund districts, Greenland. *Scand. J. dént. Res.* **80**, 169–80.

Moore, W.J. and Corbett, M.E. (1978). Dental caries experience in man: historical, anthropological and cultural diet-caries relationships, the English experience. In *Diet, nutrition and dental caries*, (ed. N.H. Rowe), pp. 3–19. University of Michigan School of Dentistry.

Mörch, T. (1961). The acid potentiality of carbohydrates: an investigation on some common dietary components in Norway. *Acta odont. Scand.* **19**, 355–85.

Mormann, J.E. and Mühlemann, H.R. (1981). Oral starch degradation and its influence on acid production in human dental plaque. *Caries Res.* **15**, 166–75.

Mühlemann, H.R. (1969). Zuckerfreie, Zahnschomende, und Nicht-kariogene Bonbons und Süssigkeiten. *Schweiz Mschr. Zahnheilk.* **79**, 117–45.

Mühlemann, H.R. and Boever, J. (1970). Radiotelemetry of the pH of interdental areas exposed to various carbohydrates. In *Dental plaque*, (ed. W.D. McHugh), pp. 179–86. Livingstone, Edinburgh.

Mühlemann, H.R. and Schneider, P. (1975). The effect of sorbose on pH of mixed saliva and inter-proximal plaque. *Helv. odont. Acta.* **19**, 76–80.

Navia, J.M. (1972). Prevention of dental caries: agents which increase tooth resistance to dental caries. *Int. dent. J.* **22**, 427–40.

Navia, J.M. and Lopez, H. (1983). Rat caries assay of reference foods and sugar-containing snacks. *J. dent. Res.* **62**, 892–8.

Navia, J.M., Di Orio, L.P., Menaker, L., and Miller, J. (1970). Effect of undernutrition during the perinatal period on caries development in the rat. *J. dent. Res.* **49**, 1091–8.

Navia, J.M., Guzman, M.A., Urrutia, J.J., Viteri, F., Gonzalez, M., and Leon, A. (1980). Retrospective evaluation of nutrition-caries interrelationships in Guatemalan children. *J. dent. Res.* **59** (spec. iss. B), 968. (Abstr. 326.)

Naylor, M.N. and Glass, R.L. (1979). A 3-year clinical trial of calcium carbonate dentifrice containing calcium glycerophosphate and sodium monofluorophosphate. *Caries Res.* **13**, 39–46.

Neff, D. (1967). Acid production from different carbohydrate sources in human plaque in situ. *Caries Res.* **1**, 78–87.

Newbrun, E. (1967). Sucrose, the arch criminal of dental caries. *Odont. Revy.* **18**, 373–86.

Newbrun, E. (1978). *Cariology*. Williams and Wilkins, Baltimore.

Newbrun, E. (1984). Diet and dental caries. In *Cariology today*, (ed.) B. Guggenheim, pp. 340–52. Karger, Basel.

Newbrun, E., Hoover, C., Mettraux, G., and Graf, H. (1980). Comparison of dietary habits and dental health of subjects with hereditary fructose intolerance and control subjects. *J. Am. dent. Ass.* **101**, 619–26.

Newman, P., MacFadyen, E.E., Gillespie, F.C., and Stephen, K.W. (1979). An indwelling electrode for 'in vivo' measurement of the pH of dental plaque. *Archs. oral Biol.* **24**, 501–7.

Nizel, A.E. (1973). Cariogenicity of honey (letter). *J. Am. dent. Ass.* **87**, 29.

Nizel, A.E. and Harris, R.S. (1964). The effects of phosphates on experimental dental caries: a literature review. *J. dent. Res.* **43**, 1123–36.

Ockerse, T. (1944). Relation of fluoride content, hardness and pH values of drinking water and incidence of dental caries. *S. Afr. med. J.* **18**, 255–8.

Ojofeitimi, E.O., Hollist, N.O., Banjo, T., and Adu, T.A. (1984). Effect of cariogenic food exposure on the prevalence of dental caries among fee and non-fee paying Nigerian schoolchildren. *Commun. Dent. oral Epidemiol.* **12**, 274–7.

Okholm, L. (1980). Dietary risk factors—industry's responsibility. *J. dent. Res.* **59** (spec. iss. D, part II), 2190–3.

Olojugba, O.O. and Lennon, M.A. (1987). Dental caries experience in 5- and 12-year-old schoolchildren in Ondo State, Nigeria in 1977 and 1983. *Commun. dent. Health.* **4**, 129–35.

Olsson, B. (1978). Dental caries and fluorosis in Arussi province, Ethiopia. *Commun. Dent. oral Epidemiol.* **6**, 338–43.

Olsson, B. (1979). Dental health situation in privileged children in Addis Ababa, Ethiopia. Commun. Dent. oral Epidemiol. **7**, 37–41.

Orland, F.J. *et al.* (1954). Use of the germ-free animal technic in the study of experimental dental caries. *J. dent. Res.* **33**, 147–74.

Osborn, T.W.B. and Noriskin, J.N. (1937). The relationship between diet and caries in South African Bantu. *J. dent. Res.* **16**, 431–41.

Osborn, T.W.B., Noriskin, J.N., and Staz, J. (1937*a*). A comparison of crude and refined sugar and cereals in their ability to produce *in vitro* decalcification of teeth. *J. dent. Res.* **16**, 165–71.

Osborn, T.W.B., Noriskin, J.N. and Staz, J. (1937*b*). Inhibition *in vitro* of decalcification of teeth. *J. dent. Res.* **16**, 545–50.

Palmer, J.D. (1971). Dietary habits at bedtime in relation to dental caries in children. *Br. dent. J.* **130**, 288–93.

Parfitt, G.J. (1954). The apparent delay between alteration in diet and change in caries incidence: a note on conditions in Norway reported by Toverud. *Br. dent. J.* **97**, 235–7.

Pearce, E.I.F. and Bibby, B.G. (1966). Protein adsorption on bovine enamel. *Archs. oral Biol.* **11**, 329–36.

Pearce, E.I.F. and Gallagher, I.H.C. (1979). The behaviour of sucrose and xylitol in an intra-oral caries test. *NZ dent J.* **75**, 8–14.

Pedersen, P.O. (1938). Investigations into dental conditions of about 3000 ancient and modern Greenlanders. *Dent. Record.* **58**, 191–8.

Persson, L-A., Stecksen-Blick, C., and Holm, A-K. (1984). Nutrition and health in childhood, causal and quantitative interpretations of dental caries. *Commun. Dent. oral Epidemiol.* **12**, 390–7.

Persson, L-A., Holm, A-K., Arvidsson, S., and Samuelson, G. (1985). Infant feeding and dental caries, a longitudinal study of Swedish children. *Swed. dent. J.* **9**, 201–6.

Price, W.A. (1936). Eskimo and Indian field studies in Alaska and Canada. *J. Am. dent. Ass.* **23**, 417–37.

Ranke, E., Ahrens, G., and Ranke, B. (1974). Beobachtungen zur Bedentung von Süssigkeitenverzehr und Zahnpflage für die Zahnkaries. *Dt. Zahnärztl.* **29**, 798–801.

Read, T.T. and Knowles, E.M. (1938). A study of the diet and habits of schoolchildren in relation to freedom from or susceptibility to dental caries. *Br. dent. J.* **64**, 185–97.

Reece, J.A. and Swallow, J.N. (1970). Carrots and dental health. *Br. dent. J.* **128**, 535–9.

Rekola, M. (1987). Approximal caries development during 2-year total substitution of dietary sucrose with xylitol. *Caries Res.* **21**, 87–94.

Retief, D.H., Cleaton-Jones, P.E., and Walker, A.R.P. (1975). Dental caries and sugar intake in South African pupils of 16 to 17 years in four ethnic groups. *Br. dent. J.* **138**, 463–9.

Reynolds, E.C. and Johnson, I.H. (1981). Effect of milk on caries incidence and bacterial composition of dental plaque in the rat. *Archs. oral Biol.* **26**, 445–51.

Richardson, A.S., Hole, L.W., McCombie, F., and Kolthammer, J. (1972). Anticariogenic effect of dicalcium phosphate dihydrate chewing gum. *J. Can. dent. Ass.* **38**, 213–18.

Richardson, A.S., Boyd, M.A., and Conry, R.F. (1977). A correlation study of diet, oral hygiene and dental caries in 457 Canadian children. *Commun. Dent. oral Epidemiol.* **5**, 227–30.

Richardson, B.D., Cleaton-Jones, P.E., McInnes, P.M., and Rantsho, J.M. (1981*a*). Infant feeding practices and nursing bottle caries. *J. Dent. Child.* **48**, 423–9.

Richardson, B.D., Sinwell, R.E., and Cleaton-Jones,, P. (1981*b*). Sweets, snacks, and dental caries, South African inter-racial patterns. *Am. J. clin. Nutr.* **34**, 1428–31.

Ripa, L.W. (1978). Nursing habits and dental decay in infants: 'nursing bottle caries'. *J. dent. Child.* **45**, 274–5.

Roberts, I.F. and Roberts, G.J. (1979). Relation between medicines sweetened with sucrose and dental disease. *Br. med. J.* **ii**, 14–16.

Roder, D.M. (1973). The association between dental caries and the availability of sweets in South Australian school canteens. *Australia dent. J.* **18**, 174–82.

Rowe, N.H., Anderson, R.H., and Wanninger, L.A. (1974). The effect of ready-to-eat breakfast cereals upon dental caries experience in adolescent children: a 3 year study. *J. dent. Res.* **53**, 33–6.

Rowe, N.H., Anderson, R.H., Wanninger, L.A., and Saari, A.L. (1975). Effect of phosphate-enriched ready-to-eat breakfast cereals on dental caries experience in adolescents: a three-year study. *J. Am. dent. Ass.* **90**, 412–17.

Rugg-Gunn, A.J. (1988*a*). Effect of Lycasin upon plaque pH when taken as a syrup or as a boiled sweet. *Caries Res.* **22**, 375–6.

Rugg-Gunn, A.J. (1988*b*). *Starchy foods and fresh fruits; their relative importance as a source of dental caries in Britain. A review of the literature.* Occasional paper No. 3. Health Education Authority, London.

Rugg-Gunn, A.J. and Edgar, W.M. (1985). Sweeteners and dental health. *Commun. dent. Health.* **2**, 213–23.

Rugg-Gunn, A.J., Edgar, W.M., Geddes, D.A.M., and Jenkins, G.N. (1975). The effect of different meal patterns upon plaque pH in human subjects. *Br. dent. J.* **139**, 351–6.

Rugg-Gunn, A.J., Edgar, W.M., and Jenkins, G.N. (1978). The effect of eating some British snacks upon the pH of human dental plaque. *Br. dent. J.* **145**, 95–100.

Rugg-Gunn, A.J., Edgar, W.M., and Jenkins, G.N. (1981). The effect of altering the position of a sugary food in a meal upon plaque pH in human subjects. *J. dent. Res.* **60**, 867–72.

Rugg-Gunn, A.J., Hackett, A.F., Appleton, D.R., Eastoe, J.E., and Jenkins, G.N. (1984*a*). Correlations of dietary intakes of calcium phosphorus and Ca P ratio with caries data in children. *Caries Res.* **18**, 149–52.

Rugg-Gunn, A.J., Hackett, A.F., Appleton, D.R., Jenkins, G.N., and Eastoe, J.E. (1984*b*). Relationship between dietary habits and caries increment assessed over two years in 405 English adolescent schoolchildren. *Archs. oral Biol.* **29**, 983–92.

Rugg-Gunn, A.J., Roberts, G.J. and Wright, W.G. (1985). The effect of human milk on plaque *in situ* and enamel dissolution *in vitro* compared with bovine milk, lactose and sucrose. *Caries Res.* **19**, 327–34.

Rugg-Gunn, A.J., Hackett, A.F., Appleton, D.R., and Moynihan, P.J. (1986). The dietary intake of added and natural sugars in 405 English adolescents. *Hum. Nutr. appl. Nutr.* **40A**, 115–24.

Rugg-Gunn, A.J., Hackett, A.F., and Appleton, D.R. (1987). Relative cariogenicity of starch and sugars in a two-year longitudinal study of 405 English schoolchildren. *Caries Res.* **21**, 464–73.

Rundegren, J., Koulourides, T., and Ericson, T. (1980). Contribution of maltitol and Lycasin to experimental enamel demineralization in the human mouth. *Caries Res.* **14**, 67–74.

Russell, A.L., Littleton, N.W., Leatherwood, E.C., Sydow, G.E., and Green, J.C. (1960). Dental surveys in relation to nutrition. *Publ. hlth. Rep.* **75**, 717–23.

Sarnat, H., Eliaz, R., Feiman, G., Flexer, Z., Karp, M., and Laron, Z. (1985). Carbohydrate consumption and oral status of diabetic and non-diabetic young adolescents. *Clin. prev. Dent.* **7**, 20–3.

Savara, B.S. and Suher, T. (1955). Dental caries in children one to six years of age as related to socio-economic level, food habits and toothbrushing. *J. dent. Res.* **34**, 870–5.

Schachtele, C.F. and Jensen, M.E. (1981). Human plaque pH studies: estimating the acidogenic potential of foods. *Cereal Foods World.* **26**, 14–18.

Scheinin, A. (1979). Influence of the diagnostic level on caries incidence in two controlled clinical trials. *Caries Res.* **13**, 91. (Abstr. 20.)

Scheinin, A. and Mäkinen, K.K. (1975). Turku sugar studies. I-XXI. *Acta odont. Scand.* **33**, Suppl. 70, 1–349.

Scheinin, A., Mäkinen, K.K., Tammisalo, E., and Rekola, M. (1975). Turku sugar studies XVIII. Incidence of dental caries in relation to 1-year consumption of xylitol chewing gum. *Acta odont. Scand.* **30**, Suppl. 70, 307–16.

Scheinin, A. *et al.* (1985*a*). Collaborative WHO xylitol field studies in Hungary I; three year caries activity in institutionalized children. *Acta odont. Scand.* **43**, 327–47.

Scheinin, A., Pienihakkinen, K., Tiekso, J., Banoczy, J., Szoke, J., and Esztari, I. (1985*b*). Collaborative WHO xylitol field studies in Hungary, VII; two year caries incidence in 976 institutionalized children. *Acta odont. Scand.* **43**, 381–7.

Schemmel, R.A., Krohn-Lutz, K., Lynch, P., and Kabara, J.J. (1982). Influence of dietary disaccharides on mouth micro-organisms and experimental dental caries in rats. *Archs. oral Biol.* **27**, 435–41.

Schroder, U. and Granath, L. (1983). Predictive value of dietary habits and oral hygiene for the occurrence of caries in 3-year-olds. *Commun. Dent. oral Epidemiol.* **11**, 308–11.

Schroder, U., and Edwardsson, S. (1987). Dietary habits, gingival status and occurrence of *Streptococcus mutans* and lactobacilli as predictors of caries in 3-year-olds in Sweden. *Commun. Dent. oral Epidemiol.* **15**, 320–4.

's-Gravenmade, E.J., Jenkins, G.N., and Ferguson, D.B. (1977). A potential cariostatic factor in cocoa beans. *Caries Res.* **11**, 138. (Abstr.)

's-Gravenmade, E.J. and Jenkins, G.N. (1986). Isolation, purification and some properties of a potential cariostatic factor in cocoa that lowers enamel solubility. *Caries Res.* **20**, 433–6.

Shallenberger, R.S. and Acree, T.E. (1967). Molecular theory of sweet taste. *Nature, Lond.* **216**, 480–2.

Shannon, I.L. (1974). Sucrose and glucose in dry breakfast cereals. *J. Dent. Child.* **41**, 347–50.

Shannon, I.L., Edmonds, E.J., and Madsen, K.O. (1979). Honey: sugar content and cariogenicity. *J. Dent. Child.* **46**, 29–33.

Shaw, J.H. (1949). Nutrition and dental caries. *Fedn. Proc. Fedn. Am. Socs. exp. Biol.* **8**, 536–45.

Shaw, J.H. (1979). Changing food habits and our need for evaluation of the cariogenic potential of foods and confections. *Pediatr. Dent.* **1**, 192–8.

Shaw, J.H. (1980). Influences of sodium, calcium and magnesium trimetaphosphates on dental caries activity in the rat. *J. dent. Res.* **59**, 614–50.

Shaw, J.H. (1986). Animal caries models—resource paper. *J. dent. Res.* **65** (spec. iss.), 1485–90.

Shaw, J.H. and Griffiths, D. (1960). Partial substitution of hexitols for sucrose and dextrin in caries producing diets. *J. dent. Res.* **39**, 377–84.

Shaw, J.H. and Ivimey, J.K. (1972). Caries in rats with starch as the only dietary carbohydrate. *J. dent. Res.* **51**, 1507.

Shaw, L. and Murray, J.J. (1980). A family history study of caries-resistance and caries-susceptibility. *Br. dent. J.* **148**, 231–5.

Sheiham, A. (1967). The prevalence of dental caries in Nigerian populations. *Br. dent. J.* **123**, 144–8.

Ship, I.I. and Mickelson, O. (1964). The effects of calcium acid phosphate on dental caries in children: a controlled clinical trial. *J. dent. Res.* **43**, 1144–9.

Shresha, B.M., Mundorff, S.A., and Bibby, B.G. (1982). Preliminary studies on calcium lactate as an anticaries food additive. *Caries Res.* **16**, 12–17.

Silver, D.H. (1987). A longitudinal study of infant feeding practice, diet and caries, related to social class in children aged 3 and 8–10 years. *Br. dent. J.* **163**, 296–300.

Silverstein, S.J., Knapp, J.F., Kircos, L., and Edwards, H. (1983). Dental caries prevalence in children with a diet free of refined sugar. *Am. J. publ. Hlth.* **73**, 1196–9.

Slack, G.L. and Martin, W.J. (1958). Apples and dental health. *Br. dent. J.* **105**, 366–71.

Slack, G.L., Duckworth, R., Sheer, B., Brandt, R.S., and Alionous, M.C. (1972). The effect of chewing gum on the incidence of dental diseases in Greek children. *Br. dent. J.* **133**, 371–7.

Smith, A.J. and Shaw, L. (1987). Baby fruit juices and tooth erosion. *Br. dent. J.* **162**, 65–7.

Sobel, A.E. and Hanok, A. (1948). Calcification of teeth, I. Composition in relation to blood and diet. *J. biol. Chem.* **176**, 1103–22.

Sobel, A.E. and Hanok, A. (1958). Calcification XVI. Composition of bones and teeth in relation to blood and diet in the cotton rat. *J. dent. Res.* **37**, 631–7.

Sobel, A.E., Shaw, J.H., Hanok, A., and Nobel, S. (1958). Calcification XXVI. Caries susceptibility in relation to composition of teeth and diet. *J. dent. Res.* **39**, 462–72.

Sognnaes, R.F. (1947). Caries conductive effect of a purified diet when fed to rodents during tooth development. *J. Am. dent. Ass.* **37**, 676–92.

Sognnaes, R.F. (1948). Analysis of wartime reduction of dental caries in European children. *Am. J. Dis. Child.* **75**, 792–821.

Sognnaes, R.F. and Shaw, J.H. (1954). Experimental rat caries IV. Effect of a natural salt mixture on the caries-conduciveness of an otherwise purified diet. *J. Nutr.* **53**, 195–206.

Sognnaes, R.F. and White, R.L. (1940). Oral conditions of children in relation to state of general health and habits of life. *Am. J. Dis. Child.* **60**, 283–303.

Sreebny, L.M. (1982). Sugar availability, sugar consumption and dental caries. *Commun. Dent. oral Epidemiol.* **10**, 1–7.

Sreebny, L.M. (1983). Cereal availability and dental caries. *Commun. Dent. oral Epidemiol.* **11**, 148–55.

Stanton, G. (1969). Diet and dental caries: the phosphate sequestration hypothesis. *NY St. dent. J.* **35**, 399–407.

Starkey, G., Kjellman, O., Hogberg, O., and Froth, L.O. (1971). Dietary composition and dental disease in adolescent diabetes. *Acta paediatr. Scand.* **606**, 461–4.

Stecksen-Blicks, C., and Gustafsson, L. (1986). Impact of oral hygiene and use of fluorides on caries increment in children during one year. *Commun. Dent. oral Epidemiol.* **14**, 185–9.

Stecksen-Blicks, C., Arvidsson, S., and Holm, A-K. (1985). Dental health, dental care and dietary habits in children in different parts of Sweden. *Acta odont. Scand.* **43**, 59–67.

Steggerda, M. and Hill, T.J. (1936). Incidence of dental caries among Maya and Navajo Indians. *J. dent. Res.* **15**, 233–42.

Steinberg, A.D., Zimmerman, S.O., and Bramer, M.L. (1972). The Lincoln dental caries study, II. The effect of acidulated carbonated beverages on the incidence of dental caries. *J. Am. dent. Ass.* **85**, 81–9.

Stephan, R.M. (1940). Changes in hydrogen-ion concentration on tooth surfaces and in carious lesions. *J. Am. dent. Ass.* **27**, 718–23.

Stephan, R.M. (1943). The effect of urea in counteracting the influence of carbohydrates on the pH of dental plaques. *J. dent. Res.* **22**, 63–71.

Stephan, R.M. (1944). Intra-oral hydrogen-ion concentration associated with dental caries. *J. dent. Res.* **23**, 257–66.

Steyn, N.P., Albertse, E.C., van Wyk Kotze, T.J., van Wyk, C.W., and van Eck, M. (1987). Sucrose consumption and dental caries in twelve-year-old children of all ethnic groups residing in Cape Town. *J. dent. Ass. S. Afr.* **42**, 43–9.

Stookey, G.K., Carroll, R.A., and Muhler, J.C. (1967). The clinical effectiveness of phosphate-enriched breakfast cereals on the incidence of dental caries in children: results after 2 years. *J. Am. dent. Ass.* **74**, 752–8.

Stralfors, A. (1964). The effect of calcium phosphate on dental caries in schoolchildren. *J. dent. Res.* **43**, 1137–43.

Stralfors, A. (1966). Inhibition of hamster caries by cocoa. *Archs. oral Biol.* **11**, 323–8.

Takahashi, K. (1961). Statistical study on caries incidence in the first molar in relation to the amount of sugar consumption. *Bull. Tokyo dent. Coll.* **2**, 44–57.

Takeuchi, M. (1960). Epidemiological study on relation between dental caries incidence and sugar consumption. *Bull. Tokyo dent. Coll.* **1**, 58–70.

Takeuchi, M. (1961). Epidemiological study on dental caries in Japanese children before, during and after World War II. *Int. dent. J.* **11**, 443–57.

Tank, G. and Storvick, C.A. (1965). Caries experience of children 1–6 years old in two Oregon communities (Corvallis and Albany) III. *J. Am. dent. Ass.* **70**, 394–403.

Tatevossian, A., Edgar, W.M., and Jenkins, G.N. (1975). Changes in the concentration of phosphates in human plaque after ingestion of sugar with and without added phosphates. *Archs. oral Biol.* **20**, 617–25.

Tehrani, A., Brudevold, F., Attarzadeh, F., van Houte, J., and Russo, J. (1983). Enamel demineralization by mouthrinses containing different concentrations of sucrose. *J. dent. Res.* **62**, 1216–17.

Thompson, M.E. and Pearce, E.I.F. (1982). The cariogenicity of experimental biscuits containing wheatgerm and rolled oats, and the effect of supplementation with milk powder. *NZ Dent. J.* **78**, 3–6.

Thompson, M.E., Dever, J.G., and Pearce, E.I.F. (1984). Intra-oral testing of flavoured sweetened milk. *NZ Dent. J.* **80**, 44–6.

Toverud, G. (1956). The influence of war and post-war conditions on the teeth of Norwegian schoolchildren. I. *Millbank Mem. Fund Q.* **34** 354–430.

Toverud, G. (1957). The influence of war and post-war conditions on the teeth of Norwegian schoolchildren II and III. *Millbank Mem. Fund Q.* **35**, 127–96; 373–459.

Toverud, G., Rubal, L., and Wiehl, D.G. (1961). The influence of war and post-war conditions on the teeth of Norwegian schoolchildren. IV. *Millbank Mem. Fund Q.* **39**, 489–539.

van der Hoeven, J.S. (1985). Effect of calcium lactate and calcium lactophosphate on caries activity in programme-fed rats. *Caries Res.* **19**, 368–70.

van Herpen, B.P.J.M. and Arends, J. (1986). Influence of the consumption frequency of filled chocolate products on the demineralization of human enamel *in vitro*. *Caries Res.* **20**, 529–33.

van Strijp, A.J.P., ten Brink, B., and Theuns, H.M. (1988). Influence of the temperature of extraoral immersions in the intraoral cariogenicity test model. *Caries Res.* **22**, 37–41.

von der Fehr, F.R., Löe, H., and Theilade, E. (1970). Experimental caries in man. *Caries Res.* **4**, 131–48.

Walker, A.R.P., Dison, E., Duvenhage, A., Walker, F., Friedlander, I., and Aucamp, V. (1981). Dental caries in South African black and white high school pupils in relation to sugar intake and snack habits. *Commun. Dent. oral Epidemiol.* **9**, 37–43.

Weaver, R. (1935). Diet and the teeth: some criticisms of Mrs Mellanby's work. *Br. dent. J.* **58**, 405–20.

Weaver, R. (1950). Fluorine and war-time diet. *Br. dent. J.* **88**, 231–9.

Wegner, H. (1971). Dental caries in young diabetics. *Caries Res.* **5**, 188–92.

Weiss, R.L. and Trithart, A.H. (1960). Between-meal eating habits and dental caries experience in preschool children. *Am. J. publ. Hlth.* **50**, 1097–104.

Westin, G. and Wold, H. (1943). 1942 års tandmönsting av inkrivningsskyldiga. *Odont. Tids.* **51**, 487–616.

Wilson, C.J. (1979). Ready-to-eat cereals and dental caries in children; a three-year study. *J. dent. Res.* **58**, 1853–8.

Winter, G.B. (1980). Problems involved with the use of comforters. *Int. dent. J.* **30**, 28–38.

Winter, G.B., Hamilton, M.C., and James, P.M.C. (1966). Role of the comforter as an aetiological factor in rampant caries of the deciduous dentition. *Archs. Dis. Childh.* **41**, 207–12.

Winter, G.B., Rule, D.C., Mailer, G.P., James, P.M.C., and Gordon, P.H. (1971). The prevalence of dental caries in pre-school children aged 1–4 years. *Br. dent. J.* **130**, 434–6.

Winter, G.B., Murray, J.J., and Goose, D.H. (1974). Prevalence of dental caries in phenylketonuric children. *Caries Res.* **8**, 256–66.

Winter, P.J. and Ridge, C.M. (1982). A scanning electron microscope study, showing that plaque does not adhere to a glass surface in the mouth. *Caries Res.* **16**, 349–52.

Yankell, S.L., Ram, C., and Lauks, I.R. (1983). *In vitro* testing of a new system for monitoring pH at multiple sites. *Caries Res.* **17**, 439–43.

Young, M. (1937). The role of nutrition as a factor in resistance to dental caries. *Br. dent. J.* **62**, 252–9.

Zita, A.C., McDonald, R.E., and Andrews, A.L. (1959). Dietary habits and the dental caries experience in 200 children. *J. dent. Res.* **38**, 860–5.

Zitzow, R.E. (1979). The relationship of diet and dental caries in the Alaskan eskimo population. *Alaska Med.* **21**, 10–14.

3

Fluorides and dental caries

M. N. Naylor and J. J. Murray

Introduction

The first of a possible connection between the fluoride ion and the prevalence of dental caries occurred towards the end of the nineteenth century when in 1892 Sir James Crichton-Brown addressed the Annual General Meeting of the Eastern Counties Branch of the British Dental Association in Downing College, Cambridge. He suggested that a specific cause of the increase of dental caries was a change in the type of bread eaten.

In as far as our own country, at any rate, is concerned, this is essentially an age of white bread and fine flour, and it is an age therefore in which we are no longer partaking to anything like the same amount that our ancestors did of the bran or husky parts of wheat, and so are deprived to a large degree of a chemical element which they received in abundance namely fluorine ... I think it well worthy of consideration whether the re-introduction into our diet of child-bearing women and of children, of a supply of fluorine in some suitable natural form ... might not do something to fortify the teeth of the next generation.

It is now over 90 years since Crichton-Browne's prophetic remarks were delivered. Today the dental literature groans under the weight of the enormous number of studies concerned with fluorides and caries. They can be divided into two main sections: the effect of fluoride taken systemically by water, or in the form of tablets and drops, or in enriched milk and salt; and the application of fluoride topically in the form of solutions, gels, mouth rinses, and toothpaste in much higher concentrations than found in water supplies. Dividing the literature into two in this way is simplistic in that those methods in the systemic group may also have a topical effect—for example, fluoride taken in the water supplies, in addition to being absorbed and incorporated into developing enamel, may also exert a topical effect both *pre-eruptively* by means of the tissue fluid contacting the maturing surface of the enamel and *post-eruptively* as the water washes over the tooth surface. Similarly with 'topical methods'—for example, fluoride in toothpaste—as well as being brushed onto the surface of the tooth is ingested to a certain degree, particularly in young children, and so fluoride from this source can be incorporated into teeth still developing within the jaws. Bearing in mind this proviso this chapter will attempt to summarize the evidence concerning the cariostatic effect of fluoride in various forms.

Water fluoridation

Historical background

Colorado stain

The man who had the greatest impact on the early history of water fluoridation was Dr Frederick McKay who arrived in Colorado Springs, Colorado in 1901, the year following his graduation from the University of Pennsylvania Dental School. He soon noticed that many of his patients, particularly those who had lived in the area all their lives, had an apparently permanent stain on their teeth which was known to the local inhabitants as 'Colorado stain'. McKay checked the lecture notes he had saved from dental school but found nothing to describe such markings, nor could he find any reference to it in any of the available scientific literature. He called the stain 'mottled enamel' and said that it was characterized by:

> Minute white flecks, or yellow or brown spots or areas, scattered irregularly or streaked over the surface of a tooth, or it may be a condition where the entire tooth surface is of a dead paper-white, like the colour of a china dish (McKay 1916*a*).

McKay decided that, first, he needed help from a recognized dental research worker and, second, he needed to define the exact geographical area of the stain—the endemic area. To attain his first objective he approached one of America's foremost authorities on dental enamel, Dr Greene Vardiman Black, Dean of the Northwestern University Dental School in Chicago. At first Black thought that McKay was mistaking the stain for something else. He could scarcely believe there could be a dental lesion affecting so many people yet which remained unmentioned in the dental literature. Black asked that some of the mottled teeth be sent to him for examination (Black 1916). He agreed to attend the Colorado State Dental Association meeting in July 1909, and promised to spend some weeks in Colorado Springs before the annual meeting.

In preparation for this visit, and as a first step in mapping out the entire endemic area, McKay and a fellow townsman, Dr Isaac Binton, examined the children in the public schools of Colorado Springs. In all they inspected 2945 children and discovered to their complete astonishment that 87.5 per cent of the children native to the area had mottled teeth (McKay 1916*b*). For the first time investigators had statistical data detailing the prevalence of the lesion in the community. This new information was given to Black when he arrived in Denver in June 1909, to tour the Colorado Springs area. Black addressed the State Dental Association meeting; he described his histological examination of the lesion and recounted his personal observations noted during the several weeks he had been touring the Rocky Mountain area. His interest together with his authority and prestige raised the study of the problem from the status of a local curiosity to that of an investigation meriting the earnest concern of all dental research workers. Black's histological findings were published in a paper: 'An endemic imperfection of the enamel of the teeth heretofore unknown in the literature of dentistry' (Black 1916).

Endemic areas of mottled teeth

Despite Black's involvement other dentists were unimpressed and showed little enthusiasm for carrying on the investigation. It was left to McKay to sustain the study by his persistent interest. His Colorado Springs survey had shown that almost nine out of ten of the native children had mottled teeth: he began searching for other endemic areas. His travels took him up and down the creek valleys of the mountainous region and out onto the nearby plains. He examined children living in Pueblo, Maniton, La Junta, Cripple Creek, Woodland Park, and Green Mountain Falls. A few trips convinced McKay that the phenomenon called 'mottling' was much more widespread than he had thought. Slowly too, McKay began to get help from dentists in other parts of the country.

The horizons were broadened still further when, in 1912 McKay discovered that people from parts of Naples in Italy also had stained teeth. He came across an article written in 1902 by Dr J. M. Eager, a United States Marine Hospital Service surgeon stationed in Italy, who reported that a high proportion of certain Italian emigrants embarking at Naples had a dental peculiarity known locally as denti di Chiaie (Eager 1902). Some of these Italians had ugly brown stains on their teeth; others had a fine horizontal black line crossing the incisor teeth. McKay heard that a young doctor, Dr J. F. McConnell from Colorado Springs, was planning a holiday in Italy, and asked him to examine some Naples children and report back. The doctor was familiar with the stain in Colorado Springs and wrote back from Naples that there was no doubt that the mottled teeth in Naples were the same as those being investigated by McKay (1916*c*).

Throughout this period the energy and enthusiasm which kept McKay going was generated by a desire to find out the cause of mottling so that some means might be found of preventing the unsightly stains on people's teeth. However, throughout his investigations, McKay was struck by the fact that caries experience was no higher in mottled teeth. This contradiction must have been in the back of McKay's mind throughout the whole period of his research. He expressed it forcibly in a paper to the Chicago Society on 17 April 1928:

> Mottled enamel is a condition in which the enamel is most obviously and unmistakably defective. In fact it is the most poorly calcified enamel of which there is any record in dental literature. If the chief determining factor governing the susceptibility to decay is the integrity or perfection of the calcification of enamel, then by all the laws of logic this enamel is deprived of the one essential element for its protection. . . . In spite of this the outstanding fact is that mottled enamel shows no greater susceptibility to the onset of caries than does enamel that may be considered to have been normally or perfectly calcified. This statement is made as a result of extensive observations and examination of several thousand cases during the past years. . . . My testimony has been supplemented by that of

others, who report that these mottled enamel cases, in the various districts are singularly free from caries. One of the first things noted by Dr Black during his first contact with an endemic locality was the singular absence of decay, and it can hardly be said that this faculty for observations was superficial (McKay 1928).

Mottled enamel—aetiological factors

In the forefront of McKay's mind all the time was the desire to determine the cause of mottled enamel. He established that the occurrence of mottled enamel was localized in definite geographical areas. Within these endemic areas a very high proportion of children were affected: only those who had been born and lived all their lives in an endemic area had mottled enamel; those born elsewhere and brought to the district when two to three years of age were not affected. The condition was not influenced by home or environment factors; families whether rich or poor were affected. This factor tended to eliminate diet as an aetiological factor. McKay observed that three cities in Arkansas where mottling occurred, although separated from each other by some miles, all received their water supply from one source, Fountain Creek. This, together with many other reports, led him to believe that something in the water supply was responsible for mottled enamel.

Further evidence supporting the water supply hypothesis came from a dentist, Dr O. E. Martin, practising in Britton, South Dakota. On reading McKay's 1916 article in Dental Cosmos, he felt that McKay's description of mottling sounded suspiciously like the blemishes he had seen in certain local children and asked for McKay's advice. McKay visited Britton in October 1916. He discovered that in 1898 Britton had changed its water supply from individual shallow wells to a deep-drilled artesian well. Without exception, McKay found that all those who had passed through childhood prior to the changing of the water supply had normal teeth, while natives who had grown up in Britton since 1898 had mottling. He concluded that some mysterious element in the water supply was responsible (McKay 1918).

A similar occurrence was reported in the town of Bauxite, a community formed in 1901 to provide homes for employees of the Republic Mining and Manufacturing Company, a subsidiary of the Aluminium Company of America (ALCOA). The first domestic water supply to Bauxite came from shallow wells and springs, but in 1909 a new source of water was obtained from a 297-foot well. A practising dentist, Dr F. L. Robertson, of nearby Benton, reported to the State Board of Health that the younger citizens of Bauxite seemed to have badly stained teeth, whereas the children living in Benton had normal teeth. The State Health Officer made a formal request to the US Public Health Service in Washington to examine the children living in Bauxite and Benton. In 1928 the US Public Health Service asked Dr McKay to accompany Dr Gromer Kempf, one of their medical officers, to carry out the examinations. They found that no mottling occurred in people who grew up on Bauxite water prior to 1909, but all native Bauxite children who used the deep well water after that date had mottled

Table 3.1. Fluoride analyses from Churchill (1931*a*)

Location of sample	Fluorine as fluoride (p.p.m.)
Deep Well, Bauxite, Ark.	13.7
Colorado Springs, Colo.	2.0
Well near Kidder, S. Dak.	12.0
Well near Lidgerwood, N. Dak.	11.0
Oakley, Idaho	6.0

teeth. No individual whose enamel developed during residence in Benton had mottled teeth. They reported that the standard water analysis of Bauxite water 'throws little light whatever on the probably causal agent' (Kempf and McKay 1930). Another piece of evidence had been gathered, but McKay seemed no closer to the solution.

Mottled enamel and fluoride concentration in the drinking water

The answer was now close at hand. In New Kensington, Pennsylvania, the chief chemist of ALCOA, Mr H. V. Churchill, read Kempf and McKay's paper and was greatly disturbed. Certain people in the United States were condemning the use of aluminium-ware for cooking. ALCOA mined most of its aluminium supply from Bauxite: if the story of the stain in Bauxite got into the hands of those who claimed that aluminium cooking utensils caused poisoning, ALCOA would have to reply to the charge. When Churchill received a sample of Bauxite water he instructed Mr A. W. Petrey, head of the testing division of the ALCOA laboratory, to look for traces of rare elements—those not usually tested for. Petrey ran a spectographic analysis and noted that fluoride was present in Bauxite water at a level of 13.7 parts per million. Churchill wrote to McKay on 20 January 1931:

> We have discovered the presence of hitherto unsuspected constituents in this water. The high fluorine content was so unexpected that a new sample was taken with extreme precautions and again the test showed fluorine in the water (Churchill 1931*a*).

He also asked McKay to send samples of water from other endemic areas with a 'minimum of publicity'. McKay quickly arranged for dentists in Britton, South Dakota, Oakley, Idaho, and Colorado Springs to send samples of the water in their areas. The results of these analyses were published in 1931 (Table 3.1). Churchill emphasized the fact that no precise correlation between the fluoride content of these waters and the mottled enamel had been established. All that was shown was the presence of a hitherto unsuspected common constituent of the waters from the endemic areas (Churchill 1931*b*).

The work of H. Trendley Dean

The study of the relationship between fluoride concentration in drinking water, mottled enamel, and dental caries was given an impetus by the decision of Dr Clinton T. Messner, Head of the US Public Health Service, in 1931, to assign a young dental officer, Dr H. Trendley Dean, to pursue full-time research on

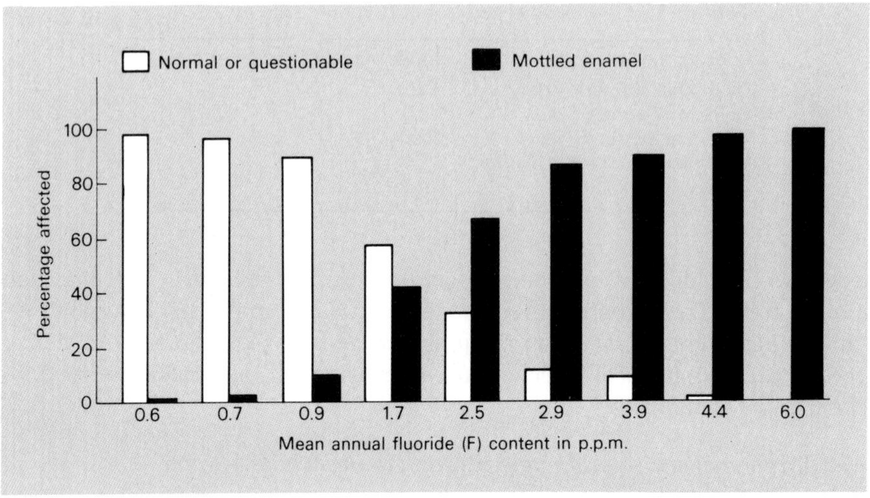

Fig. 3.1. The prevalence of mottled enamel in areas with differing concentrations of fluoride in the water supply. (From Dean (1936).) (Reproduced from *Fluride drinking waters*, edited by F. J. McClure, by kind permission of the US Department of Heatlh, Education and Welfare 1962.)

mottled enamel. Dean was responsible for the research unit within the US Public Health Service and was the first dental officer of the service to be given a non-clinical assignment. His first task was to continue McKay's work and to find the extent and geographical distribution of mottled enamel in the United States. He reported that there were 97 localities in the country where mottled enamel was said to occur and this claim had been confirmed by a dental survey. There were a further 28 areas referred to in the literature where mottled enamel was said to be endemic but no confirmatory dental surveys had yet been carried out, and there were 70 areas which had been reported by questionnaires but which had not yet been confirmed by extensive surveys (Dean 1933).

Many of these confirmatory surveys were carried out by Dean himself. He developed a standard of classification of mottling in order to record quantitatively the severity of mottling within a community (Dean 1934) so that he could relate the fluoride concentration in the drinking water to the severity of mottling in a given area. His aim was to find out the 'minimal threshold' of fluorine—the level at which fluorine began to blemish the teeth. He showed conclusively that the severity of mottling increased with increasing fluoride concentration in the drinking water (Dean and Elvove 1936; Dean 1936). His results are expressed diagrammatically in Fig. 3.1.

Dean continued his studies into the relationship between the severity of mottled enamel and the fluoride concentration in water supply. He presented additional evidence to show that amounts of fluoride not exceeding 1 p.p.m. were of no public health significance (Dean and Elvove 1936). On 25 October

1938, in conjunction with Frederick McKay, he summarized the knowledge of mottled enamel in a paper to the Epidemiology Section of the American Public Health Association. He reported that in the United States there were now 375 known areas, in 26 states, where mottled enamel of varying degrees of severity were found. He also stated that the production of mottled enamel had been halted at Oakley, Idaho, Bauxite, Arkansas, and Andover, South Dakota, simply by changing the water supply, which contained high concentrations of fluoride, to one whose fluoride concentration did not exceed 1 p.p.m. This information was 'the most conclusive and direct proof that fluoride in the domestic water is the primary cause of human mottled enamel' (Dean and McKay 1939). The publication of this information brought to a successful conclusion McKay's search for the cause of mottled enamel which began in Colorado Springs in 1902 and lasted for almost 40 years.

Dental caries prevalence in natural fluoride areas

The story of fluoridation now entered a new and, from a public health point of view, a most important phase. Dean was aware of the reports from the literature that there may be an inverse relationship between the level of mottling and the prevalence of caries in a community. He knew of McKay's observations, first made in 1916, that mottled enamel was no more susceptible to decay than normal enamel. He had read Ainswoth's report in 1933 that caries experience in the high fluoride area was markedly lower than caries experience in all other districts examined. During his study to determine the minimum threshold of mottling, Dean had, in some cities, also examined the children for dental caries. Taking a selected sample of 9-year-old children, he found that of 114 children who had continuously used a domestic water supply comparatively low in fluoride (0.6–1.5 p.p.m.) only five, or 4 per cent, were caries-free. On the other hand, of the 122 children who had continuously used domestic water containing 1.7–2.5 p.p.m. fluoride, 27 (22 per cent) were caries-free. He concluded: 'Inasmuch as it appears that the mineral composition of the drinking water may have an important bearing on the incidence of dental caries in a community, the possibility of partially controlling dental caries through the domestic water supply warrants thorough epidemiological-chemical study' (Dean 1938).

To test further the hypothesis that an inverse relationship existed between endemic dental fluorosis and dental caries, a survey of four Illinois cities was planned. The cities were Galesburg and Monmouth (water supply contained 1.8 and 1.7 p.p.m. fluoride respectively), and the nearby cities of Macomb and Quincy (water supply contained 0.2 p.p.m. F). Altogether 885 children, aged 12–14 years, were examined. The results were clear; caries experience in Macomb and Quincy was more than twice as high as that in Galesburg and Monmouth (Dean *et al.* 1939).

This study paved the way for a much larger investigation of caries experience of 7257 12–14-year-old children from 21 cities in four states. The results, (Fig.

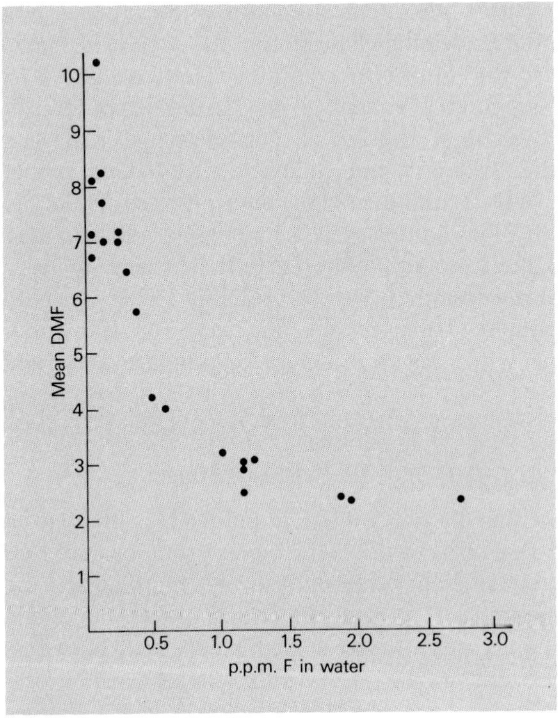

Fig. 3.2. The relation between caries experience of 7257 12–14-year-old white schoolchildren of 21 cities in the USA and the fluoride content of the water supply. (From Dean *et al.* (1942).) (Reproduced from *Fluoride drinking waters*, edited by F. J. McClure, by kind permission of the US Department of Health, Education and Welfare 1962.)

3.2) show clearly the association between increasing fluoride concentration in the drinking water and decreasing caries experience in the population. Furthermore this study showed that near maximal reduction in caries experience occurred with a concentration of 1 p.p.m F in the drinking water. At this concentration fluoride caused only 'sporadic instances of the mildest forms of dental fluorosis of no practical aesthetic significance' (Dean *et al.* 1942).

Artificial fluoridation studies in America and Canada

Grand Rapids–Muskegon study

The next crucial step was to see if dental caries could be reduced in a community by adding fluoride at 1 p.p.m. to a fluoride-deficient water supply. The US Public Health Service was ready to embark on such an experiment. In December 1942 the Service began talks with city officials of two cities in the Lake Michigan area, Grand Rapids and Muskegon. Extensive field and laboratory studies were carried out on the physiological effects of fluoride ingestion and it was concluded that not only was a fluoride concentration of 1 p.p.m. the best for caries control, but also it was well within the limits of safety (Moulton 1942).

In view of this information both city councils agreed in August 1944 to conduct the experiment, which would be carried out by Dr Dean, in conjunction

Table 3.2. Mean def in Grand rapids and Muskegon, 1953. (From Arnold *et al.* (1953))

Age	Grand Rapids		Muskegon	
	No. of children	Mean def	No. of children	Mean def
4	168	2.13	63	4.46
5	853	2.27	351	5.25
6	750	2.98	294	5.56

with the Michigan State Health Department and the University of Michigan Dental School. It was decided that Grand Rapids would be the experimental town and that Muskegon would be the control town. In September 1944 Dean and his co-workers, Francis Arnold, Philip Jay, and John Knutson, began the dental examinations of 19 680 Grand Rapids children and 4291 Muskegon children aged 4–16 years. All were continuous residents of the two cities. These baseline studies showed that caries experience in the deciduous and permanent dentitions in the Grand Rapids was similar to that of Muskegon (Dean *et al* 1950). The method used to measure caries experience was to count the number of decayed, missing and filled teeth for each child—the DMF index (Klein *et al* 1938). In addition, 5116 children continuously resident in the natural fluoride area of Aurora, Illinois (F = 1.4 p.p.m.), were examined to provide further base-line information. On 25 January 1945 sodium fluoride was added to the Grand Rapids water supply. This was an historic occasion, because for the first time a permissible quantity of a beneficial dietary nutrient was added to communal drinking water.

The effects of $6\frac{1}{2}$ years of fluoridation in Grand Rapids were reported by Arnold *et al* in 1953. The results were clear; caries experience of 6-year-old Grand Rapids children was almost half that of 6-year-old Muskegon children (Table 3.2). The city officials of Muskegon, convinced of the efficacy of fluoridation, decided to fluoridate their own water supply in July 1951, so from this date Muskegon could no longer be used as a control town. The only control left for Grand Rapids was a retrospective comparison with base-line data. Results after 10 years of fluoridation (Arnold *et al.* 1956) and 15 years of fluoridation (Arnold *et al.* 1962) are recorded in Fig. 3.3. They indicate that caries experience in 15-year-old Grand Rapids children had fallen from 12.48 DMF teeth per mouth in 1944 to 6.22 DMF teeth per mouth in 1959, a reduction of approximately 50 per cent. Furthermore, caries experience in the fluoridation community of Grand Rapids was very similar to that occurring in the natural fluoride area of Aurora. This was the experimental proof that the previously observed inverse relationship between fluoride in drinking water and dental caries experience was a cause-and-effect relationship.

The feelings that Trendley Dean and his co-workers had when they started the Grand Rapids experiment were recalled in an article by John Knutson (1970):

It is now 25 years ago that the late Trendley Dean and I journeyed by train from Wash-

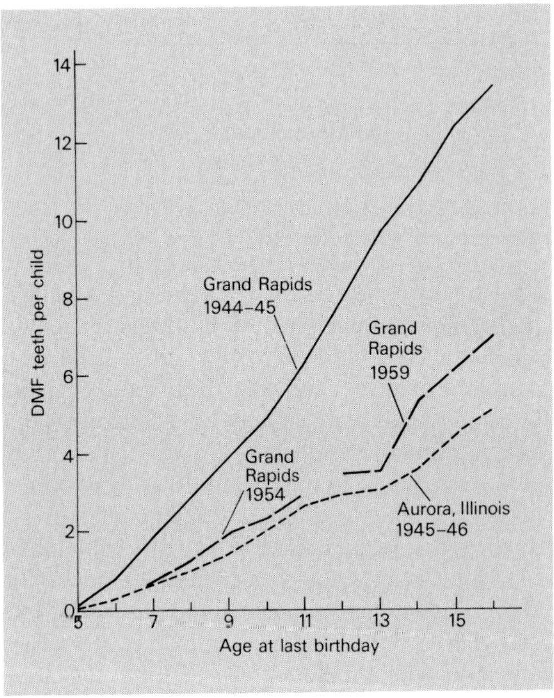

Fig. 3.3. Dental caries in Grand Rapids children after 10 and after 15 years of fluoridation. (From Arnold *et al.* (1962).) (Copyright by the American Dental Association. Reprinted by permission.)

ington D.C. to Grand Rapids, Michigan, to be joined by Philip Jay for a meeting with the mayor to gain his approval for a water fluoridation experiment. . . . There were no signs of apprehension or daring or of pioneering. There were no implications or inferences that we were being foolhardy in subjecting a population of 160,000 people to a procedure which might have either short or long-range hazards. We were merely replicating nature's best, based on an extensive background of study data in nature's laboratory, a laboratory which was extremely large. In the United States alone, some seven million people in 1,900 communities had throughout life used drinking water which was naturally fluoridated with a fluoride concentration of 0.7 ppm or greater. We knew what too much did, we knew what too little did, we knew what the optimum amount was and we had assurance that one part per million fluoride in the drinking water had the same biological effect whether it got there from flowing over rocks or from a feeding machine.

Newburgh–Kingston study

In addition to the Grand Rapids–Muskegon study two other fluoridation studies were carried out in the United States. On 2 May 1945 sodium fluoride was added to the drinking water of Newburgh, on the Hudson River. The town of Kingston, situated 35 miles away from Newburgh, was chosen as a control town. This study was directed by David B. Ast, Chief of the Dental Bureau, State of new York, Department of Health. Baseline studies were carried out in the two communities in 1944–46 (Ast *et al.* 1956). They reported that whilst caries experience in 10–12-year-old Kingston children had changed little from 1945 (23.1

per cent of teeth were carious) to 1955 (26.3 per cent), in contrast in similarly aged Newburgh children over the 10-year period the DMF rate had fallen from 23.5 per cent to 13.8 per cent, thus confirming the caries inhibitory property of fluoride drinking water.

Evanston–Oak Park study

A third American fluoridation experiment began in January 1946 in Evanston, Illinois; the nearby community of Oak Park acted as the control town. Drs J. R. Blayney, I. N. Hill, and S. O. Zimmerman of the University of Chicago Memorial Dental Clinic conducted the study and their findings after 14 years of fluoridation in Evanston were published in 1967 (Blayney and Hill 1967). Whereas the DMF values of 14-year-old Evanston children fell from 11.66 to 5.95 between 1946 and 1960 (a reduction of 49 per cent), no change was observed in the DMF values of 14-year-old Oak Park children over the intervening years. Here again was experimental proof of the caries inhibitory property of fluoride in drinking water at a concentration of 1 p.p.m. The Evanston–Oak Park study presented the most detailed data of all the fluoridation studies. In an introduction to the report Dr F. A. Arnold Jr, Chief Dental Officer, United States Public Health Service, wrote:

> Here in a single report are data on the effect of water fluoridation on dental caries so completely documented that the article is virtually a text-book for use in further research. It is an important scientific contribution towards betterment of the dental health of our nation. It is a classic in this field (Arnold 1967).

Yet the strength of the experimental proof of the caries inhibitory property of fluoride drinking water lies not only in the conclusion of one study but also in the fact that the three American studies, carried out by different investigators in different parts of the country, reached similar conclusions: addition of 1 p.p.m. fluoride in the drinking water reduced caries experience by approximately 50 per cent.

Canadian study (Brantford, Sarnia, and Stratford)

In Canada a project was undertaken in Brantford, Ontario, where fluoride was added to the water supply in June 1945. The community of Sarnia was established as the control town; in addition the community of Stratford, where fluoride was naturally present in the drinking water at a level of 1.3 p.p.m. was used as an auxiliary control. After 17 years of fluoridation in Brantford, caries experience was similar to that occurring in the natural fluoride area of Stratford and was 55 per cent lower than in the control town of Sarnia (Hutton *et al.* 1951; Brown and Poplove 1965) (Fig. 3.4).

Natural fluoride areas in the United Kingdom

McKay's work on mottled enamel had not gone unnoticed in the United King-

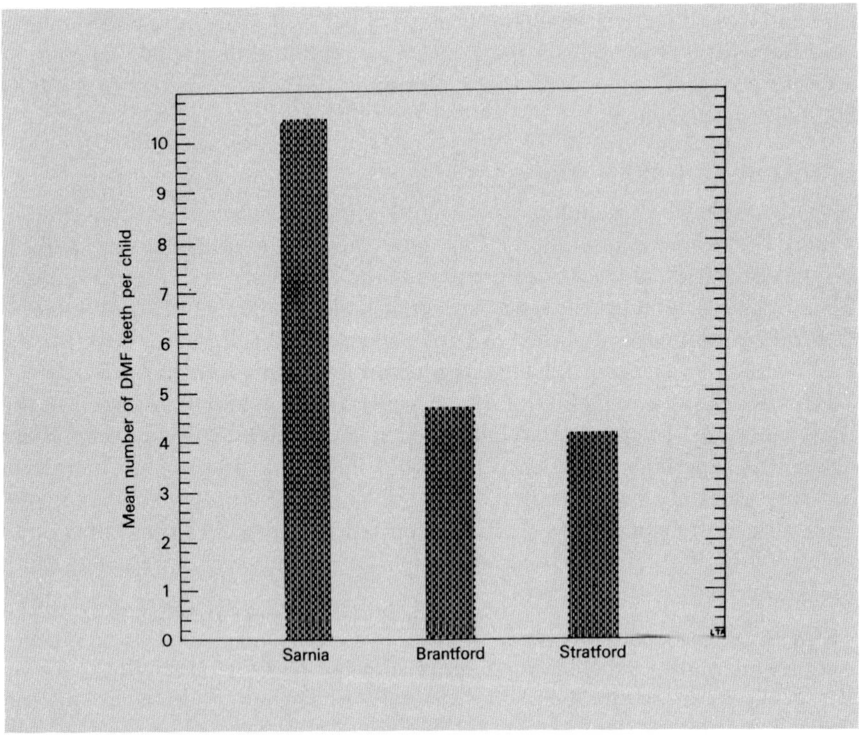

Fig. 3.4. Canadian fluoridation study. Mean DMF of 17-year-old children continuously resident in Sarnia (low fluoride area), Brantford (water fluoridated at 1 p.p.m.). (With permission of the Editor, *Journal of Canadian Dental Association.*)

dom. Reference to McKay's articles in *Dental Cosmos* of 1916 had been made in the fifth edition of Colyer's *Dental surgery and pathology* (Longmans, London) which was required reading for all dental students of that time. One such dental student was Norman Ainsworth.

Having read this [account of mottled teeth] as a dental student I regret to say that I forgot it, together with a great many other paragraphs in that volume, immediately after qualifying. When I was a student in Middlesex Hospital in 1921, I chanced to be given charge of a girl patient, aged 15, in one of the surgical wards and noticed that her teeth showed a very unusual appearance. They were curiously opaque and flecked with brownish black spots. It appeared that many other people in her home town, Maldon, Essex, were affected in the same way, and it was generally supposed that the drinking water was responsible. I fear that I had already forgotten Rocky Mountain mottled teeth, but the condition was so unusual that I made a mental note that I would look for a chance to verify the girl's statements. A year later I undertook a tour of council schools in various parts of England and Wales for the Dental Diseases Committee of the Medical Research Council, and remembering the incident I arranged that Maldon should be included (Ainsworth 1933).

The MRC report was published in 1925 (Special Report Series No. 97). Ainsworth examined 4258 children aged 2–15 years attending 36 schools in England and Wales. He visited two schools in Maldon, examining 202 children aged 5–15 years. His results showed that, taking all children, the proportion of permanent teeth with dental caries was 13.1 per cent. Ainsworth was particularly interested in the prevalence of mottling in Maldon children. He recorded that of 134 children who were lifelong residents of Maldon, 125 showed mottling. He concluded:

> The distribution of the stain ... points to an outside origin for the stain, either atmospheric or in the water, since these are precisely the surfaces most exposed to air and fluid in the acts of speaking and drinking respectively. My own view, and it is little more than a guess, is that the cause of both mottling and stain will be found in some quality or impurity of the drinking water not ascertainable by ordinary analytical methods (Ainsworth 1928).

At this time Ainsworth had not read the accounts of Black (1916) and McKay (1916*a*, *b*) concerning mottled teeth in America. When he did so he knew that the 'similarity between my own description and theirs is so striking in every detail as to leave no reasonable doubt that the conditions are identical' (Ainsworth 1933). Ainsworth read the reports by Churchill showing that water from endemic areas contains fluorides in quantities varying from 2 to 13 p.p.m. and made arrangements for the National Physical Laboratory to measure the fluoride concentration in Maldon water and also in Witham, a few miles from Maldon. They tested five samples and reported that, whereas Witham water contained 0.5 p.p.m. F, the water from the four endemic areas contained 4.5–5.5 p.p.m. (Ainsworth 1933).

The significance of Ainsworth's contribution was that he gave statistical data showing that caries experience in a fluoride area was lower than average. McKay had stressed that mottled teeth had a caries rate no higher than normal teeth.

A natural fluoride area in the North of England was discovered as a result of children being evacuated from an industrial area because of the Second World War. In 1941 Robert Weaver was told by Mr Irvine, Senior School Dentist for Westmorland, that children evacuated to the Lake District from South Shields, on the mouth of the River Tyne, 'had remarkably good teeth—much better than those of the local children'. Weaver, who was a dentist in the Ministry of Education, visited Westmorland examined 117 evacuees (average age 11 years) and found the mean DMF was 1.4 teeth. Weaver (1944) reported:

> Bearing in mind the work which had been done in America, I got in touch with Dr. Campbell Lyons, Medical Officer of Health for South Shields, and asked him if he would have the town's water analysed for fluorine. He did so, and a preliminary analysis suggested that the fluorine content might be as much as two parts per million. It was obvious that the conditions were such as to make possible a perfectly controlled investigation since North Shields, on the opposite bank of the River Tyne has an entirely different water supply.

Table 3.3. Dental caries and fluoride levels in Lincolnshire. (From Chalmers Clarke (1954))

	F in water (p.p.m.)	No. of children examined	Mean DMF
Deeping St. James	2.5	191	3.15
Heckington	0.7	188	6.18
Dorrington	0.2	39	8.0
Helpringham	0	67	8.14

(The River Tyne at this part varies in width from 350 to 500 yards and the two communities are linked by a ferry.)

At Weaver's request Dr Dawson, the Medical Officer of Health for the North Shields area, arranged for the water to be analysed and this showed a fluoride content of less than 0.25 p.p.m. Subsequently Weaver (1944) examined 1000 children on each side of the River Tyne. He reported that the mean dmf in 5-year-old children was 6.6 in North Shields and 3.9 in South Shields; the comparable figures for 12-year-old children were 4.3 and 2.4 DMF teeth. Weaver's observations were extremely important because he focused attention on the deciduous dentition as well as the permanent dentition.

Weaver (1950) repeated his studies in North and South Shields after the Second World War and also gave results for another natural fluoride area in the North East of England—West Hartlepool, which had a fluoride concentration of 3 p.p.m. He examined 500 5-year-old children and reported that the mean dmf was 1.76 and 53.6 per cent of 5-year-old children were caries free. He also examined 500 12-year-old children and reported a mean DMF of 0.96 with 60 per cent of children having no carious permanent teeth.

Another natural fluoride area Kesteven, in Lincolnshire, was reported by Chalmers Clarke in 1954. Various samples of water taken in different parts of Kesteven have shown fluoride present in amounts varying from 0 to 4 p.p.m. Dental inspections were carried out in Helpringham (0 p.p.m. F), Dorrington (0.2 p.p.m. F), Heckington (0.7 p.p.m. F) and Deeping St. James (2.5 p.p.m. F) All supplies are derived from bores which tap the Lincolnshire Limestone and are under varying degrees of artesian pressure. Children resident in Deeping St. James receive the village public water supply containing 2.5 p.p.m. F, but some children in the Deeping area consume water from private bores containing up to 4 p.p.m. F. The mean caries experience for children, aged 5–13 years, deciduous and permanent dentition combined, is recorded in Table 3.3.

Forrest (1956) expanded the knowledge of natural fluoride areas in Essex and Buckinghamshire in the South East of England by examining children in four areas, West Mersea (5.8 p.p.m. F), Burnham-on-Crouch (3.5 p.p.m. F), Harwich (1.6–2.0 p.p.m. F), and Slough (0.9 p.p.m. F). She reported that West Mersea has the highest known natural fluoride content in England and that, although Maldon had always been regarded as the classical high fluoride area in the

Table 3.4. The relation between the fluoride content of water and caries experience among children aged 12–14 years. (From Forrest (1956))

Area	Fluoride content of water (p.p.m.)	No. of children examined	Average No. of DMF teeth per child	Children caries-free (%)
West Mersea	5.8	51	2.8	24
Burnham-on-Crouch	3.5	62	1.4	50
Harwich	2.0	92	1.5	35
Slough	0.9	119	1.5	35
Saffron Walden and District, Essex	0.1	145	6.6	4
Stoneleigh and Malden West, Surrey	0.1–0.2	114	6.1	8

country, due to the work of Ainsworth, it could now not be included because the fluoride contents of its water had been reduced to under 1 p.p.m. F. Her results, summarized in Table 3.4 and Fig. 3.5, showed a markedly lower caries experience in the fluoride areas compared with two control areas, Saffron Walden in Essex, and Stonleigh and Malden West in Surrey.

Dental caries prevalence in high and low fluoride areas of East Anglia was reported by James (1961). He examined 11–13-year-old children in Norwich and Yarmouth (0.17–0.2 p.p.m. F), Chelmsford (intermittent fluoride concentration), and Colchester (1.2–2.0 p.p.m. F). Some of the children examined in Colchester resided in outlying districts and received lower levels of fluoride and therefore the Colchester children were divided into 'continuous' and 'non-continuous' residents. The results of his investigation summarized in Fig. 3.6 supported the observation that caries prevalence is lower in areas where fluoride occurs in drinking water above levels of 1 p.p.m., especially among life-long residents of the area.

The effect of life-long residence in Hartlepool was reported by Murray (1969*a*, *b*), who carried out a 'cradle to the grave study' of the effect of continuous residence in Hartlepool and the dental condition in children and adults. A total of 3765 children, aged 2–18 years were examined. The mean caries experience in the deciduous and permanent dentition in these children is recorded in Fig. 3.7. A similar number of children aged 5 and 15 years were examined in York, a low fluoride area, in order to compare caries experience at the beginning and end of school life between a natural fluoride area and a low fluoride area. The results of the 5-year-olds showed that the mean dmf was 4.1 in York compared with 1.5 in Hartlepool, a difference of 64 per cent. Half the children in Hartlepool had no decay at all (51.2 per cent) whereas less than a quarter of York children were caries free (22.4 per cent). Turning to the permanent dentition the mean DMF in York was 9.0 teeth and in Hartlepool it was 5.0 teeth, a difference of 44 per cent. Half the Hartlepool children had between 0 and 4 DMF teeth; half the York children had between nine and 22 DMF teeth. Twice as many first permanent molars had been extracted by the age of 15 years in York

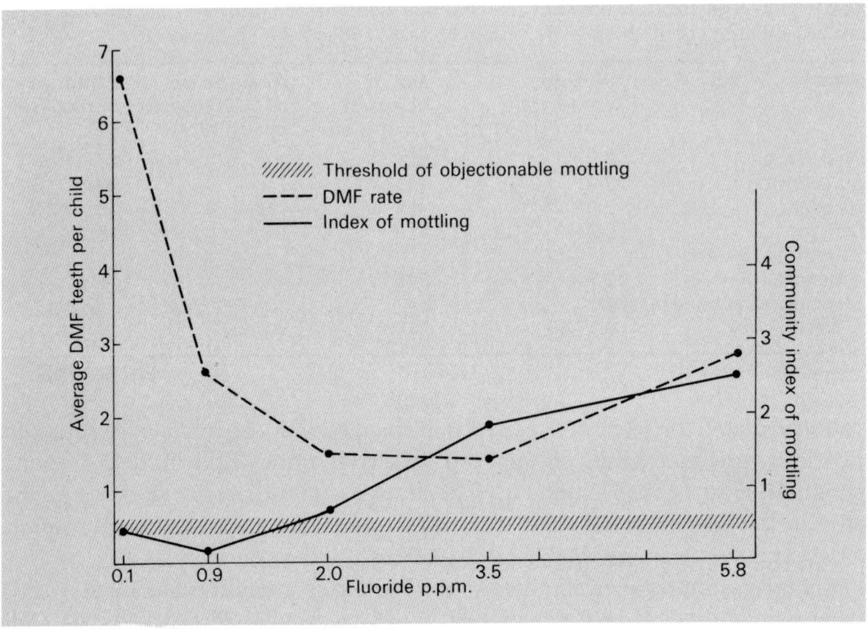

Fig. 3.5. Fluoride content of water, caries experience and enamel mottling in children aged 12–14 years. (From Forrest (1956).) (Reproduced by courtesy of the Editor, *British Dental Journal*.)

children compared with Hartlepool children (17.9 per cent as against 8.7 per cent).

Timmis (1971) reported on the caries experience of 5-year-old children living in non-fluoride and fluoride areas of Essex. The six areas with naturally fluoridated water which are in the survey were (i) Clacton, 1 p.p.m. F, (ii) Dovercourt and Harwich, 1 p.p.m. F; (iii) Colchester town, 0.7–1.0 p.p.m. F; (iv) Maldon town, 0.25–5.0 p.p.m. F; (v) Burnham-on-Crouch, 2.5–3.5 p.p.m. F; (vi) Braintree and Bocking (parts), 1.0–1.6 p.p.m. F. These included many of the towns previously surveyed by Ainsworth, Forrest, and James. Timmis used seven areas as a control, namely Harlow, Thurrock, Chigwell, Witham, Saffron Walden, Epping, and Great Baddow: 959 children were inspected in the low fluoride area and had a mean dmf of 4.9; 969 5-year-olds were examined in the high fluoride area with a mean dmf of 2.27 (Table 3.5).

An attempt was made to correlate the concentration of fluoride with the degree of caries experience. However, the small numbers of children examined in the two highest fluoride areas, Maldon and Burnham-on-Crouch, preclude the drawing of conclusions, although perhaps it is worth noting that the lowest mean dmf per child, 1.59, occurred in Burnham, which has the highest average fluoride concentration of from 2.5–3.5 p.p.m.

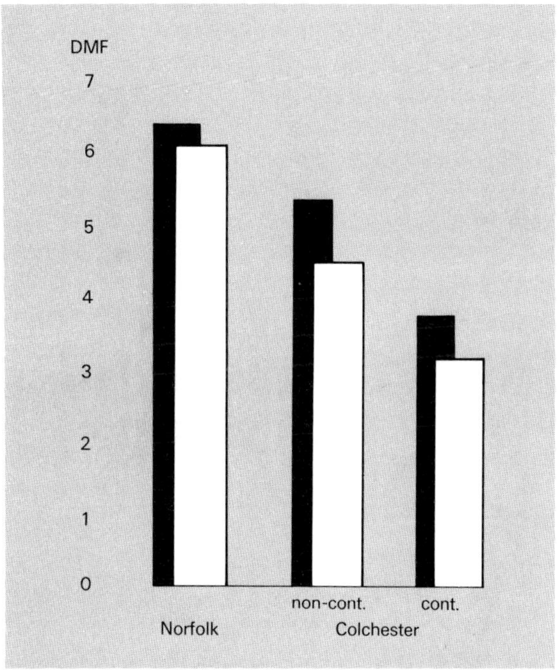

Fig. 3.6. Comparison of mean DMF of 11–13-year-old children living in Norfolk (F = 0.17–0.2 p.p.m.) and Colchester (F = 1.2–2.0 p.p.m.). Children from Colchester were divided into continuous and non-continuous residents. This shows that caries experience in children continuously resident in the natural fluoride area of Colchester was less than half that recorded in Norfolk. (With permission of the Editor, *British Dental Journal*.)

Fluoridation studies in the United Kingdom

In 1952 the British Government sent a mission to the United States of America and Canada to study fluoridation in operation. The mission concluded that fluoridation of water supplies was a valuable health measure but recommended that in this country fluoride should be added to the water supplies of some selected communities before its general adoption was considered (Report of the United Kingdom Mission 1953). Originally four areas agreed to add fluoride to their water supplies in 1955–56, namely, Andover, Watford, Kilmarnock, and part of Anglesey. However, because of opposition, the scheme in Andover was abandoned after 2 years. The control towns were Sutton, Ayr, and the remaining part of Anglesey. The results after 5 years of fluoridation (Report on Public Health and Medical Subjects No. 105, 1962) showed that caries experience in five-year-old children was 50 per cent lower in the fluoride areas than the non-fluoride areas (Table 3.6). In spite of this, fluoridation was discontinued in Kilmarnock in 1962, on instructions of the local council. However, dental examinations continued to be carried out in all areas and the findings after 11 years' fluoridation were reported in 1969 (Table 3.7). The report confirmed the main findings of 1962, that fluoridation of water supplies is a highly effective method of reducing dental decay.

In addition to demonstrating the beneficial effects of fluoridation the Report also confirmed its complete safety. 'During the eleven years under review, med-

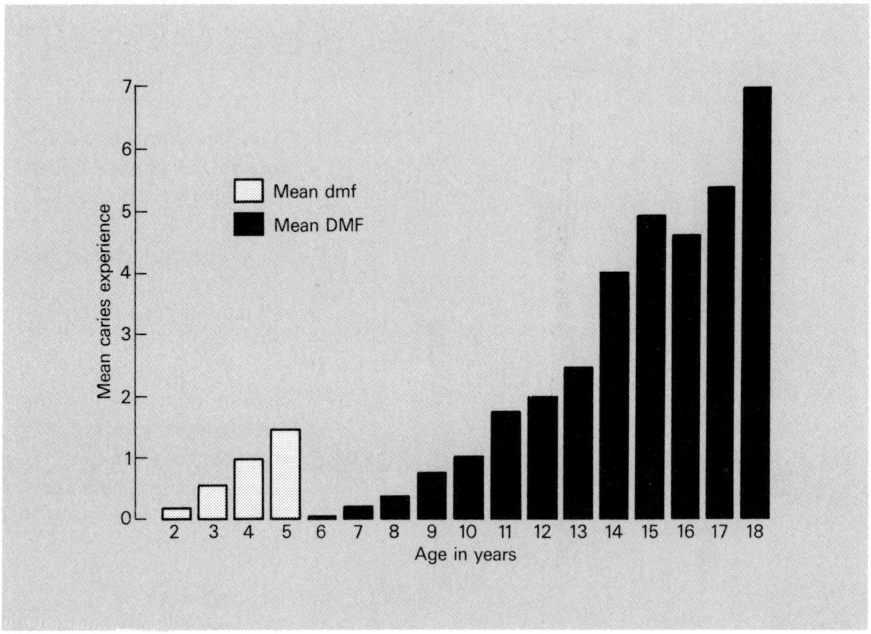

Fig. 3.7. Mean DMF of children aged 2–18 years continuously resident in the natural fluoride area of West Hartlepool (F = 1.25–2.0 p.p.m.).

Table 3.5. Summary of 5-year-old children in high and low fluoride areas in Essex. (From Timmis (1971))

	No. of children inspected	Mean dmf
Low fluoride areas		
Harlow	200	5.09
Thurrock	212	4.78
Chigwell	226	4.33
Witham	70	3.70
Saffron Walden	60	3.57
Epping	91	2.84
Great Baddow	100	2.79
Total	959	4.19
High fluoride areas		
Colchester	426	2.61
Maldon	50	2.46
Braintree	192	2.16
Dovercourt	100	2.01
Clacton	160	1.77
Burnham	41	1.59
Total	969	2.27

Table 3.6. Number of children examined and mean dmf in 1956 and 1961 for each year age group in study areas and control areas. (Department of Public Health and Social Security 1962)

Age	Study areas				Control areas			
	1956 No. of children	Mean dmf	1961 No. of children	Mean dmf	1956 No. of children	Mean dmf	1961 No. of children	Mean dmf
3*	450	3.80	388	1.29	297	3.53	329	2.32
4*	591	5.39	468	2.31	334	5.18	295	4.83
5†	785	5.81	531	2.91	461	5.66	374	5.39
6†	883	6.49	615	4.81	566	6.32	432	6.22
7†	952	7.06	593	6.05	577	7.08	446	6.89

* Full dentition.
† Canines and molars only.

ical practitioners reported only two patients with symptoms which they felt might have been associated with fluoridation. Careful investigation in both instances failed to attribute the symptoms to the drinking of fluoridated water'(Report of the Committee on Research into Fluoridation 1969). The Government is so confident of the safety of water fluoridation that it is prepared to give unlimited indemnity to any local authority in respect of actions for damages based on alleged harm to health resulting from fluoridation.

The whole of Anglesey was fluoridated in 1964 and so after this date there was no strict control for the original fluoridated part of Anglesey. Thus the British Fluoridation Studies were complicated by the fact that one of the communities stopped fluoridation after 2 years, another after 7 years, and one control area fluoridated after 9 years. Jackson *et al.* (1975*b*) examined 15-year-old children from the island of Anglesey who had received fluoridated water all their lives and compared them with children of similar age from the Bangor/ Caernarvon area, on the Welsh mainland, separated from Anglesey by the Menai Straits. Their results showed (Table 3.8) that the amount of decay was 44 per cent lower in Anglesey, the fluoridated area.

The first large community fluoridation scheme in Britain began in Birmingham in 1964. The next largest scheme started in Newcastle upon Tyne in 1968 and a number of other communities, particularly in the West Midlands, have introduced fluoridation schemes. Results have been reported from Birmingham, Newcastle, Cumbria, Leeds, and Stranraer. Beal and James (1971) reported that $5\frac{1}{2}$ years after fluoridation in Birmingham water 5-year-old children from two areas of the city showed significant reductions in their dental caries experience. A control group of children consuming unfluoridated water maintained a fairly constant level of dental caries prevalence over the same period. Rock *et al.* (1981) compared the caries experience in the permanent dentition in Birmingham and Wolverhampton children and showed that the DMF rates in Wolverhampton were approximately two and a half times those in Birmingham (Fig. 3.8). Results from Cumbria (Jackson *et al.* 1975*a*), Newcastle and Northumber-

Table 3.7. Number of children examined and mean DMF in study and control areas. (Department of Public Health and Social Security (1969))

Age	Study areas					Control areas				
	1956 No. of children	**Mean DMF**	**1967 No. of children**	**Mean DMF**	**Per cent difference**	**1965 No. of children**	**Mean DMF**	**1967 No. of children**	**Mean DMF**	**Per cent difference**
8	806	2.0	378	1.2	43	499	2.2	204	2.0	8
9	780	2.8	395	1.8	36	491	2.8	229	2.7	3
10	636	3.4	356	2.4	31	460	3.5	213	3.3	5
8–10	2222	2.8	1129	1.8	36	1459	2.8	646	2.7	5

Table 3.8. Caries and mottling in 15-year-old children. (From Jackson *et al.* (1975*b*))

	Anglesey	Mainland	Difference (%)
Mean number of decayed/missing/filled teeth per person	6.37	11.44	44
Per cent incisors attacked by decay	4.20	23.08	82
Mean number of extracted teeth per person	0.64	1.87	65
per cent children with at least one incisor mottled	35	37	not significant

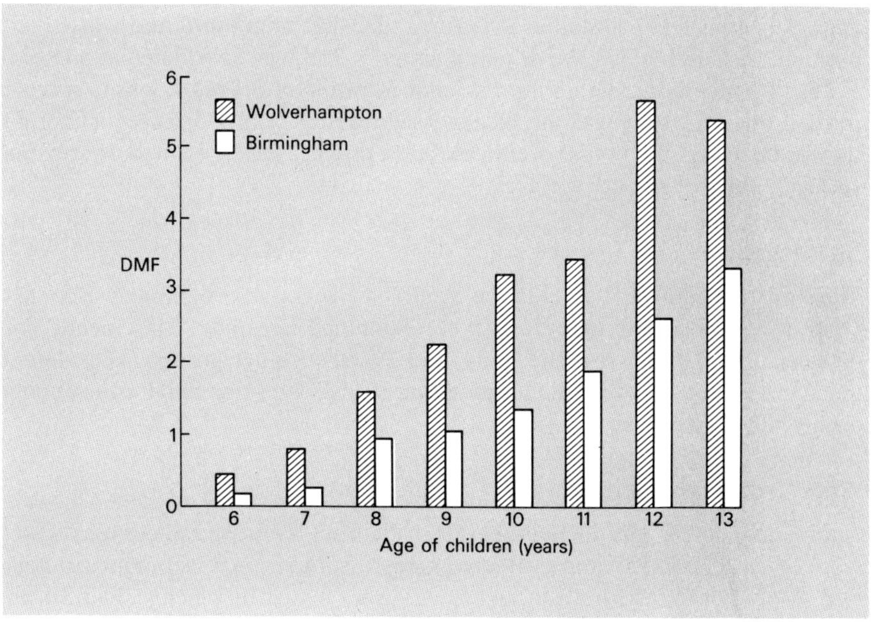

Fig. 3.8. Mean DMF of children aged 6–13 years from Birmingham (F = 1.0 p.p.m.) and Wolverhampton (low fluoride area). (With permission of the editor, *British Dental Journal*.)

land (Rugg-Gunn *et al.* 1977), Birmingham and Salford (Blinkhorn *et al.* 1981) all confirmed that caries experience was 44–57 per cent lower in the fluoridated community than in the non-fluoridated community.

Fluoridation study in the Netherlands

It is usual to compare the mean caries experience in a fluoridated area (F) with a non-fluoridated area (NF) and to express the difference between the two figures as a percentage reduction, using the figure for the non-fluoride area as the denominator [$\frac{NF-F}{NF} \times 100$]. However this method masks the fact, observed in many studies, that smooth surface caries is inhibited to a greater extent than pit and fissure caries by fluorides. Other important factors, for example the difference in the number of teeth which have to be extracted because of caries, are obscured when the composite DMF index is used. All these points can be demonstrated in the Tiel–Culemborg study in the Netherlands, which is probably the best and most detailed of all the fluoridation studies and includes a true longitudinal study over a period of 16½ years (Kwant *et al.* 1973).

Tiel and Culemborg, situated between the rivers Rhine and Maas, at a distance of 16 km from each other, were chosen for the study. The two towns were similar with respect to population structure, site, size, migration, and water composition. In March 1953 the drinking water in Tiel was fluoridated at a level of 1.1 mg/l. Culemborg, with a fluoride concentration of 0.1 mg/l, was to serve as the control. This study was specifically designed to measure the effect of fluoridation on the three main types of caries lesions, that is pits and fissures, approximal surfaces, and free smooth surfaces.

Study group

The study concentrated on children aged 7–15 years. Approximately 120–150 children in each year age group were examined annually. This meant that between 1953, the start of the study, and 1969, each age group was examined ten times and allowed a true longitudinal study (the same children examined each year) to be carried out.

Approximal surfaces

Approximal caries was diagnosed exclusively from bitewing radiographs which were taken, developed, and evaluated using a standardized technique. In addition the radiographs from the two towns were mixed by placing them in unlabelled envelopes and examined at random. The observers regularly re-scored a standard set of films to ensure a uniform diagnostic standard. Results for the number of approximal lesions, diagnosed radiographically as reaching dentine, are shown in Fig. 3.9. The mean number of proximal D lesions per child born in 1954 and examined in 1969, in premolars, molars, and maxillary incisors, was 9.7 in Culemborg and 2.3 in Tiel. The results for children born in 1944, showed that the number of proximal D lesions was similar in the two communities. The group born in 1949, who were nearly 9 years old when fluoridation started, showed that the caries experience in proximal surfaces was beginning to diverge and this trend becomes even more apparent for those children born in 1954, after the beginning of water fluoridation in Tiel. The authors concluded that this effect could have been caused partly by the fluoride enrichment of enamel during the pre-eruptive maturation of second molars, but must have been due to a post-eruptive topical effect on first molars and incisors.

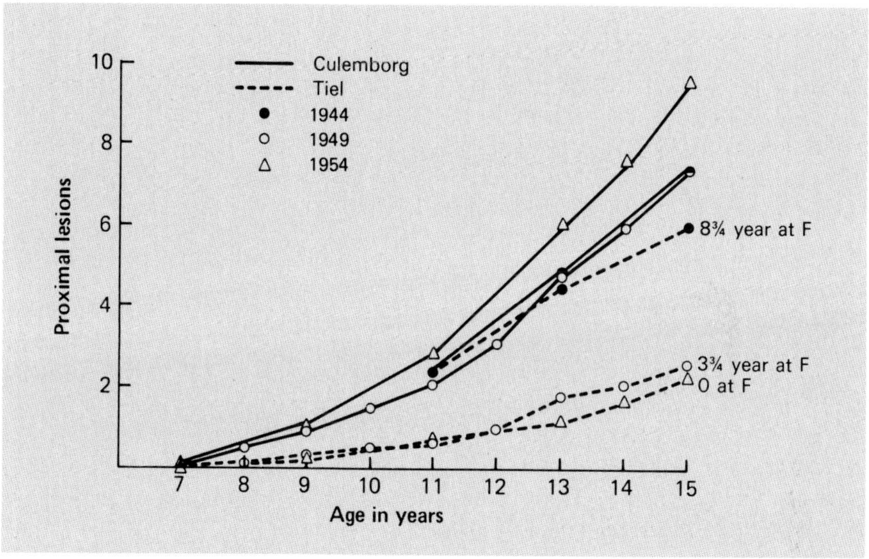

Fig. 3.9. Tiel–Culemborg study in the Netherlands. Mean number of proximal lesions per child in children born in 1944, 1949, and 1954, derived from a longitudinal study.

Pit and fissure surfaces

The fissures were cleaned and dried and the diagnosis was made with a mirror and a small light using incident and transmitted light. Caries was estimated in different grades, but only those lesions reaching dentine (D lesions) were published. Each child was examined by two dentists and the examination team alternated weekly between Tiel and Culemborg to ensure uniformity of standards. The mean number of pit and fissure cavities per child in molars and premolars is given in Fig. 3.10. For children born in 1954 and examined in 1969, the mean figures were 13.8 in Culemborg and 8.5 in Tiel. The results of these longitudinal studies show that the amount of pit and fissure caries hardly changed at all in Culemborg, for children born in 1945, 1949, or 1954, but in Tiel there was a reduced number of pit and fissure cavities with each successive year and those children born in 1954 had had the full benefits of having received fluoridated water from birth. The authors commented that the results for Tiel children born in 1954 were slightly lower than for those born in 1953, and that in the group born in 1954 all pregnancies took place during water fluoridation. The difference between the children born in 1953 and 1954 in Tiel could either be an expression of sampling error, or that fluoride has some effect on enamel formation during pregnancy. A sub-analysis showed that there was a lower caries score for the first molars than for the second molars and they concluded that the possibility of fluoride taken during pregnancy having a beneficial effect cannot be excluded and that to achieve an important preventive effect on the formation

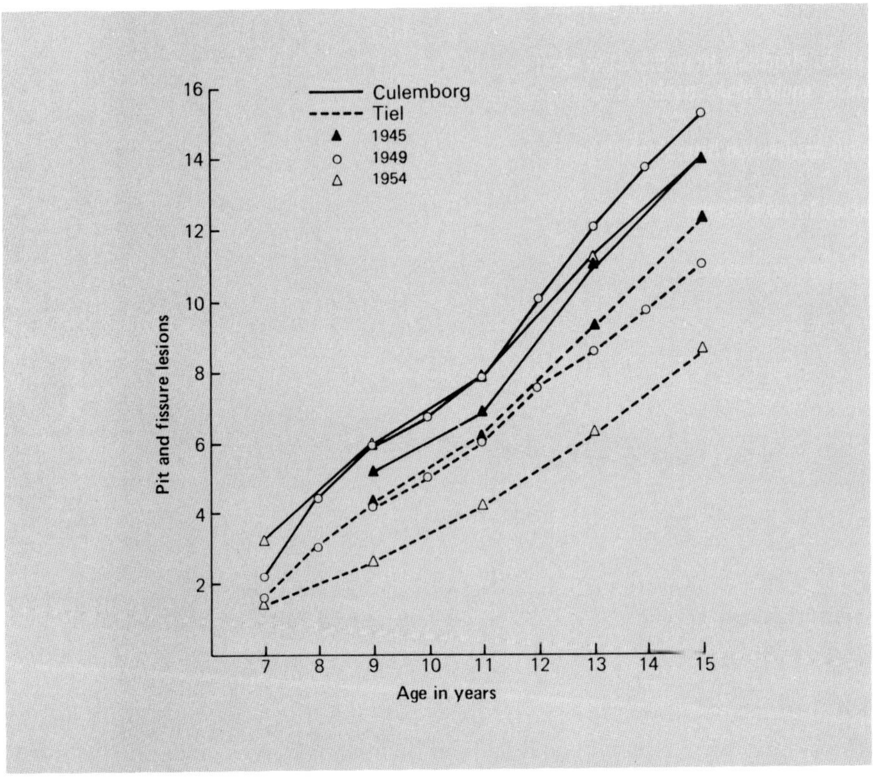

Fig. 3.10. Tiel–Culemborg study in the Netherlands. Mean numnber of pit and fissure lesions per child in molars and premolars for children born in 1945, 1949, and 1954. The water supply in Tiel was fluoridated at 1 p.p.m. in March 1953, while Culemborg, serving as the control town, kept to its natural concentration of 0.1 p.p.m. Thus the children born in 1954 in Tiel have consumed fluoridated water from birth. These results are a longitudinal study, the last clinical examination was carried out in 1969.

of pit and fissure cavities, fluoride is necessary from an early stage in enamel formation.

Free smooth surfaces

The buccal and lingual surfaces were cleansed and dried and a cavity was recorded only if a break in the enamel surface was discovered, using a Maillefer No. 6 explorer. Buccal surfaces were examined for the first time in 1957 and the lingual surfaces in 1962. The mean number of free smooth surfaces diagnosed in the two communities is given in Fig. 3.11. The mean number of free smooth cavities was 4.43 in Culemborg compared with 0.54 in Tiel, for the 15-year-old children born in 1954. In Culemborg the number of carious free smooth surfaces increased annually: for example 15-year-olds born in 1949 had on average 3.2

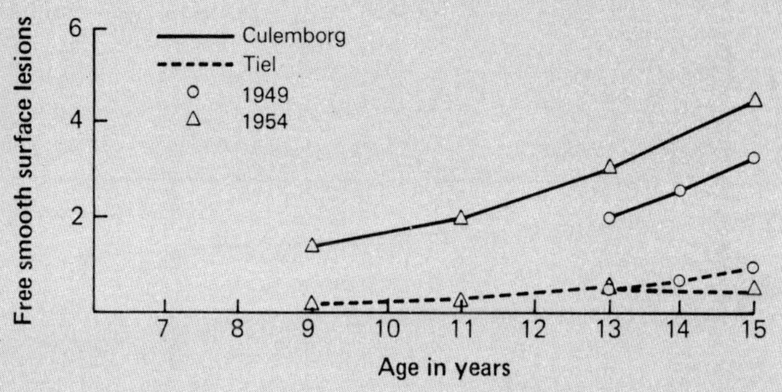

Fig. 3.11. Tiel–Culemborg study in the Netherlands. Mean number of free smooth surface lesions (gingival cavities) in children born in 1949 and 1954 in Tiel and Culemborg. Figures derived from a longitudinal study.

Table 3.9. The number of extractions per 100 children, aged 15 years examined in 1969. (From Kwant *et al.* (1973))

	Caries	Orthodontic/traumatic
Culemborg	150	18
Tiel	19	30

gingival lesions whereas those born in 1954 had 4.3 lesions. In Tiel, however, it was observed that even children born in 1945, who were 8 years old at the start of fluoridation, had significantly fewer free smooth lesions than the control group, suggesting that water fluoridation thus appears to have a significant post-eruptive caries reducing effect on these tooth surfaces.

Extractions

The number of permanent teeth extracted in 15-year-old children changed markedly in the two communities during the period 1952–1969. In the first year of the study 69 teeth had been extracted (per 100 15-year-old children) in Culemborg, compared with 83 in Tiel. The extraction rate was generally higher in Tiel than in Culemborg until 1960 when the two sets of figures started to diverge dramatically and by 1968 183 teeth had been extracted per 100 15-year-olds in Culemborg compared with 39 teeth extracted in Tiel. In 1969 the reason for extraction—either caries or orthodontic/traumatic—was ascertained. The results showed (Table 3.9) that extraction for caries was 87 per cent lower in Tiel than in Culemborg.

Table 3.10. The number of D lesions for each site separately, per 100 children, aged 15 years, examined in 1969. (From Kwant *et al.* (1973))

Sites	Culemborg	Tiel	Less in Tiel	Per cent less
Pits and fissures	1204	825	379	31
Proximal	1009	252	757	75
Free smooth surfaces	362	51	311	86
Total number of cavities	2575	1128	1447	56

Summary data

The results for all children born in 1954 and examined in 1969 are given in Table 3.10. There were 1447 fewer carious sites in Tiel than in Culemborg, per 100 15-year-old children, a reduction overall of 56 per cent. The per cent reduction varied between 31 per cent for pits and fissures and 86 per cent for free smooth surfaces. However, when considering per cent reduction, the actual number of surfaces saved must also be taken into consideration. Because pit and fissure caries is more prevalent than free smooth surface caries, the actual number of pit surfaces saved was greater than the number of free smooth surfaces.

Effect of varying concentrations of fluoride in drinking water on dental caries

The work of Dean and colleagues showing the relation between caries experience and fluoride content of the water supply to 21 cities in the United States of America showed that near maximal reduction in caries occurred at approximately 1–2 p.p.m. F. In addition, mottling of the teeth began to be noticeable when the fluoride concentration increased above 1.5 p.p.m. It was this work which formed the basis of the decision to fluoridate at 1 p.p.m. in the United States of America. Dean's original observations have been substantiated by a number of investigators. Møller (1965) showed that data from Denmark and Sweden followed the same trend as that reported by Dean *et al.* (1942) (Fig. 3.12). In addition, studies in Great Britain, Hungary, Austria, Spain, and the United States show a decrease in caries experience with increasing fluoride content of the water supply up to about 2 p.p.m.; this information is summarized in Table 3.11.

The relationship between caries experience in the deciduous dentition and the fluoride concentration in the drinking water was investigated by Rugg-Gunn *et al.* (1981). They examined 1038 5-year-old children from four areas in the North-East of England and showed a progressive decrease in caries experience with increasing concentration of fluoride in the water, up to 1.0 p.p.m. (Fig. 3.13), thus following the same trend as that reported for the permanent dentition.

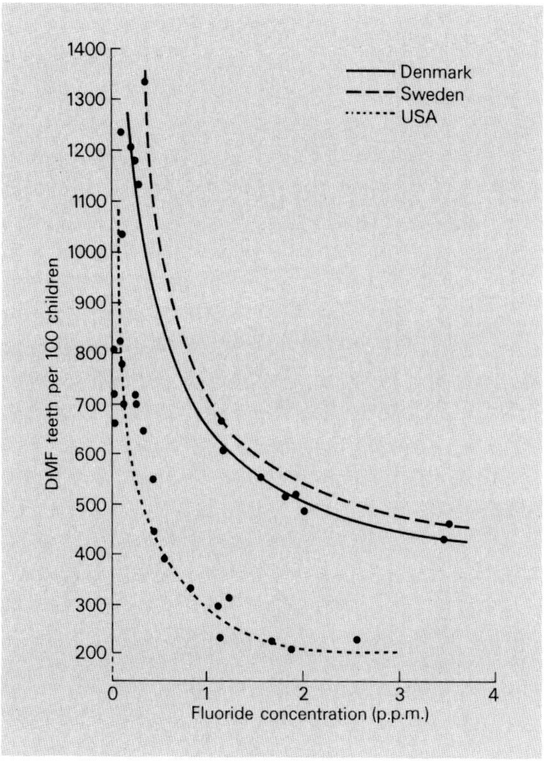

Fig. 3.12. Caries experience in 12–13-year-old children from Denmark, Sweden, and the USA in relation to concentration of fluoride in water supplies. (From Møller (1965).) (Reproduced with permission.)

Community fluoridation schemes throughout the world

After these early favourable reports appeared, many other communities decided to fluoridate their public water supplies so that by 1978 approximately 155 million people worldwide were consuming fluoridated water, in addition to the 40 million or so receiving naturally fluoride-rich water supplies. Dental health has been monitored in many of these communities, and findings in artificially fluoridated areas will be reviewed here. Such information is not readily available since reports are frequently published and written in the language of the country concerned (Table 3.12). This review will be confined to studies that report standard caries indices (i.e. deft, DMFT) (Murray and Rugg-Gunn 1982*a*, *b*).

The Americas

In addition to the studies in Grand Rapids, Newburgh, and Evanston, fluoridation has been monitored in at least 103 other communities, although some of these reports have appeared only as press articles and many are published in state health department reports and newsletters. It is inevitable, as the effectiveness of fluoridation has been demonstrated repeatedly in the United States, that

Table 3.11. Dental caries in 12–14-year-old children in communities with varying concentrations of fluoride in drinking water

Reference	Country	Town	F Supply	No. of children	Mean DMF
Dean (1942)	USA	Michigan City	0.09	236	10.37
		Elkhart	0.11	278	8.23
		Portsmouth	0.13	469	7.72
		Zanesville	0.19	459	7.33
		Middletown	0.2	370	7.03
		Quincy	0.13	330	7.06
		Lima	0.3	454	6.52
		Marion	0.43	263	5.56
		Pueblo	0.6	614	4.12
		Kewanee	0.9	123	3.43
		East Moline	1.2	152	3.03
		Colorado Springs	2.6	404	2.46
		Galesburg	1.9	273	2.36
		Waukegan	0.0	423	8.10
		Oak Park	0.0	329	7.22
		Evanstown	0.0	256	6.73
		Elgin	0.5	403	4.44
		Joliet	1.3	447	3.23
		Aurora	1.2	633	2.81
		Maywood	1.2	171	2.58
		Elmhurst	1.8	170	2.52
Arnold (1948)	USA	Nashville	0.0	662	4.6
		Key West	0.1 95	10.7	
		Clarksville	0.2	60	4.6
		Vicksburg	0.2	172	5.87
		Escanaba	0.2	270	8.8
		Hereford	3.1	60	1.47

Galagan (1953)†	USA	Yuma	0.4	29	2.45
		Tempe	0.5	45	2.82
		Tucson	0.7	167	3.48
		Chandler	0.8	42	2.45
		Casa Grande	1.0	22	2.00
		Florence	1.2	34	3.56
Nevitt *et al.* (1953)	USA	Low F	0.08–0.26	311	8.5
		Medium F	0.42–0.68	222	4.8
		High F	0.87–1.32	254	2.1
Lewis and Leatherwood (1959)	USA	Macon	0.11	1182	6.33
		Savanah	0.37	1188	5.22
		Moultrie	0.75	136	3.15
Gillooly *et al.* (1954)	Low F	0.1–0.3	114	3.65	
		Medium F	0.5	109	2.80
		High F	0.8–1.6	88	1.41
Klein (1948)	USA	Williamstown and Clayton	0.1	81	7.2
		Woodstown, Glassboro, and Pitman	1.3–2.2	176	1.9
Forrest (1956)	UK	Saffron Walden and district	0.1	145	6.6
		Stoneleign and Maldon West	0.1–0.2	114	6.1
		Slough	0.9	119	2.6
		Harwich	2.0	92	1.5
		Burnham-on-Crouch	3.5	62	1.4
		West Mersea	5.8	51	2.8
Adler (1951)	Hungary	Sarretudvari	0.20	166	4.25
		Öcsöd	0.21	222	2.09
		Bekesszentandras	0.21	177	2.43
		Biharnagybajom	0.33	143	3.06
		Kumszentmarton farms	0.72	86	1.29
		Szekszard	0.76	292	0.91
		Kunszentmarton village	0.99	283	1.02
		Komadi	1.09	343	1.31
Binder (1065)	Austria	Low F towns	0.0	90	4.9
		Umhansen, Silz, and Mallnitz	1.0–1.8	82	1.2

Table 3.11.—*continued*

Reference	Country	Town	F Supply	No. of children	Mean DMF
Sellman *et al.* (1957)	Sweden	Malmö	0.3–0.5	145	13.3
		Nyvang	1.0		
		Astorp	1.3	149	6.8
		Simrishamm	1.3		
Møller	Denmark	Vejen	0.05	148	12.5
		Aalestrup	0.2	52	12.2
		St. Heddinge	0.25	43	11.7
		Slagelse	0.34	424	11.2
		Naestved H	1.2	157	6.2
		Praestø	1.6	43	5.5
		Naestved N	1.8	42	5.2
		Naestved G	1.9	150	5.2
		Stroby Egede	2.0	12	4.9
		Tappernøje and Strøby By	3.4	14	4.2
Vines and Clavero (1968)*	Spain	Aezcoa	0.1	34	6.25
		Valle de Erro	0.1	22	6.02
		Tafalla	0.5	149	5.64
		Pitillas	0.7	21	5.14
		Pamplona	0.7	670	5.03
		Mueillo et Fruito	0.75	37	5.01
		Funes	0.65	66	4.91
		Falces	0.65	93	4.57
		Potasas	0.6	70	4.56
		Tudela	0.6	192	4.49
		Murcia	0.8	462	3.41
		Abanilla	1.5	47	2.35

* 10–12-year-old children.
† These studies were carried out in Arizona, which has a very high mean annual temperature.

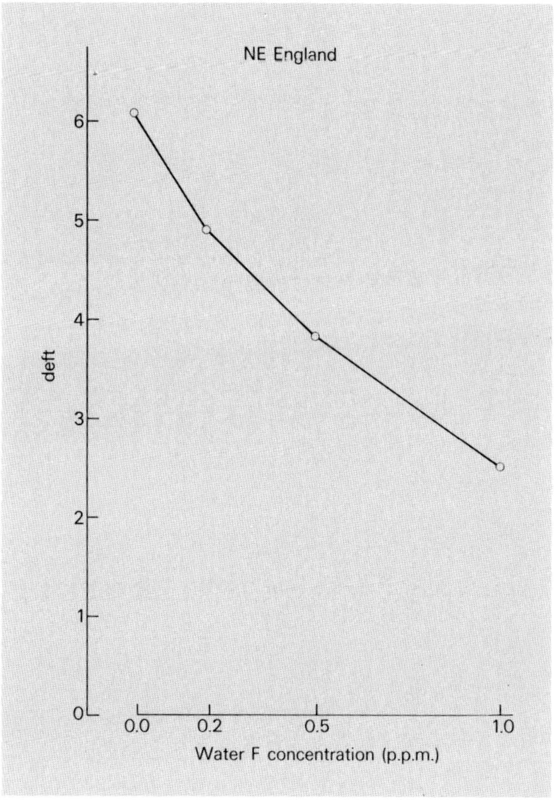

Fig. 3.13. The relationship between caries experience (deft) in 1038 5-year-old children living in four areas of NE England and the fluoride concentration in their drinking water. (Rugg-Gunn *et al.* (1981).) (Reproduced by courtesy of the Editor of the *British Dental Journal.*)

results of fresh surveys will be published less frequently. This review is therefore incomplete so far as the United States is concerned.

Approximately 6.6 million people in Canada have fluoridated water. The results of the Brantford–Sarnia–Stratford study are well known. Caries experience was also monitored in Brandon, which fluoridated in 1955, and in Toronto, which fluoridated in 1963. The Toronto survey is one of the best investigations into the effectiveness of water fluoridation as a public health measure and should serve as a guide to other cities that are operating, or planning to introduce, water fluoridation schemes.

Fluoridation has been fairly widespread in Central and South America, with 10.3 per cent of the population on piped water supplies receiving fluoridated water in 1968. The highest proportion occurred in Paraguay (100 per cent) although only a tenth of the population received a piped supply. About half the people of Chile are on a piped supply, and 56 per cent of these received fluoridated water. Fluoridation is also widespread in Panama and Nicaragua. In Brazil, where 1.5 million people received fluoridated water in 1968, Viegas and Viegas studied the effect of 10 years' fluoridation in Campinas City, Sau Paulo.

Table 3.12. Studies on the effectiveness of fluoridation in communities throughout the world.* (From Murray and Rugg-Gunn (1982*a*, *b*))

Fluoridation community	Country	Year fluoridation began	Year of study	Age of subjects (years)	Caries index	Non-fluoridated community caries experience	Caries reduction %
Grand Rapids	USA	1945	1951	5	deft	5.3	57
Grand Rapids	USA	1945	1960	15	DMFT	12.4	50
Newburgh	USA	1945	1955	6–9	DMFT	2.3	58
Marshall	USA	1945	1956	10	DMFT	4.3	67
Evanston	USA	1945	1961	14	DMFT	11.7	49
Antigo	USA	1919–1960	1966	5–6	deft	5.3	53
Newark	USA	1950	1955	6	DMFT	1.1	82
New Britain	USA	1950	1961	10	DMFT	3.9	48
Athens	USA	1951	1957	6	DMFT	1.2	85
Tuscaloosa	USA	1951	1959	6	deft	5.6	52
Tuscaloosa	USA	1951	1959	8	DMFT	2.3	73
Fort Wayne	USA	1951	1962	10	DMFT	3.7	50
Columbus	USA	1951	1962	10	DMFT	3.3	47
Grand Junction	USA	1951	1962	6	deft	5.3	50
Norway	USA	1952	1955	7	DMFT	2.1	71
Maryland	USA	1952	1959	5	deft	2.8	65
Maryland	USA	1952	1959	7	DMFT	1.1	77
Easton	USA	1952	1962	5	deft	5.0	71
Easton	USA	1952	1962	10	DMFT	3.6	53
Amery	USA	1952	1962	9	DMFT	3.8	29
Roundup	USA	1952	1962	10	DMFT	4.0	60
Cleveland, Tenn.	USA	1952	1963	11	DMFT	7.6	63
Hagerstown	USA	1952	1963	11	DMFT	4.2	62
Providence	USA	1952	1972	13	DMFT	8.4	63
Richmond	USA	1952	1962	9	DMFT	2.6	46
Richmond	USA	1952	1972	13	DMFT	7.2	50
Milwaukee	USA	1953	1959	5	deft	3.6	35
Milwaukee	USA	1953	1965	10	DMFT	3.6	56
Mystic-Stonington	USA	1953	1964	11	DMFT	4.4	35
Corvallis	USA	1953	1962	5	deft	6.0	45

Puerto Rico	USA	1953	1958	6	DMFT	1.2	66
Philadelphia	USA	1954	1967	5	deft	3.2	50
Philadelphia	USA	1954	1969–1970	15	DMFT	9.3	52
St. Louis	USA	1955	1961	7	DMFT	0.8	50
Kingsport	USA	1955	1965	10	DMFT	3.9	62
Albert Lea	USA	1955	1969	6	deft	5.7	42
Albert Lea	USA	1955	1969	12	DMFT	6.2	53
Cleveland	USA	1956	1962	5–6	deft	3.4	62
Lebanon	USA	1956	1964	6	deft	5.4	47
Lebanon	USA	1956	1964	8	DMFT	2.4	68
Fayette	USA	1957	1969	19	DMFT	5.1	63
Mobile	USA	1958	1965	6	deft	5.6	32
Mobile	USA	1958	1965	7	DMFT	2.0	72
Silver Bay	USA	1958	1968	5	deft	4.6	46
Silver Bay	USA	1958	1968	10	DMFT	3.6	45
Winona	USA	1965	1976	5	deft	4.0	74
Winona	USA	1965	1976	10	DMFT	3.4	57
Cudahy	USA	1966	1971	5	deft	3.9	56
Brantford	Canada	1945	1959	15	DMFT	8.0	51
Brandon	Canada	1955	1962	6–8	deft	6.5	41
Brandon	Canada	1955	1962	6–8	DMFT	2.0	74
Toronto	Canada	1963	1975	5	deft	3.9	56
Toronto	Canada	1963	1975	11	DMFT	3.6	35
Prince George	Canada	1955	1968	12–14	DMFT	11.2	60
Anglesey	UK	1955	1965	5	deft	4.8	40
Watford	UK	1956	1967	5	deft	2.8	43
Kilmarnock	UK	1956	1961	5	deft	6.9	42
Anglesey	UK	1956	1974	15	DMFT	11.4	44
Balsall Heath	UK	1964	1970	5	deft	5.2	62
Northfield	UK	1964	1970	5	deft	4.9	50
Birmingham	UK	1964	1977	5	deft	3.6	54
Birmingham	UK	1964	1977	12	DMFT	4.0	45
Cumbria	UK	1969	1975	5	deft	4.4	46
Newcastle on Tyne	UK	1969	1975	5	deft	6.1	57
Northumberland	UK	1969	1975	5	deft	6.1	67
Dublin	Ireland	1964	1969	5	deft	5.8	65
Cork	Ireland	1965	1969	5	deft	6.4	45
Tiel	Netherlands	1953	1969	15	DMFT	13.9	51
Kuopio	Finland	1959	1968	7	DMFT	3.1	55

Table 3.12.—*continued*

Fluoridation community	Country	Year fluoridation began	Year of study	Age of subjects (years)	Caries index	Non-fluoridated community caries experience	Caries reduction %
Basel	Switzerland	1962	1972	10	DMFT	5.0	44
Karl-Marx-Stadt	GDR	1959	1966	5	deft	2.9	76
Karl-Marx-Stadt	GDR	1959	1972	12	DMFT	4.1	66
Tabor	Czechoslovakia	1958	1964	6–7	deft	5.3	36
Wroclaw	Poland	1967	1972	5	deft	5.5	38
Wroclaw	Poland	1967	1972	7	DMFT	1.4	50
Tirgu-Mures	Romania	1960	1965	5	deft	3.6	37
Tirgu-Mures	Romania	1960	1971	10	DMFT	3.3	52
Murmansk	USSR	1966	1976	10	DMFT	3.0	50
Monchegorsk	USSR	1966	1976	8	DMFT	2.7	54
Ivano-Frankovsk	USSR	1966	1970	8	DMFT	2.2	55
Leningrad	USSR	1969	1974	5	deft	4.9	29
Campinas	Brazil	1962	1972	5	deft	5.5	68
Campinas	Brazil	1962	1972	10	DMFT	5.1	55
Singapore	Singapore	1956	1968	7–9	deft	10.7	31
Singapore	Singapore	1956	1968	7–9	DMFT	2.9	31
Yamashina	Japan	1952	1963	11	DMFT	3.6	33
Tamworth	Australia	1963	1969	5	deft	5.7	48
Tamworth	Australia	1963	1971	8	DMFT	3.2	48
Canberra	Australia	1964	1974	5	deft	5.0	71
Canberra	Australia	1964	1974	10	DMFT	4.4	51
Townsville	Australia	1965	1975	6	deft	5.3	57
Townsville	Australia	1965	1975	10	DMFT	4.8	54
Kalgoorlie	Australia	1968	1973	6	deft	6.3	40
Hastings	NZ	1954	1964	5	deft	8.4	52
Hastings	NZ	1954	1970	15	DMFT	16.8	49
Lower Hull	NZ	1959	1969	5	deft	8.0	47
Lower Hull	NZ	1959	1969	10	DMFT	6.2	42

*Whenever possible age groups five years for deciduous teeth and 15 years for permanent teeth are given. Tooth scores (deft and DMFT) only are given since surface scores were less frequently reported.

Europe

In addition to studies in the United Kingdom, in Ireland fluoridation became mandatory in 1960 and, by 1975, 57 per cent of the population were receiving fluoridated water supplies. As fluoridation is widespread, the choice of control towns was difficult; but the effectiveness of fluoridation has been assessed in the two largest cities, Cork and Dublin.

In Belgium the town of Assesse fluoridated in 1956, embracing 0.4 million people by 1974, but the effect has not been monitored. In West Germany a pilot scheme of water fluoridation began at Kassel-Wahlershausen in 1952 but stopped; in 1978 there was no water fluoridation in that country. Full data on the effectiveness of fluoridation in Kassel have not been given, although 28 per cent caries reduction was reported. Likewise, in Sweden the town of Norrkoping was fluoridated only from 1952 to 1962; nevertheless, there was a 52 per cent caries reduction in 7-year-old children after 7 years' fluoridation.

One of the best scientific studies into the effect of water fluoridation was conducted in Holland, where Tiel fluoridated in 1953. Fluoridation ceased in 1974, at a time when 2.7 million Dutch people (20 per cent of the population) were receiving fluoridated water.

The only Finnish community to fluoridate has been Kuopio, where fluoridation began in 1959 with Jyväskylä as control. Although the first Swiss community to fluoridate was Aigle in 1960, the effect of fluoridation has been studied more thoroughly in Basel (1962).

By 1972 ten cities in East Germany had fluoridated, with planned extension to half the population by the middle 1980s. The effectiveness of this measure has been thoroughly studied in Karl-Marx-Stadt by Kunzel. Fluoridation began in 1959 with the city of Plauen as a control; but this was lost in 1971, when Plauen itself fluoridated. Examinations were conducted in alternate years on children 3–18 years of age. Kunzel also gives data for each tooth type separately for each age group, confirming that incisor teeth benefit most.

In Hungary attempts to introduce fluoridation have not been successful; it was started in the town of Szolnok in 1962 but abandoned one year later. One report states that 63 per cent of the population of Bulgaria was drinking fluoridated water in 1974, but no data on its effectiveness have been found. The effectiveness of water fluoridation in Czechoslovakia, Poland, and Romania, however, has been documented. In Czechoslovakia, Tabor was the main test town, fluoridating in 1958, with Pisek as control. In addition to the 36 per cent caries reduction in Tabor, a small reduction was observed in children in Bialystok after 6 years' fluoridation and a 70 per cent reduction in Brumm after 3 years. By 1972, 36 Czech communities had fluoridated, reaching 10 per cent of the population.

Progress in fluoridation has been slower in Poland, where, by 1974, 3.7 per cent of the population (1.3 million) was receiving fluoridated water. The effect is being monitored in the city of Wroclaw, which commenced fluoridation in 1967.

The town of Tirgu-Mures in Romania fluoridated its water supplies in 1960, and in 1972 it was the only fluoridated community in that country. From 1962 onward, caries experience has been monitored in 3–14-year old Tirgu-Mures children. Owing to technical difficulties, however, fluoridation was not continuous and occurred on only 64 per cent of the total possible number of days between 1960 and 1971.

Fluoridation of public water supplies has advanced rapidly in the USSR since it commenced in Norilsk in 1958. By 1972, 13 million people were receiving fluoridated water in 24 communities, rising to 20 million in 1977. After 7 years of fluoridation dental caries in Norilsk 7-year-olds had decreased by 43 per cent, with an overall reduction in the cost of filling materials in Norilsk of 30 per cent despite the fact that fluoridation was said to be intermittent. Fluoridation began in 1966 in Ivano-Frankovsk with Dolina as control, and in Leningrad in 1969 with surrounding areas as control. One comprehensive Russian study was undertaken by the Central Research Institute of Stomatology (CRIS), Moscow, in collaboration with WHO monitored fluoridation in Murmansk (1966) and Monchegorsk (1968) in the Arctic regions.

Asia

By 1975 only one Malaysian state, Johore, had fluoridated its water supplies. Results of dental surveys carried out before and after 7 years of fluoridation in the towns of Johore Bahru and Kluang indicated reductions of 60 and 75 per cent respectively in caries experience. Fluoridation began in Singapore in 1956, covered the entire water system by 1958, and supplied two million people in 1970. No data have been found on the effectiveness of fluoridation in Hong Kong, where 3.6 million people receive fluoridated water.

There is at present no fluoridation in Japan. The only town to fluoridate, Yamashina, began in 1952 but fluoridation has now ceased.

Australasia

Fluoridation has been widely introduced in Australia. By 1971, 4.9 million Australians were drinking fluoridated water. Tamworth began fluoridating in 1963, but one of the most thorough investigations into fluoridation effectiveness was conducted in Canberra. Areas of Western Australia fluoridated in 1968, and Medcalf reports on its effect upon caries experience in the Kalgoorlie area after six years. The city of Townsville, Queensland, fluoridated in 1965; data from 16 neighbouring low-fluoride towns acted as negative control, and four naturally fluoridated areas as positive control. The survey was in 1975 after 10 years' fluoridation.

Hastings was the first New Zealand city to fluoridate, and reports of the effectiveness of its programme are well known. The high caries experience found in New Zealand has meant that, in real terms, a larger number of teeth were prevented from becoming carious in New Zealand, for a given per cent reduction, than in other communities. The mean DMFT for Hastings 15-year-olds in 1954 was 16.8, which fell to 8.5 by 1970, a reduction of 49 per cent or 8.3 teeth. The

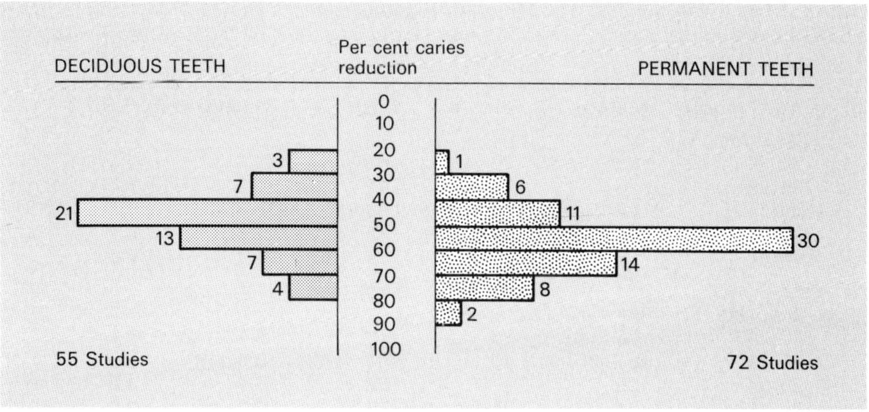

Fig. 3.14. Percentage caries reduction observed in 95 studies into the effectiveness of artificial fluoridation in 20 countries. Fifty-five studies gave results for the deciduous dentition (dmft) and 73 studies for the permanent dentition (DMFT).

corresponding figures for tooth surfaces were 42.5 DMFS in 1954 and 17.4 in 1970, a 59 per cent reduction or the large difference of 25 tooth surfaces.

Summary

The per cent caries reductions in these various studies for deciduous teeth and permanent teeth are recorded in Fig. 3.14. For deciduous teeth the per cent reduction varied from 20–80 per cent and for permanent teeth from 20–90 per cent. However, for both dentitions the vast majority of the studies reported a reduction of between 40–70 per cent.

Fluoridation and adult dental health

Although many studies have shown conclusively that water fluoridation is effective in reducing caries in the permanent teeth of children, some doubts have been raised as to whether the observed reductions are due to a delay in the onset of clinical dental caries in the permanent dentition, or whether water fluoridation is having a truly long-term caries-preventive effect. Studies by Deatherage (1943) and Forrest *et al.* (1951) showed that continuous residence in a high fluoride area was associated with lower caries experience in adults, but both these studies involved highly selected groups—white national service selectees in America (Deatherage) and pregnant and nursing mothers in England (Forrest *et al.*). Three studies have attempted to obtain a more representative sample, bearing in mind that one necessary qualification must be that people included in this type of investigation must have resided for the greater part of their lives in a natural fluoride area. The first study (Russell and Elvove 1951) measured the effect of fluoride on dental caries experience in adults from Colorado Springs,

Table 3.13. Mean number of DMF teeth together with its standard deviation (SD) in adults from Boulder and Colorado Springs (excluding third molars). (From Russell and Elvove (1951))

Age (years)	Male	Female	Both	Mean DMF	±SD
Boulder					
20–24	22	29	51	14.0	4.9
25–29	26	15	41	16.5	5.5
30–34	17	12	29	18.3	5.2
35–39	8	14	22	21.8	5.1
40–44	6	6	12	21.7	6.0
20+	79	76	155	17.2	
Colorado Springs					
20–24	36	36	72	5.4	5.1
25–29	61	40	101	6.5	5.0
30–34	55	27	82	7.1	4.9
35–39	51	24	75	9.2	7.0
40–44	36	19	55	10.3	6.4
20+	239	146	385	7.5	

selected for investigation because of the long and reliable fluoride history of this town; the water supply contained 2.55 p.p.m. F. Nearby Boulder, Colo. was utilized as a control; in this town there was only a trace of fluoride in the drinking water. For the purpose of this study 'continuous residence' was defined as 'residence unbroken except for periods not exceeding 60 days during the time of development and eruption of the permanent teeth—thereafter more than half the life had to be spent in the respective community. The results of this study are recorded in Table 3.13. Russell and Elvove concluded that total rates for decayed, missing or filled permanent teeth were about 60 per cent lower in Colorado Springs than in Boulder for each age group. Caries inhibition apparently continued undiminished up to at least 44 years. Boulder residents had lost three or four times as many teeth from dental caries as had those of Colorado Springs.

The second study (Englander and Wallace 1962) compared a larger sample of adults who had continuously resided in a city having approximately 1 p.p.m. F in its domestic water with a similar sample of adults in a nearby city who had consumed water low in fluoride. The communities chosen for study were Aurora, Illinois (F = 1.2 p.p.m.), and Rockford, Illinois (fluoride-free). The main purpose concerned the effect of fluoride on periodontal disease and hence only persons with at least 10 natural teeth present were examined. A total of 896 continuous residents in Aurora and 935 residents in Rockford were examined. Women constituted 61 per cent of the sample in Aurora and 63 per cent of the sample in Rockford. The number in each age group, and the DMF values, for Aurora and for Rockford, are given in Table 3.14. Overall reduction in DMF teeth for Aurorans over residents of Rockford was 40 per cent approximately.

The third study was carried out in 1968–69 when 4774 adults from Hartlepool and York were examined to try and measure in greater detail the long-term effects of fluoride in drinking water (Murray 1971*a*). The County Borough of

Table 3.14. Mean DMF values against age for residents in Aurora (1.2 p.p.m. F) and Rockford (np F). (After Englander and Wallace (1961))

Age group	Aurora		Rockford	
	No. in group	Mean DMF	No. in group	Mean DMF
18–19	162	6.05	120	11.27
20–29	188	8.78	223	16.92
30–39	255	11.03	342	17.65
40–49	205	12.41	191	18.00
50–59	86	12.58	59	13.34
All ages	896	10.13	935	16.78

Hartlepool, population 100 000, is situated in the south-east corner of County Durham, some 12 km north of the River Tees. Domestic water is supplied to Hartlepool by the Hartlepool Water Company, founded in 1841; it is a private company and its pipelines are not connected to any of the surrounding local authority water boards. The fluoride concentration in the drinking water is 1.5–2.0 p.p.m.

The City of York was used as a control town. Domestic water is supplied to it by the York Water Company which obtains its water from the River Ouse. The fluoride content of the water varies between the limits of 0.15 p.p.m. and 0.28 p.p.m., depending on whether or not the river is in spate. The mean fluoride concentration is 0.2 p.p.m. The population of York is 105 000, very similar to that of Hartlepool.

The following definition of 'continuous residence' was adopted: a person who had been born in Hartlepool, had lived all his/her school life in the town (except for holidays) and had been away from the town during his/her life for no more than 6 years. This meant that all those people termed 'continuous residents' had been exposed to fluoride drinking water during birth and childhood and had spent nearly all, of not all, of their adult life in the town. The definition was sufficiently flexible to allow people attending college, or working in other areas for short periods, or those who had done military service, to be included in the sample.

In order to obtain a sample of Hartlepool adults, large establishments were approached and asked to co-operate in the study. The aims of the project were discussed with the management and respresentatives of the work force in order to obtain as much co-operation as possible. Once approval had been given, a letter was sent to each person in the factory or establishment explaining the reason for the survey and asking for his/her co-operation. Subsequently arrangements were made for those people who had been born in Hartlepool, and who had agreed to a dental examination, to be seen in the place of work. A similar procedure to that used in Hartlepool was adopted in York to obtain a population sample of a low fluoride area.

The mean DMF values for all people examined, including edentulous persons, is shown in Fig. 3.15. Unfortunately, the DMF index is not an accurate measure

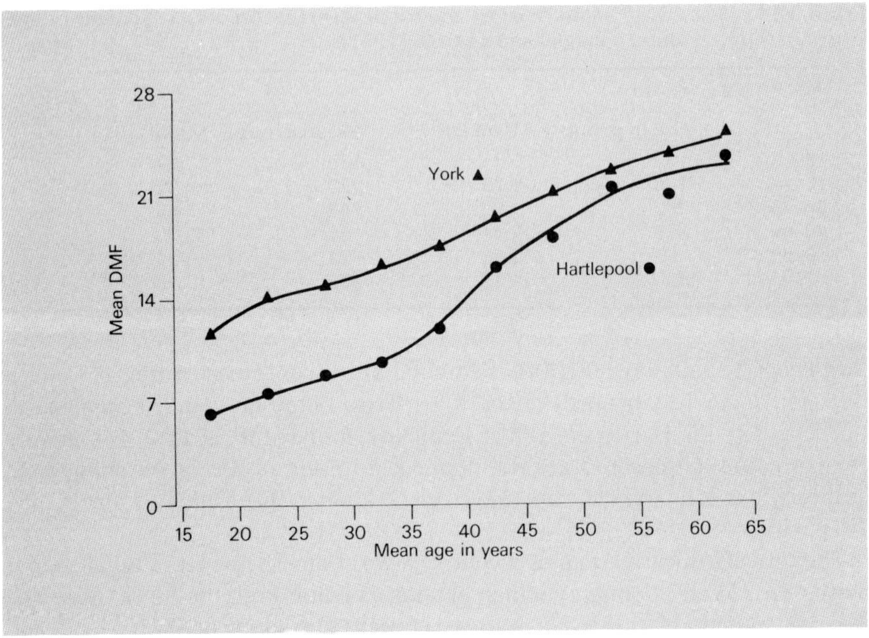

Fig. 3.15. Mean DMF values in adults from Hartlepool and York, including edentulous persons. From Murray (1971*a*).) (Reproduced by courtesy of the Editor of the *British Dental Journal*.)

of caries experience in adults because of the increasing number of caries-free teeth which are extracted (for periodontal and prosthetic reasons) as age advances. In order to try to measure the full caries inhibitory effect of fluoride in drinking water, it is essential to try to measure more accurately caries experience in an adult population in fluoride and non-fluoride areas. Russell and Elvolve (1951) attempted to compensate for the inaccuracy of the DMF index in adults by recording the primary reasons for extraction based upon a history of signs and symptoms. Apart from the fact that subjective evidence of this nature is unreliable, a tooth removed for any reason other than caries may have suffered caries attack also. Unless reliable life records are available, an accurate assessment of the cumulative incidence of dental caries over a wide range would seem to be impossible.

Three different approaches were made in the Hartlepool–York study to try to overcome this problem. First, it can be argued that the greatest error in the DMF index when used in adults is the inclusion of edentulous people in the DMF count, because it is these people who will have had the greatest proportion of caries-free teeth extracted in order to wear full dentures. On the other hand, those people who want to keep their teeth will have had relatively few caries-free teeth extracted and thus a more accurate measure of caries experience would be

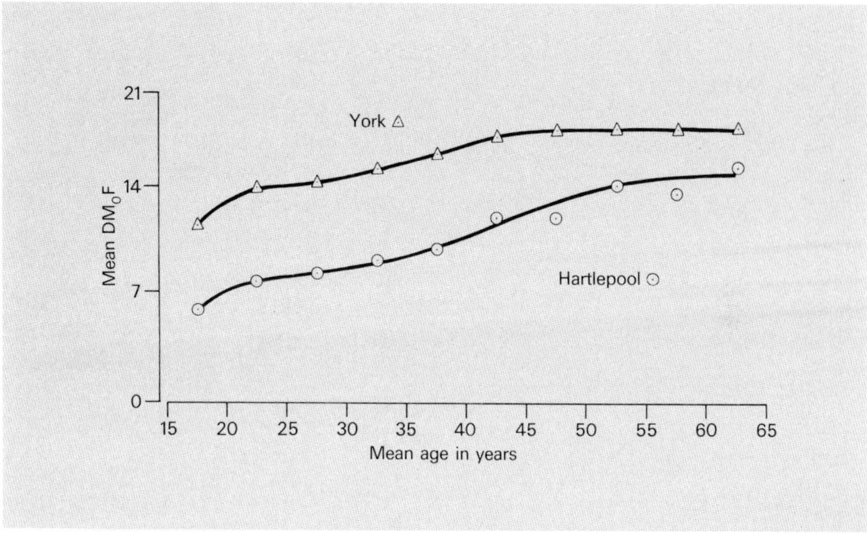

Fig. 3.16. Mean DMF values in adult from Hartlepool and York, excluding edentulous persons. (From Murray (1971*a*).) (Reproduced by courtesy of the Editor of the *British Dental Journal*.)

to calculate the observed DMF ($DM^{o}F$) in dentate persons (Fig. 3.16). Comparing Figs. 3.15 and 3.16 it will be seen that, using the latter index, the difference between the communities is much more clear-cut.

A second approach is to use the method put forward by Jackson (1961) who suggested that if, by a sampling survey, the percentage number of extracted teeth which were carious was known for any specific community it would appear reasonable to apply correction factors of the M fraction of the DMF value at each age group, in order to obtain a more accurate measurement of caries experience in an adult population. This procedure was adopted in order to obtain 'correction factors' for the Hartlepool–York data.

All seven dental practitioners in Hartlepool and 19 of the dental practitioners in York agreed to co-operate in the study by collecting teeth extracted in their surgeries, over a specific period of time. Ten polythene bottles marked according to the quinquennial age groups used in the study (15–19 years, 20–24 years, and so on) were supplied to each practitioner. In Hartlepool only those teeth extracted from people who had been born and lived most of their lives in Hartlepool were collected. This part of the study extended from March 1968 to April 1969 in York and from January 1968 to September 1969 in Hartlepool. The teeth were separated according to age and type and examined for dental caries. A probe was used if caries was not obvious to the naked eye. All filled teeth were presumed to have been carious. In all 7933 extracted teeth were collected in York and 2958 teeth were collected in Hartlepool. The correction factors for

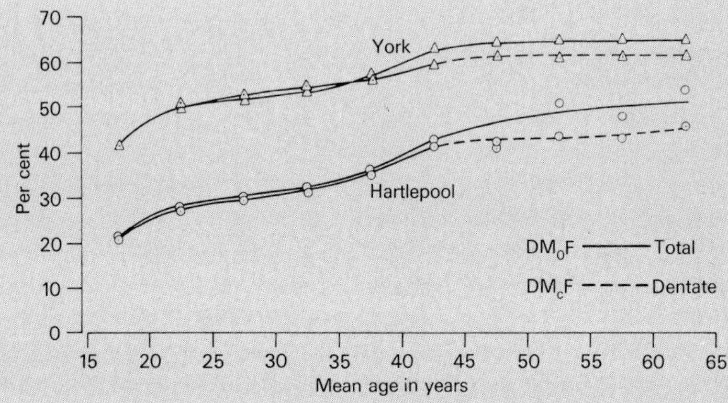

Fig. 3.17. Comparison of corrected DMF values (total population) with observed values of the dentate population. (From Murray (1971*b*).) (Reproduced by courtesy of the Editor of the *British Dental Journal*.)

each tooth type and the corrected DMF values (DM_cF) for the total population (including the endentulous) were calculated (Murray 1971*b*).

The DM_cF valued at any year age group can only be an approximation of true caries experience in the whole population. As a check on the validity of the correction factors, the DM_cF values for the total population were compared with the DM_cF values for the dentate population in each community (Fig. 3.17). (The dentate population includes only those people with at least one natural tooth). The DM_cF values (tooth population) were effectively identical with the DM_oF values (dentate population) up to the age of 45 years in both communities. Thereafter the DM_oF (dentate) values were slightly higher than the DM_cF (general values; this is to be expected because even in a dentate population one would imagine that a small proportion of caries-free teeth would have to be extracted for periodontal, prosthetic, or surgical reasons. The ceiling DM_cF value in Hartlepool was 45.6 per cent and in York it was 61.0 per cent; this means that the maximum DMF in Hartlepool was 25 per cent lower than it is in York.

Unfortunately, the DMF index gives no indication of the number of surfaces affected by caries. Thus the third approach is to ignore missing teeth altogether and not attempt to apply correction factors or assume that a missing tooth should be counted as three or five surfaces. Instead the number of decayed or filled surfaces in teeth present in the mouth can be measured and this method gives perhaps the most accurate measure of the extent of caries in adults in different communities. Three types of tooth sites were considered: smooth surface sites (mesial, distal, and buccal cervical), occlusal surfaces and pit sites (Jackson

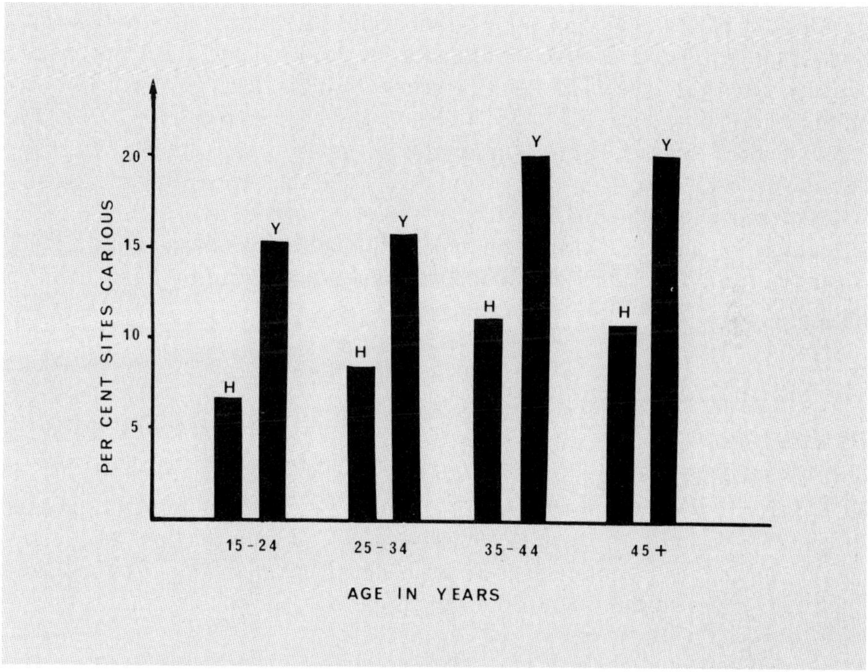

Fig. 3.18. The percentage number of decayed/filled sites in teeth present in the mouth of Hartlepool and York adults. (From Murray (1974).) (Reproduced by courtesy of the Editor of *Community Health*.)

et al. 1973). The increment in caries was virtually nil in persons aged 45 years and above. Thus in this age group permanent differences between Hartlepool and York can be observed. In persons aged 45 years and above 36 678 specified sites in the York population were examined; of these 7182 or approximately 20 per cent were carious. In Hartlepool 17 422 specified sites were examined and of these 1909 or approximately 11 per cent were carious. Thus in dentate persons aged 45 years and above the number of carious sites was 44 per cent lower in Hartlepool than it was in York. Data for the number of DF sites instanding teeth in 10-year age groups for the two communities is recorded diagrammatically in Fig. 3.18. Taking this information as a whole, it can be stated that fluoride in drinking water does not have a merely short-term delaying effect on the appearance of dental caries, but has substantial life-long caries-preventive effects.

Fluoridation and the law

Legislation authorizing water fluoridation is of two types. It may be mandatory, requiring a Ministry of Health or communities of a certain size to fluoridate their public water supplies, or the legislation may be permissive or enabling, giving the Ministry of Health or a local government the authority to institute fluoridation. Such legislation does not automatically bring about fluoridated water supplies but paves the way for health officials or units of local government to act on the matter.

Mandatory laws requiring fluoridation of public water supplies that are fluorine-deficient have been enacted in Brazil, Bulgaria, Greece, Ireland, and five states of the United States of America.

Examples of countries with enabling legislation are several states of the USA, Australia, German Democratic Republic, Israel, New Zealand, Canada, United Kingdom (Roemer 1983).

The Strathclyde fluoridation case

Background

In 1978 Strathclyde Regional Council, as a statutory water authority in Scotland, agreed to co-operate with local Health Boards by fluoridating water supplies for which they were responsible. Mrs Catherine McColl, a Glasgow citizen, applied for an interdict to restrain Strathclyde Regional Council from implementing its decision. The interdict was based on four main grounds:

1. Fluoridation would be *ultra vires*, i.e. beyond the legal powers of the Regional Council.
2. It would be a nuisance and, being a toxic substance, harmful to consumers, particularly in relation to cancer.
3. It would be a breach of the Water Act in that the Council would be failing in their duty to provide a supply of wholesome water.
4. It would be unlawful in that the Council would be providing a medicinal product for a medicinal purpose without having a product licence.

The hearings, held in the Court of Session, Edinburgh, commenced on 23 September 1980 and continued (after a few breaks) until 26 July 1982. The court sat on 201 days making it the longest and costliest case in Scottish legal history. The judge, Lord Jauncey, took almost 12 months to consider the massive evidence and gave his verdict on 29 June 1983. His judgement was contained in a 400 page document. He summarized his conclusions, in relation to the general topics which were canvassed in evidence, as follows.

Summary

'Before turning to consider the law it may be convenient to summarise my conclusions in relation to the general topics which were canvassed in evidence.

1. Fluoride at a concentration of 1 p.p.m. is not mutagenic.
2. No biochemical mechanism has been demonstrated whereby fluoride at a concentration of 1 p.p.m. is likely to cause cancer or accelerate existing cancerous growth.

3. No association between fluoridation of water supplies and increased CDRs (cancer death rates) in the consumers has been demonstrated.
4. There is no reason to anticipate that fluoride at a concentration of 1 p.p.m. is likely to have an adverse effect upon the migration of leucocytes in the consumer.
5. There is no reasonable likelihood that CRF (chronic renal failure) patients drinking water fluoridated to 1 p.p.m. will suffer harm.
6. Fluoridation of water supplies in Strathclyde would be likely to reduce considerably the incidence of caries.
7. Such fluoridation would be likely to produce a very small increase in the prevalence of dental mottling which would only be noticeable at very close quarters and would be very unlikely to create any aesthetic problems.
8. The present low levels of fluoride in the water supplies in Strathclyde do not cause caries.

I am not therefore prepared to make a finding that the present concentration of fluoride in the water in Strathclyde causes caries. However, I have no doubt that increasing the present concentrations to 1 p.p.m. would considerably reduce the incidence of that disease.'

(Opinion of Lord Jauncey, pp. 326–63)

He then dealt with the four questions of Law. Namely, (1) *ultra vires*; (2) nuisance; (3) breach of the Water (Scotland) Act 1980; and (4) breach of the Medicines Act 1968. He repelled the last three legal arguments but upheld that part of her case which claimed that water fluoridation was *ultra vires*.

The Judge's opinion on the legal point of *ultra vires* centred around the meaning of the work 'wholesome'. The relevant section of the Act provided 'it shall be the duty of every local authority to provide a supply of wholesome water in pipes to every part of their district where a supply of water is required for domestic purposes and can be provided at reasonable cost'.

The Judge considered in detail the judgement in the Lower Hutt Case in New Zealand, which had ruled in favour of fluoridation. He decided that

'the question is a narrow and difficult one but I consider that there are material differences between the circumstances in the Lower Hutt case and the present. . . . In my view the word 'wholesome' falls properly to be constructed in the more restricted sense advocated by the petitioner as relating to water which was free from contamination and pleasant to drink. It follows that fluoridation which in no way facilitates nor is incidental to the supply of such water is out with the powers of the respondents. The petitioner therefore succeeds on this branch of her case.'

The UK Government's response

The Government's response was given by the Secretary of State for Social Services.

'Fluoridation has been supported by successive Governments as a safe and effective public health measure and we consider that Lord Jauncey's opinion amply demonstrates that the Government should continue to support fluoridation as a positive means to promote good dental health. It is therefore the Government's intention, when the Parliamentary timetable permits, to bring forward legislation which will clarify the power of water authorities in Scotland to add fluoride to the water supply on the recommendation of the appropriate Health Boards.'

The Fluoridation Bill was laid before Parliament in February 1985. It passed through its last stage on 30th October 1985, supported by the leaders of all the main political parties, and received the Royal Assent. This legislation enables a health authority to make arrangements with a 'statutory water undertaker' to add fluoride to the water supply. The Bill requires the health authority, before implementing their proposal, to inform the public by publishing details in a newspaper and informing every local authority whose area falls wholly or partly within the area affected by the proposal.

Fluoridation and cancer: a review of the epidemiological evidence

A general review of the evidence on the health effects of the fluoridation of the water supplies was undertaken in the United Kingdom by the Committee of the Royal College of Physicians of London in 1976. The review concluded that fluoridation is safe, and in particular that there is no evidence that fluoride increases the incidence of mortality in any organ. Since the College Committee reported the results a number of new epidemiological investigations have become available, and the authors of some of the studies have claimed that increased cancer rates are associated with fluoridation. The Department of Health and Social Security set up a working party under the Chairmanship of Professor Knox 'to reappraise the published and other available data and conclusions on cancer incidence and mortality amongst populations whose drinking water is either artificially fluoridated or contains high levels of fluoride from natural sources.' The report was published in 1985 (Knox, 1985).

The study reviewed data from twelve countries and concluded:

(1) 'We have found nothing in any of the major classes of epidemiological evidence which could lead us to conclude that either fluoride occurring naturally in water, or fluoride added to water supplies, is capable of inducing cancer, or of increasing the mortality from cancer. This statement applies both to cancer as a whole, and to cancer at a large number of specific sites. In this we concur with the great majority of scientific investigators and commentators in this field. The only contrary conclusions are in our view attributable to errors in data, errors in analytical technique, and errors in scientific logic.

(2) The evidence permits us to comment positively on the safety of fluoridated water in this respect. The absence of demonstrable effects on cancer rates in the face of long-term exposures to naturally elevated levels of fluoride in water: the absence of any demonstable effect on cancer rates following the artificial fluoridation of water supplies: the large human populations observed: the consistency of the findings from many different sources of data in many different countries: lead us to conclude that in this respect the fluoridation of drinking water is safe.'

Fluoride tablets and drops

There is no doubt that when a central piped water supply serves a large population it is simple and inexpensive to fluoridate the drinking water. However, when there are a multiplicity of sources the implementation of water fluoridation may not be practicable. In addition, there are many communities throughout the world which do not have piped water supplies. Other vehicles for fluoride, particularly tablets and drops, have been recommended for over 40 years.

Over fifty reports on the effectiveness of fluoride tablets or drops have appeared in the literature, although some of these are difficult to interpret because of the small size of the test group, the short experimental period, or inadequate reporting. The remaining investigations fall into two groups: first, those where the fluoride supplements were given daily at home and were started before school age; and second, those where tablets have been distributed in school, on school days only, usually without additional supplementations during holidays or before school age. The effectiveness of the use of fluoride tablets at home is very much harder to investigate because it is difficult to choose a comparable control group and there is frequently a marked fall off in co-operation; these difficulties do not usually arise in school-based trials. An excellent review of the effectiveness of fluoride tablets is given by Driscoll (1974) and Tables 3.15 and 3.16 are based on this report, but with additional recent data.

Deciduous teeth

Summaries of 20 trials into the effect of fluoride tablets on the deciduous dentition are given in Table 3.15. Twelve were conducted in Europe, five in the United States, and three in Australia. Sodium fluoride was used in all but one study (although the compound used was not stated in a further one study), sometimes in combination with vitamins.

The initial age of the subjects and the length of time the tablets were taken varied considerably, making it difficult to draw accurate conclusions on effectiveness. Nevertheless, it would appear that a caries-preventive effect was consistently observed (about 50–80 per cent reduction) in studies where the initial age was 2 years or younger. In the three studies in which no effect was found, the children were initially aged 3 years or older. In a more thorough analysis of effectiveness in relation to the age at which ingestion of tablets began, Granath *et al.* (1978) suggested that while buccolingual surfaces may benefit if the commencement age is over 2 years, the effect on approximal surfaces is very much less if the commencement age is 2 years or over. This suggests that the topical effect is greater on the more exposed buccolingual surfaces than on the less accessible approximal surfaces.

The study of Hennon *et al.* (1977) is the only clinical trial of fluoride tablets conducted in an area with an almost optimal water fluoride level (0.6–0.8 p.p.m. F) although the observations of Glenn (1979) were on children living

Table 3.15. Caries-preventive effects of fluoride tablets/drops in deciduous teeth. (Based on some references from Driscoll (1974) and Binder *et al.* (1978))

Reference	F compound	Daily dosage (mg)	Initial age of subjects (years)	Number of subjects in F group	Duration of F intake (years)	Caries reduction (%) deft	Caries reduction defs	Statistical significance
Arnold *et al.* (1960)	NaF	0.5–1	birth–6	121	1–12	'comparable to water F'		NR
Pollak (1960)‖	NaF + V	1	3	100	2	80		NR
	NaF + V	1	4	111	2	20		NR
Ziemnowicz-Clowaka (1960)‖	NaF	0.8	3	139	2		26	S
Lutomska and Kominska (1962)‖	Naf	0.6	3–4	154	2	'no significant effect'		NR
Kamocka *et al.* (1964)‖	NaF	0.75*	3	64	3	0		NS
	NaF	0.75*	4	79	3	0		NS
Leonhardt (1965)‖	NaF + V	1 +	3	?	2	38		NR
	NaF + V	1 +	4	?	2	30		NR
Hennon *et al.* (1966, 1967, 1970)	NaF + V	0.5–1	birth–5½	85	3		63	S
	NaF + V	0.5–1	birth–5½	54	4		68	S
	NaF + V	0.5–1	birth–5½	60	5		66	S
Margolis *et al.* (1975)	NaF + V	0.5–1	birth	149	4–6	76		S
	NaF + V	0.5–1	4	77	0–2	29		NS
Hoskova (1968)	NaF	0.25–1	prenatal	78	4	93		S
	NaF + V	0.25–1	birth–1	151	4	54		S
Kailis *et al.* (1968)	NaF	?	prenatal	50	4–6	82		S
	NaF	?	birth	92	4–6	56		S
Stolte (1968)‖	?	1	3	130	3	11		NR

Pritchard (1969)	NaF	?	prenatal	176	6–8	70		S
	NaF	?	birth	282	6–8	40		S
Hamberg (1971)	NaF + V (drops)	0.5	birth	342	3	57		NR
	NaF + V (drops)	0.5	birth	342	6	49		NR
Kraemer (1971)‖	CaF_2	1	4	170	2	22		NR
	CaF_2	1	5	82	2	18		NR
Schutzmannsky (1971)	NaF	1	prenatal	100	<1	13	S	
	NaF	0.25–1	prenatal	100	9	30		S
	NaF	0.25–1	birth	100	9	14		S
Aasenden and Peebles (1974)	NaF + V†	0.5–1	birth	87	8–11		78	S
Fanning *et al.* (1975)	NaF	?	<1	581	5	33		NR
Andersson and Grahnen (1976)	NaF	0.25–0.5	1	127	5†	31		S
Hennon *et al.* (1977)§	NaF + V	0.5–1	<1	44	5		47	S
	NaF + V	0.5	<1	47	5		37	S
Granath *et al.* (1978)	NaF	0.25–0.5	<2	48	2–4		46 BL	NS
							51 AP	S
	NaF	0.25–0.5	2–3	123	1–2		33 BL	NS
							−1 AP	NS

V = vitamins; S = statistically significant; NS = statistically non-significant; NR = no statistical test reported; BL = buccolingual; AP = approximal surfaces.

* Tablets given only on school days.

† A NaF + V combination was given up to three years of age. Beyond this age, some children received NaF + V while others received only NaF.

‡ Aged 8–10 at examination.

§ In F area (0.6–0.8 p.p.m. F).

‖ Quoted by Driscoll (1974).

Table 3.16. Caries-preventive effects of fluoride tablets on permanent teeth. (Based on some references from Driscoll (1974) and Binder *et al.* (1978))

Reference	F compound	Daily dosage (mg)	Initial age of subjects (years)	Number of subjects in F group	Duration of F intake (years)	Caries reduction (%) DMFT	DMFS	Statistical significance
Stones *et al.* (1949)	NaF	1.5	6–14	125	2	0		NS
Bibby *et al.* (1955)	NaF	1	5–14	133	1		Nil	NR
	NaF	1	5–14	119	1		tentative finding: 'possible'	NR
Niedenthal (1957)§	NaF	1*	6–7	251	3	22		NR
Wrzodek (1959)§	NaF	1*	6–9	8381	3	21		NR
	NaF	1*	6–9	13 585	4	22		NR
Arnold *et al.* (1960)	NaF	0.5–1	birth–6	121	1–15	'comparable to water F'		NR
Krusic (1960)§	CaF_2	?	8–15	480	1–3	70		NR
Pollak (1960)§	NaF + V	1	6–7	300	2	38		NR
Ziemnowicz-Glowaka (1960)§	NaF	0.8*	3–6	704	2		33	S
	NaF	0.8*	5–6	204	3		28	S
Jez (1962)§	CaF_2	?	7–11	7200	$2\frac{1}{2}$	0		NR
Krychalska-Karwan and Laskowa (1963)§	NaF	?	grammar school	134	4		5	NR
Minoguchi *et al.* (1963)	NaF + V	0.25	birth–6	75	6	36		NR
Grissom *et al.* (1964)	NaF	1*	6–11	178	2		34	S
Kamocka *et al.* (1964)§	NaF	0.75*	3	64	3	17		NS
	NaF	0.75*	4	79	3	60		S
Leonhardt (1964)	NaF	1	6	398	4	32		NR
	NaF	1	7	429	3	25		NR
Hippchen (1965)§	?	1	6	500	3	32		NR

Schützmannsky (1965)	NaF	0.75*	6	580	4		25	NR
	NaF	0.75*	6	197	6		27	NR
Berner *et al.* (1967)	NaF	0.5–1*	5–7	105	3		84 (except 1st molar)	NR
							33 (1st molar)	NR
	NaF	1*	7–9	158	4	16		NR
	NaF	1*	7–9	160	6	20		NR
	NaF	1*	7–9	109	7	24		NR
De Paola and Lax (1968)	APF	1*	6–8	130	2		23	S
Girardi-Vogt (1968)§	NaF	1	6	?	3	31		NR
Stolte (1968)§	?	1	3	150	3	69		NR
Marthaler (1969)	NaF	0.5–1*	7	450	1–8	36	47	S
Hamberg (1971)	NaF + V	0.5	birth	342	7	70		NR
Schützmannsky (1971)	NaF	1	prenatal	100	<1	6		NS
	NaF	0.25–1	prenatal	100	9	43		S
	NaF	0.25–1	birth	100	9	39		S
Aasenden *et al.* (1972)	APF	1*	8–11	109	3		30	S
	NaF	1*	8–11	114	3		27	S
Plasschaert and Konig (1974)	NaF	1	7	208	2		38	S
Aasenden and Peebles (1974)	NaF + V†	0.5–1	birth	100	8–11		80	S
Binder (1974)	NaF	0.25–1	birth–14	3084	8–14	43		S
Margolis *et al.* (1975)	NaF + V	0.5–1	birth	56	7–10	58		S
	NaF + V	0.5–1	4	31	3–6	14		NS
Andersson and Grahnen (1976)	NaF	0.25–0.5	1	127	5‡		40	S
Stephen and Campbell (1978)	NaF	1*	5½	54	3		81	S
Driscoll *et al.* (1978)	APF	1*	6–7	150	6		28	S
	APF	2*	6–7	135	6		29	S

V = vitamins; S = statistically significant; NS = statistically non-significant; NR = no statistical test reported.
* Tablets given only on school days.
† A NaF + V combination was given up to three years of age. Beyond this age, some children received NaF + V while other received only NaF.
‡ Aged 8–12 at examination.
§ Quoted by Driscoll (1974).

in a fluoridated community. A substantial preventive effect was observed by Henon *et al.* in the children taking fluoride tablets, in addition to the benefit that could be expected to be derived from living in an area with a moderate water fluoride level. In their study one group of children received 0.5 mg F from birth throughout the 5 year trial period while another group received 0.5 mg F up to 3 years of age and 1 mg for the remaining 2 years. The effect was slightly greater (47 per cent reduction compared with 37 per cent) in the latter group.

Permanent teeth

Summaries of investigations into the effectiveness of fluoride tablets in preventing caries in the permanent dentition are given in Table 3.16; again, most of the studies are European. The initial age of the subjects and the duration of fluoride tablet intake varied widely. In only four of the studies (Hamberg 1971; Schützmannsky 1971; Aasenden and Peebles 1974; Margolis *et al.* 1975) were fluoride tablets taken from birth for at least 7 years. Reductions ranged from 39 per cent in Schützmannsky's trial to 80 per cent in the trial of Aasenden and Peebles. In the trial of Margolis *et al.* the children who started taking fluoride tablets at birth showed a 58 per cent reduction in DFT compared with only a 14 per cent reduction in the group of children who started at the age of 4 years, suggesting the importance of ingestion in the first few years of life, before the permanent teeth erupted.

In the four studies conducted in school (initial age 6–7 years) and lasting at least 5 years, the following reductions in caries have been reported: 27 per cent (Schützmannsky 1965), 20–24 per cent (Berner *et al.* 1967), 36 per cent (Marthaler 1969), and 28–29 per cent (Driscoll *et al.* 1978). The only study conducted in the United Kingdom was by Stephen and Campbell (1978) where an 81 per cent reduction was reported after a 3 year trial in Glasgow children initially aged 5½ years.

Pre-natal

Six trials have investigated the effectiveness of the ingestion of pre-natal fluoride tablets, although results of only four of these are given in Tables 3.15 and 3.16, because in the remaining two (Feltman and Kosel 1961; Glenn 1979) insufficient data were reported. In all these trials the per cent caries reduction was greater in the children whose mothers received fluoride tablets in pregnancy. But in spite of the apparent greater benefit of pre-natal fluoride, Hoskova (1968) concluded that fluoride administration should begin as soon after birth as possible, attributing the greater benefit to better home conditions in the pre-natal group. Feltman and Kosel (1961) compared the caries experience of 672 children who had received (i) only pre-natal supplements (162 children); (ii) pre- and post-natal supplements (228 children); and (iii) only post-natal tablets from varying ages (282 children). Pre-natal fluoride appeared to confer benefit additional to that derived from post-natal fluoride exposure. The trial of Schützmannsky (1971) was better reported and also had three groups: a pre-natal fluoride-only group, a pre- and post-natal (for 9 years) group, and a post-natal fluoride only group (also for 9 years). The per cent reductions for deciduous teeth were 13, 30, and 14 per cent respectively (Table 3.15) and 6, 43, and 39 per cent respectively for permanent teeth (Table 3.16), suggesting that a small benefit may be derived from pre-natal fluoride ingestion particularly in the deciduous dentition.

Summary of effectiveness of fluoride tablets and drops

From the results of published trials it would seem that there is no doubt that the use of fluoride tablets or drops are effective in preventing dental caries in both the deciduous and permanent dentitions. The effectiveness would seem to be greater the earlier the child began to take the fluoride supplement—from 40–80 per cent reduction being expected in both deciduous and permanent dentitions if supplementation was commenced before 2 years of age. For school-based schemes the effectiveness would appear to be lower and more variable (30–80 per cent reduction). NaF would appear to be the compound of choice, but the data are insufficient to judge whether the size of the daily dose influences effectiveness.

Results of the home-based trials have to be interpreted with caution, for the attitude to dental health of the mothers who gave their children supplements from birth is likely to be more favourable than mothers who began supplementation later or who formed the control group.

It has to be admitted that daily administration of tablets at home from birth (or pre-natally) requires a very high level of parental motivation, and campaigns to get parents to give their children fluoride supplements have not been successful in the United Kingdom. Smyth and Withnell (1974) reported that when parents of 3500 pre-schoolchildren in Gloucestershire were asked to give their chidren fluoride tablets, only 759 (22 per cent) entered the scheme and only 70 of these (2 per cent of those originally invited) were still giving tablets at the end of 9 months, despite widespread publicity and subsidy of the cost of the tablets. Silver (1974, 1982) found that only 6–10 per cent of 3 year-olds in Hertfordshire were consuming fluoride tablets despite their widespread recommendation and availability. The acceptability of school-based tablet or programmes would appear to be much better (Driscoll *et al.* 1977; Poulsen *et al.* 1981).

School-water fluoridation

Two advantages of water fluoridation are that, no effort is required by the recipients and, secondly, that the cost per person is low. However, the cost per person increases as the size of the population served by each fluoridation plant decreases. It was therefore of interest to see whether fluoridation of a school's water supply was effective and economical. Unlike other school-based preventive programmes no action is required by the children. As yet school water fluoridation has been tested only in the United States where 40 million people live in areas without community water supplies and many rural schools are supplied by their own well. By the end of 1976, 125 000 children attending 400 schools in 13 states were benefiting from school fluoridation programmes (Jenny and Heifetz 1978).

The first investigations began in 1954 in the Virgin Islands with fluoridation of the water supply at two schools at a level of 2.3 p.p.m. F. Because one of the schools was altered and enlarged during the study and operation of the machinery was intermittent and eventually broke down, the study cannot be considered satisfactory. In 1962, 7–13-year-old children in the school receiving the more consistent supply of fluoridated water (for 8 years) were examined together with children attending the fluoridated school and had about 22 per cent less DMFT than the control children, at least indicating that school-water fluoridation might be beneficial (Horowitz *et al.* 1965).

Since then three major studies each planned to last 12 years have been undertaken in mainland United States. The first two, in Pike County (Kentucky) and Elk Lake (Pennsylvania) began in 1958, while the third, in Seagrove (North Carolina), began in 1968 with final examinations planned for 1980. In Elk Lake, the final examinations (after 12 years) took place in 1970, but this was not possible in Pike County where the organization at the two test schools changed and school fluoridation ceased after the 8-year follow-up examination in 1966.

In the Pike County Schools, water was fluoridated at 3.0 p.p.m. (or 3.3 times the optimum level for public water supplies in the same area), while in the Elk Lake schools the water fluoride level was 5 p.p.m. (or 4.5 times the optimum public water supply level). These levels were chosen because children consume only part of their daily water intake as school and only attend school a maximum of about 200 days per year. In addition children do not enter school before 6 years, an age when incisor teeth can be considered no longer at risk of developing mottled enamel. As no objectionable mottling was observed in any teeth in the children attending the Pike County and Elk Lake schools, a higher fluoride level (6.3 p.p.m. or seven times the optimal community water fluoride level) was tested in the third American study in Seagrove. In all three of these studies children in the test schools were examined before fluoridation of the school's water supply began, and the results of these base-line examinations then served as control data for comparison with the results of the surveys after 4, 8 and 12 years school fluoridation.

Results after 8 years of school fluoridation in Pike County and Elk Lake (Horowitz *et al.* 1968) showed that children who had continually attended schools in the two study areas had very similar reductions in DMFT of about 33 and 35 per cent respectively compared with similarly aged children who attended these schools before fluoridation began.

In summary, fluoridation of school water supplies is technically feasible, results in a substantial reduction in caries experience in school-children, and the cost of this public health measure is low (about US $1.5 per person per year) (Horowitz and Heifetz 1979). In the opinion of Heifetz *et al.* (1978), from the results so far, the slightly bigger benefit achieved with 6.3 p.p.m. F is not suffi-

Table 3.17. Caries experience (deft) for 6-year-old children living in test and control communities in Hungary after 8 years salt fluoridation (at 250 mg F/kg). (From Toth (1976))

	Experimental	Control
1966	6.8	8.6
1974	4.1	9.2
Difference	−2.7 (−39.5%	+0.6 (+7.1%)

ciently greater than that observed with 5 p.p.m. F to warrant the higher fluoride level, and they therefore recommend school fluoridation at the lower level of 5 p.p.m. F, or 4.5 times the optimum level of fluoridation of community water supplies in that locality.

Fluoridized salt

As a dietary vehicle for ensuring adequate ingestion of fluoride, domestic salt comes second to drinking water. The enrichment of salt with iodide already provides an effective means of preventing goitre. Indeed it was a medical practitioner concerned with the prevention of goitre in Switzerland who, over 30 years ago, pioneered the addition of fluoride to salt as a caries preventive measure (Wespi 1948, 1950). Fluoridated salt has been on sale in Switzerland since 1955, and, by 1967, three-quarters of domestic salt sold in Switzerland was fluoridated at 90 mg F/kg salt (or 90 p.p.m. F). However, it was soon accepted that the original estimates of salt intake, upon which calculations of fluoride concentrations in salt were based, were too high and the ingestion of fluoride too low. In more recent investigations the level of fluoride has been raised to 200, 250, and 350 mg F/kg salt, with enhanced effectiveness. Toth (1976, 1980) has suggested that the urinary fluoride concentration is the most accurate guide for estimating fluoride intake in communities using fluoridated salt. From these results he concluded that, in Hungary, 250 mg F/kg provides too low a fluoride intake compared with optimally fluoridated water and is therefore currently testing 350 mg F/kg salt.

Despite the widespread use of fluoridized salt in Switzerland, its effectiveness is not easily measured because, in many Swiss communities, other preventive programmes have been introduced in addition to fluoridated salt. However, Marthaler *et al.* (1977, 1978) concluded that the caries-preventive effectiveness of 250 mg F/kg salt used in the Swiss canton of Vaud was greater than the 25 per cent or so reduction observed following the addition of 90 mg F/kg in other Swiss Cantons (Marthaler and Schenardi 1962).

Toth (1976) reported the effectiveness of 250 mg F/kg salt fluoridized in Hungary after 8 years use. The results (Table 3.17) indicated a reduction of 39 per cent in deft in 6-year-old children in the test community, while caries experience increased by 7 per cent in the control community children over the same period. Although there was an imbalance in caries experience between the two

Table 3.18. Caries experience (DMFT) for 8-year-old children living in three test communities and one control community in Columbia, South America, after 8 years. (From Mejia *et al.* (1976))

	NaF salt	CaF_2 salt	Water F	Control
1964	3.7	3.8	3.8	4.3
1972	1.4	1.1	0.8	3.8
Difference	2.3	2.7	3.0	0.5
	(61%)	(72%)	(78%)	(13%)

communities at the start of the experiment in 1966, this alone could not explain the differences observed in 1974. After 10 years exposure to fluoridized salt, Toth (1979) observed that 4–6-year-olds in the same test community had 2.8 deft, compared with 6.0 deft in the control community, and 1.4 deft in children of the same age living in an area with fluoridated water. These 10-year results indicated that a substantial caries reduction occurred after the introduction of fluoridized salt but this was less than occurred with water fluoridation. No results are yet available from the studies testing 350 mg F/kg salt in Hungary.

In 1964, a well-planned study was initiated in four Colombian communities (Mejia *et al.* 1976). In the village of Montebello, sodium fluoride was added to domestic salt (at 200 mg F/kg), while in Armenia calcium fluoride was added to domestic salt (at 200 mg F/kg), in San Pedro drinking water was fluoridated (at 1 p.p.m. F), and Don Matias remained as the control community. At the end of the project, after 8 years, reductions in caries prevalence and experience in 8-year-old children were large in the three communities receiving fluoride in salt or water, although a small reduction was also observed in the control town (Table 3.18). When all children aged 6–14 years were included in the data analyses, the reduction in DMFT between 1964 and 1972 was 50 per cent in Montebello (NaF in salt), 48 per cent in Armenia (CaF_2 in salt), 60 per cent in San Pedro (water F), and 5 per cent in the control town Don Matias.

The caries preventive effectiveness of fluoridated salt is substantial, although it appears to be slightly less than that observed with fluoridated water. This view is based on a comparatively small number of studies, compared with the data on water fluoridation, and which have lasted for a maximum of 10 years. From urinary analyses data, it is possible that doses tested so far (up to 250 mg F/kf) are sub-optimal and results of trials of higher doses are awaited with interest to see whether the effectiveness approaches that achieved by water fluoridation. Salt appears to be a safe vehicle for fluoride administration (Mühlemann 1967; Ruzicka *et al.* 1976). Fluoridized salt uses only 3 per cent of the quantity of fluoride required for water fluoridation (Toth 1978) but has the same advantage that no personal effort is needed by the public.

Fluoridized milk and fruit juices

Both bovine and human milk contain low levels of fluoride—about 0.03 p.p.m. F

(Ericsson and Ribelius 1971). Because milk is recommended as a good food for infants and children, it was considered, over 20 years ago, to be a suitable vehicle for supplementing children's fluoride intake in areas with fluoride-deficient water supplies. Ericsson (1958) showed that fluoride was absorbed in the gut just as readily from milk as from water, refuting the suggestion that the high calcium content of milk would render the fluoride unavailable. However, the binding of added fluoride to calcium or protein might reduce the topical fluoride effect in the mouth compared with fluoride in water (Duff 1981).

Despite its potential promise, only three studies have been reported. Although all three indicated that the addition of fluoride to milk might have a caries-preventive effect, the first two studies can be criticized in certain respects. The study of Rosoff *et al.* (1962) involved 171 children aged 6–9 years from two schools in Louisiana, USA. Children from one school received $\frac{1}{2}$ pint of homogenized milk daily fortified with 2.2 mg NaF (yielding 1 mg F). Children in the control group received homogenized milk without fluoride. This pilot study lasted $3\frac{1}{2}$ years, when 65 children aged 9–12 years remained in the fluoride group, and 64 children of similar age in the control group. Unfortunately the two groups were not well balanced with respect to first-molar caries experience at the beginning of the experiment. The DMFT in second molars and first and second premolars, after $3\frac{1}{2}$ years consumption of fluoridated milk, was 0.34 in the fluoride group and 1.70 in the control group. However, because of the considerable divergence in caries attack on first molars between groups before the study and the small size of the groups, the lower caries rate in the experimental children must be viewed with caution. The data indicated that some of the effect was likely to be topical.

Ziegler (1962) reported his attempts to introduce fluoridized milk in Winterthur, Switzerland. The results of clinical surveys indicated that dental caries was lower in children who had consumed the fluoridated milk for 6 years, compared with control children (Wirz and Ziegler 1964, quoted in WHO 1970).

Davis (1975) has reported that clinical studies of fluoridized milk have been conducted in Germany and Japan, but as yet no details of these studies are available. In an abstract, Stephen *et al.* (1981) reported that consumption of 200 ml of milk containing 1.5 mg F each school day for 4 years reduced the occurrence of caries in first permanent molars in Glaswegian primary schoolchildren by 34 per cent. The 49 test children had a mean of 1.7 DMFT (first permanent molars) at the age of 9 years, compared with 2.4 DMFT in the 59 control children who also drank 200 ml of milk each school day but with no added fluoride.

In warm climates, fluoridized fruit juices may be a practical alternative to fluoridated milk. Gedalia *et al.* (1981) have recently reported a 28 per cent reduction in DMFS increment in 6–9-year-old Israeli children who consumed 1 mg F in 100 ml of pure orange juice (= 10 p.p.m. F) each school day for 3 years. The 111 test group children developed 2.5 DMFS over 3 years compared with 3.5 DMFS in the 111 control children who had no beverage. However, interpretation of the results was complicated by the observation that a third group of similarly aged children, who consumed 100 ml of orange juice with no added fluoride, developed 2.9 DMFS over the 3 year period. It would appear, therefore, that the fluoride *per se* might have been responsible for only part of the difference between the fluoride-drink group and the no-drink group.

In summary, although milk and fruit juices are possible vehicles for fluoride, clinical data are limited. In addition, intake of milk varies widely and methods previously tested have required parental or school effort. It would therefore seem that fluoridized salt would appear to be a more promising alternative to water fluoridation in areas unable to implement the latter.

Topical fluoride

For over 40 years fluorides applied topically to the teeth in a variety of ways have been regarded as important caries-preventive measures. Amongst the vehicles employed to apply the fluoride compounds, aqueous solutions, gels, and dentifrices are the most commonly used. Many studies have been carried out in numerous parts of the world to measure the caries-preventive effect of these compounds. Widely differing findings have been reported, largely due to the differences in experimental design, study population, methods of administration of the agent, and to examiner variability. However, it is reasonable to accept that topical applications of fluoride do not match the efficiency of fluoridated drinking water consumed during the period of tooth development and maturation. Many studies designed to test topical fluoride effectiveness express the findings in terms of percentage reductions. For obvious reasons such a method of expression can be grossly misleading in terms of the actual number of tooth surfaces protected. For example, a 50 per cent reduction occurs when the caries increment falls from 10 to 5 and when it falls from 1 to 0.5. Clearly the former reduction is clinically relevant, whereas the latter is probably not.

The value of topical fluorides was first suggested by Miller (1938) before the definitive studies of Dean and his colleagues had been fully reported. Miller, using a rat-caries model, demonstrated that caries in already erupted teeth was inhibited by fluoride incorporated into the diet. Volker and his colleagues (1940) carried out laboratory experiments which showed that enamel and fluoride ions reacted together chemically and by so doing significantly reduced the solubility of the enamel in acid solution. Soon afterwards Volker and Bibby (1941) noted a reduction in caries of anterior teeth washed by fluoride-containing water, and argued that the added protection was due to an increased uptake of fluoride associated with the more intimate contact of these teeth with the F ion. This observation led Bibby (1942) to carry out the first clinical study to assess the value of topical fluoride applications.

Topical fluorides fall into two categories: those applied by the dentist in the surgery and those applied by the patient at home. In practice those employed by the dentist are of high fluoride concentration and are applied generally at regular but infrequent intervals, perhaps twice a year. Those used by the patient are of low fluoride levels and are applied at frequent intervals, often daily.

Fluorides applied by the dentist

Such fluoride agents mainly include simple aqueous solutions of sodium fluoride and stannous fluoride, and low pH solutions and gels of an acidulated phosphate fluoride system. Other agents comprise fluoride prophylaxis pastes and fluoride-containing varnishes.

Sodium and stannous fluoride solutions

The first clinical study in this group was reported by Bibby (1942) in which a 0.1 per cent aqueous solution of sodium fluoride was applied to cleaned and dried teeth of one quadrant for 7–8 minutes three times a year. After 2 years the caries increments in the test quadrant was of the order of 35 per cent less than in the untreated control quadrant.

A number of further trials using sodium fluoride were carried out during and immediately after the Second World War, which culminated in the classical studies by Knutson and his colleagues (1946, 1948). These involved use of the much higher concentration of 2 per cent sodium fluoride applied repeatedly at ages in a child's life which coincided with eruption of teeth. In practice the 'Knutson technique' included thorough cleaning and drying of the teeth followed by four 3-minute applications of the solution at weekly intervals at ages 3, 7, 10, and 13 years. Reductions in new caries when control and experimental groups were compared were in the order of 30 per cent. Subsequent studies using the Knutson technique generally confirmed this beneficial effect although the level of reduction varied from 4.9 per cent (Jordon *et al.* 1946) to 58 per cent (Davies 1958). Despite a further interesting study by Galagan and Knutson (1948), which showed that a 1 per cent solution of sodium fluoride was just as effective as the 2 per cent solution, it is the 2 per cent aqueous solution that enjoyed widespread acclaim. As is the case in virtually all clinical studies designed to test the efficiency of a topical fluoride procedure, the finding applies only to the short periods of time. There is no reliable evidence of the value of these procedures over periods in excess of 4 years at the most. It is not known whether the preventive effect gradually diminishes nor whether they merely postpone the onset of disease by say 3 or 4 years.

At the same time that Knutson and his colleagues were completing their sodium fluoride studies, Muhler and his colleagues were carrying out studies *in vitro* in an attempt to identify more effective topically applied fluoride compounds. Amongst the findings which emerged from these experiments was that stannous fluoride was three times more effective than sodium fluoride in inhibiting enamel dissolution by weak acids. Further it was shown that rats fed on specific caries-producing diets developed fewer cavities when drinking water containing 10 p.p.m. stannous fluoride than when drinking water containing

10 p.p.m. sodium fluoride (Muhler and Day 1950). During the 1950s and 1960s a number of clinical studies were carried out by several groups of workers which attempted to evaluate regimens of topically applied 8 and 10 per cent stannous fluoride solutions. There was considerable disparity in the reported findings, which varied from a 51 per cent reduction in caries over a 1 year period (Mercer and Muhler 1961) to a zero reduction over 2 years (Horowitz and Lucye 1966). Direct comparison of the various studies is ill-advised as generally they differ in such fundamental aspects as number and age of subjects, experimental and control regimens, and diagnostic criteria.

One major disadvantage associated with stannous fluoride is its chemical instability in solution, which requires a fresh solution to be made each time an application is carried out. A further disadvantage of stannous fluoride is that it causes a brown extrinsic stain to be formed on the teeth especially in association with margins of restorations and areas of enamel hypocalcification. Such stain is mildly disfiguring and in clinical studies could be responsible for the introduction of examiner bias.

Acidulated agents

The fact that fluoride uptake by enamel is enhanced by lowering the pH was first reported by Bibby (1947). However, it was not until 1963 that Brudevold and his colleagues confirmed that prolonged exposure of enamel to a 1.23 per cent fluoride solution acidulated by means of acid sodium phosphate enhanced the uptake of fluoride by enamel. Initial clinical studies (Wellock *et al.* 1963, 1965) produced highly favourable results with caries reductions matching those found in the case of water fluoridation. Indeed, at the conclusion of a 2-year study employing annual applications of the 1.23 per cent acidulated phosphofluoride solution a 67 per cent reduction in DMF teeth and 70 per cent reduction in DMF surfaces compared with the untreated control group were reported. In a further report by the same group, (Parmeijer *et al.* 1963), it was shown that application of orthophosphate acidulated fluoride solution to one half of a mouth caused 50 per cent fewer cavities than in the other half which had been treated with neutral sodium fluoride. Thus it would appear that the superiority of the acidulated fluoride solution over the neutral solution was established.

Further studies generally confirmed the caries-preventive effectiveness of acidulate phosphofluoride solutions but the extent of the reductions demonstrated did not match the original levels shown by Brudevold and his colleagues. In the development of caries-preventive agents this is by no means unique. Part explanation may be that in an original study the test group is small, comprising subjects who co-operate fully and so allow meticulous execution of the technique of application, whereas, in a full study, the numbers will be larger, some of the subjects will be less co-operative and the technique of application may fall short of ideal. It is the difference between a study conducted under laboratory conditions and a study carried out in the community at large. A major clinical problem in the use of topical fluoride solutions in young children is the control of the salivary flow during the recommended 4-minute period when the teeth have to remain soaked in the fluoride solution. This is especially difficult with APF solution which, because of its acidic nature, stimulates profuse salivary flow. Furthermore, accidental swallowing of even small volumes of solution can initiate a feeling of nausea or even vomiting. To attempt to overcome these problems various trays have been designed involving use of absorbent linings to carry the solution to the teeth. Such trays certainly help and have the added advantage that one arch rather than a single quadrant can be treated at a time. However, they are cumbersome and one can never be certain that the solution is reaching the areas where it is most needed, i.e. the approximal surfaces. Many of the problems associated with solutions were overcome by the introduction of gels which involved the addition to the solution of a gelling agent such as methyl or hydroxyethyl cellulose. In order to produce a 'smooth' gel it is essential to employ the correct grade of cellulose. The APF gel is a much simpler agent to use and, if it is used in a personalized tray, several advantages pertain. First, the gel does not spill into the mouth and cause excess salivation and nausea; second, the gel, which has thixotropic properties, can be forced into the less accessible areas of the tooth such as the approximal surfaces; and third, less gel is used, thus achieving an economy in the use of an expensive agent.

A considerable number of clinical studies have tested the efficacy of acidulated phosophofluoride gels. Almost all demonstrate a beneficial effect, though the magnitude of the reductions varied markedly. The reason for these variations is almost certainly multifactorial, depending *inter alia* on the age of the subjects, the quality of technique employed, the duration of the study, the frequency of application, and the level of disease experience in the community from which the subjects were taken. In general terms, however, one might reasonably expect caries reductions in the area of 20–40 per cent, with annual or semi-annual applications.

Fluoride varnishes

Based on the premise that a longer duration and more intimate contact between fluoride ions and enamel leads to a higher fluoride uptake by the enamel, a series of lacquers and varnishes containing fluoride in various forms has been formulated. Three materials have been used in clinical trials: Duraphat, Elmex Protector, and Epoxylite 9070.

Duraphat, was first used by Heuser and Schmidt (1968). This fluoride varnish yields 2.26 per cent F^- from a suspension of sodium fluoride in an alcoholic solution of natural varnish substances. The manufacturers claim that it is remarkably water-tolerant, so that it covers even moist teeth with a well-adhering film of varnish. Riethe and Weinmann (1970), using 75 Osborne–Mendel rats, reported that both Duraphat and an amine fluoride gel showed similar short-term caries inhibitory properties. Amine fluoride 297, similar to that used in Reithe and Weinmann's study, had a self-polymerizing polyurethane varnish added to it and was marketed under the name of Elmex Protector. Although amine fluoride has been shown to have caries-inhibitory properties when incorporated in a tooth paste (Marthaler 1968), no large-scale clinical studies have been carried out to determine whether Elmex Protector has a caries-preventive effect. Rock (1974), in a 2-year study involving 100 children aged 11–13 years, concluded that this material was ineffective as a caries-preventive agent; after 2 years, 19.3 per cent of test teeth and 20.5 per cent of control teeth became carious.

Epoxylite 9070 has been described as a long-lasting topical fluoride coating. The type of fluoride used in this preparation is disodium monofluorophosphate, which is incorporated into a soft, flexible, polyurethane-based adhesive coating. Rock (1972), in a 1-year study of 11–13-year-old children, reported that Epoxylite 9070 produced no significant reduction in the incidence of occlusal caries between test and control group.

Following the early work on Duraphat by Heuser and Schmidt (1968), the clinical potential of this material has been tested in two main ways. The fluoride content of surface enamel after topical application of Duraphat has been measured *in vitro* and *in vivo*, and the inhibition of caries in children taking part in clinical trials where Duraphat has been applied annually or semi-annually has been assessed. This combination of both clinical and laboratory investigation can be regarded as a microcosm of the research activity into topical fluoride therapy.

In an *in vitro* study, Koch and Petersson (1972) measured the uptake of fluoride by enamel treated with Duraphat for 1–12 hours, using 20 non-carious premolars extracted for orthodontic reasons. The highest concentrations of fluoride were found in the outermost layer. In the experimental group the mean concentration in this layer ranged between 3800 and 2250 p.p.m. F compared with about 1150 p.p.m. F for the control group. After exposure of the enamel to the varnish for 6–12 hours, the concentrations in all the layers down to a depth of 80 p.p.m. were significantly higher than the corresponding values in the control parts. Result of *in vitro* studies of Duraphat on deciduous teeth (Edenholm *et al.* 1977) reported a high fluoride leakage 1 week after application and that a depth of 15 μm no difference between study and control groups was found. Other workers, using a variety of *in vitro* and *in vivo* techniques, have reported an increase in the fluoride content of enamel after application of Duraphat varnish (Stamm 1974; Bang and Kim 1975; Petersson 1975).

The first clinical study was by Heuser and Schmidt (1968), who treated 224 children aged 13–14 years and reported a 30 per cent reduction in the incidence of caries 15 months after a single administration of Duraphat as compared with the caries increment in 163 controls. A contrary result was reported by Maiwald and Geiger (1973), who tested the same material in 179 children aged 11 years; 174 children of similar age acted as a control. After 23 months they reported that the varnish had no effect on caries incidence if applied once a year, but obtained a reduction of 45 per cent when used every 4 months.

Hetzer and Irmisch (1973) determined the effect of five applications of Duraphat over a 3-year period on 72 children aged 9½ years (group 1) and 67 chil-

Table 3.19. Duraphat—Summary of clinical studies on deciduous teeth

Author	Year	Country	No. of Patients	Age	No. of Applications per year	Duration of study	% caries reduction
Hochstein *et al.*	75	GDR	94	3–4	1.5	2 yr	34
Murray *et al.*	77	England	302	5–6	2	2 yr	7.4
Holm *et al.*	79	Sweden	225	3	2	2 yr	44
Treide *et al.*	80	GDR	110	Pre-school	4	21 m	26
Ulvestad*	78	Norway	103	7–11	2	2 yr	56*
Petersson	83	Poland	322	3	2	2 yr	9
Clark *et al.*	85	Canada	703	6–7	3	20 m	7

* Includes first permanent molars—% reduction of approximal surfaces only.

dren aged 10½ years (group 2), with 137 children of comparable ages acting as controls. The children in the test group were given oral hygiene instruction and parental involvement was encouraged. Children brushed their own teeth before being treated at the local clinic; in this way 35 children were treated in 60–70 minutes. It is not known whether bitewing radiographs were taken. In group 1 there was an 18 per cent reduction in DMFS scores over untreated controls (5.0 DMFS as against 6.1 DMFS) and in group 2 a 43 per cent reduction in DMFS scores was reported (4.3 as against 7.6).

Koch and Petersson (1975) studied the effect of semi-annual applications of Duraphat to the teeth of 60 15-year-old children over a period of 1 year. In the test group, the mean DMFS score was 31.0 at baseline and this increased to 31.9 at the first-year examination. The baseline score for the control group (27.4) was lower than for the test group, but increased to 31.3 by the end of the first year. The mean reduction in caries increment was approximately 75 per cent. The percentage reduction on occlusal surfaces was similar to that recorded on approximal and free smooth surfaces. The authors suggested that the excellent effects on the occlusal surfaces might be the result of the adhesiveness of the varnish and concluded that the short time needed for application, and the low application frequency, make the varnish practical as a preventive measure.

The caries-inhibitory effect of applying Duraphat every 6 months for 2 years to the teeth of 5-year-old children has been reported (Murray *et al.* 1977). A half-mouth technique was used involving two varnishes supplied by the manufacturers. Over the 2-year trial period 694 new dmf surfaces were recorded on deciduous molars treated with the placebo compared with 643 new dmf surfaces on teeth treated with Duraphat, a reduction of 7.4 per cent. In addition 124 surfaces were affected on first permanent molars treated with the placebo compared with 80 carious surfaces on teeth coated with Duraphat—a reduction of 37 per cent.

Overall, the results of clinical trials with Duraphat varnish suggest that it is at least as effective as fluoride solutions and gels. Summaries of the clinical trials with Duraphat varnish (deciduous and permanent teeth separately) are given in

Table 3.20. Duraphat varnish—summary of clinical studies on permanent teeth.

Author	Year	Country	No. of Patients	Age	No. of Applications per year	Duration of study	% caries reduction
Heuser	68	FRG	224	13–14	1	15 m	30
Maiwald	73	GDR	82	11	1	23 m	10
			97	11	3	23 m	46
Hetzer	73	GDR	139	9–10	2	3 yr	18–43
Winter	75	FRG	165	6	1	2 yr	37
Koch	75	Sweden	60	15	2	1 yr	75
Murray *et al.*	77	England	302	5–6	2	2 yr	37
Leiser	77	FRG	366	10–12	2	3 yr	58
Maiwald *et al.*	78	Cuba	350	6–12	2	4½ yr	39
Koch	79	Sweden	200	14	2	2 yr	30*
Seppa *et al.*	82	Finland	62	11–13	2	3 yr	30
Holm	84	Sweden	109	5	2	2 yr	56**
Tewari *et al.*	84	India	645	6–12			73

* 30 per cent reduction compared with a positive control group using a 0.2% NaF mouthrinse weekly.
** 65 per cent reduction in fissure caries in first permanent molars.

Tables 3.19 and 3.20, and suggest that it is at least as effective as fluoride solutions and gels.

Self-applied fluoride agents

Fluoride dentifrices

Without question the most widely used method of applying fluoride topically is by means of dentifrice. In countries where dentifrices are used over 95 per cent on sale contains a fluoride compound. Indeed, in Western countries it is only with difficulty that a non-fluoride dentifrice can be purchased. The first attempt to determine the value of a fluoride dentifrice was by Bibby (1945) who, in a 2-year study in which 0.1 per cent sodium fluoride was added to a conventional formulation and used unsupervised, failed to show any anti-caries effect. No formulation details are given in Bibby's report, but it is reasonable to speculate that the fluoride added to the conventional paste combined with one or more of the original constituents and was thus inactivated. Indeed, one of the major problems in the manufacture of fluoride dentifrices is preventing the fluoride component reacting with other ingredients, notably the abrasive system. Because of the attractiveness of conveying fluoride to enamel surfaces by means of a dentifrice, considerable attention has been given to finding active fluoride compounds and compatible abrasive systems. The first fluoride dentifrice thus formulated contained 0.2 per cent sodium fluoride with an abrasive system comprising a heat-treated calcium orthophosphate (calcium pyrophosphate). The reductions reported (Muhler *et al.* 1955) were of neither clinical nor statistical significance. Other studies by Kyes *et al.* (1961) and Brudevold and Chilton (1966) failed to establish real clinical benefits.

During this time Ericsson and his colleagues in Sweden were actively studying the compatibility of a number of fluoride compounds with the various dentifrice constituents. They demonstrated that sodium fluoride was inactivated by calcium carbonate and calcium phosphate, both common abrasive systems. Following this work Torell and Ericsson (1965) tested a 0.2 per cent sodium fluoride-containing dentifrice in a sodium bicarbonate base and after 2 years showed a statistically significant reduction of questionable clinical relevance. In 1967 Goran Koch reported an extensive clinical study of a dentifrice in which conventional abrasive systems were discarded and replaced by acrylic resin particles that were not only compatible with the fluoride compound but in addition conferred upon the formulation very low abrasiveness. The fluoride was the sodium salt at 0.22 per cent and over the 3-year period of the study, in which the subjects brushed under supervised conditions, an overall reduction of 50–58 per cent was reported. In practical terms the cumulative reductions over 3 years represented 7 surfaces in the younger age group and 10 surfaces in the older ones.

Whilst the studies with dentifrices containing sodium fluoride were continuing, Muhler and his colleagues in Indiana were transposing to the dentifrice field their findings with topical applications of stannous fluoride. The final formulation was marketed first in 1955 under the brand name 'Crest' and contained 0.4 per cent stannous fluoride in a calcium pyrophosphate base into which was incorporated 1 per cent stannous pyrophosphate. After this formulation development, a formidable series of clinical trials ensued in which the dentifrice was tested using various age groups and under differing conditions of usage. The design and conduct of many of these studies are open to serious critisism by present-day standards, but the validity of the findings were sufficiently convincing for the Council of Dental Therapeutics of the American Dental Association in 1964 to grant the dentifrice Grade A certification. This graded the formulation as being of proven preventive value.

Studies carried out in other parts of the world, notably in the United Kingdom, Australia, and Canada, have tested stannous fluoride formulations. Some have involved the Crest formulations as marketed whilst others have included different abrasive systems including insoluble sodium metaphosphate. The findings of the United Kingdom studies have been reviewed by Duckworth (1968). The difference in design and method of conduct of these studies make valid comparison impossible. However, there can be no doubt that regular usage led to a reduced caries experience though generally the reductions were less than those demonstrated in the early United States studies.

Despite the undoubted clinical efficacy, stannous fluoride-containing dentifrices have one major disadvantage in that they lead to unsightly black/brown extrinsic staining of tooth surfaces, especially around the margins of anterior restorations. The enamel stain can easily be removed but the discoloration of filling margins may often require replacement of the restorations. The discoloration is probably due to precipitation on the acquired pellicle of oxides and sulphides of tin. Crest is now no longer on the market, having been replaced by an entirely new formulation containing sodium fluoride with an abrasive system based on silicon dioxide. This means that no clinically tested and proven stannous fluoride dentifrices is now available in the market place of the world. This new dentifrice is marketed as 'Crest +' and has been clinically tested by Beiswanger *et al.* (1981) and Zacherl (1981), who demonstrated a significant superiority over the previous stannous fluoride formulation.

Since sodium fluoride was introduced into Crest + in 1981 some investigations have compared sodium fluoride with sodium monofluorophosphate (NaMFP) and also investigated the effect of increasing the fluoride concentration in toothpaste. Lu *et al.* (1987) used three toothpastes (1100 p.p.m. F as NaF, 2800 p.p.m. F as NaMFP, 2800 p.p.m. F as NaF) in a 3-year study of 4500 children, aged 7–15 years. The NaF toothpaste at 2800 p.p.m. F provided a significant 11 per cent reduction in DMFS increment compared with the NaMFP toothpaste (Table 3.21).

The authors claimed that the NaF dentifrice was more effective than the SMFP paste and that increasing the concentration of NaF in a dentifrice from 1100 p.p.m. F. to 2800 p.p.m. F. resulted in a statistically significant improve-

Table 3.21. Effect of high fluoride dentifrices on dental caries in children. (Lu *et al.* (1987))

Dentifrice	No. of Children	3 year DMFS increment		
		Mean	SEM	Per cent Reduction
1100 p.p.m. F as NaF	703	4.40	0.195	—
2800 p.p.m. F as SMFP	673	4.37	0.207	0.7
2800 p.p.m. F as NaF	679	3.88	0.186	11.8

ment in reducing new carious lesions. However the high F concentration used in two of these test products was almost twice the limit set by the EEC cosmetics directive, and also higher than in a study by Hargreaves and Chester (1973), who used an MFP toothpaste yielding 2200 p.p.m. F.

By far the greatest number of dentifrices on sale in the world today have as their active ingredient sodium monofluorophosphate, the caries inhibitory value of which was established over 30 years ago (Zipkin and McClure 1951). There is, however, uncertainty regarding its mode of action. Ericsson (1963) on the one hand believes that the MFP ion is incorporated into the hydroxyapatite crystal lattice with a subsequent slower release of fluoride ion which then replaces hydroxyl groups to form fluorapatite. On the other hand it has been suggested by Ingram (1972) that it is the MFP ion itself which is incorporated into the apatite crystal by means of a substitution reaction with one or more of the phosphate groups. This being the case, the transfer mechanism is not pH dependent. Apart from the fact that sodium monofluorophosphate does not require an acid pH, it is also compatible with the most commonly used chalk-based abrasive systems.

A large number of clinical studies have been reported in which MFP-containing dentifrices have been compared with non MFP-containing control formulations. Virtually all studies have demonstrated a clinically relevant anticaries effect though, as in previous dentifrice studies, differences in design of the trials make direct comparisons of findings invalid. In general terms reductions in caries increments were of the order of 30 per cent. MFP dentifrices have a neutral or slightly alkaline pH, and do not stain enamel surfaces or the margins of restorations.

During recent years there have been attempts by research workers to improve further the caries-preventive action of MFP dentifrices. These enhancements have involved the addition of calcium glycerophosphate (Mainwaring and Naylor 1983) and sodium fluoride (Hodge *et al.* 1981). In the latter case the total level of fluoride present was increased to approximately 1450 p.p.m., just short of the limit set by the EEC cosmetics directive. Both dentifrices have been shown by clinical studies to have an enhanced performance. However, concern is being expressed regarding the availability of higher fluoride-level dentifrices especially when used by children during the age range when enamel development and maturation are taking place, because of the possibility of causing mild fluorosis.

Amongst a number of dentifrice formulations containing other fluoride compounds as the active ingredient, the one which has envinced great interest contains amine fluoride. *In vitro* studies by Irwin *et al.* (1957) demonstrated that aliphatic monoamine compounds prevented acid demineralization of enamel. Further *in vitro* work by Mühlemann *et al.* (1957) showed that a number of amine fluoride compounds were more effective in reducing enamel solubility than inorganic fluorides. This finding led to further studies in which a direct antimicrobial effect was shown (Hermann and Mühlemann 1958), and that when formulated with an insoluble sodium metaphosphate abrasive agent the system was stable (König and Mühlemann 1961). A group of clinical trials were reported by Marthaler (1965, 1968) using single or compound amine fluorides in conjunction with abrasive systems comprising insoluble metaphosphate or barium sulphate. These studies can be criticized on the basis of certain aspects of their design, but in general it was demonstrated that up to 30 per cent statistically significant reduction in caries may be expected with the insoluble metaphosphate abrasive system. The low abrasive system based on barium sulphate did not produce significant reductions. Clearly, these clinical studies need to be confirmed by other workers.

Fluoride dentifrices, properly formulated and tested to show chemical stability and clinical efficacy, are clearly an important component of any caries-preventive programme. Such dentifrices not only deliver fluoride in relatively low non-toxic concentrations to the tooth surfaces but, in addition, when used with a brush they contribute to the removal of microbial plaque. Indeed, the decline in dental caries prevalence recently reported from many western countries has been attributed in part at least to the widespread use of fluoride-containing dentifrices. The future of fluoride dentifrices will be interesting for there is no doubt that manufacturers are striving to enhance the efficacy of their product formulations.

Mouth rinses

The first reported study on the use of fluoride rinses was by Bibby *et al.* (1946), who instructed dental students to rinse at least three times a week with a 0.01 per cent sodium fluoride solution, the pH of which had been adjusted to 4.0 by means of an acetate–acetic acid buffer system. The control group used a non-fluoride rinse. After one year no benefits were reported. This study can be criticized on a number of grounds, notably that the number of subjects in the trial was unacceptably low, that dental students are highly motivated in terms of plaque control and dental health generally, and that they are of an age group when new caries is low. Appreciating these shortcomings, Bibby and his colleagues (Roberts *et al.* 1948) carried out a much larger study comprising 500 sixth-grade children, rinsing twice per week with the same test and control solutions as in the earlier study. After 1 year 356 subjects remained in the study but no significant difference between test and control groups was demonstrated. In fact, the fluoride group developed more new caries than the control! Serious criticisms of this study are the short duration of the trial and the fact that different examiners carried out the base-line and 1-year examinations.

The main thrust in the development of fluoride mouth rinses came from Scandinavia during the 1960s. A series of fluoride solutions at varying concentrations were tested by Torell and his colleagues in Sweden. A study involving 9-year-old children rinsing at fortnightly intervals with 0.2 per cent sodium fluoride solutions produced significant caries reduction (Fjaestad-Seger *et al.* 1961). In the same study, iron fluoride was also found to be effective. Torell and Siberg (1962) investigated the effect of monthly rinsing with sodium fluoride and potassium fluoride, both at 0.2 per cent concentrations. In this study the 3-minute rinse was supervised, and drinking and eating was forbidden for half an hour following. Because of the unusual method of analysis of the findings these Swedish studies are difficult to interpret. For example, the differences in caries increments referred only to lesions on the approximal surfaces of anterior teeth and the control group data were obtained from a sample of subjects of the same age as the test group but a year prior to the beginning of the rinsing. Thus the important double-blind feature of the study was missing. The authors, however, concluded that rinsing with sodium fluoride once per month reduced caries in anterior teeth and was of particular value to 'caries-active' children—defined as those who have at least one cavity in anterior teeth. Potassium fluoride is again difficult to evaluate because of the unique design of the study, but overall, it would seem to be less useful than sodium fluoride.

In 1965 Torell and Ericsson reported a multi-group study in which a number of topical applications were tested. Such a study, while presenting a range of administrative, design, and statistical problems, can be extremely useful in providing vital comparative information on the relative efficacy of various agents and procedures. This study comprised nine groups and at the initial examination each group contained between 174 and 210 children, aged 10 years. Groups which rinsed included one which rinsed daily with 0.05 per cent sodium fluoride and one which rinsed fortnightly with 0.2 per cent sodium fluoride. Comparisons between groups were made on the basis of clinically recognized lesions, bitewing radiographs, and fillings inserted by the end of the study. This 2-year study demonstrated that daily use of a 0.05 per cent sodium fluoride halved the number of new carious lesions when compared with the control group, and that of the various topical agents tested, which included dentifrices, the daily rinse was the most effective. The fortnightly rinse reduced the level by about one-third.

In a further even larger multigroup study, Koch (1967) tested the efficacy of fluoride dentifrices and fluoride rinses. The rinses used were 0.5 and 0.05 per cent sodium fluoride. One group rinsed fortnightly with 0.5 per cent sodium fluoride; one group rinsed fortnightly with 0.05 per cent sodium fluoride; two other groups each rinsed with 0.5 per cent sodium fluoride and 0.05 per cent sodium fluoride on the occasion of their regular visits to the school dentist, which averaged 3–4 times per year. The subjects were aged 7–10 years at the beginning of the study and its main part extended over 3 years. The results show significant reductions of 23 per cent in respect of DMFS in 10-year-old subjects rinsing fortnightly with the 0.5 per cent solution. Seven-year-old children who rinsed 3–4 times per year showed a 25 per cent reduction in DMFS, but 7–9 year-olds rinsing with 0.05 per cent solution failed to show any significant reductions. Further examinations, carried out 1 and 2 years after completion of the study and after treatments had ceased, showed that the preventive effects of the rinsing were not maintained. This was in contradiction to the findings of Naylor and Glass (1978) who, in a dentifrice study, reported significant differences between test and control groups 1 year after cessation of the treatment regimes. However, in this case it is likely that subjects continued to brush with residual supplies of the study dentifrices or purchased fluoride dentifrices.

Soon after the publication of the Swedish findings, a series of studies were undertaken in the United States, mainly by workers from the National Institute for Dental Research. These included studies of neutral sodium fluoride, acidulated sodium fluoride, and stannous fluoride; a number have been associated with the much-publicized National Caries Program. These studies have included a 20-month study by Horowitz *et al.* (1971) involving weekly 1-minute rinses of 0.2 per cent NaF solution by children at school which, despite a wastage rate of almost 50 per cent of the subjects, demonstrated significant reductions in the older children, notably on newly erupted teeth. By the early 1970s the use of professionally applied acidulated phosphofluoride solutions and gels had become established and the question arose whether there was any advantage in providing acidulated fluoride solutions for self-administered home use. Frankl and his colleagues (1972) carried out the first such study, using a 0.02 per cent acidulated phosphofluoride solution. The study extended over 2 years and included 500 14-year-old subjects. The solution used was flavoured with lime and was pH 4. Each rinse comprised 5 ml of solution and was used daily for 1 minute. After 2 years the DFS incremental difference between the test and non-fluoride control groups was 1.94, which represented a 22 per cent reduction in new diseased surfaces.

An interesting and important comparative study of the relative efficacy of a neutral sodium fluoride solution and an acidulated phosphofluoride solution (pH 4.0) was undertaken by Aasenden *et al.* (1972). In this 3-year study children, aged 8–11 years at the beginning of the trial, rinsed daily with 5 ml of a solution containing 200 p.p.m. fluoride ions; at the conclusion of the rinse the solution was swallowed, thus providing a dietary supplement of approximately 1 mg F. The control group similarly used a placebo rinse which contained neither fluoride nor phosphate. At the conclusion of the study both rinsing groups showed significantly lower caries increments than the placebo control group, but the differences between the two test groups were very small, and certainly not statistically significant. Again in relative terms the reductions were greatest for teeth which erupted during the study; for all teeth the reduction was of the order of 25 per cent whilst for newly erupted teeth the reduction approached 35 per cent. A similar comparative study was carried out by Heifitz *et al.* (1973) involving almost 1000 subjects, aged 10–12 years at the start of the investigation. In this trial the neutral and acidulated phosphofluoride (pH 4.0) solutions both had fluoride ion concentrations of 0.3 per cent and were used weekly at school. The control group rinsed similarly with a fluoride and phosphate-free placebo solution. The rinsing procedure was strictly supervised by teachers in the classroom and comprised two successive 1-minute rinses, each with 8 ml of solution. Originally the study was scheduled to last for more than 2 years but because of erosion of the original sample due to movement of subjects away from the study area and objection to the taste of the solution, analysis of data collected after the 2-year point was abandoned. The findings, based on both clinical and radiographic data, confirmed those of Aasenden *et al.* (1972) that the benefits obtained by neutral and acidulated fluoride solutions are similar and are of the order of one surface saved per year. Expressed in relative terms the reduction is of the order of 25 per cent.

Mouth rinsing studies carried out in the United Kingdom include a 21-month trial by Brandt *et al.* (1972) in which 300 11-year-old subjects rinsed twice per week at school for 1 minute with 10 ml of either a slightly alkaline (pH 8.8) 0.2 per cent solution of sodium fluoride or a NaCl solution of pH 8.2. At the end of the study 246 subjects fulfilled the criterion of having rinsed 60 times but unfortunately the distribution of losses between the test and control group caused the mean initial DMFS at the base-line examination of subjects who completed the study to be significantly different. This is a common hazard to clinical trial studies and, although the problem can be overcome by use of specialized statistical methods, such an occurrence is disappointing for the investigator. In this case Brandt and his colleagues carried out a retrospective matched-pair analysis with 94 pairs of subjects precisely matched for base-line sex, age, and initial DMFS. In this way, over 21 months, a saving of 0.8 surfaces or 22 per cent in the sodium fluoride rinse group was demonstrated. This difference was not statistically significant but, when the analysis was confined to radiological assessment of the mesial and distal surfaces of posterior teeth only, the difference in the number of new lesions was 48 per cent. This finding added further confirmation to the view that topical fluorides provide protection more effectively to smooth surfaces than pits and fissures. In another United Kingdom study, Rugg-Gunn *et al.* (1973) carried out a clinical study of classical design involving 434 12-year-old children at the beginning of the study. The study population were divided into two groups with the test group following the Torrell and Ericsson (1965) regime and rinsing with 0.05 per cent neutral sodium fluoride once per day. The control group used daily a non-fluoride placebo rinse. Statistically significant reductions in DMFS were reported, demonstrating that the fluoride rinse caused a saving of 3.65 surfaces (35.7 per cent) over 3 years. Again the predilection for smooth surfaces was shown.

Combinations of fluoride therapy

Not surprisingly dental practitioners increasingly have been prescribing 'preventive packages' which, in addition to dietary counselling on the controlled consumption and pattern of eating of sucrose-containing foods and advice on plaque-removal techniques, have included systemic intake and topical-application fluorides in various forms. For example, the use of fluoride tablets to achieve an optimal daily systemic intake may well be prescribed in association with topical applications of a professionally applied fluoride solution or gel, regular rinsing at home with a dilute fluoride solution, and use of a fluoride-containing dentifrice. To test the efficacy of such a regimen would be logistically almost impossible. However, a number of studies have been carried out which do give some indication of the value of multiple procedures.

A very important basic question relates to the value of topical fluoride procedures in areas where the drinking water supplies contain fluoride at the optimum level. Radike *et al.* (1973) carried out a 20-month study which compared the efficacy of mouth rinsing with 0.1 per cent stannous fluoride solution and a non-fluoride placebo solution on alternative days. Residents of the area in which this study was conducted had been receiving water containing 1 p.p.m. F for 17 years. This study demonstrated that the stannous fluoride rinsing group received a small but significant added protection over and above that provided by the fluoridated drinking water. Peterson (1979) evaluated the effect of two monofluorophosphate dentifrices when used under supervised conditions at school by 16–12-year-old children living in communities provided with optimally fluoridated drinking water. When compared with a group using a non-fluoride control dentifrice, it was shown that the dentifrice containing sodium monofluorophosphate in a calcium carbonate base caused a small but significant additional benefit. However, a monofluorophosphate dentifrice with an insoluble sodium metaphosphate base failed to provide any added protection.

Heifitz *et al.* (1979) carried out a study to assess the value of the combined effect of acidulated phosphate fluoride gel applications made on five consecutive days three times per year plus weekly 1-minute rinses of 0.2 per cent neutral sodium fluoride solution. The control group rinsed only with a non-fluoride solution. Both control and test groups had received optimally fluoridated water since birth. After 30 months there were small but significant differences between test and control groups, the relative differences in DMFS increments being greatest in respect of newly erupted teeth. From these and other studies it would seem reasonable to conclude that use of topical fluoride appliactions will further enhance the caries inhibition provided by fluoridated drinking water.

The combined use of systemically administered fluoride in the form of an acidulated 1 mg F tablet, which daily was chewed, swished, and swallowed, with the weekly use of a 0.2 per cent sodium fluoride rinse, was evaluated by Horowitz *et al.* (1979) as part of a long-term preventive programme in Nelson County Va, a low fluoride area. This was a retrospective study in which there was no conventional control group as in the more common longitudinal clinical trial. Indeed, the performance of the prescribed regimen in the participating subjects was assessed by comparing the disease increments with those of children of similar age and previous caries experience at the initial examination but who did not participate in the programme. After 4 years there was a 35 per cent overall reduction in DMFS, the preventive effect being demonstrated in respect of all types of surfaces, i.e. approximal, buccolingual, and occlusal. This study is interesting not only because of the treatment regimen tested but also because it is an evaluation of a community health programme rather than a purpose-designed clinical trial. Further it is interesting to speculate on the relative merits of the two components of the regime and to question the need actually to swallow the tablet, particularly in children of the older age group where the value of systemic fluoride is severely diminished. It must also be remembered that these children were using a fluoride dentifrice at home. In 1983 dental examinations of children aged 6–17 years, who had continuously participated in the program for 1 to 11 years, showed a mean prevalence of 3.12 DMFS which was 65 per cent lower than the corresponding score of 9.02 DMFS for children of the same age at the base line examinations (Horowitz *et al.* 1986).

In the United Kingdom, Ashley *et al.* (1977) investigated the supervised daily use at school of a 0.01 per cent acidulated phosphate fluoride mouthwash and a sodium monofluorophosphate dentifrice used alone and in combination. This was a four-group study in which one group was a control, using both a fluoride-free rinse and dentifrice; another rinsed with the test solution and used a fluoride-free dentifrice; another used a placebo rinse and the fluoride dentifrice; the fourth group used both fluoride rinse and fluoride dentifrice. After 2 years there were statistical significant reductions in new caries when the three groups using fluoride dentifrice and fluoride rinse were compared with the control group. However, there were no statistically significant differences between the three test groups indicating that under the conditions of this study at least, daily use of a fluoride mouthwash is no more effective than a fluoride dentifrice, and that the combined use of the fluoride rinse and the dentifrice does not confer added benefits. In a study of similar design, Mainwaring and Naylor (1978) determined the separate and combined effects of twice annual, professionally aplied, acidulated phosphofluoride gel and the unsupervised use at home of a sodium monofluorophosphate calcium carbonate-based dentifrice. This study extended over 3 years and, as in the previously described investigation, the effect of topically applied gel and use of the fluoride dentifrice alone and together significantly reduced the caries increments compared with the control group, but again there were no significant differences between the groups receiving topical fluoride in the form of a fluoride gel or a dentifrice or both in combination.

From this group of studies it would seem reasonable to conclude that fluorides administered topically do enhance the effect of systemically administered fluoride especially if the latter has been given since early life. However, there is no clear evidence that the use of a multi-regimen of topical agents provides significant added benefits. Under these circumstances it must be agreed that because a sound and effective brushing technique aimed at regular removal of plaque is the basis of all preventive procedures, and because for cosmetic and social reasons a dentifrice is invariably used, the most certain and most cost-effective method of administering topical fluoride is by means of clinically tested fluoride-containing dentifrice of proven value.

Conclusion

The study of the systemic and topical efects of fluoride has produced a tremendous outpouring of research, particularly over the last 50 years, and our knowledge of dental epidemiology, clinical trials, community dental health, dental plaque, physiology, and biochemistry has increased enormously as a result. The incorporation of fluoride in its various forms as a caries-preventive agent for both the individual and the community, is one of the most important factors responsible for the decrease in dental caries in children observed in many Western countries over the last 10 years.

A conference in 1982 on the appropriate use of fluorides for human health, under the auspices of the International Dental Federation, the Kellogg Foundation, and the World Health Organization, reached the following conclusions and recommendations (WHO, 1986).

1. The International Conference on Fluorides reviewed the findings of recent experimental, clinical, and epidemiological research on the use of fluorides in promoting dental health. While welcoming the reports of declining caries experience in many developed countries, it was greatly concerned about the sharp increase in dental caries in some developing countries. As there is no possibility of treating so many decayed teeth with the dental resources at present available in the developing countries, the only hope is to contain the caries problem by preventive measures.

2. The Conference agreed that community water fluoridation is an ideal public measure for the prevention of dental caries in countries with well-developed, centralized public water supplies. It was in agreement with the view of the FDI, WHO, and the medical and dental professions throughout the world that community water fluoridation is an effective, safe, and inexpensive preventive measure, which has the virtue of requiring no active compliance on the part of the persons benefitted. The Conference recommended that community water fluoridation by introduced and maintained wherever possible.

3. Unfortunately, the vast majority of the world's population live in rural and urban areas with few large water installations. In these situations, community water fluoridation is not feasible and alternative strategies need to be adopted. There is evidence from three long-term studies in both developing and industrialized countries that salt fluoridation may be nearly as effective as water fluoridation in reducing the incidence of dental caries. Consequently, the Conference stressed the need for more long-term field trials of salt fluoridation.

4. There is no justification for using more than one systemic fluoride measure at any one time.

5. Various topical fluoride methods, or combinations of such methods, may be beneficial in communities that have a source of systemic fluoride that is used widely.

6. Wherever possible, when combinations of fluoride therapy are considered, it is best to choose those that are self-administered or group-administered because they are less expensive.

7. Professionally applied fluorides are particularly appropriate for individuals who have been identified as at high risk of dental caries.

8. The conference was concerned about the problems of dental fluorosis in areas with high concentrations of fluoride in the public water supply and urged research to develop effective, simple, and economical defluoridation methods for water supplies of varying sizes. It recommended that, in children under the age of 6 years, brushing with a fluoride toothpaste should be supervised in order to prevent excessive ingestion. For similar reasons, fluoride mouth rinsing should not be considered for children under 5 years.

9. Current knowledge of the effectiveness of various methods of using fluorides led the Conference to conclude that each country should review its own dental needs and take legislative action to adopt those methods of using fluorides that best suit its needs in different regions. In view of the proven value of fluorides in promoting dental health, their use should be extended without further delay to all populations throughout the world.

References

Aasenden, R. and Peebles, T.C. (1974). Effects of fluoride supplementation from birth on human deciduous and permanent teeth. *Archs. oral Biol.* **19**, 321–6.

Aasenden, R., de Paola, P.F., and Brudevold, F. (1972). Effects of daily rinsing and ingestion of fluoride solutions upon dental caries and enamel fluoride. *Archs. oral Biol.* **17**, 1705–14.

Adler, P. (1951). The connections between dental caries experience and water-borne fluorides in a population with low caries incidence. *J. dent. Res.* **30**, 368–81.

Ainsworth, N.J. (1928). Mottled teeth. *R. dent. Hosp. Mag.* February.

Ainsworth, N.J. (1933). Mottled teeth. *Br. dent. J.* **60**, 233–50.

Arnold, F.A. Jr. (1948). Fluorine in drinking waters. Its effect on dental caries. *J. Am. dent. Ass.* **36**, 28–36.

Arnold, F.A. Jr. (1967). Foreword to fluorine and dental caries. *J. Am. dent. Ass.* **74**, 230.

Arnold, F.A. Jr., Dean, H.T., and Knutson, J.W. (1953). Effect of fluoridated public water supplies on dental caries prevalence. Results of the seventh year of study at Grand Rapids and Muskegon, Mich. *Publ. Hlth. Rep.* **68**, 141–8.

Arnold, F.A. Jr., Dean, H.T., Jay, P., and Knutson, J.W. (1956). Effect of fluoridated public water supplies on dental caries prevalence. 10th year of the Grand Rapids-Muskegon Study. *Publ. Hlth. Rep.* **71**, 652–8.

Arnold, F.A. Jr., Likens, R.C., Russell, A.L., and Scott, D.B. (1962). Fifteenth year of the Grand Rapids fluoridation study. *J. Am. dent. Ass.* **65**, 780–5.

Ashley, F.P., Mainwaring, P.J., Emslie, R.D. and Naylor, M.N. (1977). Clinical testing of a mouthrinse and a dentifrice containing fluoride. *Br. dent. J.* **143**, 333–8.

Ast, D.B., Finn, S.B., and McCafferty, I. (1950). The Newburgh-Kingston caries fluoride study. I, Dental findings after three years of water fluoridation. *Am. J. publ. Hlth.* **40**, 116–24.

Ast, D.B., Smith D.J., Wacks, B., and Cantwell, K.T. (1956). Newburgh-Kingston caries fluorine study XIV. Combined clinical and roentgenographic dental findings after ten years of fluoride experience. *J. Am. dent. Ass.* **52**, 314–25.

Bang, S. and Kim, Y.J. (1973). Electron microprobe analysis of human tooth enamel coated *in vivo* with fluoride-varnish. *Helv. odont. Acta* **17**, 84–8.

Beal, J.F. and James, P.M.C. (1971). Dental caries prevalence in 5 year old children following five and a half years of water fluoridation in Birmingham. *Br. dent. J.* **130**, 284–8.

Beiswanger, B.B., Gish, C.W., and Mallatt, M.E. (1981). Effect of a sodium fluoride-silica abrasive dentifrice upon caries. *J. dent. Res.* **60** (spec. iss. A), 1072. (Abstr.)

Berner, L., Fernex, E., and Held, A.J. (1967). Study on the anti-carious effect of sodium fluoride tablets (Zymafluor). Results recorded in the course of 13 years of observation. *Schweiz. Monatsschr. Zahnheilkd.* **77**, 528–39.

Bibby, B.G. (1942) A new approach to caries prophylaxis. *Tufts dent. Outlook* **15**, 4.

Bibby, B.G. (1945). Test of the effect of fluoride-containing dentifrice on dental caries. *J. dent. Res.* **24**, 297–303.

Bibby, B.G. (1947). A consideration of the effectiveness of various fluoride mixtures. *J. Am. dent. Ass.* **34**, 26.

Bibby, B.G., Zander, H.A., McKelleget, M., and Labonsky, B. (1946). Preliminary reports on the effect on dental caries of the use of sodium fluoride in a proplylactic cleaning mixture and in a mouthwash. *J. dent. Res.* **25**, 207–11.

Binder, K. (1965). Karies und fluorreiches Trinkwasser-kritische Betrachtung. *Osterr. Z. Stomat.* **62**, 14–18.

Black, G.V. (1916). Mottled teeth. *Dent. Cosmos* **58**, 129–56.

Blayney, J.R. and Hill, I.N. (1967). Fluoride and dental caries. *J. Am. dent. Ass.* **74**, 233–302.

Blinkhorn, A.S., Brown, M.D., Attwood, D., and Downer, M.C. (1981). The effect of fluoridation on the dental health of urban Scottish schoolchildren. *J. Epidemiol. Commun. Hlth.* **35**, 98–101.

Brandt, R.S., Slack, G.L., and Waller, D.F. (1972). The use of sodium fluoride mouthwash in reducing dental caries increment in 11-year old English school children. *Proc. Br. paedodont. Soc.* **2**, 23–5.

Brown, H.K. and Poplove, M. (1965). Brantford–Sarnia–Stratford fluoridation caries study: final survey 1963. *J. Can. dent. Ass.* **31**, 505–11.

Brudevold, F. and Chilton, N.W. (1966). Comparative study of a fluoride dentifrice containing soluble phosphate and a calcium-free abrasive. Second year report. *J. Am. dent. Ass.* **72**, 889–94.

Chalmers Clarke, J.H. (1954). The value of fluoridation of domestic water supplies in prevention of dental caries and dental sepsis. *Med. Off.* **92**, 39–43.

Churchill, H.V. (1931*a*). Letter to F.S. McKay in the McKay papers. Cited by McNeil (1957), p.26.

Churchill, H.V. (1931*b*). Occurrence of fluorides in some waters of the United States. *Ind. Engng. Chem.* **23**, 996–8.

Clark, D.C., Stamm, J.W., Chin Once, T., and Robert, G. (1985). results of the Sherbrooke–Lac Mégantic fluoride varnish study after 20 months. *Commun. Dent. Oral Epidemiol.* **13**, 61–4.

Crichton Browne, J. (1892). Address to the Annual General Meeting of the Eastern Counties Branch of the British Dental Association. *J. Br. dent. Ass.* **13**, 404–16.

Davies G.N. (1950). Dental caries control and the general practitioner. *NZ dent. J.* **46**, 25.

Davis, J.G. (1975) Fluoridised milk for children, part 2. *Dairy Industries* **40**, 48–51.

Dean, H.T. (1933). Distribution of mottled enamel in the United States. *Publ. Hlth. Rep.* **48**, 704–34.

Dean, H.T. (1934). Classification of mottled enamel diagnosis. *J. Am. dent. Ass.* **21**, 1421–6.

Dean, H.T. (1936). Chronic endemic dental fluorosis (mottled enamel). *J. Am. med. Ass.* **107**, 1269–72.

Dean, H.T. (1938). Endemic fluorosis and its relation to dental caries. *Publ. Hlth. Rep.* **53**, 1443–52

Dean, H.T. and Elvove, E. (1935). Some epidemiological aspects of chronic endemic dental fluorosis. *Am. J. publ. Hlth.* **26**, 567–75.

Dean, H.T. and McKay F.S. (1939). Production of mottled enamel halted by a change in common water supply. *Am. J. publ. Hlth* **29**, 567–75.

Dean, H.T., Jay, P., Arnold, F.A. Jr, and Elvove, E. (1939). Domestic water and the dental caries including cartain epidemiological aspects of oral L. acidophilus. *Publ. Hlth Rep.* **54**, 862–88.

Dean, H.T., Arnold, F.A. Jr., and Elvove, E. (1942). Domestic water and dental caries, V, additional studies of the relation of fluoride domestic waters to dental caries experience in 4425 white children aged 12–14 years, of 13 cities in 4 states. *Publ. Hlth. Rep.* **57**, 1155–79.

Dean, H.T., Arnold, F.A. Jr., Jay, P., and Knutson, J.W. (1950). Studies on mass control of dental caries through fluoridation of public water supply. *Publ. Hlth. Rep.* **65**, 1403–8.

Deatherage, C.F. (1943). Fluoride domestic waters and dental caries experience in 2026 white Illinois selective service men. *J. dent. Res.* **22**, 129–37.

Department of Public Health and Social Security (1962). The results of fluoridation studies in the United Kingdom and the results achieved after five years. *Rep. publ. Hlth. Med. Subj., Lond.* No. 105.

Department of Public Health and Social Security (1969). Report of the Committee on Research into Fluoridation. The fluoridation studies in the United Kingdom and the results achieved after eleven years. *Rep. publ. Hlth. Med. Subj., Lond.* No. 122.

Driscoll, W.S. (1974). The use of fluoride tablets for the prevention of dental caries. In *International Workshop of fluorides and dental caries prevention*, (ed. D.J. Forrester and E.M. Schulz), pp. 25–111. University of Maryland, Baltimore.

Driscoll, W.S., Heifetz, S.B., Korts, D.C., Meyers, R.J., and Horowitz, H.S. (1977). Effect of acidulted phosphate-fluoride chewable tablets in schoolchildren: results after 55 months. *J. Am. dent. Ass.* **94**, 537–43.

Driscoll, WS., Heifetz, S.D., and Korts, D.C. (1978). Effect of chewable fluoride tablets on dental caries in schoolchildren: results after six years of use. *J. Am. dent. Ass.* **97**, 820–4.

Duckworth, R. (1968). Fluoride dentifrices. A review of clinical trials in the United Kingdom. *Br. dent. J.* **124**, 505–9.

Duff, E.J. (1981). Total and ionic fluoride in milk. *Caries Res.* **15**, 406–8.

Eager, J.M. (1902). Abstract: chiaie teeth. *Dent. Cosmos.* **44**, 300–1.

Englander, H.R. and Wallace, D.A. (1962). Effects of naturally fluoridated water on dental caries in adults. *Publ. Hlth. Rep.* **77**, 887–93.

Ericsson, Y. (1958). The state of fluorine in milk. *Acta odont. Scand.* **16**, 51–77.

Ericsson, Y. (1963). The mechanism of monofluorophosphate action on hydroxyapatite and dental enamel. *Acta odont. Scand.* **21**, 341–58.

Ericsson, Y. and Ribelius, U. (1971). Wide variations of fluoride supply to infants and their effect. *Caries Res.* **5**, 78–88.

Feltman, R. and Kosel, G. (1961). Prenatal and postnatal ingestion of fluorides—fourteen years of investigation—final report. *J. dent. Med.* **16**, 190–8.

Fjaestas-Seger, A.M., Nordstedt-Larsson, K., and Torell, P. (1961). Forsok med enkla metoder for Klinisk fluorapplikation. *Sven Tandlak. Forb. Tidn.* **53**, 169–80.

Forrest, J.R. (1956). Caries incidence and enamel defects in areas with different levels of fluoride in the drinking water. *Br. dent. J.* **100**, 195–200.

Forrest, J.R., Parfitt, G.J., and Bransby, E.R. (1951). The incidence of dental caries among adults and young children in three high and three low fluoride areas in England. *Mon. Bull. Minist. Hlth* **10**, 104–11.

Frankl, S.N., Fleisch, S., and Diodati, R.R. (1972). The topical anticariogenic effect of daily rinsing with an acidulated phosphate fluoride solution. *J. Am. dent. Ass.* **85**, 882–6.

Galagan. D.J. (1953). Climate and controlled fluoridation. *J. Am. dent. Ass.* **47**, 159–70.

Galagan, D.J. and Knutson, J.W. (1948). Effects of topically applied fluoride on dental caries experience VI. Experiments with sodium fluoride and calcium chloride; widely spaced applications, use of different solution concentrations. *Publ. Hlth. Rep.* **63**, 1215.

Gedalia, I., Galon, H., Rennert, A., Biderco, I., and Mohr, I. (1981). Effect of fluoridated citrus beverage on dental caries and on fluoride concentration in the surface enamel of children's teeth. *Caries Res.* **15**, 103–8.

Gilooly, C.J., Heinz, H.W., and Eastman, P.W. (1954). A dental caries and fluoride study of 19 Nebraska cities. *J. Neb. dent. Ass.* **31**, 3–13.

Glenn, F.B. (1979). Immunity conveyed by sodium-fluoride supplement during pregnancy: part II. *J. dent. Child.* **46**, 17–24.

Granath, L.-E., Rootzen, H., Liljegren, E., Holst, K., and Kohler, L. (1978). Variation in caries prevalence related to combinations of dietary and oral hygiene habits and chewing fluoride tablets in 4-year-old children. *Caries Res.* **12**, 83–92.

Hamberg, L. (197). Controlled trial of fluoride in vitamin drops for prevention of caries in children. *Lancet* **i**, 441–2.

Hargreaves, J.A. and Chester, C.G. (1973). Clinical trial among Scottish children of an anti-caries dentifrice containing 2% sodium monofluorophosphate. *Commun. Dent. oral. Epidemiol.* **1**, 47–57.

Heifetz, S.B., Driscoll, W.S., and Creighton, W.E. (1973). The effect on dental caries on weekly rinsing with a neutral sodium fluoride or an acidulated phosphate-flouride mouthwash. *J. Am. dent. Ass.* **87**, 364–8.

Heifetz, SB., Horowitz, H.S., and Driscoll, W.S. (1978). Effect of school water fluoridation on dental caries: results in Seagrove, NC, after eight years. *J. Am. dent. Ass.* **97**, 193–6.

Heifetz, S.B., Franchi, G.J., Moseley, G.W., MacDougall, O., and Brunelle, J. (1979). Combined anticariogenic effect of fluoride gel trays and fluoride mouthrinsing in an optimally fluoridated community. *J. clin. prevent. Dent.* **6**, 21–8.

Hennon, D.K., Stookey, G.K., and Beiswanger, B.B. (1977). Fluoride-vitamin supplements: effects on dental caries and fluorosis when used in areas with suboptimum fluoride in the water supply. *J. Am. dent. Ass.* **95**, 965–71.

Hermann, U. and Mühlemann, H.R. (1958). Inhibition of salivary respiration and glucolysis by an organic fluoride. *Helv. odont. Acta.* **2**, 28–33.

Hetzer, G. and Irmisch, B. (1973). Kariesprotektion durch Fluorlack (Duraphat) Klinische ergebnisse und erfahrungen. *Dt. Stomatol.* **23**, 917–22.

Heuser, H. and Schmidt, H.F.M. (1968). Deep impregnation of dental enamel with a fluoride lacquer for prophylaxis of dental caries. *Stoma* **2**, 91.

Hochstein, H.J., Hochstein, U., and Breitung, L. (1975). Erfahrungen mit dem Fluorlack Duraphat. ZWR

Hodge, H.C., Holloway, P.J., Davies, T.G.H., and Worthington, H.V. (1980). Caries prevention by dentifrices containing a combination of sodium monofluorophosphate and sodium fluoride. *Br. dent. J.* **149**, 193–204.

Holm, A.K. (1975). Caries preventive effect of a fluoride-containing varnish (Duraphat) after 1 year's study. *Commun. Dent. Oral Epidemiol.* **3**, 262–6.

Holm, A.K. (1979). Effect of a fluoride varnish (Duraphat) in pre-school children. *Commun. Dent. Oral Epidemiol.* **7**, 241–5.

Horowitz, H.S. and Heifetz, S.B. (1979). Methods for assessing the cost-effectiveness of caries preventive agents and procedures. *Int. dent. J.* **29**, 106–17.

Horowitz, H.S. and Lucye, H.S. (1966). A clinical study of stannous fluoride in a prophylaxis paste and as a solution. *J. oral Ther. Pharmacol.* **3**, 17.

Horowitz, S.B., Law, F.E., and Pritzker, T. (1965). Effect of school water fluoridation on dental caries, St. Thomas, V.I. *Publ. Hlth. Rep.* **80**, 382–8.

Horowitz, S.B. *et al.* (1968). School fluoridation Studies In Elk Lake, Pennsylvania, and Pike County, Kentucky—results after eight years. *Am. J. publ. Hlth.* **50**, 2240–50.

Horowitz, H.S., Creighton, W.E. and McClendon, B.J. (1971). The effect on human dental caries of weekly oral rinsing with a sodium fluoride mouthwash. *Arch. oral Biol.* **16**, 609–16.

Horowitz, H.S., Heifetz, S.B., Meyers, R.J. Driscoll, W.S., and Korts, D.C. (1979). Evaluation of a combination of self administered fluoride procedures for the control of dental caries in a non-fluoride area: findings after 4 years. *J. Am. dent. Ass.* **98**, 219–23.

Horowitz, H.S., Meyers, R.J. Heifetz, S.B., Driscoll, W.S., and Li, S. (1986). Combined fluoride school-based program in a fluoride-deficient area: results of an 11-year study. *J. Am. dent Ass.* **112**, 621–5.

Hoskova, M. (1968). Fluoride tablets in the prevention of tooth decay. *Cesk. Pediatr.* **23**, 438–41.

Hutton, W.L., Linscott, B.W., and Williams, D.B. (1951). Brantford fluorine experiment. *Can. J. publ. Hlth.* **42**, 81.

Ingram, G.S. (1972). The reaction of monofluorophosphate with apatite. *Caries Res.* **6**, 1–15.

Irwin, M., Leaver, A.G., and Walsh, J.P. (1957). Further studies on the influence of surface active agents on decalcification of the enamel surface. *J. dent. Res.* **36**, 166–72.

Jackson, D. (1961). An epidemiological study of dental caries prevalence in adults. *Arch. oral Biol.* **6**, 80–93

Jackson, D., Murray, J.J., and Fairpo, C.G. (1973). Lifelong benefits of fluoride in drinking water. *Br. dent. J.* **134**, 419–22.

Jackson, D., Gravely, J.F., and Pinkham, I.O. (1975*a*). Fluoridation in Cumbria. *Br. dent. J.* **139**, 319–22.

Jackson, D., James, P.M.C., and Wolfe, W.G. (1975*b*). Fluoridation in Anglesey. *Br. dent. J.* **138**, 165–71.

James, P.M.C. (1961). Dental caries prevalence in high and low fluoride areas of East Anglia. *Br. dent. J.* **110**, 165–9.

Jauncey. (1983). *Opinion of Lord Jauncey* in causa *Mrs. Catherine McColl against Strathclyde Regional Council*. The Court of Session, Edinburgh.

Jenny, J. and Heifetz, S.B. (1978). Prevention update. *Dent. Hyg.* **52**, 18–94.

Jordon, W.A., Wood, O.B., Allison, J.A., and Irwin, V.D. (1946). Effect of various numbers of topical applications of sodium fluoride. *J. Am. dent. Ass.* **33**, 1385–91.

Kempf, G.A. and McKay, F.S. (1930). Motted enamel in a segregated population. *Publ. Hlth. Rep.* **45**, 2923–40.

Kempler, D., Anaise, J., Westreich, V., and Gedalia, I. (1977). Caries rate in hamsters given non-acidulated and acidulated tea. *J. dent. Res.* **56**, 89.

Klein, H. (1948). Dental effects of accidentally fluoridated waters—dental caries experience in deciduous and permanent teeth of school age children. *J. Am. dent. Ass.* **36**, 443–53.

Klein, H., Palmer, G.E., and Knutson, J.W. (1938). Studies on dental caries: (1) Dental status and dental needs of elementary schoolchildren. *Publ. Hlth. Rep.* **53**, 751–65.

Knox, E.G. (1985). *Fluoridation of water and cancer: a review of the epidemiological evidence.* Report of a Working Party. HMSO, London.

Knutson, J.W. (1948). Sodium fluoride solutions: technic for application to the teeth. *J. Am. dent. Ass.* **36**, 37–9.

Knutson, J.W. (1970). Water fluoridation after 25 years. *Br. dent. J.* **129**, 297–300.

Knutson, J.W. and Armstrong, W.D. (1946). The effect of topically applied sodium fluoride on dental caries experience III. Report of findings for the third study year. *Publ. Hlth. Rep.* **61**, 1683.

Koch, G. (1967). Effect of sodium fluoride in dentifrice and mouthwash on the incidence of dental caries in school children. *Odont. Revy.* **18**, 48–71.

Koch, G. and Petersson, L.G. (1972). Fluoride content of enamel surface treated with a varnish containing sodium fluoride. *Odont. Revy.* **23**, 437.

König, K.G. and Mühlemann, H.R. (1961). caries inhibiting effect of amino fluoride-containing dentifrices tested in an animal experiment and a clinical study. In *The present status of caries prevention by fluoride-containing dentifrices*, (ed. H.R. Mühlemann and K.G. König). Huber, Berne.

Kwant, G.W. Houwink, B., Backer Dirks, O., Groeneveld, A., and Pot, T.J. (1973). Artificial fluoridation of drinking water in the Netherlands; results of the Tiel-Culemborg experiment after $16\frac{1}{2}$ years. *Neth. dent. J.* **80**, (suppl. 9), 6–27.

Kyes, F., Overton, N.J., and McKean, T.W. (1961). Clinical trials of caries inhibitory dentifrices. *J. Am. dent. Ass.* **63**, 189–93.

Lewis, F.D. and Leatherwood, E.C. Jr (1959). Effects of natural fluorides on caries incidence in three Georgia cities. *Publ. Hlth. Rep. Wash.* **74**, 127–31.

Lieser, O. and Schmidt, H.F.M. (1978). Karies prophylaktische Wirkung von Fluorlack nach mehrjahriger Anwendung in der Jugendzahnpflege. *Dt. Zahnärztl. Zfs.* **33**, 176–8.

Lu, K.H., Ruhlman, C.D., Chung, K.L., Sturzenburger, O.P., and Lehnhoff, R.W. (1987). A three year clinical comparison of a sodium monofluorophosphate dentifrice with sodium fluoride dentifrices on dental caries in children. *J. Dent. Child.* 241–4.

McKay, F.S. (1916*a*). An investigation of mottled teeth (I). *Dent. Cosmos* **58**, 477–84.

McKay, F.S. (1916*b*). An investigation of mottled teeth (III). *Dent. Cosmos* **58**, 781–92.

McKay, F.S. (1918). Progress of the year in the investigation of mottled enamel with special reference to its association with artesian water. *J. Am. dent. Ass.* **5**, 721–50.

McKay, F.S. (1928). The relation of mottled teeth to caries. *J. Am. dent. Ass.* **15**, 1429–37.

Mainwaring, P.J. and Naylor, M.N. (1978). A three-year clinical study to determine the separate and combined caries-inhibiting efects of a sodium monofluorophosphate toothpaste and an acidulated phosphate fluoride gel. *Caries Res.* **12**, 202–12.

Mainwaring, P.J. and Naylor, M.N. (1983). A four-year clinical study to determine the caries inhibiting effect of calcium glycerophosphate and sodium fluoride in calcium carbonate base dentifrices containing sodium monofluorophosphate. *Caries Res.* **17**, 267–76.

Maiwald, J.H. and Geiger, L. (1973). Topical application of a fluoride protective varnish for caries prophylaxis. *Dt. Stomatol.* **23**, 56.

Maiwald, H.J., Miyares, S.R., and Banos, F.D. (1978). Result del estudio de aplicación de laca de flúor. *Rev. Cub. Est.* **15**, 109–14.

Margolis, F.J., Reames, H.R., Freshman, E., Macauley, J.C., and Mehaffey, H. (1975). Fluoride—ten year prospective study of deciduous and permanent dentition. *Am. J. Dis. Child.* **129**, 794–800.

Marthaler, T.M. (1965). The caries inhibiting effect of amine fluoride dentifrices in children during 3 years of unsupervised use. *Br. dent. J.* **124**, 510–15.

Marthaler, T.M. (1968). Caries inhibiting after seven years of an amine fluoride dentifrice. *Br. dent. J.* **124**, 510–15.

Marthaler, T.M. (1969). Caries-inhibiting effect of fluoride tablets. *Helv. odontol. Acta.* **13**, 1–13.

Marthaler, T.M. and Schenardi, Ç. (1962). Inhibition of caries in children after $5\frac{1}{2}$ years use of fluoridated table salt. *Helv. odontol. Acta* **6**, 1–6.

Marthaler, T.M., De Crousaz, Ph., Meyer R., Regolati, B., and Robert, A. (1977). Frequence globale do la carie dentaire dans le canton de Vaud, apres passage de la fluoruration par comprimes a la fluoruration du sel alimentaire. *Schweiz. Machr. Zahnheilk.* **87**, 147–58.

Marthaler, T.M., Mejia, R., Toth, K., and Vines, J.J. (1978). Caries-preventive salt fluoridation. *Caries Res.* **12**, Suppl. 1, 15–21.

Medical Research Council (1925). *The incidence of dental disease in children.* MRC Special Report Series, No. 97, London.

Mejia, D.R., Espinal, F., Velez, H., and Aguire, S.M. (1976). Use of fluoridated salt in four Columbian communities VIII. Results achieved from 1964 to 1972. *Bol. Sanit. Panam.* **80**, 205–19.

Mercer, V.H. and Muhler, J.C. (1961). Comparison of single application of stannous fluoride with a single application of sodium fluoride or two applications of stannous fluoride. *J. Dent. Child.* **28**, 84.

Miller, B.F. (1938). Inhibition of experimental dental caries in the rat by fluoride and iodoacetic acid. *Proc. Soc. exp. Biol. Med.* **39**, 389.

Møller, I.J. (1965). *Dental fluorose og caries.* Rhodes International Science Publishers, Copenhagen.

Moulton, F.R. (1942). *Fluorine and dental health.* American Association for the Advancement of Science, Washington, DC.

Mühlemann, H.R. (1967). Fluoridated domestic salt; a discussion of dosage. *Int. dent. J.* **17**, 10–17.

Mühlemann, H.R., Schmid, H., and Konig, F.G. (1957). Enamel solubilty reduction studies with inorganic and organic fluorides. *Helv. odont. Acta.* **1**, 23–33.

Muhler, J.C. and Day, H.C. (1950). Effects of SnF_2, NaF on incidence of dental lesion in rats fed caries producing diets. *J. Am. dent. Ass.* **41**, 528.

Muhler, J.C., Radike,A.W., Nebergall, W.H., and Day, H.G. (1955). A comparison between the anticariogenic effect of dentifrices containing stannous fluoride and sodium fluoride. *J. Am. dent. Ass.* **51**, 556–9.

Murray, J.J. (1969*a*). Caries experience of five-year-old children from fluoride and non-fluoride communities. *Br. dent. J.* **126**, 352–4.

Murray, J.J. (1969*b*). Caries experience of 15-year-old children from fluoride and non-fluoride communities. *Br. dent. J.* **127**, 128–31.

Murray, J.J. (1971*a*). Adult dental health in fluoride and non-fluoride areas. *Br. dent. J.* **131**, 391–5.

Murray, J.J. (1971*b*). Adult dental health in fluoride and non-fluoride areas. Part 2. Caries experience in each tooth type. *Br. dent. J.* **131**, 437–42.

Murray, J.J. and Rugg-Gunn, A.J. (1982*a*). Water fluoridation update. In *Pediatric dentistry*, (ed. R.E. Stewart, T.K. Barber, K.C. Troutman and S.H.Y. Wei). Mosby, St. Louis.

Murray, J.J. and Rugg-Gunn, A.J. (1982*b*). *Fluorides in caries prevention*, 2nd edn. Wright, Bristol.

Murray, J.J., Winter, G.B., and Hurst, C.P. (1977). Duraphat fluoride varnish: a 2-year clinical trial in 5-year-old children. *Br. dent. J.* **143**, 11–17.

Naylor, M.N. and Glass, R.L. (1979). Persistant cariostatic effects of $CaCO_3$ based MFP dentifrices with and without calcium glycerophosphate. *J. dent. Res.* **58** (spec. Iss. C), 1262. (Abstr.)

Nevitt, G.A., Difenbach, V., and Presnell, C.E. (1953). Missouri's fluoride and dental caries study. A study of the dental caries experience and the fluoride content of the drinking water of 3,206 white children in nine selected cities in Missouri. *J. Mo. State dent. Ass.* **33**, 10–26.

Parmeijer, J.H.N., Brudevold, F., and Hunt, E.E. (1963). A study of acidulated fluoride solutions, III. The cariostatic effect of repeated topical sodium fluoride applications with and without phosphate. A pilot study. *Archs. oral. Biol.* **8**, 183.

Peterson, J.K. (1979). A supervised brushing trial of sodium monofluorophosphate dentifrice in a fluoridated area. *Caries Res.* **13**, 68–72.

Petersson, L.G. (1975). On topical application of fluorides and its inhibiting effect on caries. *Odont. Revy.* **26**, Suppl. 34.

Poulsen, S., Larsen, M.J., and Larson, R.H. (1976). Effect of fluoridated milk and water on enamel fluoride content and dental caries in the rat. *Caries Res.* **10**, 227–33.

Poulsen, S., Gradegaard, E., and Mortensen, B. (1981). Cariostatic effect of daily use of a fluoride-containing lozenge compared to fortnightly rinses with 0.2% sodium fluoride. *Caries Res.* **15**, 236–42.

Radike, A.W., Gish, C.W., Peterson, J.K., and Segreto, V.A. (1973). Clinical evaluation of stannous fluoride as an anti-caries mouth rinse. *J. Am. dent. Ass.* **86**, 404–8.

Report of United Kingdom Mission (1953). Caries inhibition with fluoride gel and fluoride varnish in rats. *Caries Res.* **4**, 63.

Roberts, J.F., Bibby, B.G., and Wellcok, W.D. (1948). The effect of an acidulated fluoride mouthwash on dental caries. *J. dent. Res.* **27**, 497–500.

Rock, W.P. (1972). Fissure sealants: further results of clinical trials. *Br. dent. J.* **136**, 317.

Rock, W.P., Gordon, P.H., and Bradnock, G. (1981). Dental caries experience in Birmingham and Wolverhampton school children following the fluoridation of Birmingham water in 1964. *Br. dent. J.* **150**, 61–6.

Roemer, R. (1983). Legislation on fluorides and dental health. *Int. Dig. hlth. Legislation.* **34**, 3–31.

Rugg-Gunn, A.J., Holloway, P.J., and Davies, T.G.H. (1973). Caries prevention by daily fluoride mouth rinsing. *Br. dent. J.* **135**, 353–60.

Rugg-Gunn, A.J., Edgar, W.M., Jenkins, G.N., and Cockburn, M.A. (1976). Plaque F. and plaque acid production in children drinking milk fluoridated to 1 and 5 ppm F. (Abstr.) *J. dent. Res.* **55**, D143.

Rugg-Gunn, A.J., Carmichael, C.L., French, A.D., and Furness, J.A. (1977). Fluoridation in Newcastle and Northumberland: a clinical study of 5-year-old children. *Br. dent. J.* **142**, 359–402.

Rugg-Gunn, A.J., Nicholas, K.E., Potts, A., Cranage, J.D., Carmichael, C.L., and French, A.D. (1981). Caries experience of 5 year old children living in four communities in N.E. England receiving differing water fluoride levels. *Br. dent. J.* **150**, 9–12.

Rosoff, L.L., Konikoff, B.S., Frye, J.B., Johnston J.E., and Frye, W.W. (1962). Fluoride addition to milk and its effect on dental caries in school children. *Am. J. clin. Nutr.* **11**, 94–107.

Russell, A.L. and Elvove, E. (1951). Domestic water and dental caries, VII. A study of the fluoride dental varies relationship in an adult population. *Publ. Hlth. Rep.* **66**, 1389–401.

Ruzicka, J.A., Mrklas, L., and Rokytova, K. (1976). The influence of salt intake on the incorporation of fluoride into mouse bone. *Caries Res.* **10**, 386–9.

Schützmannsky, G. (1965). Further results of our tablet fluoridation in Halle. *Dt. Stomatol.* **15**, 107–14.

Schützmannsky, G. (1971). Fluorine tablet application in pregnant females. *Dt. Stomatol.* **21**, 122–9.

Sellman, S., Syrrist, A., and Gustafson, G. (1957). Fluorine and dental health in Southern Sweden. *T. Odont. Tskr.* **65**, 61–93.

Seppa, L., Tuutti, H., and Luoma, H. (1982). Three year report on caries prevention using fluoride varnish for caries risk children in a community with fluoridated water. *Scand. J. dent. Res.* **96**, 89–94.

Silver, D.H. (1974). The prevalence of dental caries in 3-year-old children. *Br. dent. J.* **137**, 123–8.

Silver, D.H. (1982). Improvements in the dental health of 3-year-old Hertfordshire children after 8 years. *Br. dent. J.* **153**, 179–82.

Smyth, J.F.A. and Withnell, A. (1974). Daily fluoride tablets. *Hlth. soc. Sci. J.* **84**, 419–23.

Stamm, J.W. (1974). Fluoride uptake from topical sodium fluoride varnish measured by an *in vivo* enamel biopsy. *J. Can. dent. Ass.* **40**, 501–5.

Stephen, K.W. and Campbell, D. (1978). Caries reduction and cost benefit after 3 years of sucking fluoride tablets daily at school. *Br. dent. J.* **144**, 202–6.

Stephen, K.W., Campbell, D., and Boyle, I.T. (1981). A double-blind caries study with fluoridated school milk—five year data from a vitamin D deficient area. *Caries Res.* ORCA Congress, Erfurt, 1981, Abstr. 71.

Tewari, A., Chawla, H.S., and Utreja, A. (1984). Caries preventive effect of three topical fluorides ($1\frac{1}{2}$ years clinical trial in Chandigarh schoolchildren of North India). *J. int. Ass. Dent. Child.* **15**, 71–81.

Timmis, J.C. (1971). Caries experience of 5-year-old children living in fluoride and non-fluoride areas of Essex. *Br. dent. J.* **130**, 278–83.

Torell, P. and Ericsson, Y. (1965). Two year clinical tests with different methods of local caries prevention. Fluoride application in Swedish school children. *Acta odont. Scand.* **16**, 329–41.

Torrell, P. and Siberg, A. (1962). Mouthwash with sodium fluoride and potassium fluoride. *Odont. Revy.* **13**, 62–72.

Toth, K. (1976). A study of 8 years of domestic salt fluoridation for prevention of caries. *Commun. Dent. oral Epidemiol.* **4**, 106–10.

Toth, K. (1978). Some economic aspects of domestic salt fluoridation. (Abstr.) *Caries Res.* **12**, 110.

Toth, K. (1979). 10 years of domestic salt fluoridation in Hungary. (Abstr.) *Caries Res.* **13**, 101.

Toth, K. (1980). Factors influencing the urinary fluoride level in subjects drinking low fluoride water. (Abstr.) *caries Res.* **14**, 168.

Treide, A., Hebenstreit, W., and Gunther, A. (1980). Kollective Kariespravention in Vorchulatter unter Verwendung eines Fluoridhaltingenlackes. *Stomat.* DDR **30**, 734.

Ulvestad, H. (1987). Preventive effect of semi-annual applications of a 2% NaF solution and of a fluoride varnish over a two year period, relating to approximal caries in primary and first permanent molars. *Scand. J. dent. Res.*

Vines, J.J. and Clavero, J. (1968). Investigacion de la relacion entre la incidencia de caries y contenido del ion fluor en las agnas de abastecimiento. *Rev. San. E. Hig. Pub.* **42**, 401–31.

Volker, J.F. and Bibby, B.G. (1941). The action of fluoride on limiting dental caries. *Medicine* **20**, 211.

Volker, J.F., Hodge, H.C., Wilson, H.J., and Von Voorhis, S.N. (1940). The absorption of fluoride by enamel dentine bone, and hydroxyapatite as shown by radioactive isotope. *J. biol. Chem.* **134**, 543.

Water (Fluoridation) Act (1985). *An Act to make provision with respect to the fluoridation of water supplies.* Chapter 63, 30 October. HMSO, London.

Weaver, R. (1944). Fluorosis and dental caries on Tyneside. *Br. dent. J.* **76**, 29–40.

Weaver, R. (1950). Fluorine and wartime diet. *Br. dent. J.* **88**, 231–9.

Wellock, W.D. and Brudevold, F. (1963). A study of acidulated fluoride solutions II. The caries inhibiting effect of single annual applications of an acid fluoride and phosphate solution. A 2 year experience. *Archs. oral. Biol.* **8**, 179–82.

Wellock, W.D., Maitland, A., and Brudevold, F. (1965). Caries increments, tooth discoloration, and state of oral hygiene in children given single annual applications of acid phosphate fluoride gel and stannous fluoride. *Archs. oral. Biol.* **10**, 453.

Wespi, H.J. (1948). Gedanke zuer Frage der optimalen Ernahrung in der Schwangerschaft. Salz and Brot als Trager zusatzlicher Nahrungsstoffe. *Schweiz. med. Wschr.* **78**, 153–5.

Wespi, H.J. (1950). Fluoriertes Kochsalz zur Cariesprophylaxe. *Schweiz. med. Wschr.* **80**, 561–4.

Whittle, J.G. and Downer, M.C. (1979). Dental health and treatment needs of Birmingham and Salford schoolchildren. *Br. dent. J.* **147**, 67–71.

Winter, K. (1975). Kariesprophylaxe durch Lokalapplikation von Natrium fluoride-Lack. *Zahnärtztl. Mitt.* **65**, 215.

World Health Organization (1970). *Fluorides and human health*, WHO Monogr. Ser. No. 59, WHO, Geneva.

World Health Organization (1986). *Appropriate use of fluorides for human health*. WHO, Geneva.

Zacherl, W.A. (1981). A three-year clinical caries evaluation of the effect of a sodium fluoride-silica abrasive dentifrice. *Pharmacol. ther. Dent.* **6**, 1–7.

Ziegler, E. (1962). Milk fluoridation. *Bull. Schweiz. Akad. Med. Wiss.* 18.

Zipkin, I. and McClure, F.J. (1951). Complex fluorides: caries reduction and fluoride retention in the bones and teeth of white rats. *Publ. Hlth. Rep.* **66**, 1523–32.

4

Oral cleanliness and dental caries

PHILIP SUTCLIFFE

THIS exploration of the relationship between oral cleanliness and caries begins with the widely accepted premise that dental caries occurs only after plaque has accumulated on susceptible tooth surfaces in individuals who eat sugar frequently. The process is slow and all three factors must occur together. Epidemiological corroboration of the theory lacks consistency and as a result the intrinsic value of oral hygiene practices against the initiation of caries has been vigorously challenged (Bibby 1966).

The interdependence of plaque, sugar, tooth susceptibility, and time has been well demonstrated in Tristan du Cunha and Hopewood House where susceptible populations with heavy accumulations of plaque remained relatively free from dental caries as long as only small amounts of sugar were eaten. In 1938 no one under the age of 20 years in Tristan da Cunha had a carious first permanent molar, even though the standard of oral cleanliness was poor. The average daily consumption of sugar, confectionery, preserves, and sweets totalled 2.5 g per person. By 1962 this had risen to 244 g (Fisher 1968) and 50 per cent of first permanent molars were found to be carious in a sample of 64 islanders aged between 6 and 20 years. The standard of oral cleanliness had remained poor (Holloway *et al.* 1963).

Hopewood House was established in New South Wales, Australia, to look after needy children. The diet, which was lactovegetarian, consisted mainly of uncooked vegetables and was notable for an almost complete absence of sugar. The food was adequate in essential nutrients and the general health of the children compared well with that of other children in New South Wales except for dental caries where the Hopwood House children were much better off. The standard of oral cleanliness was poor. Thirteen-year-olds in Hopewood House had a mean of 1.1 DMF teeth compared with 10.7 in children of similar age attending state schools (Sullivan and Harris 1958; Gillham and Lennon 1958).

Studies of the relationship between caries and oral cleanliness may be divided into four approaches: point-prevalence surveys of total caries experience and oral cleanliness; longitudinal retrospective studies of oral cleanliness and increments in caries experience; reported tooth-brushing frequency and total caries experience; and finally prospective studies of improved oral cleanliness and increments in caries experience. The fundamental difficulty with the first three approaches is that good oral hygiene habits may be accompanied by other practices that help to preserve the teeth. It is extremely difficult to disentangle the effect of these habits retrospectively and frequently this has not been attempted.

Fluoride has a proven effect against caries and dentrifices are becoming an increasingly important method of topical application. Except where a specific note is made this review is confined to fluoride-free, unmedicated toothpastes.

Point-prevalence surveys (Table 4.1)

Oral cleanliness is usually described by a qualitative plaque index, and caries experience by the DMFT and DMFS indices. The combined use of these indices in a single investigation may be inappropriate because of the transient nature of plaque deposits. Plaque indices refer strictly to the standard of oral cleanliness at the moment of the examination whilst caries indices give the total caries experience accumulated from the time of tooth eruption. Thus an investigation into the permanent dentitions of 12-year-olds assumes that the standard of oral cleanliness has remained the same for roughly 6 years. This assumption may be more valid when only the children with extreme standards of oral cleanliness are selected for comparison.

The reported studies appear to have been conducted almost exclusively on children between the ages of 3 and 15 years, and mainly with older children. Where mean DMFT or DMFS values may be identified the results of the studies are summarized in Table 4.1

Trubman (1963) studied 397 children from Jackson, Missouri, aged between 12 and 14 years, and found a weak negative and statistically insignificant correlation between caries experience and oral cleanliness. The children with the cleanest oral hygiene scores had a mean of 15.0 DMF surfaces compared with 14.2 in the worst group.

McHugh *et al.* (1964) found no significant correlation between oral hygiene scores and the mean numbers of DMF teeth in 2905 children aged 13 years from Dundee, Scotland. Similar results have been reported from Finland and Canada. Parviainen *et al.* (1977) studied 365 13- to 15-year-olds from three Finnish communities with varying amounts of fluoride in the drinking water. In none of the communities was a correlation found between visible plaque index scores and DMF caries scores. Richardson *et al.* (1977) found no significant correlation between oral hygiene indices and caries when they examined a total of 457 7- and 13-year-old Canadian children. In this study of first- and seventh-grade children, refined and total carbohydrate consumption was also measured. It was found that the children with high caries indices did not have the poorest oral hygiene nor consume the most carbohydrates. The children with low caries indices did not have the cleanest teeth nor consume lesser amounts of carbohydrates.

Table 4.1. Prevalence studies of caries and oral cleanliness

Reference	Age of subjects	Index of oral cleanliness	No. of subjects	Mean caries experience	% Increase	Significance
McCauley and Frazier (1957)	6–10	Oral hygiene score				
		(good) 4.0	983	2.4 DMFT		Not given
		3.0–3.9	1238	2.9	21	
		2.0–2.9	247	3.5	46	
		(poor) 1.0–1.9	30	4.4	83	
Mansbridge (1960)	12–14	Good	146	9.6 DMFT		
		Fair	162	10.2	6	$p<0.05$
		Neglected	1[illegible]8	11.5	20	$p<0.01$
Trubman (1963)	12–14	Oral hygiene index				
		(good) 0.0–0.4	99	15.0 DMFS		$r = -0.07$
		0.5–0.9	142	15.9	6	$p>0.05$
		1.0–1.4	80	14.6	−3	
		1.5–1.9	37	11.1	−26	
		(poor) 2.0+	39	14.2	−5	
McHugh *et al*. (1964)	13	Oral hygiene index				
		(good) Under 5	341	9.6 DMFT		n.s.
		6–7	730	9.7	1	
		8–9	859	10.3	7	
		(poor) 10–12	955	9.9	3	
Sutcliffe (1977)	3–4	Simplified debris				
		(good) 0.0–0.5	259	1.6 dmft		$p<0.001$
		(poor) 1.5+	236	3.6 dmft	125	
Bjertness *et al*. (1986)	35 (1973)	OHI-S 0.00–0.99	35	81.7 DMFS		
		1.00–1.99	54	86.1	11	
		2.00+	27	95.6	17	$0.05>p>0.01$
	35	OHI-S 0.00–0.99	47	80.3 DMFS		
		1.00–1.99	62	89.8	12	
		2.00+	35	82.9	3	$0.05>p>0.01$

The authors commented that the lack of correlation between caries and carbohydrate consumption may have been due to the limitations of self-recorded diet surveys and to the problem of correlating indices with different time bases. However, in a study of the dental health of 1015 schoolchildren, aged 11 to 12 years, living in South Wales, Addy *et al.* (1986) reported highly statistically significant but low Pearson correlation coefficients between plaque scores ad DMFT ($r = 0.14$) or DMFS ($r = 0.09$).

In an earlier and broadly similar study of 12- to 14-year-olds from Miami the diet and oral cleanliness of 46 caries-free children was contrasted with data from 40 caries-active children. Diet scores, based upon the frequency and quality of sugar eating, were found to be significantly associated with caries experience. However a negligible inverse relationship between caries and oral cleanliness was found that may have occurred because many children who normally did not brush their teeth did so because they expected the dental examination (Duany *et al.* 1972).

Bay and Ainamo (1974) adopted a slightly different approach: 293 7-year-old Copenhagen children were ranked according to caries experience, and the PLG plaque index scores were compared between 89 low caries-risk children (4 or fewer affected tooth surfaces) and 56 high caries-risk children (22 or more affected tooth surfaces). The first group had a mean plaque score of 1.9 and the second group 2.2. Although this difference was significant ($p<0.05$), the authors commented that it was of no clinical importance. Additional analysis did reveal that most of the heavy plaque scores were in the high caries group.

In two studies of random samples of 35-year-old Oslo citizens carried out in 1973 and 1984 the participants were grouped together according to their simplified oral hygiene index scores (*Bjertness et al.* 1986). The mean numbers of DMFS surfaces were then compared between each of the three oral hygiene groups. In each survey a statistically significant increase in caries experience was found with increase in the OHI-S score. In the 1973 survey there was a 17 per cent increase in DMF surfaces between the low and high oral-hygiene score groups; in 1984 the increase was 3 per cent. These average differences amounted to 13.9 and 2.6 DMF surfaces respectively.

McCauley and Frazier (1957), Mansbridge (1960), and Sutcliffe (1977) found that poorer standards of oral cleanliness in children were accompanied by an increase in the total caries experience. When the results of the three studies are taken together and only the 'best' and 'worst' children are compared then it can be seen that the greatest increase was found in the youngest children (3- and 4-year-olds), and the smallest increase in the oldest subjects (12- to 14-year-olds).

Kleemola-Kujala (1978) examined the relationship between the amount of plaque that had accumulated on groups of teeth and caries experience in a total of 806 5-, 9- and 13-year-old Finnish children. The results showed an increase in caries experience of all tooth types with increasing plaque at all ages, although only slight increases were found in permanent molar teeth. Mansbridge (1960) came to a similar conclusion when he compared the 12- to 14-year-olds with 'good' and 'neglected' oral hygiene. He found that the differences in caries experience were greatest in the premolar and incisor teeth, and smallest in molars. Similarly a greater response to poor oral cleanliness was found in deciduous incisor and canine teeth, rather than molar teeth, in 4-year-olds (Sutcliffe 1977).

In a further report on Finnish children in low fluoride areas the relative contribution of increased plaque accumulation and sugar consumption to the total load of caries was assessed (Kleemola-Kujala ans Rasanen 1982). A total of 543 children, aged 5, 9 and 13 years, took part in the study. They were divided into three groups of plaque level according to their plaque indices, and into three groups of sugar consumption assessed by a 24-hour recall method. Caries experience was expressed as the proportion of tooth surfaces examined which were found carious or filled.

The results suggest that when oral hygiene is poor, even a relatively low total sugar consumption can promote decay in caries-susceptible primary and young permanent teeth. The association between the amount of plaque and dental caries was statistically significant at all levels of sugar consumption. With increasing total sugar consumption the risk of caries increased significantly only when oral hygiene was simultaneously poor.

Retrospective longitudinal studies (Table 4.2)

Data collected during clinical trials have been used to look back upon the relationship between successive estimations of oral cleanliness and the increase in caries that has occurred over the same period. This approach goes some way to-towards avoiding the combined use of indices with different time bases, but children recruited to take part in clinical trials are selected for their qualities of co-operation and motivation, and may not be typical of all children.

In a 3-year study with adolescents, Holloway and Teagle (1976) compared mean caries increments in 63 subjects with good oral cleanliness at annual examinations with the increment measured in 52 subjects with poor oral cleanliness throughout. Although lower increments were found in those with good oral cleanliness the difference, which amounted to only one attacked tooth surface in 3 years, did not attain statistical significance.

In a similar 3-year study, Sutcliffe (1973) compared the caries increments between 42 children who had good oral cleanliness at annual examinations and 107 children with poor oral cleanliness. The children were initially aged between 11 and 12 years. Those children with clean teeth at each examination had the smallest mean increment, but the difference was rather less than 0.5 DMFT and was not statistically significant.

The dry weight of plaque collected from one side of the mouth at intervals of 1, two, and three years after baseline examinations had been completed was compared with the 3-year increment in DF surfaces in 51 boys, aged between 11 and 14 years. All of the coefficients of correlation showed a weak, positive associ-

Table 4.2. Retrospective longitudinal studies of caries increments and oral cleanliness

Reference	Initial age of subjects	Duration of study	Index of oral cleanliness	Number of subjects	Mean caries increments	% increase	Significance
Sutcliffe (1973)	11–12	3 years	Good	Boys 8	3.00 DMFT		n.s.
			Fair	131	3.17	6	
			Poor	78	3.47	16	
			Good	Girls 34	4.21 DMFT		n.s.
			Fair	118	3.97	−6	
			Poor	29	4.52	7	
Tucker *et al.* (1976)	11	3 years	Good.	184	4.25 DMFT		$p < 0.05$
			Poor	192	4.96	17	
			Good	184	8.35 DMFS		n.s.
			Poor	192	9.27	11	
Beal *et al.* (1979)	11–12	3 years	Clean	59	7.59 DMFS	36	$p < 0.05$
			Not clean	101	10.29		

ation but only the correlation for first-year plaque was significant (Ashley and Wilson 1977). The correlation between the 3-year DF surface increment and the mean dry weight of plaque from the three samples was also weak and positive and was again not statistically significant.

Tucker *et al.* (1976) examined the relationship between the 3-year increment in caries experience in 184 children with 'good' and 192 with 'poor' oral cleanliness measured at three annual intervals. Initially the children were between 11 and 12 years old. Children with good oral cleanliness had mean increments of 4.3 DMFT or 8.4 DMFS, the mean values in children with 'poor' oral cleanliness were greater by 0.7 DMFT or 0.9 DMFS respectively. Only the difference between DMF teeth was statistically significant ($p<0.05$). The results were more clear-cut for teeth which had erupted during the trial. The mean caries increment in teeth which were unerupted at the base-line examination was 1.3 DMFT or 1.6 DMFS in those with good oral cleanliness, and 1.9 DMFT or 2.5 DMFS in those with poor oral cleanliness. These differences were highly statistically significant ($p<0.001$).

Beal *et al.* (1979) also contrasted the 3-year increment in caries experience in children initially aged 11 to 12 years whose dental status was consistantly clean or not clean. There were 59 children with consistently clean mouths with a mean increment of 7.59 DMFS compared with a mean of 10.29 DMFS in 101 children with consistently unclean mouths—the difference was statistically significant ($p<0.05$).

In a prospective 2-year study involving 405 English children, initially aged 11.5 years, the results of 3-day diet records, collected on five occasions, were compared with the increments in caries experience (Rugg-Gunn *et al.* 1984). Correlations between caries increment and dietary factors were low due to the low caries increments observed and the large error associated with dietary data where analyses attempt to discriminate between individuals. The highest correlation was between caries increment and weight of daily intake of sugars ($+0.143, p<0.01$). At each annual examination the level of gingival inflammation was used as a measure of plaque accumulation for each child. Of the non-dietary variables studied (sex, social class, gingival index, and tooth-brushing frequency) only gingival index significantly increased the correlation between weight of sugars and caries increment. This interesting result parallels the finding by Kleemola-Kujala and Rasanan (1982) of an interaction between increased plaque accumulation and sugar consumption.

The frequency of tooth-brushing and dental caries (Table 4.3)

The reported frequency of tooth-brushing has also been used to investigate the relationship between oral cleanliness and dental caries. This indirect method has considerable limitations because those who frequently brush their teeth are probably those who are most likely to carry out other procedures to improve their dental health such as restricting sugar eating and seeking regular dental

Table 4.3. Studies of caries and frequency of tooth-brushing

Reference	Age of subjects	Daily brushing frequency	Number of subjects	Mean caries experience	% Increase	Significance
Smith and Striffler (1963)	18–44	Twice or more yesterday	1043	9.51 DMFT		n.s.
		Once yesterday	752	7.57	−20	
		Did not brush yesterday	171	5.73	−40	
Dale (1969)	17–29	Three times	31	17.19 DMFT		n.s.
		Twice	188	19.11	11	
		Once	327	19.47	13	
		Less than once	67	18.67	9	
Miller and Hobson (1961) Miller (1961)	12	Regular	115	5.8 DMFT		$p < 0.05$
		Irregular	264	5.0	−14	
		None	357	5.0	−14	
				3 year increment		
Tucker *et al.* (1976)	11–14	Twice or more	187	4.29 DMFT		$p < 0.05$
		Less than twice	189	4.94	15	

check-ups. An additional complication is that dental attenders have been found to have higher mean numbers of DMF teeth than irregular attenders (Todd 1975; Todd and Walker 1980). Regular adult tooth-brushers have also been found to have a lower mean number of decayed, that is untreated teeth, than regular brushers (Dale 1969; Ainamo 1971). This may be seen as evidence of the relationship between regular brushing and other tooth-preserving habits. Finally a direct relationship between tooth-brushing and oral hygiene status has not always been found (Tucker *et al.* 1976). Frequent tooth-brushing need not necessarily lead to freedom from plaque if the brushing is inefficient. An exaggerated claim for frequent brushing may be checked by an oral examination (Miller and Hobson 1961).

In a study of 555 children, aged between 1 and 5 years, from Camden in London, parents were asked whether or not they brushed their child's teeth each day. Two hundred and ninety-five children (53 per cent of the total study population) were reported to have daily tooth-brushing. Eighty four per cent of these children were caries-free compared with 89 per cent among those who did not clean daily. This small difference was not statistically significant (Holt *et al.* 1982).

In the study of Danish 7-year-olds already referred to, Bay and Ainamo (1974) found no difference in frequency of tooth-brushing between the low- and high-caries risk groups. A correlation was not found between the frequency of tooth-brushing and DFS scores in 13- to 15-year-old Finnish children (Ainamo and Parviainen 1979).

One hundred and fifteen 12-year-old English children who brushed once a day and who were also found to have clean teeth had a mean of 5.8 DMF teeth, which was significantly greater ($p<0.05$) than the mean of 5.0 found in 621 children who brushed less than once a day (Miller 1961; Miller and Hobson 1961).

In their 3-year retrospective study, Tucker *et al.* (1976) reported that the increment in caries experience was 4.3 DMF teeth in those who brushed their teeth as least twice daily compared with a mean of 4.9 DMF teeth in those who brushed less frequently. The difference was significant ($p<0.05$).

This type of investigation has also been carried out on adults. The reported frequency of tooth-brushing was not found to be related to the mean DMFT in 1976 adults aged 18 to 44 years from New Mexico (Smith and Striffler 1963). No relationship was found between tooth-brushing frequency and DMFT in 613 regular servicemen aged between 17 and 29 years from Sydney, Australia (Dale 1969).

In an interesting study Rajala *et al.* (1980) tried to disentangle the influence of behaviours associated with tooth-brushing upon caries experience. Information was obtained from 212 male employees at a Finnish paper mill. Potential risk indicators other than tooth-brushing were controlled by stratification using a multivariate confounder summarizing score. The variates included in the model were number of teeth, education, sucrose consumption, previous fluoride exposure, income, and use of dental services. In general it was found that caries experience was consistently higher for sporadic tooth-brushers. The authors also commented that their results indicated that the positive association between reported daily tooth-brushing and low caries experience may be more pronounced in groups with higher overall risk status, e.g. in the strata where education and income was low, frequency of dental visits irregular, number of teeth small, use of sucrose high, and fluoride exposure low. This finding suggests that in situations where the 'base-line prevention' is weak, tooth-brushing may be useful in caries prevention, or vice versa, the true effect of tooth-brushing may be hidden by other, perhaps more powerful, means of caries prevention.

Prospective studies (Table 4.4)

The most satisfactory method of examining the relationship between oral cleanliness and caries is by means of controlled prospective studies in which randomly assigned test subjects experience an improved standard of oral cleanliness. The improvement may be achieved by either encouraging the participants to thoroughly clean their teeth under supervision or by cleaning the teeth professionally.

Self-cleaning studies

Fosdick compared the 2-year caries increment in 423 students who continued with their customary oral hygiene habits, with the increment in 523 test subjects who undertook to brush their teeth thoroughly within 10 minutes after eating food or sweets or, when brushing was impossible, to rinse the mouth thoroughly with water. A significantly smaller increment was recorded in the test group but deficiences in the design of this early study complicate an overall assessment of the result (Fosdick 1950; Smith and Striffler 1963).

Alice M. Horowitz and her colleagues studied the effect of an intensive school-based plaque-removal programme on children initially aged from 10 to 13 years. A fluoride-free dentifrice was used. Children from the same school were randomly placed in the test or control group. For 32 months the subjects in the treatment group carried out tooth-brushing and flossing each school day. Of the 481 children initially examined, 295 remained in the study for 32 months. Of these, 279 were present at all of the six examinations, 111 in the treatment group and 168 in the control group. Data were reported for these children only. Most of the children found the system of cleaning boring, the school staff became increasingly less co-operative, and the supervising personnel commented that the programme was very demanding. After 32 months only the test-group girls showed a significant reduction in plaque score ($p < 0.01$) although the boys showed some improvement. Both boys and girls showed a significant improvement in gingival health ($p < 0.01$). Losses of subjects during the trial resulted in an imbalance in the initial mean caries experience of the children seen at every examination and adjusted mean incremental DMFS scores are presented in the results. The adjusted mean increment in the treatment group was 4.3 DMF sur-

Table 4.4. Prospective studies of caries increments and improved oral cleanliness

Reference	Age of subjects	Duration of study	Group	Number of subjects	Mean caries increment	% Decrease	Significance
Horowitz *et al.* (1980)	10–13	32 months	Self-cleaning	111	4.27 DMFS	13	n.s.
			Control	168	4.89		
Silverstein *et al.* (1977)	12	29 months	Montera				
			self-cleaning	42	4.17 DMFS	−157	n.s.
			control	45	1.62		
			Lowell				
			self-cleaning	76	6.51 DMFS	7	n.s.
			control	73	7.00		
Ashley and Sainsbury (1981)	11	3 years	Professional cleaning	119	4.83 DFS	−11	n.s.
			Control	102	4.34		
Wright *et al.* (1979)	5.8	20 months	Professionally flossed		New proximal lesions		
			surfaces	Group 1. 44	13	55	$p = 0.004$
			Control	44	29		
			Professionally flossed				
			surfaces	Group 2. 44	12	52	$p = 0.014$
			Control	44	25		

faces and 4.9 DMF surfaces in the control group. This 13 per cent reduction was not significant. The biggest reduction of 26 per cent or 0.7 DMF surfaces was seen in proximal sites but this was not statistically significant (Horowitz *et al.* 1980).

Another study from the United States produced broadly similar results (Silverstein *et al.* 1977, and personal communication). At each of two junior high schools in Oaklands, California, 393 12-year-olds were randomly allocated to control and test groups. The treatment groups brushed without a dentifrice and flossed every school day under supervision. At the fifth and final examination after 29 months, 227 children remained in the study. In one school significant reductions in plaque and gingivitis scores were measured in the test children but in the other school only a reduction in gingivitis scores were recorded. Caries examinations at both schools showed no significant differences in DMFS increments. In this study the control group experienced only slightly smaller improvements in gingivitis and plaque deposits than those in the test group, perhaps as a result of peer pressure from the test-group children.

The value of limited self-flossing under supervision in schools has also been investigated. The aim was to test a very simple style of flossing, which was achieved by pulling the waxed floss once up and down through each contact point. A half-mouth technique was adopted for the evaluation and 140 Swedish children aged between 12 and 13 years flossed the right or the left lateral region once every school day for 2 years. The children were stratified according to their dietary and oral hygiene habits. After 2 years no statistically significant differences were found in caries increments between the flossed and unflossed surfaces. The authors commented that this was probably due to the inadequate flossing technique (Granath *et al.* 1979).

Professional tooth-cleaning

In order to investigate the value of more thorough flossing against proximal caries, Wright and his co-workers carried out two successive short studies each of 20 months duration. The combined results from the two studies are referred to here. The first-grade Canadian children had an initial mean age of 5.8 years. A half-mouth technique was used in which quadrants were assigned randomly to test and control groups. Initially 118 children took part in the study yielding 528 pairs of contralateral surfaces. To qualify for inclusion the pairs of surfaces had to be initially caries-free and in contact with the adjacent tooth. Six surfaces were studied, from the distal of the deciduous canine tooth to the mesial of the first permanent molar. Caries assessments depended upon a combination of mirror and probe examinations supplemented by radiographic data. Drop outs and losses at individual examinations reduced the number of participants to 88 Research assistants flossed the test surfaces each school day and no other oral hygiene procedure or instruction was provided. The 20-month study period included a 4-month summer vacation when flossing was discontinued. The study yielded 374 test and 374 control surfaces. After 20 months, 25 of the test surfaces had developed caries compared with 54 control surfaces. The difference in the incidence of new proximal lesions was significant ($p = 0.014$).

The authors concluded that professionally applied flossing reduces proximal caries but also added that the results were produced under strictly controlled circumstances that could not necessarily be found in an individual or community flossing programme (Wright *et al.* 1979). It is also appropriate to comment that a clinical trial of 20 months duration is rather short. It is impossible to set out precise guidelines but a test period of 2 years for teeth erupting during a trial has been recommended (Horowitz 1968).

The effect of a 3-year school-based plaque-control programme with English girls initially aged 11 years has been reported (Ashley and Sainsbury 1981). Initially 261 children agreed to take part in the study and 221 were seen at the final examination, 119 in the experimental group and 102 in the control group. The children all attended the same school but the classes were randomly assigned to experimental or control groups. Girls in the experimental group visited a dental hygienist, based at the school, every 2 weeks during term time and, following disclosing, brushing, and oral hygiene reinforcement, received a professional prophylaxis using a fluoride-free polishing paste. Girls in the control group received oral hygiene instruction during the first term of the base-line year only. All participants received a new toothbrush each term and were encouraged to use a fluoride-containing toothpaste at home. Caries was assessed clinically supplemented by bitewing radiographs of posterior teeth. Mean dry weights of plaque are given for the first 2 years of the study.

The baseline mean number of DF surfaces in the 119 experimental group of children was 6.8 compared with 7.0 in the 102 control group girls. The 3-year mean increments in DF surfaces were 4.8 and 4.3 respectively; the difference was not statistically significant. The authors commented that a 'spill-over effect' from the experimental group regime to the control group may have influenced the results; there is some evidence of this from the changes in gingival health in both groups of participants. At the end of the first and second years the experimental group of girls had fewer inflamed gingival sites but by the end of the third year there was only a slight difference in favour of the experimental group which did not reach statistical significance. A second factor may have been the effect of selecting girls for the study since they have a higher dental awareness than boys. Even the most unkempt girls may not have accumulated sufficient quantities of plaque to permit an evaluation on the initiation of caries. However, at the end of the first and second years the experimental group had a significantly smaller mean dry weight of plaque. Home use of fluoride dentifrice in both groups may have obscured benefits arising from the professional cleaning. Twelve months after the end of the study 109 children from the experimental group and 93 from the control group were re-examined. The experimental group still had significantly less plaque than the control group. However no significant differences were observed in caries increments between the groups, indicating that the programme had no delayed effect on caries experience. (Ashley and Sainsbury 1982).

A number of Scandinavian studies have shown remarkable reductions in caries increments in children who have received regular professional prophylaxis combined with some form of fluoride therapy (Lindhe *et al.* 1975; Badersten *et al.* 1975; Hamp *et al.* 1978). The individual contributions of the effects of the prophylaxis and of fluoride to the reductions in caries increments remains speculative. The result of a cross-over study has been published, which was designed to measure the relative effects of fluoride and plaque control. Initially 164 13- to 14-year-old Swedish children were randomly assigned to one of four groups. The value of chlorhexidine gel, mechanical tooth-cleaning with and without fluoride, rinsing with fluoride solution or distilled water, and the use of fluoride or placebo dentifrices were all evaluated over a 2-year period with changes in the regimes after 1 year. The authors found that the results of the trial revealed the overall importance of regularly repeated inter-proximal plaque elimination in the prevention of proximal surface caries in children (Axelsson *et al.* 1976). However, 1 year is probably too short a time to judge the effect of a regime on mean caries increment.

In a review of 22 studies of the effectiveness of frequent professional prophylaxis, Ripa (1985) commented that although this technique can apparently significantly reduce dental caries incidence in both children and adults, a wide range of preventive techniques had been employed in the investigations. He observed that in the studies that did not employ a fluoride-containing prophylaxis paste or in which the children were not making use of fluoride, statistically significant differences in the caries increments between control and treatment groups were not achieved.

Discussion

As a starting point three ways of investigating the relationship between caries and oral cleanliness have been described. About half of the prevalence studies reviewed earlier have shown a positive association between plaque and caries (McCauley and Frazier 1957; Mansbridge 1960; Bay and Ainamo 1974; Sutcliffe 1977; Kleemola-Kujala 1978; Bjertness *et al.* 1986). The remaining studies revealed no relationship (McHugh *et al.* 1964; Nordling and Ainamo 1977; Richardson *et al.* 1977) or a weak negative relationship (Trubman 1963; Duany *et al.* 1972). The list of prevalence studies is not exhaustive but those selected are sufficient to show the pattern of results. All of the retrospective studies showed a positive trend with an increase in caries experience associated with poorer standards of oral cleanliness although the results seldom reached significance (Sutcliffe 1973; Holloway and Teagle 1976; Tucker *et al.* 1976; Ashley and Wilson 1977; Beal *et al.* 1979).

Studies of the relationship between brushing frequency and caries represent the least satisfactory approach because of the indirectness of the method and most of the results showed no relationship (Smith and Striffler 1963; Dale 1969; Bay and Ainamo 1974; Ainamo and Parviainen 1979; Holt *et al.* 1982). One study showed a significant negative relationship (Miller 1961). Two studies showed a positive relationship (Tucker *et al.* 1976; Rajala *et al.* 1980).

The consensus of the results of the more preferable prevalence and retrospective studies point towards the presence of a weak positive association between plaque and caries. As possessing clean teeth may be associated with other caries-preventing behaviours it is important to establish if oral cleanliness alone has a direct relationship with caries. This is best achieved by clinical trials of a least two, and preferably three years' duration, in which caries-susceptible subjects are randomly assigned to control and test groups that are initially well balanced. Because the presence of plaque, as measured in epidemiological studies, is likely to have only a weak influence on caries increments, other powerful preventive agents such as fluoride should preferably be absent. A treatment-controlled study is also preferable since a high level of restorative care provided outside the control of the investigators may obscure a preventive effect (Jackson and Sutcliffe 1967). None of the prospective studies that have been described completely fulfil these criteria. This in itself is an indication of the difficulty of conducting such studies.

Unfortunately the well-designed study by Horowitz and her co-workers suffered losses that upset the initial balance of the groups, and the final caries increment data was adjusted to accommodate the influence of the losses. The effect of this adjustment on the final overall conclusion of a positive but statistically insignificant relationship between plaque and caries is not clear.

In the similar study conducted by Silverstein and his colleagues the control group experienced marked reductions in gingivitis and plaque as the trial continued, possibly as a result of peer pressure. It is a fundamental requirement in self-cleansing studies that the experimental group should have measurably less plaque after the base-line examinations and the absence of this difference, particularly at one of the schools makes it difficult to interpret the final result of no significant differences in caries increments between the control and experimental groups.

The problem of ensuring that the participants maintain high levels of oral cleanliness is eliminated if teeth are cleaned professionally. The clearest indication that daily interproximal cleaning reduces the incidence of proximal surface caries in the deciduous dentition comes from a study conducted by Wright *et al.* (1979). It is tantalizing that the study continued for only 20 months.

Both the control and experimental groups of girls in the school-based plaque-control programme described by Ashley and Sainsbury (1981) were encouraged to use a fluoride-containing toothpaste at home and it is possible that this was sufficient to mask the effect of the fortnightly disclosing, brushing, and fluoride-free professional prophylaxis.

Thus there is no unequivocal evidence that good oral cleanliness reduces caries experience, nor is there sufficient evidence to condemn the value of good oral cleanliness as a caries preventive. When the effects of a number of variables upon caries experience were studied the results indicated that poor standards of oral cleanliness enhance the cariogenicity of sucrose in the diet (Kleemola-Kujala and Rasanen 1982; Rugg-Gunn *et al.* 1984). Fortunately there is no conjecture about the advice that may be given to patients. Fluoride toothpastes are capable of reducing the incidence of caries and their regular and frequent use is recommended.

References

Addy, M., Dummer, P.M.H., Griffiths, G., Hicks, R., Kingdom, A., and Shaw, W.C. (1986). Prevalence of plaque, gingivitis and caries in 11–12 year old children in South Wales. *Commun. Dent. oral Epidemiol.* **14**, 115–18.

Ainamo, J. (1971). The effect of habitual toothcleansing on the occurrence of peridontal disease and dental caries. *Proc. Finn. dent. Soc.* **67**, 63–70.

Ainamo, J. and Parviainen, K. (1979). Occurrence of plaque, gingivitis and caries related to self reported frequency of toothbrushing in fluoride areas in Finland. *Commun. Dent. oral Epidemiol.* **7**, 142–6.

Ashley, F.P. and Sainsbury, R.H. (1981). The effect of a school based plaque control programme on caries and gingivitis. *Br. dent. J.* **150**, 41–5.

Ashley, F.P., and Sainsbury, R.H. (1982). Post study effects of a school based plaque control programme. *Br. dent. J.* **153**, 337–8.

Ashley, F.P. and Wilson, R.F. (1977). Dental plaque and caries, a three year longitudinal study in children. *Br. dent. J.* **142**, 85–91.

Axelsson, P., Lindhe, J., and Waseby, J. (1976). The effect of various plaque control measures on gingivitis and caries in schoolchildren. *Comm. Dent. oral Epidemiol.* **4**, 232–9.

Badersten, A., Egelberg, J., and Koch, G. (1975). Effect of monthly prophylaxis on caries and gingivitis in schoolchildren. *Commun. Dent. oral Epidemiol.* **3**, 1–4.

Bay, I. and Ainamo, J. (1974). Caries experience among children in Copenhagen. -*Commun. Dent. oral Epidemiol.* **2**, 75–9.

Beal, J.F., James, P.M.C., Bradrock, G., and Anderson, R.J. (1979). The relationship between dental cleanliness, dental caries incidence and gingival health. *Br. dent. J.* **146**, 111–14.

Bibby, B.G. (1966). Do we tell the truth about preventing caries? *J. Dent. Child.* **33**, 269–79.

Bjertness, E., Eriksen, H.M., Hansen, B.F. (1986). Caries prevalence of 35 year old Oslo citizens in 1973 and 1984. *Commun. Dent. oral Epidemiol.* **14**, 277–82.

Dale, J.W. (1969). Toothbrushing frequency and its relationship to dental caries and peridontal disease. *Australia dent. J.* **14**, 120–3.

Duany, L.F., Zinner, D.D., and Jablon, J.M. (1972). Epidemiologic studies of caries free and caries active students: II. Diet, dental plaque, and oral hygiene. *J. dent. Res.* **51**, 727–33.

Fisher, F.J. (1968). A field survey of dental caries, peridontal disease and enamel defects in Tristan da Cunha. *Br. dent. J.* **125**, 398–401; 447–53.

Fosdick, L.S. (1950). The reduction of the incidence of dental caries I. Immediate toothbrushing with a neutral dentifrice. *J. Am. dent. Ass.* **40**, 133–43.

Gillham, J. and Lennon, D. (1958). The biology of the children of Hopewood House, Bowral, N.S.W. II. Observations extending over five years (1952–1956 inclusive). 4. Dietary survey. *Australia dent. J.* **3**, 378–82.

Granath, L.E., Martinsson, T., Matsson, L., Nilsson, G., Schröder, U., and Söderholm, B. (1979). Intraindividual effect of daily supervised flossing on caries in schoolchildren. *Commun. Dent. oral Epidemiol.* **7**, 147–50.

Hamp, S.E., Lindhe, J., Fornell, J., Johansson, L.A., and Karlsson, R. (1978). Effect of a field programme based on systematic plaque control on caries and gingivitis in schoolchildren after 3 years. *Commun. Dent. oral Epidemiol.* **6**, 17–23.

Holloway, P.J. and Teagle, F. (1976). The relationship between oral cleanliness and caries increment. *J. dent. Res.* **55** (spec. iss. D), Abstr. No. 1.

Holloway, P.J., James, P.M.C., and Slack, G.L. (1963). Dental disease in Tristan da Cunha. *Br. dent. J.* **115**, 19–25.

Holt, R.D., Joels, D., and Winter, G.B. (1982). Caries in pre-school children, the Camden study. *Br. dent. J.* **153**, 107–9.

Horowitz, A.M., Suomi, J.D., Peterson, J.K., Mathews, B.L., Voglesong, R.H., and Lyman, B.A. (1980). Effects of supervised daily dental plaque removal by children after 3 years. *Commun. Dent. oral Epidemiol.* **8**, 171–6.

Horowitz, H.S. (1968). In *Art and science on dental caries research*, (ed. R.S. Harris), p. 179. Academic Press, New York.

Jackson, D. and Sutcliffe, P. (1967). Clinical testing of a stannous fluoride-calcium pyrophosphate dentifrice in Yorkshire schoolchildren. *Br. dent. J.* **123**, 40–8.

Kleemola-Kujala, E. (1978). Oral hygiene and its relationship to caries prevalence in Finnish rural children. *Proc. Finn. dent. Soc.* **74**, 76–85.

Kleemola-Kujala, E. and Rasanan, L. (1982). Relationship of oral hygiene and sugar consumption to risk of caries in children. *Commun. Dent. oral Epidemiol.* **10**, 224–33.

Lindhe, J., Axelsson, P., and Tollskog, G. (1975). Effect of proper oral hygiene on gingivitis and dental caries in Swedish schoolchildren. *Comm. Dent. oral Epidemiol.* **3**, 150–5.

McCauley, H.B. and Frazier, T.M. (1957). Dental caries and dental care needs in Baltimore school children (1955). *J. dent. Res.* **36**, 546–51.

McHugh, W.D., McEwen, J.D., and Hitchin, A.D. (1964). Dental disease and related factors in 13-year-old children in Dundee. *Br. dent. J.* **117**, 246–53.

Mansbridge, J.N. (1960). The effects of oral hygiene and sweet consumption on the prevalence of dental caries. *Br. dent. J.* **109**, 343–8.

Miller, J. (1961). Relationship of occlusion and oral cleanliness with caries rates. *Archs. oral Biol.* (spec. suppl.) **6**, 70–9.

Miller, J. and Hobson, P. (1961). The relationship between malocclusion, oral cleanliness, gingival conditions and dental caries in school children. *Br. dent. J.* **111**, 43–52.

Parviainen, K., Nordling, H., and Ainamo, J. (1977). Occurrence of dental caries and gingivitis in low, medium and high fluoride areas in Finland. *Commun. Dent. oral Epidemiol.* **5**, 287–91.

Rajala, M., Selkainaho, K., and Paunio, I. (1980). Relationship between reported toothbrushing and dental caries in adults. *Commun. Dent. oral Epidemiol.* **8**, 128–31.

Richardson, A.S., Boyd, M.A., and Conry, R.F. (1977). A correlation study of diet, oral hygiene and dental caries in 457 Canadian children. *Commun. Dent. oral Epidemiol.* **5**, 227–30.

Ripa, L.W. (1985). The roles of prophylaxes and dental prophylaxis pastes in caries prevention in *Clinical uses of fluorides*, (ed. S.H.Y. Wei). Lea and Febiger, Philadelphia.

Rugg-Gunn, A.J., Hackett, A.F., Appleton, D.R., Jenkins, G.N., and Eastoe, J.E. (1984). Relationship between dietary habits and caries increment assessed over two years in 405 English adolescent school children. *Archs. oral Biol.* **29**, 983–92.

Silverstein, S., Gold, D., Heilbron, D., Nelms, D., and Wycoff, S. (1977). Effect of supervised deplaquing on dental caries, gingivitis and plaque. *J. dent. Res.* **56** (spec. iss. A) A85. Abstr. 169.

Smith, A.J. and Striffler, D.F. (1963). Reported frequency of toothbrushing as related to the prevalence of dental caries in New Mexico. *Publ. Hlth. Dent.* **23**, 159–75.

Sullivan, H.R. and Harris, R. (1958). The biology of children of Hopewood House, Bowral, N.S.W.2. Observations on oral conditions. *Australia dent. J.* **3**, 311–17.

Sutcliffe, P. (1973). A longitudinal clinical study of oral cleanliness and dental caries in school children. *Archs. oral Biol.* **18**, 765–70.

Sutcliffe, P. (1977). Caries experience and oral cleanliness of 3 and 4 year old children from deprived and non-deprived areas in Edinburgh, Scotland. *Commun. Dent. oral Epidemiol.* **5**, 213–19.

Todd, J.E. (1975). *Children's dental health in England and Wales*, 1973. HMSO, London.

Todd, J.E. and Walker, A.M. (1980). *Adult dental health*. Vol. 1. *England and Wales 1968–1978*. HMSO, London.

Trubman, A. (1963). Oral hygiene: its association with periodontal disease and dental caries in children. *J. Am. dent. Ass.* **67**, 349–51.

Tucker, G.J., Andlaw, R.J., and Birchell, C.K. (1976). The relationship between oral hygiene and dental caries incidence in 11-year-old children. *Br. dent. J.* **141**, 75–9.

Wright, G.Z., Banting, D.W., and Feasby, W.H. (1979). The Dorchester dental flossing study: final report. *Clin. prevent. Dent.* **1**, 23–6.

5

Fissure sealants

P. H. Gordon

Introduction

Fissure sealants are materials which are designed to prevent pit and fissure caries. They are applied mainly to the occlusal surfaces of the teeth in order to obliterate the occlusal fissures, and remove the sheltered environment in which caries may thrive.

Fissure sealing is a very conservative way of tackling the problem of occlusal caries, and involves a minimum of operative treatment, usually no more than polishing the teeth in order to remove plaque and food debris. The application of the resin is a straightforward matter, which involves etching the tooth enamel and painting the sealant resin on to the tooth. Most children have no difficulty in accepting treatment along these lines.

On the face of it, fissure sealants are such a good idea, and the reaction of the patients is so favourable, that it is difficult to understand why these materials have not gained widespread acceptance, and why they are not in general use. A look at the history of fissure sealing, and the impact made by the development of new techniques and new materials, will help to explain how this situation has arisen.

Early materials

There was a surge of interest in fissure sealing in the early part of the decade starting in 1970, and a casual observer could be forgiven for assuming that fissure sealing was a new and exciting development. In fact there had been a long-standing interest in sealing as a method of preventing occlusal caries ever since the early part of the century, when a number of workers had attempted to prevent the onset of decay by applying silver nitrate (Miller 1905; Prime 1937; Klein and Knutsen 1942; Miller 1950), nitrocellulose (Gore 1939), and zinc chloride (Ast *et al.* 1950). Miller's paper (1905) was not the result of a scientific study, but rather a report that he had used silver nitrate to prevent the onset of occlusal caries and had found it useful. The other studies did not demonstrate any detectable benefit from the materials under test.

Silver nitrate, and other materials mentioned above, would not work by physical occlusion of the fissure. They would exert their effect, if they worked at all, by altering the composition of the enamel in the depths of the fissure, to make it more resistant to bacterial action. The work was carried out at a time when the proteolytic theory of the initiation of caries was in fashion, and it was hoped that by precipitating inorganic material on to the tooth surface, it would be possible to block organic pathways into the tooth.

A different approach had been by other researchers (Hyatt 1923; Miller 1950). They attempted to fill the occlusal fissure with a sealant material which, by blocking up the fissure, would prevent bacteria and their substrate from coming into contact with that part of the tooth. Clearly, if successfully retained on the tooth, this would have a good chance of preventing caries of the underlying enamel. The difficulty was to ensure the retention of the sealing material.

Hyatt recommended that the occlusal fissure of the erupting tooth should be sealed with zinc phosphate cement, as soon as possible, and that when the tooth was sufficiently erupted a minimal Class I cavity should be prepared, and the tooth filled with amalgam before it became carious. There was considerable resistance to his proposals from the dental profession, which objected to cutting cavities in caries-free teeth. One might also expect a certain amount of 'consumer resistance' to the idea of having a tooth filled before it had a cavity in it. From the patient's point of view it was well to wait until caries developed, because the operative procedures were the same. Hyatt's argument was that it was almost inevitable that the first permanent molar would develop occlusal caries. One should fill the tooth before progression of this caries made restoration difficult, and there was no time like the present. Hyatt's concept, sometimes called 'prophylactic odontotomy', never gained wide acceptance, probably because the procedure involved drilling the child's teeth.

Miller (1950) tested the preventive action of black copper cement when used as a fissure sealant. The copper cement was compared with silver nitrate, and neither material was found to be effective in preventing caries when contrasted with a group of control teeth that received no treatment. The copper cement was not retained on the occlusal surfaces.

Acid-etch retained materials

While investigating different methods of improving the edge-seal of acrylic resin filling materials, Buonocore decided to test the effect of etching the tooth surface with an acid solution before applying the filling material (Buonocore 1955). This alteration in technique had a dramatic effect on the adhesion of the resin to the tooth, and acid-etch techniques were soon introduced into the field of fissure sealing. When the cyanoacrylate resins became available a number of research workers reported on the use of these materials as fissure sealants, and most used an acid-etch technique as part of the application procedure (Takeuchi *et al.* 1966, 1971; Cueto and Buonocore 1967; Ripa and Cole 1970). The results of

Table 5.1. Cyano-acrylate studies

Reference	Retention of resin	
	at 6 months (%)	at 12 months (%)
Cueto and Buonocore (1967)	80	71
Ripa and Cole (1970)	68	32
Parkhouse and Winter (1971)	resin lost before 6 month recall	

their studies are shown in Table 5.1, where it can be seen that they quote good retention figures for the materials they were testing. A respectable number of teeth in the studies retained the sealant resin on the occlusal surface. These were essentially short-term studies, and as such were not designed to detect a reduction in the incidence of caries. These promising results encouraged other research workers to take an interest in cyano-acrylate resins as fissure sealing materials (Parkhouse and Winter 1971), but the outcome of the subsequent trial did not inspire confidence in the material.

Rock (1974) reported on the use of two polyurethane materials as fissure sealants: one was retained by an acid-etch, the other was applied directly to the enamel with no etch to prepare the surface. Neither material was retained on the tooth, and it appeared that any effect on caries was minimal, despite the incorporation of a fluoride compound in to the resins in the hope that this would have some local effect as an anti-caries agent.

Following the introduction of the bis-glycidyl-methacrylate (GMA) resins, there were several studies carried out in quick succession, testing the suitablilty for use as fissure sealants (Buonocore 1970, 1971; Rock 1972, 1973; Ibsen 1973; McCune *et al.* 1973). The results from these studies are presented in Table 5.2, and it can be seen that these researchers obtained very satisfactory retention rates from the materials they were using. These results reawakened interest in fissure sealing, and more trials were undertaken, but once again it soon became apparent that there were considerable differences in the results obtained by different workers. The promising results reported in the early trials were not always repeated in subsequet studies, and Table 5.3 shows that the retention figures obtained in these follow-up clinical trials varied to a considerable degree.

Table 5.2. Early trials with bis-GMA resins

Reference	Retention of resin (%)	Duration of trial (months)
Buonocore (1970)	9	12
Buonocore (1971)	87	24
Rock (1972)	56	12
Ibsen (1973)	100	12
McCune *et al.* (1973)	85	12
Rock (1973)	86	12

Table 5.3. Fissure sealing of first permanent molars. Clinical trials of one year duration, published in 1976

Reference	Retention on 1st molars (%)	Initial age of subjects (years)
Brooks *et al.* (1976)	95	6– 8
Going *et al.* (1976)	78*	10–14
Harris *et al.* (1976)	81*	6–14
Higson (1976)	32*	6– 8
Leake and Martinello (1976)	65*	6– 8
Leske *et al.* (1976)	76*	6– 8
Stephen *et al.* (1976)	2	6

* The material used was 'Nuva-Seal'.

The results of clinical trials

There are several possible explanations for this variation: for example, the different workers may have used slightly different materials; they may have sealed different teeth (premolars as opposed to molars); possibly they were working under different conditions; and they were certainly working on different groups of children. In addition, there may have been variations in the application technique. To what extent are these different factors responsible for the varying results obtained in clinical trials?

The first obvious possibility is that the different studies may have been testing different materials. Modern sealant studies have been conducted on a variety of materials, the cyano-acrylates, the polyurethanes, the GMA resins and the glass ionomer cements forming the main groups. The GMA resins and the glass ionomer cements have produced the most consistent results, with retention figures generally better than the cyano-acrylates and polyurethane. However, even if we consider only one particular material, 'Nuva Seal', and look at some of the many trials conducted on this product, there is a lot of variation in the results obtained (Table 5.3). It is apparent that while differences between materials may account for some of the variation in the results of clinical trials, there must be other factors involved.

Variation in application technique may account for some of these differences. The majority of studies do not give a detailed account of the application technique, simply stating that the material was applied according to the manufacturer's instructions. There is seldom any mention of the degree of difficulty experienced by the operators in complying with these instructions. In particular, only a very few reports indicate whether or not children were discarded from the trial if the operator found it difficult to maintain a dry working field when applying the resin to the child's teeth. This very important aspect of the protocol under which the trials were conducted is hardly ever mentioned directly, though there are oblique references to difficulties that have been encountered: '... the clinical studies of fissure sealants are, in reality, a study of the proficiency of the operators ... best results are achieved when the sealants are applied under conditions approaching the ideal of private practice, and (the resins) are less effective when applied under conditions of mass prophylaxis' (Ibsen 1973). Good results, as in other areas of paediatric dentistry, require the co-operation of the child, and although this is relatively easy to obtain when using fissure sealants, there will always be a number of children who find it difficult to contribute this necessary factor.

Application technique

It quickly became apparent that application technique is very important to the success of a fissure sealant, but it is difficult, using clinical data, to decide which aspects of the application technique are most important. Most of the research work carried out on the strength of the bond between resin and tooth, and the effect of changing various aspects of the application technique, has been done in the laboratory, where it is easier to test the effect of changing one factor in isolation.

The application procedure is more or less the same for all the modern materials, which depend on an acid etch for their retention. The manufacturer will usually recommend that the tooth concerned is first polished, then isolated, and etched with the material provided (usually phosphoric acid) for a specific time. The acid is then rinsed off the tooth, keeping the tooth isolated from contact with saliva, and the tooth dried, using compressed air. The sealing material is placed on the occlusal surface, which must be kept isolated until the material has polymerized. Laboratory tests indicate that the most critical parts of the application procedure are rinsing the etched enamel, drying the tooth surface, and maintaining the isolation of the teeth until the sealant material had polymerized.

Variation in the concentration of the etching material appears to have little effect: provided that the concentration of *ortho*-phosphoric acid (which is the most widely used etching material) lies between 30 and 50 per cent by weight, small variations in the concentration do not appear to effect the quality of the etched surface (Silverstone 1974).

Variation in the time during which the tooth enamel is exposed to etching solution is more important, but provided the enamel is exposed to the etching material for 20 s, there will be sufficient demineralization to allow adequate retention of the sealant. Even in areas where there is an optimal level of fluoride in the water supply, it appears there is little to be gained by increasing the etching time (Beech and Jalaly 1980; McCabe and Storer 1980; Barkmeier *et al.* 1985). Laboratory studies indicate it may be more difficult to gain adequate retention by etching the enamel of deciduous teeth, but clinical studies (Simonsen 1979) suggest it may not, in fact, be necessary to increase the etching time when sealing deciduous molars, as perfectly adequate retention figures are obtained using the same sort of etching times as are recommended for permanent teeth.

Relatively small variations in the time for which the etched enamel is rinsed have a more marked effect on the strength of the bond between resin and enamel (Williams and von Frauenhofer 1977), and the operator applying sealant resins should take particular care over the rinsing and drying of the tooth surface, before applying the resin. It would appear that the enamel should be rinsed for a full 20–25 s before being dried.

As a final comment on the difficulties of assessing the effectiveness of application technique, it is ironic to note that in a trial in which the operators graded the ease with which the resin was applied, there was no relationship between the retention of the resin and the operator's assessment of the level of the child's co-operation (Rock and Evans 1982).

Further clinical trials

After the early studies that have already been mentioned, there has come a flood of reports of clinical trials of fissure sealants. For reasons that are discussed later, attention should be focussed on the first permanent molars, and Table 5.4 shows the results of some of the clinical trials that have considered the extent to which fissure sealants are retained on these teeth. The first permanent molar, shortly after eruption, is a severe testing ground for any fissure sealant. The children are young, the teeth are only partly erupted and right at the back of the mouth, and if the resin will stay on this tooth, it has done all that can reasonably be expected.

The mass of results tabulated here shows that the sealant resins do indeed stay on the great majority of these teeth, and for a considerable time. Resin material is progressively lost from the tooth surface as time goes by. The loss of resin is most marked in the first 6 months, but there is a further progressive loss of about 10 per cent per annum (Horowitz *et al.* 1977). More recent trials generally report better retention rates than earlier studies, perhaps reflecting an increasing familiarity on the part of the operators with the use of acid-etch retained materials.

The use of fissure sealants

It is entirely proper that any new material should be examined critically before being accepted into general use, and this principle applies especially in cases where a whole new technique is being introduced, rather than a new material. Arguments have been put forward that fissure sealants will be ineffective in general use, due to failure of retention, or that the operator will inadvertently damage the tooth by sealing in caries, or that the teeth may be more liable to caries following loss of the sealant resin because the enamel surface has been damaged by etching. These arguments cannot simply be ignored, and we should now consider to what extent these reservations are justified.

As to whether or not fissure sealant will be effective in general use, it is worth noting that the most frequently used design of clinical trial does not test the material in the way in which it would, in fact, be used. The usual procedure adopted in sealant studies has been to apply the material to the occlusal surfaces

Table 5.4. Clinical trials and fissure sealants applied to first permanent molars

	Per cent of teeth retaining sealant	Age of children
Duration 6 months		
Burt *et al.* (1975)	36	5–17
Charbeneau *et al.* (1977)	91	5–8
Cueto and Buonocore (1967)	75	5–17
Dorignac (1987)	98	6–8
Eidelman *et al.* (1984)	99	5.5–6.5
Ferguson (1980)	78	3–16
	62	3–16
Harris *et al.* (1976)	81	6–14
Helle (1975)	100	5–7
Higson (1976)	64	6–8
Hinding and Buonocore (1974)	100	10.2 mean
Leake and Martinello (1976)	84	6–8
Li *et al.* (1981)	94	5–16
	88	5–16
Luoma *et al.* (1973)	100	7 mean
Raadal (1978)	95	5–7
	93	5–7
Ripa and Cole (1970)	72	5–10
Rock *et al.* (1978)	51	6–7
	80	6–7
Rock and Evans (1982)	81	7–8
	84	7–8
Shekholeslam and Houpt (1978)	97	6–10
Stephen *et al.* (1978)	97	6–10
Stephen *et al.* (1981*a*)	100	6–7
	99	6–7
Stephen *et al.* (1981*b*)	90	6–11
	98	6–11
Stephen *et al.* (1985)	100	5–8
	94	6.8 mean
Duration 12 months		
Alvesalo *et al.* (1977)	74	6–7
Bokanini *et al.* (1976)	91	6–8
Brooks *et al.* (1976)	95	6–8
Brooks *et al.* (1976)	83	6–8
Charbeneau *et al.* (1977)	79	5–8
Collins *et al.* (1985)	71	>9
	79	5–8
Cueto and Buonocore (1967)	63	5–17
Dorignac (1987)	96	6–8
Eidelman *et al.* (1984)	99	5.5–6.5
Ferguson (1980)	72	3–16
	60	3–16
Fuks *et al.* (1982)	28	6–10
Going *et al.* (1976)	78	10–14
Harris *et al.* (1976)	72	6–14
Helle (1975)	96	5–7
Higson (1976)	32	6–8

Table 5.4.—*continued*

	Per cent of teeth retaining sealant	**Age of children**
Hinding and Buonocore (1974)	92	10.2 mean
Leake and Martinello (1976)	65	6–8
Leske *et al.* (1976)	77	6–8
Li *et al.* (1981)	91	5–16
	73	5–16
McCune *et al.* (1973)	72	5–14
McCune *et al.* (1979)	92	6–8
Poulsen *et al.* (1979)	82	kindergarten
Raadal (1978)	90	5–7
	88	5–7
Richardson *et al.* (1978)	80	7–8
Ripa and Cole (1970)	36	5–10
Risager and Poulsen (1974)	69	6–8
Rock *et al.* (1978)	41	6–7
	75	6–7
Rock and Evans (1982)	76	6–7
	75	7–8
Sheykholeslam and Houpt (1978)	92	6–10
Stephen *et al.* (1976)	2	6
Stephen *et al.* (1978)	93	6–10
Stephen *et al.* (1981*a*)	100	6–7
	99	6–7
Stephen *et al.* (1981*b*)	86	6–11
	93	6–11
Stephen *et al.* (1985)	100	5–8
	95	5–8
Duration 18 months		
Charbeneau *et al.* (1977)	74	5–18
Collins *et al.* (1985)	66	5–8
	68	>9
Dorignac (1987)	96	6–8
Harris *et al.* (1976)	60	6–14
Helle (1975)	91	5–7
Higson (1976)	16	6–8
Leake and Martinello (1976)	54	6–8
Li *et al.* (1981)	88	5–16
	65	5–16
Meurman *et al.* (1975)	98	7 mean
Poulsen *et al.* (1979)	78	kindergarten
Raadal (1978)	85	5–7
	85	5–7
Stephen *et al.* (1981*b*)	71	6–11
Stephen *et al.* (1985)	925–8	
	93	5–8
Duration 24 months		
Alvesalo *et al.* (1977)	40	6–7
Bagramian *et al.* (1977)	15	6–7
	35	14

Table 5.4.—*continued*

	Per cent of teeth retaining sealant	Age of children
Ball (1981)	91	various
Brooks *et al.* (1979*a*)	84	<8
	58	<8
Brooks *et al.* (1988)	79	5–14
	86	5–14
	92	5–14
Burt (1977)	20	5–12
Burt *et al.* (1977)	19	5–17
Charbeneau and Dennison (1979)	71	5–8
Colins *et al.* (1985)	48	5–8
	54	>9
Dorignac (1987)	92	6–8
Going *et al.* (1976)	58	10–14
Harris *et al.* (1976)	50	6–14
Higson (1976)	3	6–8
Hinding and Buonocore (1974)	89	10.2 mean
Horowitz *et al.* (1974)	48	5–14
Leake and Martinello (1976)	43	6–8
Leske *et al.* (1976)	50	6–8
Li *et al.* (1981)	88	5–16
	69	5–16
McCune *et al.* (1979)	89	6–8
Poulsen *et al.* (1979)	58	kindergarten
Raadal (1978)	82	5–7
	84	5–7
Richardson *et al.* (1978)	86	7–8
Richardson *et al.* (1977)	51	6–20
Sheykholeslam and Houpt (1978)	85	6–10
Simonsen (1980*b*)	59	3–15
Stephen *et al.* (1980*b*)	70	6–11
	81	6–11
Stephen *et al.* (1985)	91	5–8
	92	5–8
Thystrup and Poulsen (1978)	60	7
Ulvestad (1976)	98	6–9
Vrbic (1986)	86	6.8 mean
Williams *et al.* (1978)	98	6–8
	50	6–8
	62	6–8
Williams *et al.* (1986)	16	7.5 mean
	77	7.5 mean
	80	7.5 mean
Duration 30 months		
le Bell and Forsten (1980)	93	7–8
	88	7–8
Dorignac (1987)	81	6–8
Harris *et al.* (1976)	48	6–14
Raadal (1978)	84	5–7
	75	5–7

of a number of teeth, and then observe the children over a period of time in order to determine how many teeth retain the resin, and for how long. If a sealant was being used as part of a programme to prevent dental caries, and it was noticed at a recall appointment that the sealant had been lost from any particular surface, then the resin would be re-applied and the tooth would not be left without its protective covering. When this approach has been adopted, the results have been very encouraging (Bagramian *et al.* 1978; Rantala 1979; Isler *et al.* 1980, 1981).

What would happen if a tooth were sealed when it already had a carious lesion? This is an obvious possibility; the accurate diagnosis of early occlusal caries is very difficult, and there are bound to be occasions on which the operator has difficulty in deciding whether or not a tooth has already been attacked. Fortunately, clinical research indicates that if a tooth with early occlusal caries, or even more advanced dentinal caries, is treated with a fissure sealant, then one might reasonably hope for a favourable outcome (Jeronimus *et al.* 1975; Handelman *et al.* 1976; Harris *et al.* 1976; Thielade *et al.* 1977; Going *et al.* 1978; Jensen and Handelman 1980; Handelman *et al.* 1981, 1986; and Mertz-Fairhurst *et al.* 1986). These studies show that there is a decrease in the number of viable organisms in the effected dentine, and that the metabolic activity of the remaining bacteria is reduced. It appears that, providing the sealant layer remains intact, the cavity will not progress to any significant extent. The evidence in this respect is now so persuasive that the conscientious practitioner should be encouraged to adopt the maxim 'when in doubt, seal', rather than the alternative 'when in doubt, fill'.

Some of the clinical trials quoted in the tables and in the bibliography give figures for caries reductions obtained by the use of sealants. These data should be interpreted with caution, particularly in the case of the shorter 1- or 2-year trials, as the diagnosis of early occlusal caries is very liable to error. Some sealant studies, however, have run for several years, and these studies indicate that teeth which lose the sealant resin are not more likely to become carious than the control teeth that were never sealed. It appears that the acid etch applied to the enamel in the process of sealing the tooth does not make the tooth more susceptible to decay.

The cost-effectiveness of sealants

It is difficult to be dogmatic about whether or not fissure sealants are 'cost-effective' (Houpt and Shey 1980). This is a difficult question to answer in a straightforward way because the answer depends on the value, in money terms, that is placed on intangible benefits such as the prevention of pain and suffering, the adoption of a reversible, non-traumatic procedure for the treatment of 'sticky fissures', and a change in attitude on the part of the public at large (Mitchell and Murray 1987).

If we work on the basis of sealing every tooth that has an occlusal surface, than fissure sealing does become more expensive than the alternative approach, which is the restoration of carious teeth with amalgam (Horowitz 1980; Klock 1980; Eklund 1986). The process of applying the resin is not particularly time-consuming, and the resin itself is not expensive—the difficulty lies in the fact that if every premolar and molar tooth is sealed, then a lot of teeth are sealed unnecessarily, because they are not going to decay in the first place. Far fewer teeth are treated if treatment is confined to the teeth that do develop caries, but who can say in advance which teeth are going to decay, and which are not? It is the treatment of all these extra teeth that increases the cost. To avoid this potential cost, treatment should be confined to the particular teeth that are most likely to decay at any given time. We know which teeth are liable to decay, and at what age, because this information is available from epidemiological studies, and it is evident that the first permanent molar, shortly after eruption, emerges as the prime target for fissure sealants.

If fissure sealants are used on the first permanent molars, shortly after the eruption of these teeth, the procedure soon becomes 'cost-effective', even when we allow for the fact that in a proportion of cases the resin will have to be re-applied. There is no doubt that it can be very difficult to keep the teeth isolated when using the resin on young children, and the retention of the resin does depend very much on this particular aspect of the technique but, as with most other skills, one can expect some improvement with practice. In one study, (Rantala 1979), fissure sealants were applied to the first permanent molars, as part of an overall programme of caries prevention. After about 2 years, sealing all the first molars had become cheaper, simply in terms of money, than filling those teeth that would have become carious. There were, of course, all the additional benefits arising from the use of a procedure that was very acceptable to the children involved.

Naturally, the amount of money saved as a result of the sealing depends on the number of teeth that would otherwise have become carious. According to some studies, 50 per cent of first molars are decayed within 1 year of their eruption (Miller 1953; Jackson 1965), 80 per cent are carious within 2 years (Hargreaves and Chester 1973; Lewis and Hargreaves 1975), and 90 per cent are carious within 4 years (Berman and Slack 1972). More recent work indicates that the condition of first permanent molars has improved, and the high incidence of caries quoted by the earlier workers is no longer found (Mansson 1977; Holm 1978; Todd 1975; King *et al.* 1980; Rock *et al.* 1981*a*; Todd and Dodd 1985; Dummer *et al.* 1988). Possibly the standards of diagnosis have changed, or else the condition of the teeth has improved. Even so, there is no doubt that the first permanent molar is still liable to suffer occlusal caries in the first few years after its eruption. The diagram reproduced here as Fig. 5.1 was published in one of these later studies, and it gives an indication of the rate at which first molars are affected by caries, in fluoride and non-fluoride areas. In the non-fluoride area approximately half the first molars were decayed by the age of 9,

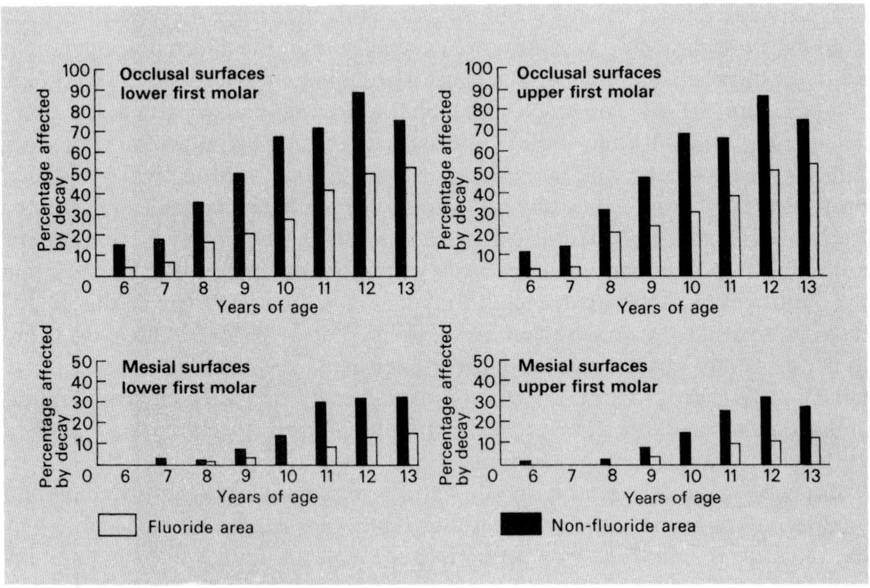

Fig. 5.1. Caries in first permanent molars. (After Rock *et al.* (1981*b*).)

while in the fluoride area the children had reached the age of 12 before half the teeth were affected. Virtually all the affected teeth suffered from occlusal caries.

With regard to the onset of approximal caries, at the age of 13, 30 per cent of first permanent molars in the non-fluoride area had mesial cavities or restorations, while only 10 per cent of mesial surfaces of the first molars in the fluoride area were similarly affected. The effectiveness of fissure sealing is reduced unless some measures are taken to reduce the incidence of approximal caries. Both fissure sealing and some form of fluoride supplement should be employed in any programme designed to prevent caries. The use of either measure in isolation will provide only partial benefit.

Improvements in the cost-effectiveness of fissure sealants can be obtained if the technique is employed in the care of particular target groups—for example: children with medical conditions which make the prevention of dental caries particularly important, or children whose previous dental history indicates they are susceptible to caries. Ancillary staff may be trained to apply fissure sealants, and can achieve retention rates similar to those obtained by dentists (Stiles *et al.* 1976; Stephen *et al.* 1978). Clearly the choice of staff employed to apply the resin will have an impact on the cost-effectiveness of the procedure.

Comparisons with amalgam

When considering the cost-effectiveness of fissure sealing, the durability of sealants should not be considered in isolation; what about the failure rate of the alternative procedure, namely the amalgam restoration? As with sealants, the durability of amalgam restorations has been shown to improve as the age of the patient increases (Walls *et al.* 1985). Fissure sealants are best used in newly erupted first permanent molars, and therefore a comparison should be made with amalgam restorations in young children, at the age at which first permanent molars develop occlusal caries.

There have been relatively few studies which have considered the life expectancy of amalgam restorations in this age group. Walls *et al.* (1985) found a median survival time of 26 months for amalgam restorations in children aged 5–7 years when the restoration was provided. This means that half the restorations had failed after 26 months. The median survival time for amalgam restorations placed in 7–9-year-old children was 33 months. If a local anaesthetic had not been used, these survival times were reduced by 23 per cent. Similar figures are quoted by Hunter (1985), who found a median survival time of 26 months for amalgam restorations placed in a group of children aged 8 years or younger.

Mitchell and Murray (1987) used a type of analysis similar to that employed by Walls *et al.* (1985) and examined data from a similar group of children. They found a median survival time of 27 months for fissure sealants used on first permanent molars in a group of 5- to 8-year-old children.

These figures suggest that there is no greater difference between the survival of fissure sealants and amalgams in this age group, provided that a local anaesthetic is employed when a cavity is prepared for amalgam. The type of analysis used (median survival times from life-table analysis) is likely, however, to be operating to the disadvantage of the sealant group. The children in the amalgam studies were followed up for 12 years (Walls) and 20 years (Hunter). The sealant group was followed up for 5.5 years. This means that no sealant had the opportunity to last longer than 5.5 years, while some of the amalgam restorations could have lasted for 12 or 20 years.

The preventive resin restoration

One approach that has been employed to deal with the problem of early fissure caries is to use a procedure which employs a minimal composite restoration (Raadal 1978; Simonsen 1980*a*; Houpt *et al.* 1984; Walls *et al.* 1988). The technique involves making a very small, local cavity preparation in the immediate area of the fissure system at which the presence of caries is suspected. No attempt is made to extend the cavity beyond the immediate area affected by caries. Exposed dentine is protected with a calcium-hydroxide lining material, and the occlusal surface of the tooth etched in the conventional way. The defect in the occlusal surface is restored with sealant, or with a composite resin filling material, according to the size of the defect. Following this, the occlusal surface of the tooth is sealed, the sealant being applied over the top of any composite resin.

The advantage of this approach is that the absolute minimum of tooth substance is removed. Walls *et al.* (1988) reported that the occlusal amalgam restorations in this study occupied, on average, 25 per cent of the occlusal surface of the tooth, compared with 5 per cent for the minimal composite resin. In addition, the procedure avoids the unfortunate consequences of an error in diagnosis. If a healthy tooth is investigated, little harm is done, for it quickly becomes evident that there is no caries present and the resulting cavity is very small. If the caries is more extensive than was originally supposed, then this will become apparent during the procedure and appropriate action can be taken.

The results of clinical trials which have included this type of restoration would suggest that the durability of preventive resin restorations is similar to the durability of fissure sealants. The composite restorations are small and are positioned at the bottom of a pit or fissure. These factors, taken together, minimize any potential problems arising from wear of the composite.

Conclusion

The early history of fissure sealing is littered with accounts of techniques and procedures that were recommended by a variety of authorities, and found to be useless when it came to providing a practical method of preventing caries. The ray of hope offered by the cyano-acrylate adhesives came to nothing, and the polyurethane materials were found to be ineffective. The introduction of the bis-GMA resins was greeted with an understandable reserve, and the good results of early trials were attributed to dedication on the part of a few, committed research workers. This gloomy point of view was reinforced when later clinical trials showed some variation in the results obtained by different operators. However, the importance of meticulous operating technique is now accepted, and the more recent clinical trials report consistently good retention figures.

The United States NIH Concensus Development Conference (National Institute of Health 1984) reported that 'Sealants are highly effective in preventing pit and fissure caries'. The British Paedodontic Society (1987) 'strongly supports the use of fissure sealants as a primary preventive measure'. Despite these recommendations, Cohen and Sheiham (1988) report the results of a survey of General Dental Practitioners in Great Britain, which show that, on average, only 13.4 per cent of the child patients receive sealants. In view of the continuing pressure from professional bodies involved in the dental care of children, and the ready acceptance of sealants by patients and parents, it seems likely that this figure will increase.

References

Alvesalo, L., Brummer, R., and le Bell, Y. (1977). On the use of fissure sealants in caries prevention. A clinical study. *Acta odont. Scand.* **35**, 155–9.

Ast, D.B., Bushel, A., and Chase, H.C. (1950). A clinical study of caries prophylaxis with zinc chloride and potassium ferrocyanide. *J. Am. dent. Ass.* **41**, 427–42.

Bagramian, R.A., Graves, R.C., and Srivastava, S. (1977). Sealant effectiveness for children receiving a combination of preventive methods in a fluoridated community: Two-year results. *J. dent. Res.* **56**, 1511–19.

Bagramian, R.A., Graves, R.C., and Srivastava, S. (1978). A combined approach to preventing dental caries in schoolchildren: caries reductions after 3 years. *Commun. Dent. oral Epidemiol.* **6**, 166–71.

Bagramian, R.A., Srivastava, S., and Graves, R.C. (1979). Pattern of sealant retention in children receiving a combination of caries preventive measures: Three-year results. *J. Am. dent. Ass.* **98**, 46–50.

Ball, I.A. (1981). Pit and fissure sealing with Concise Enamel Bond. *Br. dent. J.* **151** 220–2.

Barkmeier, W.M., Gwinnett, A.J., and Shaffer, S.E. (1985). Effects of enamel etching time on bond strength and morphology. *J. clin. Orthod.* **19**, 36–8.

Beech, J.L. and Jalaly, T. (1980). Bonding of polymers to enamel: influence of deposits formed buring etching, etching time and period of water immersion. *J. dent. Res.* **59**, 1156–62.

le Bell, Y. and Forsten, L. (1980). Sealing of preventively enlarged fissures. *Acta odont. Scand.* **38**, 101–4.

Berman, D.S. and Slack, G.L. (1972). Caries experience relative to individual susceptibility. *Br. dent. J.* **135**, 68–70.

British Paedodontic Society (1987). A policy document for fissure sealants. *Br. dent. J.* **163**, 42–3.

Bojajini, J., Garces, H., McCune, R.J., and Pineda, A. (1976). Effectiveness of pit and fissure sealants in the prevention of caries. *J. prev. Dent.* **3**(6), 31–4.

Brooks, J.D. *et al.* (1976). A comparative study of the retention of two pit and fissure sealants: one-year results. *J. prev. Dent.* **3**, 43–6.

Brooks, J.D. *et al.* (1979*a*). A comparative study of two pit and fissure sealants: two-year results in Augusta, Ga. *J. Am. dent. Ass.* **98**, 722–5.

Brooks, J.D. *et al.* (1979*b*). A comparative study of two pit and fissure sealants: three-year results in Augusta, Ga. *J. Am. dent. Ass.* **99**, 42–6.

Brooks, J.D., Pruhs, J.J., Azhadari, S., and Ashrafi, M.H. (1988). A pilot study of three tinted unfilled pit and fissure sealants: 23-month results in Milwaukee, Wisconsin. *Clin. Prev. Dent.* **10**, 18–22.

Buonocore, M.G. (1955). A simple method of increasing the adhesion of acrylic filling materials to enamel surfaces. *J. dent. Res.* **34**, 849–53.

Buonocore, M.G. (1970). Adhesive sealing of pits and fissures for caries prevention, with use of ultra-violet light. *J. Am. dent. Ass.* **80**, 324–8.

Buonocore, M.G. (1971). Caries prevention in pits and fissure sealed with an adhesive resin polymerised by ultra-violet light: a two-year study of a single adhesive application. *J. Am. dent. Ass.* **82**, 1090–3.

Burt, B.A. (1977). Tentative analysis of the efficiency of fissure sealants in a public program in London. *Commun. Dent. oral Epidemiol.* **5**, 73–7.

Burt, B.A., Berman, D.S., Gelbier, S., and Silverstone, L.M. (1975). Retention of a fissure sealants six months after application. *Br. det. J.* **138**, 98–100.

Burt, B.A., Berman, D.S., and Silverstone, L.M. (1977). Caries retention and effects on occlusal caries after 2 years in a public program. *Commun. Dent. oral Epidemiol.* **5**, 15–21.

Charbeneau, G.R. and Dennison, J.B. (1979). Clinical success and potential failure after a single application of a pit and fissure sealant: a four-year report. *J. Am. dent. Ass.* **98**, 559–64.

Charbeneau, G.T., Dennison, J.B., and Ryge, G. (1977). A filled pit and fissure sealant: 18 months results. *J. Am. dent. Ass.* **95**, 299–306.

Cohen, L. and Sheiham, A. (1988). The use of pit and fissure sealants in the General Dental Service in Great Britain and Northern Ireland. *Br. dent. J.* **165**, 50–3.

Collins, W.J.N. *et al.* (1985). Experience with a mobile fissure sealing unit in the greater Glasgow area: results after three years. *Commun. dent. Hlth.* **2**, 195–202.

Cueto, E.I. and Buonocore, M.G. (1967). Sealing of pits and fissures with an adhesive resin: its use in caries prevention. *J. Am. dent. Ass.* **75**, 121–8.

Dorignac, G.F. (1987). Efficacy of highly filled composites in the caries prevention of pits and fissures: two and one half years of clinical results. *J. Pedodont.* **11**, 139–45.

Dummer, P.M.H., Addy, M., Oliver, S.J., and Shaw, W.C. (1988). Changes in the distribution of decayed and filled tooth surfaces and the progression of approximal caries in children between the ages of 11–12 years and 15–16 years. *Br. dent. J.* **164**, 277–82.

Eidelman, E., Shapira, J., and Houpt, M. (1984). The retention of fissure sealants using twenty-second etching time. *J. Dent. Child.* **51**, 422–4.

Eklund, S.A. (1986). Factors affecting the cost of fissure sealants: a dental insurer's perspective. *J. Public Health Dent.* **46**, 133–40.

Ferguson, F.S. (1980). Retention of two sealant systems applied by inexperienced operators: results after 6 months and 12 months. *J. prev. Dent.* **7**, 355–8.

Fuks, A.B. *et al.* (1982). A comparison of the retentive properties of two filled resins used as fissure sealants. *ASDC J. Dent. Child.* **49**, 127–30.

Gibson, G.B., Richardson, A.S., and Waldman, R. (1982). The effectiveness of a chemically polymerized sealant in preventing occlusal caries: five-year results. *Pediatr. Dent.* **4**, 309–10.

Going, R.E. *et al.* (1976). Two-year clinical evaluation of a pit and fissure sealant Part 1: Retention and loss of substance. *J. Am. dent. Ass.* **92**, 388–97.

Going, R.E. *et al.* (1977). Four-year clinical evaluation of a pit and fissure sealant. *J. Am. dent. Ass.* **95**, 972–81.

Going, R.E. *et al.* (1978). The viability of microorganisms in carious lesions five years after covering with a fissure sealant. *J. Am. dent. Ass.* **17**, 455–62.

Gore, J.T. (1939). Etiology of dental caries. Enamel immunization experiments. *J. Am. dent. Ass.* **26**, 958–9.

Handleman, S.L., Washburn, F., and Wopperer, P. (1976). Two-year report of the sealant effect on bacteria in dental caries. *J. Am. dent. Ass.* **93**, 967–70.

Handelman, S.L. *et al.* (1981). Use of adhesive sealants over occlusal carious lesions: radiographic evaluation. *Commun. Dent. oral Epidemiol.* **9**, 256–9.

Handelman, S.L., Leveratt, D.H., Espeland, M.A., and Curzon, J.A. (1986). Clinical radiographic evaluation of sealed carious and sound tooth surfaces. *J. Am. dent. Ass.* **113**, 751–4.

Hargreaves, J.A. and Chester, C.G. (1973). Clinical trial among Scottish children of an anti-caries dentifrice containing 2 per cent sodium monofluorophosphate. *Commun. Dent. oral Epidemiol.* **1**, 47–57.

Harris, N.O. *et al.* (1976). Adhesive sealant clinical trial: effectiveness in a school population of the U.S. Virgin Islands. *J. prev. Dent.* **3**, 27–37.

Helle, A. (1975). Two fissure sealants tested for retention and caries reduction in Finnish children. *Proc. Finn. dent. Soc.* **71**, 91–5.

Higson, J.F. (1976). Caries prevention in first permanent molars by fissure sealing: a 2-year study in 6–8 year old children. *J. Dent.* **4**, 218–22.

Hinding, J.H. and Buonocore, M.G. (1974). The effects of varying the application protocol on the retention of pit and fissure sealant: a two-year clinical study. *J. Am. dent. Ass.* **89**, 127–31.

Holm, A-K. (1978). Dental Health in a group of Swedish 8-year-olds followed since the age of 3. *Commun. Dent. oral Epidemiol.* **6**, 71–7.

Horowitz, H.S. (1980). Pit and fissure sealants in private practice and public health programmes: analysis of cost-efectiveness. *Int. dent. J.* **30**, 117–26.

Horowitz, H.S., Heifetz, S.B., and McCune, R.J. (1974). The effectiveness of an adhesive sealant in preventing occlusal caries: findings after two years in Kalispell, Montana. *J. Am. dent. Ass.* **89**, 885–90.

Horowitz, H.S., Heifetz, S.B., and Poulsen, S. (1976). Adhesive sealant clinical trial: an overview of results after four years in Kalispell, Montana. *J. prev. Dent.* **3**, 38–49.

Horowitz, H.S., Heifetz, S.B., and Poulsen, S. (1977). Retention and effectiveness of a single application of an adhesive sealant in preventing dental caries: final report after five years of a study in Kalispell, Montana. *J. Am. dent. Ass.* **95**, 1133–9.

Houpt, M.I. and Shey, Z. (1980). Cost-effectiveness of fissure sealant placement. *J. prev. Dent.* **6**, 7–10.

Houpt, M. and Shey, Z. (1983). The effectiveness of a fissure sealant after six years. *Pediatr. Dent.* **5**, 104–6.

Houpt, M., Eidelman, E., Shey, Z., Fuks, A., Chosak, A., and Shapira, J. (1984). Occlusal restoration using fissure sealant instead of extension for prevention. *J. Dent. Child.* **51**, 270–3.

Hunter, B. (1985). Survival of dental restorations in young patients. *Commun. Dent. oral Epidemiol.* **13**, 285–7.

Hyatt, T.P. (1923). Prophylactic odontotomy. The cutting into the tooth for the prevention of disease. *Dent. Cosmos* **65**, 234–41.

Ibsen, R.L. (1973). Use of a filled diacrylate as a fissure sealant: one-year clinical study. *J. Am. Soc. prev. Dent.* **3**, 60–5.

Isler, S.L. and Doline, S.L. (1981). Practical application of pit and fissure sealants. A seven year retrospective study. *Clin. prev. Dent.* **3**, 18–20.

Isler, S.L., Malecz, R., and Ruff. J. (1980). A pedodontic preventive dentistry practice. Part 1. Pit and fissure sealants: a 5-year clinical evaluation. *J. prev. Dent.* **6**, 201–14.

Jackson, D. (1965). The mortality of permanent teeth. *Br. dent. J.* **118**, 158–62.

Jensen, O.E. and Handelman, S.L. (1980). Effect of an autopolymerizing sealant on viability of microflora in occlusal dentine caries. *Scand. J. dent. Res.* **88**, 382–8.

Jeronimius, D.J., Till, M.J., and Sveen, O.B. (1975). Reduced viability of microorganisms under dental sealants. *J. Dent. Child.* **42**, 275–80.

King, N.M, Shaw, L., and Murray, J.J. (1980). Caries susceptibility of the permanent first and second molars in children aged 5–15 years. *Commun. Dent. oral Epidemiol.* **8**, 151–8.

Klein, H. and Knutson, J.W. (1942). Studies on dental caries XIII. Effect of ammoniacal silver nitrate on caries in the first permanent molar. *J. Am. dent. Ass.* **29**, 1420–6.

Klock, B. (1980). Economic aspects of a caries preventive program. *Commun. Dent. oral Epidemiol.* **8**, 97–102.

Leake, J.L. and Martinello, B.P. (1976). A four-year evaluation of a fissure sealant in a public health setting. *Can. dent. Ass.* **42**, 409–15.

Leske, G.S., Pollard, S., and Cons, N. (1976). The effectiveness of dental hygienist teams in applying a pit and fissure sealant. *J. prev. Dent.* **3**, 33–6.

Lewis, D.W. and Hargreaves, J.A. (1975). Epidemiology of dental caries in relation to pits and fissures. *Br. dent. J.* **138**, 345–8.

Li, S.H. *et al.* (1981). Evaluation of the retention of two types of pit and fissure sealants. *Commun. Dent. oral Epidemiol.* **9**, 151–8.

Luoma H. *et al.* (1973). Retention of a fissure sealant with caries reduction in Finnish children after six months. *Scand. J. dent. Res.* **81**, 510–12.

McCabe, J. and Storer, R. (1980). Adaptation of resin restorative materials to etched enamel and the interfacial work of fracture. *Br. dent. J.* **148**, 155–8.

McCune, R.J. *et al.* (1973). Pit and fissure sealants: one-year results from a study in Kalispell, Montana. *J. Am. dent. Ass.* **87**, 1177–80.

McCune, R.J., Bojanini, J., and Abodeely, R.A. (1979). Effectiveness of a pit and fissure sealant in the prevention of dental caries: three-year clinical results. *J. Am. dent. Ass.* **99**, 619–23.

Mansson, B. (1977). Caries progression in the first permanent molars: a longitudinal study. *Swed. dent. J.* **1**, 185–91.

Mertz-Fairhurst, E.J., Fairhurst, C.W., Williams, J.E., Della-Giustina, V.E., and Brooks, J.D. (1984). A comparative clinical study of two pit and fissure sealants: 7-year results. *J. Am. dent. Ass.* **109**, 252–5.

Mertz Fairhurst, E.J., Schuster, G.S., and Fairhurst, C.W. (1986). Arresting caries by sealants: results of a clinical study. *J. Am. dent. Ass.* **112**, 194–7.

Meurman, J.H. and Helminen, S.K.J. (1976). Effectiveness of fissure sealant after 3 years after application. *Scand. J. dent. Res.* **84**, 218–23.

Meurman, J.H. *et al.* (1975). Caries reduction 1.5 years after application of a fissure sealant as related to dietary habits. *Scand. J. dent. Res.* **83**, 1–6.

Meurman, J.H., Helminen, S.K.J., and Luoma, H. (1978). Caries reduction over five years from a single application of a fissure sealant. *Scand. J. dent. Res.* **86**, 153–6.

Miller, J. (1950). A clinical investigation in preventive dentistry. *Dent. Practit.* **1**, 66–75.

Miller, J. (1953). Observations in clinical preventive dentistry. *Br. dent. J.* **94**, 7–9.

Miller, W.D. (1905). The preventive treatment of teeth with special reference to nitrate of silver. *Dent. Cosmos* **47**, 913–22.

Mitchell, L. and Murray, J.J. (1987). The durability of fissure sealants placed in children attending a dental hospital. *Br. dent. J.* **163**, 353–6.

National Institutes of Health (1984). Consensus development conference statement on dental sealants in the prevention of tooth decay. *J. Am. dent. Ass.* **108**, 233–6.

Parkhouse, R.C. and Winter, G.B. (1971). A fissure sealant containing methyl-2-cyanoacrylate as a caries preventive agent. *Br. dent. J.* **130**, 16–19.

Poulsen, S. *et al.* (1979). Evaluation of a pit-and-fissure sealing program in a public dental health service after 2 years. *Commun. Dent. oral Epidemiol.* **7**, 154–7.

Prime, J.M. (1937). Controlling dental caries. *J. Am. dent. Ass.* **24**, 1950–61.

Raadal, M. (1978). Follow-up study of sealing and filling with composite resins in the prevention of occlusal caries. *Commun. Dent. oral Epidemiol.* **6**, 176–80.

Rantala, E.V. (1979). Caries incidence in 7–9-year-old children after fissure sealing and topical fluoride therapy in Finland. *Commun. Dent. oral Epidemiol.* **7**, 213–17.

Richardson, A.S., Waldman, R., and Gibson, G.B. (1978). The effectiveness of a chemically polymerised sealant in preventing occlusal caries: 2 year results. *Can. dent. Ass. J.* **44**, 269–72.

Richardson, A.S., Gibson, G.B., and Waldman, R. (1980*a*). Chemically polymerised sealant in preventing occlusal caries. *Can. dent. Ass. J.* **46**, 259–60.

Richardson, A.S., Gibson, G.B., and Waldman, R. (1980*b*). The effectiveness of a chemically polymerised sealant: four-year results. *Pediatr. Dent.* **2**, 24–6.

Richardson, B.A., Smith, D.C., and Hargreaves, J.A. (1977). Study of a fissure sealant in mentally retarded Canadian children. *Commun. Dent. oral Epidemiol.* **5**, 220–6.

Richardson, B.A., Smith, D.C., and Hargreaves, J.A. (1981). A five-year clinical evaluation of the effectiveness of a fissure sealant in mentally retarded Canadian children. *Commun. Dent. oral Epidemiol.* **9**, 170–4.

Ripa, L.W. and Cole, W.W. (1970). Occlusal sealing and caries prevention: results 12 months after a single application of adhesive resin. *J. dent. Res.* **49**, 171–3.

Risager, J. and Poulsen, S. (1974). Fissure sealing with Nuva-Seal in a public health program for Danish schoolchildren after 12 months observation. *Scand. J. dent. Res.* **82**, 570–3.

Rock, W.P. (1972). Fissure sealants. Results obtained with two different sealants after one year. *Br. dent. J.* **133**, 146–51.

Rock, W.P. (1973). Fissure sealants. Results obtained with two different bis-GMA type sealants after one year. *Br. dent. J.* **134**, 193–6.

Rock, W.P. (1974). Fissure sealants. Further results of clinical trials. *Br. dent. J.* **136**, 317–21.

Rock, W.P. and Evans, R.I.W. (1982). A comparative study between a chemically polymerised fissure sealant resin and a light-cured resin. *Br. dent. J.* **152**, 232–4.

Rock, W.P. and Evans, R.I.W. (1982). A comparative study between a chemically polymerised fissure sealant resin and a light-cured resin: three-year results. *Br. dent. J.* **155**, 344–6.

Rock, W.P., Gordon, P.H., and Bradnock, G. (1978). The effect of operator variability and patient age on the retention of fissure sealant resin. *Br. dent. J.* **145**, 72–5.

Rock, W.P., Gordon, P.H., and Bradnock, G. (1981*a*). Dental caries experience in Birmingham and Wolverhampton school children following the fluoridation of Birmingham water in 1964. *Br. dent. J.* **150**, 61–6.

Rock, W.P., Gordon, P.H., and Bradnock, G. (1981*b*). Caries experience of West Midland school children following fluoridation of Birmingham water in 1964: caries of first permanent molars. *Br. dent. J.* **150**, 269–73.

Sheykholeslam, Z. and Houpt, M. (1978). Clinical effectiveness of an auto-polymerised fissure sealant after 2 years. *Commun. Dent. oral Epidemiol.* **6**, 181–4.

Silverstone, L.M. (1974). Fissure sealants, laboratory studies. *Caries Res.* **8**, 2–26.

Simonsen, R.J. (1979). Fissure sealants in primary molars: retention of coloured sealants with variable etch times at 12 months. *J. Dent. Child.* **46**, 382–4.

Simonsen, R.J. (1980*a*). Preventive resin restorations: three-year results. *J. Am. dent. Ass.* **100**, 535–9.

Simonsen, R.J. (1980*b*). The clinical effectiveness of a colored pit and fissure sealant at 24 months. *Pediatr. Dent.* **2**, 10–16.

Simonsen, R.J. (1987). Retention and effectiveness of a single application of white sealant after 10 years. *J. Am. dent. Ass.* **115**, 31–6.

Stephen, K.W., Sutherland, D.A., and Trainer, J. (1976). Fissure sealing by practitioners. First year retention data in Scottish 6-year-old children. *Br. dent. J.* **140**, 45–51.

Stephen, K.W. *et al.* (1978). Fissure sealing of first permanent molars. An improved technique applied by a dental auxilliary. *Br. dent. J.* **144**, 7–10.

Stephen, K.W., Kirkwood, M., Campbell, D., Young, K.C., Gillespie, F.C., and Boyle, P. (1981*a*). Fissure sealing with Nuva-Seal and Alpha-Seal: two-year data. *J. Dent.* **9**, 53–7.

Stephen, K.W. *et al.* (1981*b*). A clinical comparison of two filled fissure sealants after one year. *Br. dent. J.* **150**, 282–4.

Stephen, K.W., Campbell, D., Kirkwood, M., and Strang, R. (1985). A two-year visible light/UV light filled sealant study. *Br. dent. J.* *159*, 404–5.

Stiles, H.M. *et al.* (1976). Adhesive sealant clinical trial: comparative results of application by a dentist or dental auxilliaries. *J. prev. Dent.* **3**, 8–11.

Takeuchi, M. *et al.* (1966). Sealing of the pit and fissure with resin adhesive II. Results of nine months' field work, an investigation of electrical conductivity of teeth. *Bull. Tokyo dent. Coll.* **7**, 50–9.

Takeuchi, M. *et al.* (1971). Sealing of the pit and fissure with resin adhesive IV. Results of 5 year field work and a method of evaluation of field work for caries prevention. *Bull. Tokyo dent. Coll.* **12**, 295–320.

Theilade, E. *et al.* (1977). Effect of fissure sealing on the microflora in occlusal fissures of human teeth. *Archs. oral Biol.* **22**, 251–9.

Thylstrup, A. and Poulsen, S. (1978). Retention and effectiveness of a chemically polymerised pit and fissure sealant after two years. *Scand. J. dent. Res.* **86**, 21–4.

Todd, J.E. (1975). *Children's dental health in England and Wales, 1973*. HMSO, London.

Todd, J.E. and Dodd, T. (1985). Children's dental health in the United Kingdom 1983. HMSO, London.

Ulvestad, H. (1976). A 24-month evaluation of fissure sealing with a diluted composite material. *Scand. J. dent. Res.* **84**, 51–5.

Vrbic, V. (1986). Five-year experience with fissure sealing. *Quintessence Int.* **17**, 371–2.

Walls, A.W.G., Wallwork, M.A., Holland, I.S., and Murray, J.J. (1985). The longevity of occlusal amalgam restorations in first permanent molars of child patients. *Br. dent. J.* **158**, 133–6.

Walls, A.W.G., Murray, J.J., and McCabe, J.F. (1988). The management of occlusal caries in permanent molars. A clinical trial comparing a minimal composite restoration with an occlusal amalgam restoration. *Br. dent. J.* **164**, 288–92.

Williams, B. and von Frauenhofer, J.A. (1977). The influence of the time of etching and washing on the bond strength of fissure sealants applied to enamel. *J. oral Rehab.* **4**, 139–43.

Williams, B. and Winter, G.B. (1981). Fissure sealants. Further results at 4 years. *Br. dent. J.* **150**, 183–7.

Williams, B., Price, R., and Winter, G.B. (1978). Fissure sealants. A 2-year clinical trial. *Br. dent. J.* **145**, 359–64.

Williams, B., Ward, R., and Winter, G.B. (1986). A two-year clinical trial comparing different resin systems used as fissure sealants. *Br. dent. J.* **161**, 367–70.

6

The carious lesion in enamel

Edwina Kidd

Nearly a hundred years ago a remarkable American dentist, Dr G. V. Black, was studying the problem of dental caries. He wrote extensively on the pathology of the disease (Black, 1908) and based on his observations he laid the foundations for the operative management of the disease. He wrote, 'The complete divorcement of dental practice from studies of the pathology of dental caries, that existed in the past, is an anomaly in science that should not continue. It has the apparent tendency plainly to make dentists mechanics only.'

In the intervening years a mass of information has been gathered about this sugar-dependent, infectious disease. It is now appreciated that dental caries is not a simple process of demineralization but is characterized by alternating periods of destruction and arrest or even repair. When the destructive forces predominate the disease will progress. Conversely, preventive measures, such as dietary control, effective plaque removal, and judicious use of fluoride, can arrest the disease and provided it is caught in its early stages, even partial repair is possible.

Part of this chapter will describe the pathology of enamel caries as this is the scientific basis on which the management strategies rest. In addition the clinical detection of enamel carious lesions will be discussed, for without accurate diagnosis it is not possible to formulate a sensible approach to the management of the disease.

Macroscopic features of the early enamel lesion

The earliest macroscopic evidence of enamel caries is known as the 'white spot lesion'. The lesions form in areas of plaque stagnation, such as enamel pits and fissures in the occlusal surface of molars and premolars, approximal enamel smooth surfaces just cervical to the contact point (Fig. 6.1), and the enamel of the cervical margin just coronal to the gingival margin. The lesion is best seen on dried teeth where the opaque, white appearance distinguishes it from the adjacent sound enamel. At this stage the enamel is still hard and shiny. Sometimes the lesion may appear brown in colour, the so-called 'brown spot lesion'. Even-

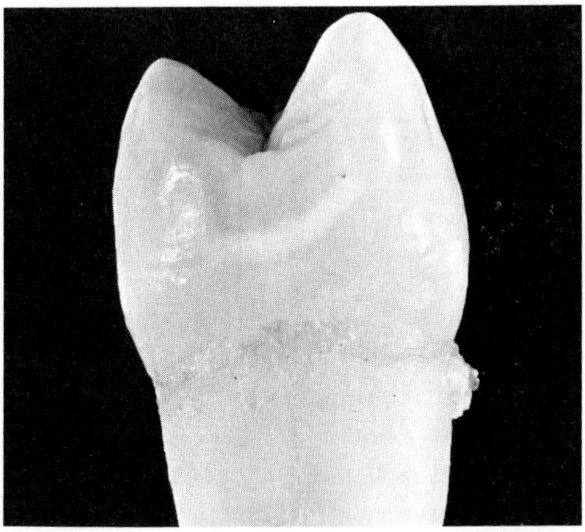

Fig. 6.1. Premolar showing a white spot lesion on the approximal tooth surface.

tually, if the lesion progresses, the intact surface breaks down (cavitation) and a hole is formed (a cavity).

Although the white spot lesion is the earliest visual sign of the disease it has been preceded by destructive processes which are not discernible macroscopically. Research workers have used the scanning electron microscope to observe the early enamel reaction to acids produced by bacteria in the dental plaque. At this ultrastructural level direct dissolution of the outer enamel surface can be seen (Thylstrup and Fejerskov 1986). This involves partial dissolution of the crystal peripheries leading to an enlargement of intercrystalline spaces. In addition the tissue immediately beneath the outer microsurface appears more porous than the microsurface itself. Eventually these changes, involving an increase in porosity of the tissue, become macroscopically visible after air-drying.

It is perhaps worth considering why air-drying makes these changes easier to see. The explanation concerns the refractive indices of hydroxyapatite (1.62), water (1.33), and air (1.0). When the tissue is dried, air will replace the water in the intercrystalline spaces. The difference between the refractive index of hydroxyapatite and air is now so large that the porous tissue loses its translucency and appears opaque. Lesions which appear opaque without air-drying are more demineralized than those which are only apparent on a dry surface. Thus to pick up early demineralization visually, teeth must be both clean and dry.

Microscopic features of the early enamel lesion

To examine carious enamel in the light microscope, ground sections are required. On a smooth surface the lesion is usually triangular in shape, the apex of the triangle pointing towards the enamel–dentine junction (Plate 6.1). The small lesion has been divided into zones based upon its histological appearance when longitudinal ground sections are examined with the light microscope. Four zones may be distinguished. There is a translucent zone at the inner advancing front of the lesion, while a dark zone may be found just superficial to this. The body of the lesion is the third zone, lying between the dark zone and the apparently undamaged surface enamel. This is the zone that makes up the major part of the lesion and shows the most marked demineralization. The relatively unaffected surface zone, superficial to the lesion, is the fourth zone.

While each of these zones may be seen in plain transmitted light, the lesion is particularly clear when examined with polarized light. In addition, the microscope may be used quantitively to deduce the degree of demineralization of carious enamel.

Polarized light and enamel caries

Silverstone (1973) described the technique of polarized light microscopy in the following manner. Mature human dental enamel consists of crystallites of apatite packed closely together in the tissue and aligned approximately along the length of the prism. Between the crystallites are minute spaces which contain the organic component of the tissue and an aqueous phase. The mineral component of enamel, like most biological structures and non-cubic crystals, can resolve a beam of plain polarized light into two rays travelling at different velocities. Such a structure is termed 'birefringent' because it has two refractive indices (RI) related to the two planes of transmission within the crystal. A sign of birefringence is given to the structure determined by the path taken by the slower (+) and faster (−) rays in relation to the morphology of the crystal. The sign of birefringence of enamel has been described as 'negative' with respect to prism length. This is known as the 'intrinsic birefringence' of the tissue. Enamel thus has a negative intrinsic birefringence, relative to prism direction. The sign of birefringence of the organic component of enamel is positive with respect to prism length but, as the organic component in mature human enamel is very small, its birefringence has been disregarded.

Apart from the mineral and organic components of enamel there are minute 'spaces' in the tissue. During carious dissolution there is an increase in the total volume of these spaces or pores, which themselves give rise to an additional type of birefringence. This birefringence has been called 'form birefringence'. It is produced when the spaces contain a medium having a refractive index different from that of the enamel crystals (1.62). Whereas intrinsic birefringence is negative with respect to prism length, form birefringence is positive.

Carious enamel will therefore show a negative intrinsic birefringence due to its oriented crystallite component, and a positive form birefringence due to the intercrystallite spaces. The observed birefringence will be the summation of the two. Only when the spaces or pores are filled with a medium having the same refractive index as enamel will form birefringence be eliminated.

When ground sections are examined in polarized light, it is usual to place the section in a liquid; this liquid is called an 'inhibition medium'. Two inhibition media will be referred to in the description that follows—water and quinoline.

Enamel has a refractive index of 1.62. Water, however, has a different refractive index of 1.33. When carious enamel is examined after imbibition with water, positive form birefringence will be produced if the holes created in the tissue are large enough to admit water. Quinoline, on the other hand, has a refractive index of 1.62, the same as enamel. Thus, if quinoline enters the pores created by dental caries, no form birefringence will be seen. The appearance of each of the four zones of enamel caries in polarized light will now be described.

Zone 1: the translucent zone

The translucent zone of enamel caries lies at the advancing front of the lesion and is the first recognizable zone of alteration from normal. This zone is only seen when a longitudinal ground section is examined in a clearing agent, such as quinoline, having the same refractive index (1.62) as that of enamel. The translucent zone appears structureless, the tranlucency being demarcated from normal enamel on its deep aspect and the dark zone on its superficial aspect (Plate 6.1).

The translucent zone is a more porous region than sound enamel, the pores having been created by the demineralization process. Sound enamel has a pore volume of about 0.1 per cent. The translucent zone, however, has a pore volume of approximately 1 per cent. The pores are probably located at junctional sites such as prism borders, cross-striations, and striae of Retzius (Silverstone 1966). Once these areas are imbibed with quinoline these structural markings are lost, due to the penetration of a medium having an identical refractive index to that of enamel apatite.

A translucent zone is not present in all lesions and may sometimes only be observed on the lateral aspects of a lesion, close to the enamel surface.

Zone 2: the dark zone

If a translucent zone is present at the advancing front of a lesion when examined in quinoline, the dark zone is the second zone of alteration from normal and lies just superficial to the translucent zone. The zone appears dark or positively birefringent after imbibition with quinoline (Plate 6.1). The dark zone may show considerable variation in its width and is not present in all lesions (Plate 6.2).

The dark zone is more porous than the translucent zone, having a pore volume of 2–4 per cent. The explanation of why the dark zone appears dark, or positively birefringent, is an intriguing one. It would seem that in this zone the pores are of varying sizes, large and small. Quinoline is a large molecule and cannot enter the small pores, which remain filled with air (Darling *et al.* 1961). Because the refractive index of air is remote from that of enamel, positive-form birefringence is produced. Thus, some of the pores of the dark zone act as a 'molecular sieve', excluding large molecules such as quinoline.

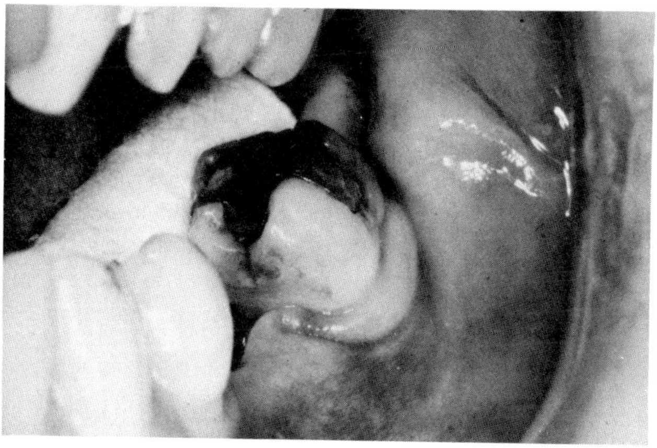

Fig. 6.2. Arrested caries on the mesial surface of the lower second molar.

There are two theoretical ways in which these small pores may have formed. They may have been created by demineralization, that is by an opening up of sites not previously attacked. Alternatively, the small pores could represent areas of healing where mineral has been redeposited. There is now considerable evidence to support the view that the dark zone can represent an area of remineralization. If arrested lesions that have been present clinically for many years (Fig. 6.2) are examined histologically (Kidd 1983), they show wide, well-developed dark zones at the front of the lesion, within the body of the lesion, and at the surface of the lesion (Plate 6.3).

Attempts have been made to remineralize enamel lesions in the laboratory using human saliva and calcifying fluids prepared from synthetic hydroxyapatite with added fluoride (Silverstone 1973). After such exposure there were changes in the histological appearance of the lesions including significant broadening of the dark zones (Plates 6.4 and 6.5).

Zone 3: the body of the lesion

The body is the largest proportion of carious enamel in the small lesion. It lies superficial to the dark zone and deep to the relatively unaffected surface layer. When a longitudinal ground section is examined in quinoline in polarized light, the area appears translucent, negatively birefringent, and the striae of Retzius may be well marked (Plates 6.1 and 6.2).

The body of the lesion is particularly clearly seen if the ground section is examined after imbibition with water. The body now shows as an area of positive birefringence in contrast to the negative birefringence of sound enamel and the rest of the lesion (Plates 6.6 and 6.7). The region has a minimum pore volume of 5 per cent at its periphery, increasing to 25 per cent or greater in the centre. After imbibition with water the striae of Retzius are often particularly clear.

The area appears positively birefringent because the water (RI 1.33) enters the pores in the tissue and positive-form birefringence is produced.

Several workers have described natural enamel lesions that show bands of well-mineralized tissue passing through the body of the lesion (Kostlan 1962; Crabb 1966; Silverstone 1970). Histologically this appearance may be found in 'old' or 'chronic' lesions (Plate 6.8). This feature may represent a lesion which has developed very slowly with alternating periods of de- and re-mineralization, or a lesion which having developed has arrested and partially healed.

Zone 4: the surface zone

One of the important characteristics of enamel caries is that the greatest degree of demineralization occurs at a subsurface level. The small lesion remains covered by a surface layer which appears relatively unaffected by the attack. When such a lesion is examined in polarized light after imbibition with water, the porous subsurface region is positively birefringent while the surface zone retains a negative birefringence (Plate 6.7).

The appearance of a surface zone as being one of the zones of caries, and not just the resistant sound enamel surface, was first described by Silverstone (1968), who defined it as the negatively birefringent zone seen after imbibition with water. This relatively unaffected surface zone is usually some 30 μm in depth and has a pore volume of approximately 1 per cent. If the lesion progresses, this surface layer is eventually destroyed and a cavity forms.

The subsurface demineralization that characterizes the enamel lesion has intrigued research workers for many years. Some have suggested that the formation of this relatively unaffected surface layer is associated with the special properties of surface enamel, which shows a high degree of mineralization, a higher fluoride content, and possibly a greater amount of insoluble protein than subsurface enamel. However, in the laboratory, artificial caries-like lesions can be produced in enamel when the original surface has been ground away. Consequently the existence of surface enamel with 'special' characteristics cannot be entirely responsible.

The surface zone has also been attributed to the presence of a layer of plaque over the lesion. The plaque may act as a diffusion trapping calcium, phosphate, and fluoride ions released by subsurface dissolution or from saturated solution in plaque. These ions may then reprecipitate into the surface enamel. This suggestion implies that the surface zone of enamel caries may, in part, be a manifestation of remineralization.

Fissure caries

Occlusal fissures and buccal pits are obvious stagnation areas where plaque can form and mature, anatomically protected from the toothbrush bristle by the dimensions of the fissure.

PLATES

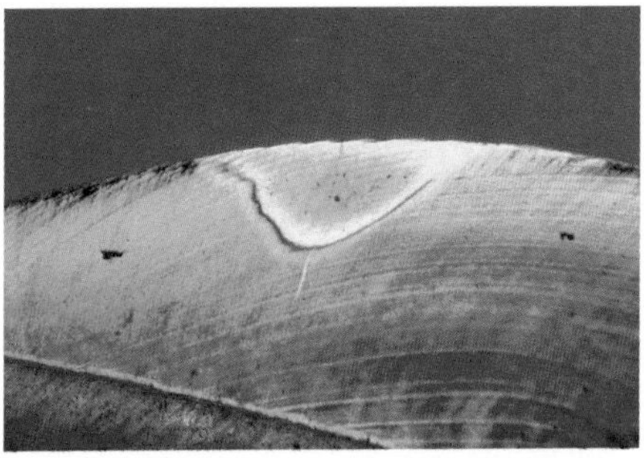

Plate 6.1. Longitudinal ground section through a small lesion of enamel caries examined in quinoline with polarized light. The translucent zone is clearly differentiated from sound enamel and the dark zone shows positive birefrigence. The striae of Retzius are well marked within the body of the legion. × 50.

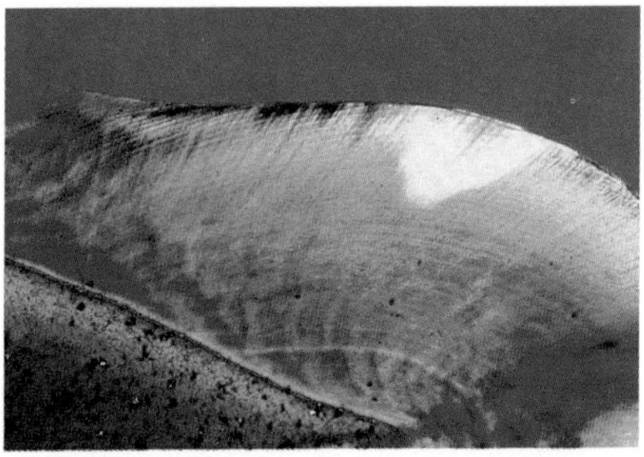

Plate 6.2. Longitudinal ground section through a small lesion of enamel caries examined in quinoline with polarized light. The body of the lesion is seen as a translucent area. No dark zone is present in this specimen. × 50.

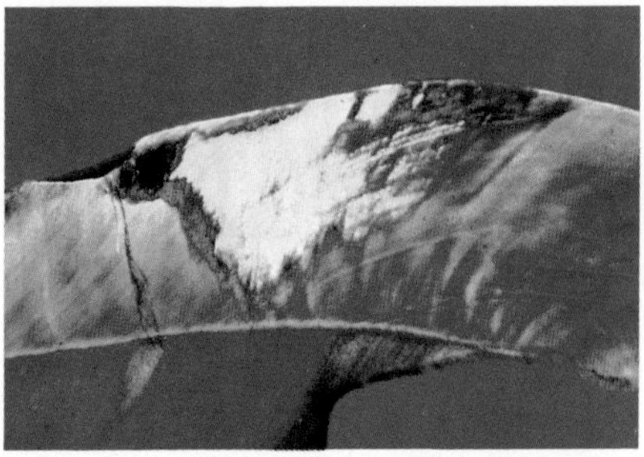

Plate 6.3. Longitudinal ground section of a natural carious lesion in a tooth extracted from a patient aged 70 years, examined in quinoline with polarized light. Wide, well-developed dark zones are obvious at the advancing front of the lesion, within the body of the lesion, and at the surface of the lesion. × 50.

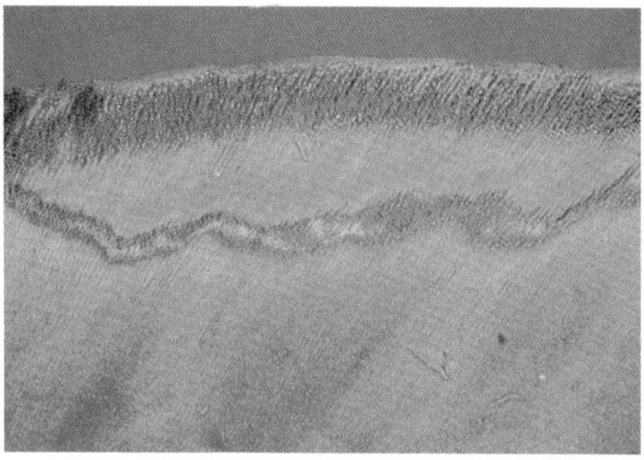

Plate 6.4. Longitudinal ground section of a small lesion examined in quinoline with polarized light before exposure to a calcifying fluid. The advancing front of the lesion shows a translucent zone and a positively birefringent dark zone. × 50. (From Silverstone (1977), by courtesy of *Caries Research*).

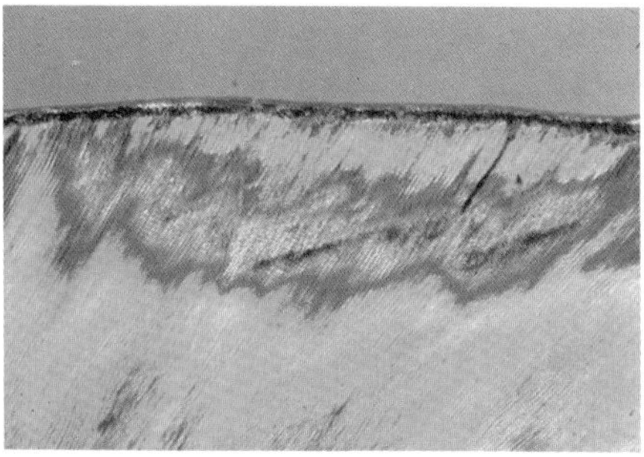

Plate 6.5. The same section as in Plate 6.4 after exposure to a synthetic calcifying fluid. The section is again examined in quinoline. The dark zone appears much broader than prior to the experiment. Whilst its deep border is approximately at the original position, its superficial boundary has extended towards the enamel surface into the region previously identified as the body of the lesion. This region of 'new' dark zone has a pore volume of between 2 and 4 per cent and shows a negative birefringence in water. This region previously had been demineralized to a stage exhibiting a pore volume of between 5 and 20 per cent. × 50. (From Silverstone (1977), by courtesy of *Caries Research*).

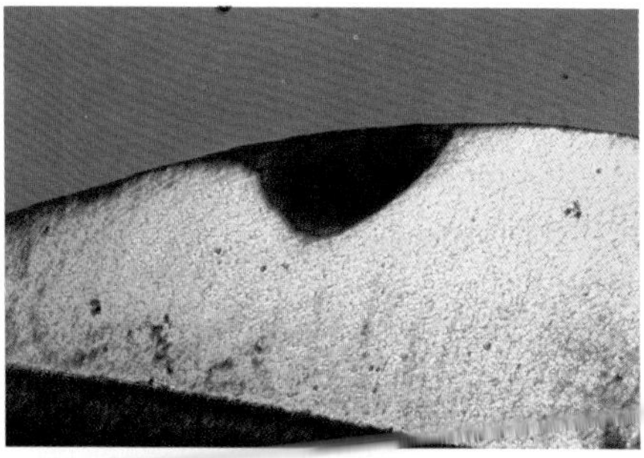

Plate 6.6. The same section as in Plate 6.1 now examined in water with polarized light. The body of the lesion shows as an area of positive birefringence. × 50.

Plate 6.7. The same section as in Plate 6.2 now examined in water with polarized light. The body of the lesion, positioned in the subsurface enamel, shows positive birefringence. The surface overlying the lesion exhibits a negative birefringence. × 50.

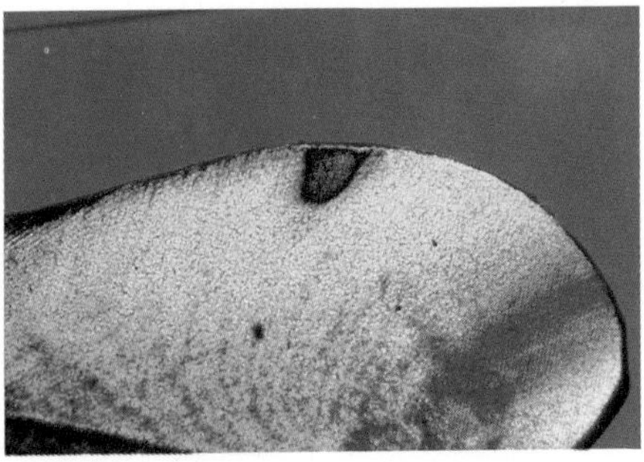

Plate 6.8. The same section as in Plate 6.3 now examined in water with polarized light. Well-mineralized laminations are obvious within the body of the lesion, particularly on its occlusal aspect. × 50.

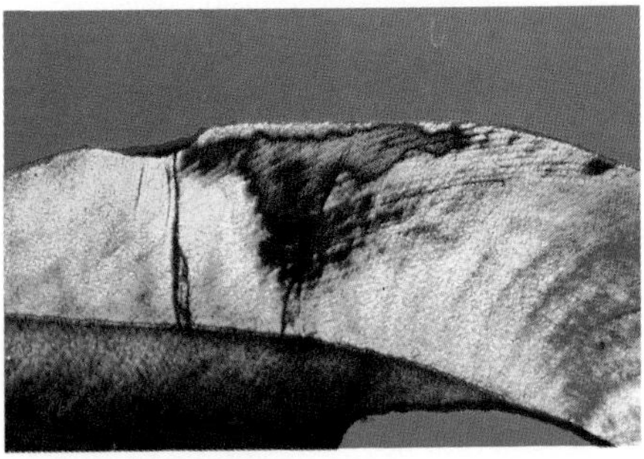

Plate 6.9. Longitudinal ground section through a deciduous molar tooth examined in quinoline with polarized light. The lesion is seen as a translucent area, there being no evidence of a dark zone in this specimen. × 50.

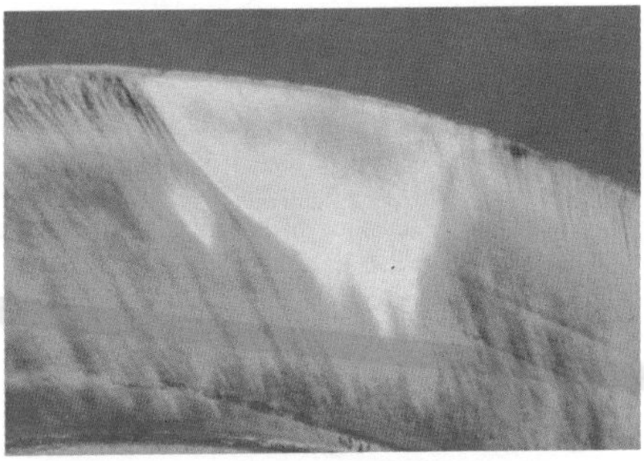

Plate 6.10. The same section as in Plate 6.9 now examined in water with polarized light. The body of the lesion shows as an area of positive birefringence beneath an intact, negatively birefringent, surface zone. × 50.

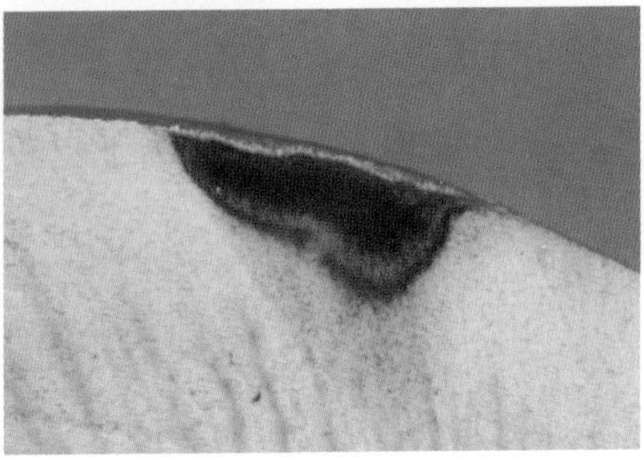

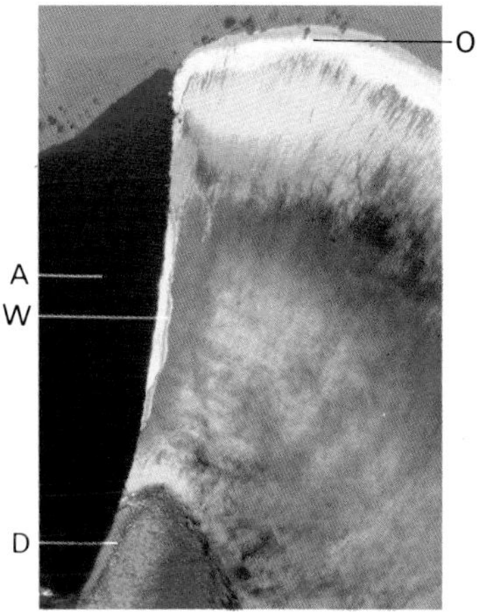

Plate 6.11. Longitudinal ground section of a natural secondary carious lesion. The ground section is in quinoline and viewed with polarized light. An amalgam restoration is present (A). The wall lesion is seen as a translucent zone (W). Dentine involvement is obvious (D). An outer lesion, caused by primary attack on the enamel surface, is also present (O). × 50. (By courtesy of *Dental Update*.)

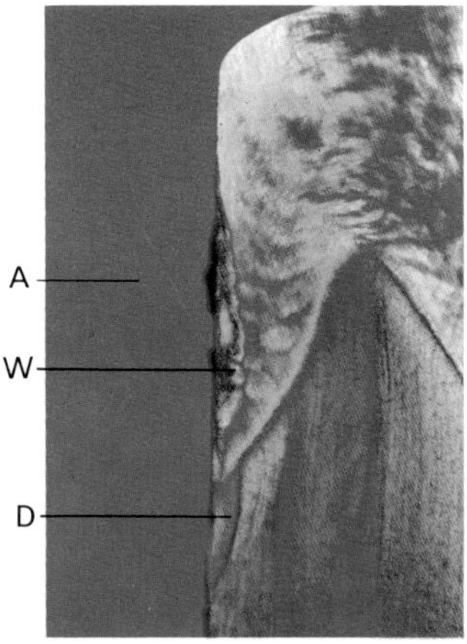

Plate 6.12. Longitudinal ground section of a natural secondary carious lesion. The ground section is in quinoline and viewed with polarized light. An amalgam restoration was present but lost during section preparation (A). The wall lesion is seen as a dark zone (W) Dentine involvement is obvious (D). × 50. (By courtesy of *Dental Update*).

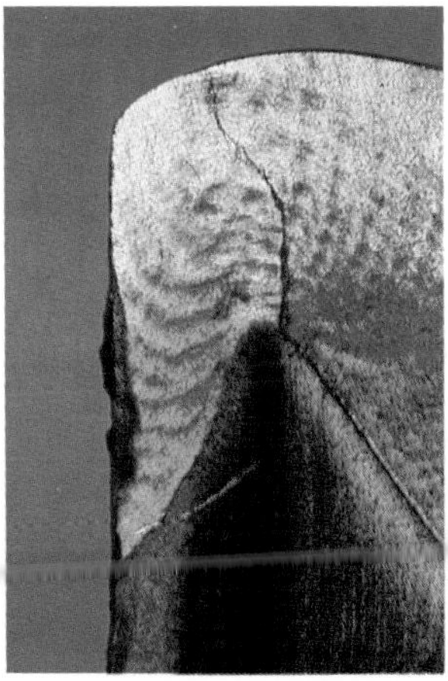

Plate 6.13. The same section as in Plate 6.12 now viewed in water with polarized light. The wall lesion is now seen as an area of positive birefringence indicating a demineralization in excess of 5 per cent. × 50.

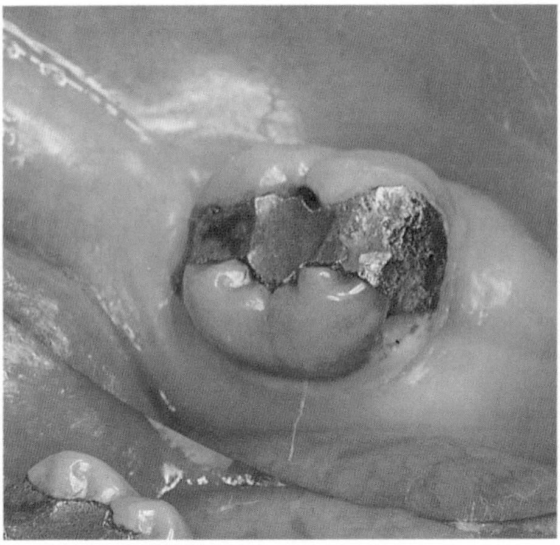

Plate 6.14. A cavitated lesion adjacent to a restoration.

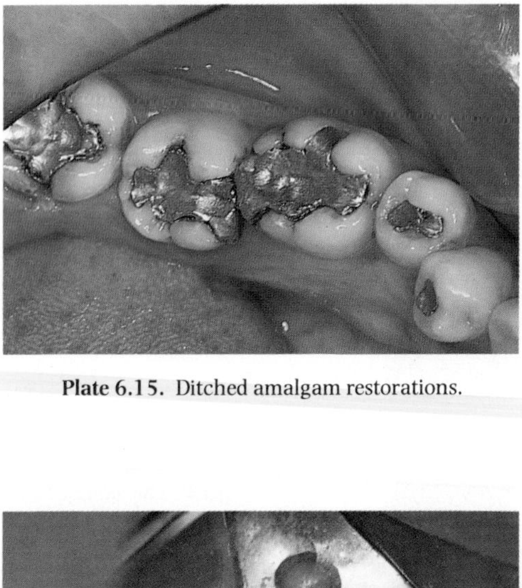

Plate 6.15. Ditched amalgam restorations.

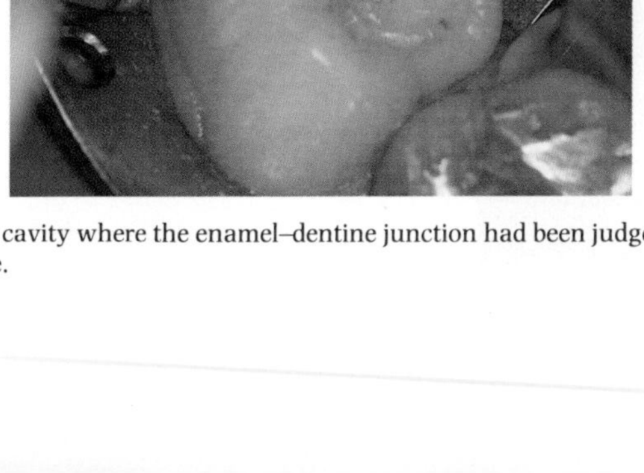

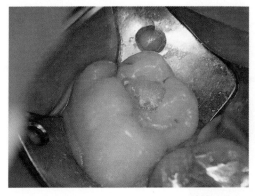

Plate 6.16. A cavity where the enamel–dentine junction had been judged to be clinically caries-free.

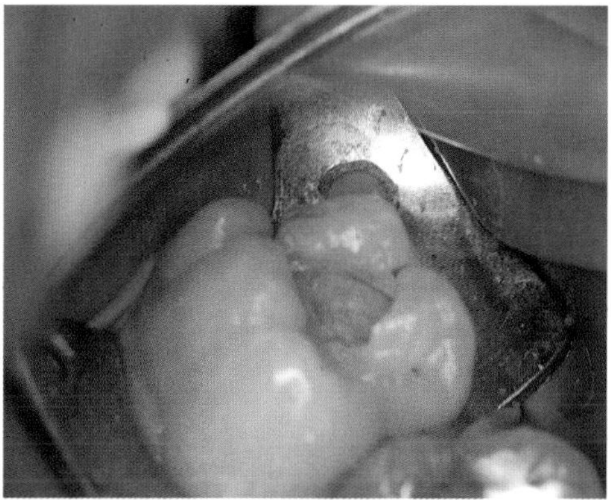

Plate 6.17. The same cavity as in Plate 6.16 after use of the caries detector dye. Note areas of red stain at the enamel–dentine junction.

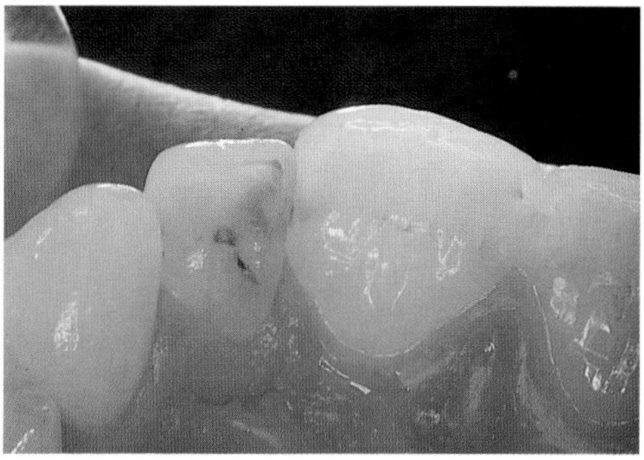

Plate 6.18. Caries is present beneath the restoration on the mesial aspect of the lateral incisor.

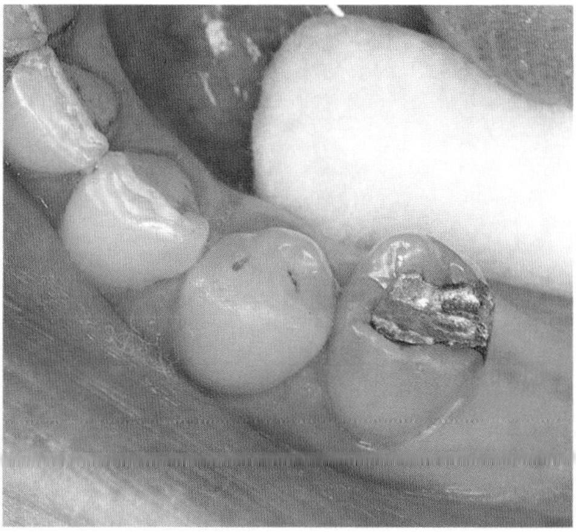

Plate 6.19. Discoloration around the margin of an amalgam restoration. Is this caries or corrosion products?

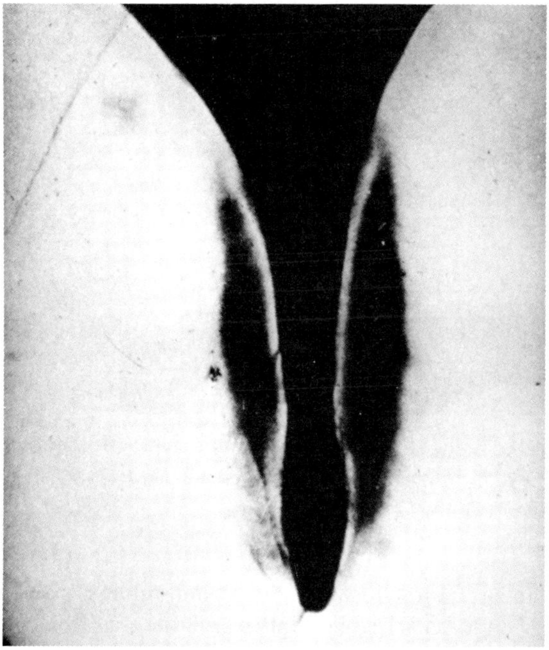

Fig. 6.3. Microradiograph of fissure caries showing lesion formation on either side of the fissure walls. × 30. (From Mortimer (1964), by courtesy of *Caries Research.*)

The histological features of fissure caries are similar to those already described for smooth surfaces. The lesion forms on either side of the fissure walls, giving the appearance of two small, smooth surface lesions (Fig. 6.3) (Mortimer 1964). Eventually the lesions increase in size, coalescing at the base of the fissure. The enamel lesion broadens as it approaches the underlying dentine, guided by prism direction. With lateral spread at the enamel–dentine junction, the area of involved dentine is larger than with smooth surface lesions.

The early lesion in deciduous teeth

The histological features of enamel caries in deciduous teeth are essentially similar to those already described in permanent enamel (Plates 6.9 and 6.10). All of the four zones described for the classical lesion of caries in permanent enamel may be present in the lesion of primary enamel (Silverstone 1970). However, the enamel in deciduous teeth is much thinner than in permanent teeth and the pulps are relatively large. Thus, early diagnosis of the incipient lesion in primary enamel is of particular importance.

Microradiography

In the laboratory it is possible to take a radiograph of a ground section. This is called a microradiograph and may be examined in the light microscope.

Microradiography is sufficiently sensitive to demonstrate demineralization in

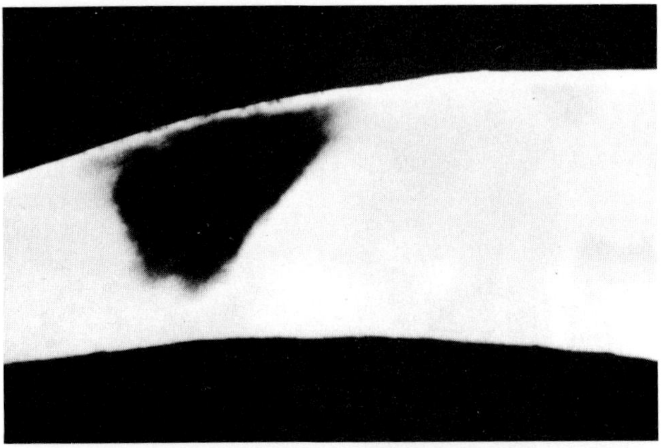

Fig. 6.4. Microradiograph of an early carious lesion in a deciduous molar tooth. The body of the lesion, in the subsurface enamel, shows marked radiolucency in contrast to the surface of the tooth, which remains well mineralized. × 70.

excess of 5 per cent as a radiolucent area whose size corresponds almost exactly with the body of the lesion as seen in polarized light after imbibition with water (Fig. 6.4). The striae of Retzius and prism structure are often well marked. Superficially the radiolucent region is limited by the presence of a well-mineralized radiopaque layer at the surface of the lesion, which may or may not coincide with the presence of a surface zone.

Electron microscopy

The *scanning electron microscope* has been used to examine the surface of white spot lesions (Thylstrup and Fejerskov 1981). On interproximal surfaces the contact facet has a smooth appearance without perikymata. In the active lesion the opaque surface of the enamel cervical to the facet shows numerous irregular holes which represent deepened and more irregular Tomes' processes pits and an increased number of eroded focal holes. These areas may merge together to form larger areas of irregular cracks or microcavities. Thus, although polarized light shows that the early lesion is principally a subsurface demineralization, the scanning electron microscope shows a distinct disintergration of the very surface.

The first evidence of a change from sound enamel that can be recognized with the *transmission electron microscope* appears to coincide with the body of the lesion as seen in the light microscope. Demineralization of enamel is diffuse, affecting both intra- and inter-prismatic enamel. Prism junctions would appear to be sites of preferential dissolution, with narrow channels occurring between prisms (Fig. 6.5) (Johnson 1967*a*, *b*). In these areas, crystallites larger than those in sound enamel may be seen, which probably represent areas of recrystal-

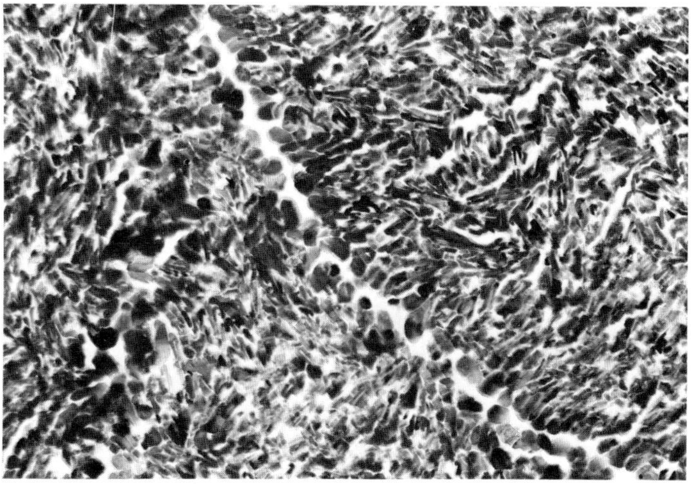

Fig. 6.5. Electronmicrograph showing parts of two transversely sectioned prisms from carious enamel. Inter-crystallite space containing embedding material can be differentiated from artefact. A double row of enlarged, polyhedral cells is present at the prism junction lining a channel which is largely artefact, but which does contain Araldite. This is seen where it forms a halo to the crystals. The majority of crystals are irregular flattened hexagons with central deficiencies. ×42 500. (By courtesy of Professor N. W. Johnson.)

lization. Carious destruction of individual crystals results in loss of crystal centres and in surface damage.

Dental caries and the organic matrix of enamel

As enamel mineralizes much of its organic contents disappear so that the mature tissue contains relatively little organic material.

For many years there has been argument as to whether the initial lesion of enamel caries was caused by demineralization or by alteration of the organic matrix. Microdissection techniques have been developed which allow the various histological zones of enamel caries, as seen with the light microscope, to be dissected out and analysed chemically. Such experiments have shown that mineral is lost from the translucent zone with no evidence of change in the organic matrix (Hallsworth *et al.* 1972). Thus, it is now thought that demineralization precedes organic destruction.

However, the role of the organic matrix in the initiation and progress of caries is not fully known. It has been shown by microchemical studies that the composition of interior enamel is variable with pockets of high and low mineral content (Robinson *et al.* 1971). Mineral content has been found to correlate inversely with protein distribution. It might be thought that areas of comparatively low mineralization and increased protein would be more susceptible to acid attack. However, enamel protein could be protective by preventing the spread of the small ions responsible for dissolving mineral. It is known that fluorosed enamel, which is relatively poorly mineralized, is remarkably resistant to acid attack. (Kidd *et al.* 1978). This could be related to its high protein content. Alternatively, the high level of fluoride in the tissue may be the important factor.

It is thought that the organic content of carious enamel is greater than that of sound tissue. The organic material is of exogenous origin, bacterial or salivary, but little is known of the effect this has on the carious process.

Arrested lesions

It is important to realize that enamel lesions do not automatically progress and the clinician will frequently see arrested carious lesions. These are particularly common on proximal surfaces where the adjacent tooth is missing (Fig. 6.2). Such lesions commonly are heavily stained and it has been suggested that extraction of the adjacent tooth changes the environment so that the lesion becomes more cleansable and accessible to saliva.

Another situation where arrested lesions are commonly seen is cervically where bands of demineralized enamel, which formed during tooth eruption, are left 'high and dry' as passive eruption occurs. This arrest of the carious process may allow some redeposition of mineral (remineralization) within the lesion, which probably explains why these chronic lesions in old teeth appear quite different histologically from acute lesions. Sometimes this healing may appear clinically to be complete in that a white spot lesion can actually disappear. A well-known example of this is found in the work of Backer-Dirks (1966), who studied 184 buccal surfaces of maxillary first molars in the same children at age 8 and again at age 15. Of 72 surfaces with white spots at age 8, 37 appeared sound at age 15.

Evidence of remineralization from experimental caries in man

The concept of arrest and partial remineralization of the carious lesion has attracted a great deal of research interest, and several experiments have been carried out *in vivo*.

When blocks of enamel, covered with Teflon gauze to facilitate bacterial colonization, were mounted in removable bridges in the mouths of human subjects, the enamel blocks showed surface softening as detected by micro-hardness testing. When the gauze was removed, to expose the enamel to the saliva *in vivo*, an increase in hardness occurred in the test blocks. This increase in hardness was thought to be due to remineralization (Koulourides 1966).

In subsequent work with the same method (Koulourides *et al.* 1980), fluoride solutions were used to encourage remineralization. Subsequently the 'healed' lesions were again covered with gauze to create a cariogenic environment. The enamel which had remineralized was now found to be more resistant to dental caries than an adjacent area of sound enamel which had not previously been exposed. It thus seems possible that a remineralized white spot lesion may be more resistant to carious attack than sound enamel.

Other experiments have been carried out on teeth destined for extraction. Plates or bands were placed on the teeth to induce plaque accumulation and thus produce a cariogenic environment. Once lesions had formed, the plates or bands were removed to expose the enamel to the oral fluids. Remineralization occurred and the lesions either disappeared or remained as hard, discoloured areas. It was thought that the disappearance of the lesions was associated with deposition of new mineral in the demineralized area (von der Fehr 1965, Holmen *et al.* 1987).

Experimental caries has also been induced with sucrose mouth rinses in human subjects over a 23-day period. After this time, oral hygiene procedures were recommended and the subjects used daily mouth rinses with 0.2 per cent sodium fluoride solutions for 1 month. Caries scores showed regression of 'healing' of the experimental lesions during the fluoride mouth-rinsing regime (von der Fehr *et al.* 1970).

The clinical relevance of arrest and remineralization

As caries progression is not inevitable an important role for the dentist is the early diagnosis of caries. The dentist can then show the patient how to arrest the disease by dietary control, judicious use of fluorides, and effective plaque removal. These diagnostic and preventive efforts are just as much *treatment* of the disease as is operative dentistry, and should be recognized and rewarded as such.

It is important to realize that once cavitation occurs, remineralization will not 'fill up the hole'. Indeed the cavity will favour progression rather than arrest if it hinders effective plaque removal. This does not mean, however, that cavitated lesions will automatically progress, because if they are cleansable and if the diet is modified, the disease can still be arrested.

Clinical detection of the enamel lesion (Kidd and Joyston-Bechal 1987)

The diagnosis of caries requires good lighting and dry, clean teeth. If heavy deposits of plaque or calculus are present the mouth should be cleaned before attempting accurate diagnosis.

Free smooth surfaces

Enamel lesions are easily seen on free, smooth surfaces and can be diagnosed at the stage of the white or brown spot lesion, before cavitation has occurred, pro-

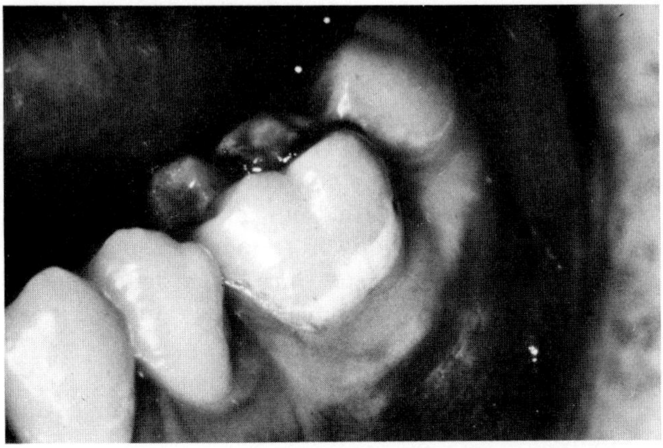

Fig. 6.6. White spot lesions on the buccal aspect of first and second molars.

vided the teeth are clean, dry and well lit (Fig. 6.6). Traditionally, sharp probes have also been used to detect the 'tacky' feel of early cavitation. However, this approach should *not* be used because the sharp probe can physically damage an incipient carious lesion.

Pits and fissures

While caries on free smooth surfaces is easy to see, caries in pits and fissures is difficult to diagnose at this early stage because, histologically, the white spot lesion forms on the walls of the fissure. Thus, the fissure which looks clinically caries-free may histologically show signs of an early lesion. In addition, the fissure that is sticky to a sharp probe may not be carious histologically. The stickiness may relate to the fissure shape or the pressure exerted rather than caries, and indeed a sharp probe can actually damage an incipient carious lesion. The probe should be used to remove any plaque from the fissure to allow sharp eyes to pick up discoloration, cavitation, and the grey appearance of enamel undermined by caries in the dentine beneath.

Bitewing radiographs are also important in the diagnosis of occlusal caries although by the time a lesion can be seen on radiograph it is well into dentine.

Thus the early diagnosis of caries in pits and fissures is difficult and is giving rise to considerable concern among practitioners. However, help may be on the way in the form of an electronic caries detector (Rock and Kidd 1988). The principle behind this machine is that the spaces in the porous tissue fill with fluid and therefore the electrical conductivity increases with increasing demineralization. A machine has been produced commercially (Vanguard Electronic Caries Detector) where a battery-generated current is applied to the fissure through a probe (Fig. 6.7). The probe is placed co-axially in an air tube which dries the tooth surface, and the machine gives a digital read-out varying from 0 to 9,

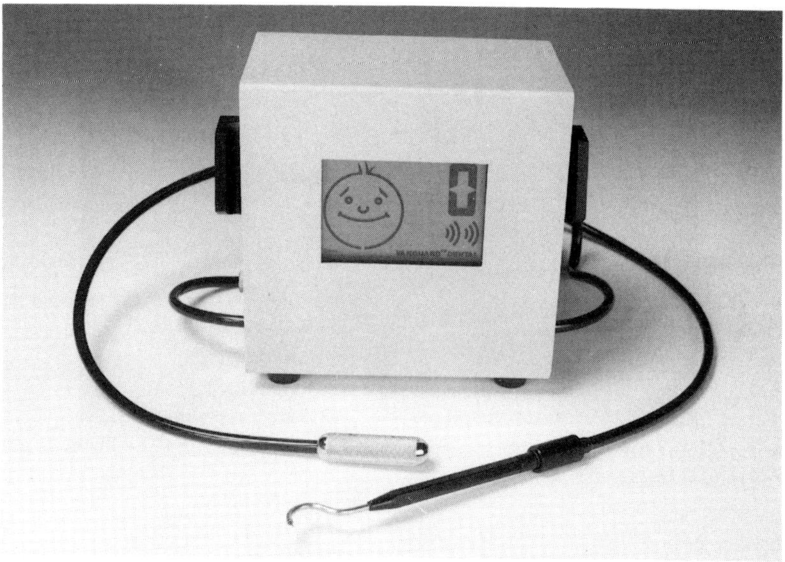

Fig. 6.7. The Vanguard electronic caries detector.

representing increasing degrees of demineralization. The possibility may well exist for monitoring progression or arrest of early enamel fissure lesions in this way.

Approximal surfaces

As with the fissure, it will be difficult to see the enamel lesion on an approximal surface. Vision is obscured by the adjacent tooth. The lesion is discovered visually at a relatively late stage when it has already progressed into dentine and is seen as a pinkish grey area shining up through the marginal ridge.

It is, however, possible to insert circles of elastic between teeth to separate them. This technique is extensively used in orthodontic treatment when bands are to be placed on teeth. An interdental gap of 0.5–1.0 mm is readily produced in 48 hours. The method is non-destructive, reversible, and inexpensive, and may be a useful aid in the diagnosis and management of some lesions (Pitts 1987).

Visual diagnosis can be aided by the use of transmitted light. The technique consists of shining light through the contact point. A carious lesion has a lowered index of light transmission and therefore appears as a dark shadow that follows the outline of the decay through the dentine. This technique has been used for many years in the diagnosis of approximal lesions in anterior teeth. Light is reflected through the teeth using the dental mirror and the carious lesions are seen readily in the mirror. In posterior teeth a stronger light source is required and fibre-optic lights, with the beam reduced to 0.5 mm in diameter,

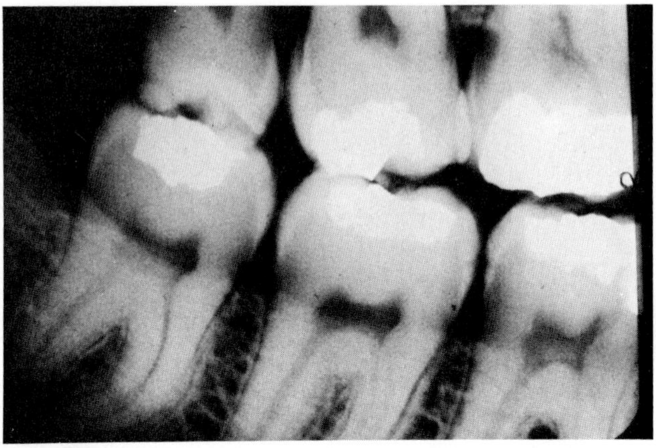

Fig. 6.8. A bitewing radiograph showing early carious lesions on the distal surface $\overline{6|}$ and the mesial surface $\overline{7|}$.

have been used (Mitropoulus 1985). However, the technique is unreliable in the diagnosis of the enamel lesion although once the caries is in dentine, reliability improves.

The bitewing radiograph is still the most important diagnostic tool for approximal caries but the technique is relatively insensitive and is not able to detect early subsurface demineralization. The earliest radiographic sign of approximal caries is seen on a bitewing radiograph as a small, triangular radiolucent area just cervical to the contact point (Fig. 6.8). Although the lesion appears confined to the outer enamel, histological examination shows that it penetrates into the underlying dentine. At this stage the lesion may, or may not, be cavitated.

Unfortunately, in spite of rigorous attempts to standardize all aspects of the radiographic method and viewing techniques, visual estimates of lesion size remain subjective and liable to considerable error. In an attempt to improve the situation a television-based image analysis technique has been developed (Pitts 1984), which can both detect and measure approximal enamel radiolucencies. Currently the system is only available as a research tool but in the future it may be developed further for use in practice.

The relevance of the diagnostic information to the management of the disease

The preceding section has discussed the clinical methods available for the detection of the enamel lesion. How should this information be used clinically? First of all it is important to remember that clinical and radiographic diagnoses may be inaccurate. No one can be sure of recording the same caries diagnosis on different occasions on one patient and even the trained epidemiologist is only 70 to

80 per cent reliable. When the disease is at an early stage, diagnoses are more likely to be incorrect.

Once such lesions have been recognized, consideration should be given to what these appearances mean in the particular mouth being examined. In a young child or young adult this appearance may be indicative of active and progressive disease. Unless preventive measures are instituted, cavitation will occur as the disease progresses. A similar appearance in the mouth of an older person might indicate a period of active disease some years earlier. Alternatively, this same picture could indicate a recent change in diet, such as sweets substituted for cigarettes, and active disease which will progress unless prevented.

As with all clinical problems, a careful history from the patient is of obvious importance. In addition, knowledge of the mouth as it was months and years previously is invaluable. The scientific basis for the popular six-monthly dental examination has been questioned (Sheiham 1977), as it is known that dental caries in the permanent dentition is a very slow disease, taking about 2 to 4 years to progress through the enamel. However, there is now considerable evidence to show that it may only be possible to remineralize a lesion where the damage is minimal. Thus, it would appear that from the point of view of arresting disease before treatment is required, the six-monthly examination has much to recommend it.

If the clinician detects white spot lesions and decides that these represent active disease, the correct treatment is to institute prevention and observe the lesions rather than to attack them immediately with the dental drill. Plaque control and dietary advice are of obvious importance. As the fluoride ion appears so important in remineralization, some form of topical fluoride therapy should be begun. It would appear that the remineralization effect requires the presence of the fluoride ion in the fluid environment of the tooth surface. For this reason, frequent, low-dose, topical applications such as fluoridated water, toothpastes, mouth rinses, and tablets, would seem particularly useful. On occlusal surfaces a fissure sealant is a sensible additional preventive measure.

Finally, because dental caries is an infectious disease involving specific microorganisms, microbiological monitoring of disease activity may be sensible (Krasse 1985). There is now some evidence that individuals with a high level of *Streptococcus mutans* infection may be at risk to dental caries. In addition there is some evidence that a high level of lactobacilli is associated with a cariogenic diet. High levels of this organism are also associated with multiple open cavities and such cavities should be excavated and temporarily dressed before determining the level of lactobacillus infection.

Strep. mutans and lactobacillus counts can be carried out on paraffin wax-stimulated saliva. The saliva sample is collected and some of it is transferred to a transport vial, containing transport fluid, using a syringe or pipette. The sample is then taken to the laboratory where it is homogenized, diluted quantitatively, and cultivated on selective media for *Strep. mutans* and lactobacilli. In most laboratories *Strep. mutans* is cultivated on mitis salivarius agar containing sucrose and bacitracin. For cultivation of lactobacilli, SL agar is generally used. The number of typical colonies at a suitable dilution is counted and the figure obtained is multiplied by the dilution factor. This gives the number of *Strep. mutans* and lactobacilli respectively for each millilitre of saliva.

High value > 1 000 000 *Strep. mutans* > 100 000 lactobacilli
Low value < 100 000 *Strep. mutans* < 1 000 lactobacilli

Commercially available kits are now available, making it feasible for these tests to be carried out in the surgery.

Secondary caries

Dentists spend a considerable amount of their time and derive a substantial part of their income from replacing restorations in teeth. One in three restorations present at any time is unsatisfactory and has failed to meet the clinical criteria commonly used to define success (Elderton 1976). Secondary caries is often the single most important factor given by dentists for the replacement of restorations (Healey and Phillips 1949; Richardson and Boyd 1973; Lavelle 1976; Dahl and Eriksen 1978; Mjor 1981; 1985; Qvist *et al.* 1986*a*, *b*) and yet dentists vary widely in their treatment planning (Elderton and Nuttall 1983). This must call into question the ability of dentists to diagnose caries within restored teeth.

Histological features of the early lesion

When a filling is placed, the adjacent enamel may be considered in two planes: the surface enamel and the enamel of the cavity wall. For this reason, a secondary carious lesion has been described as occurring in two parts; an 'outer lesion' formed on the surface of the tooth as a result of primary attack and cavity 'wall lesion', which will only be seen if hydrogen ions can pass between the restoration and the cavity wall (Hals *et al.* 1974, Hals and Kvinnsland 1974).

The early secondary carious lesion in enamel is most clearly seen in polarized light when ground sections are imbibed with quinoline. In this medium the wall lesion appears as either a translucent zone or a dark zone extending along the cavity wall. If the lesion reaches the enamel–dentine junction, it spreads laterally to involve the dentine on a wider front (Plates 6.11 and 6.12). An outer lesion may also be present (Plate 6.11). Examination of sections after imbibition with water will reveal areas of enamel demineralization in excess of 5 per cent as positively birefringent (Plate 6.13).

The prevention of secondary caries

It appears that the interface between a restoration and the dental tissue is susceptible to demineralization whenever leakage of bacteria, fluids, molecules, or ions can occur between a cavity wall and the restorative material applied to it. This clinically undectable leakage around restorations has come to be referred to as 'microleakage' and has been extensively investigated over the last 25 years (see review by Kidd 1976).

Many techniques have been devised to test the cavity sealing properties of restoration both *in vitro* and *in vivo*. These include the use of dyes, radioactive isotopes, air pressure, bacteria, neutron activation analysis, scanning electron microscopy, and artificial caries. The salient point in all this work is that all filling materials leak and therefore, in a caries-prone mouth, all restorations may potentially fail because of recurrent caries. Thus restorations cannot be regarded as a treatment for dental caries. Fillings merely replace missing tissue with a poor substitute for unblemished enamel and dentine. The management of dental caries, be it primary or secondary, rests with assessing risk and reducing the rate of caries progression by dietary control, judicious use of fluorides, and plaque control.

However, there are measures the clinician can take during the restoration of teeth which make secondary caries less likely (Elderton 1987; Kidd and Joyston-Bechal 1987) and these measures will now be discussed.

Plaque control and restorative technique

It is well known that caries forms in areas of plaque stagnation. The junction between a restoration and a tooth is a potential plaque trap and it is important that this area can be cleaned easily. For many years it was held that cavity margins be finished in 'self-cleansing' areas but it is now known that 'self-cleansing' is an unreliable method of plaque control. Thus cavity margins should normally allow access for tooth-brush filaments, dental floss, or interdental wood points. This implies that on occlusal surfaces, cavity margins should not be finished in deep fissures where plaque would tend to collect unless these fissures are sealed, as in the sealant (preventive resin) restoration (Simonsen 1978).

Approximally, the bucco-axial and linguo-axial margins of the Class II cavity should not be finished at the contact point but brought into the embrasure so that they may be cleaned with a toothbrush. It could, of course, be argued that if patients were routinely to use dental floss this would not be necessary. However, finishing these margins in a cleansable area has the added advantage that the dentist is able to see the margin to check it at subsequent visits. Cavity margins should also be placed coronal to gingival margin wherever possible, because subgingival margins encourage plaque accumulation and therefore recurrent caries and periodontal disease.

Ditching is a particular problem with amalgam restorations (Fig. 6.9) which predisposes to plaque retention and therefore secondary caries. As early as 1895, G. V. Black noted this appearance and attributed it to deformation under the stress of mastication. Recent research has confirmed this observation as it has been shown that those amalgams with the lowest creep rate display the least incidence of marginal breakdown. The high copper content alloys show a significant reduction in creep rate in comparison with conventional alloys and in addition are more resistant to corrosion. Jorgensen (1965) has suggested that

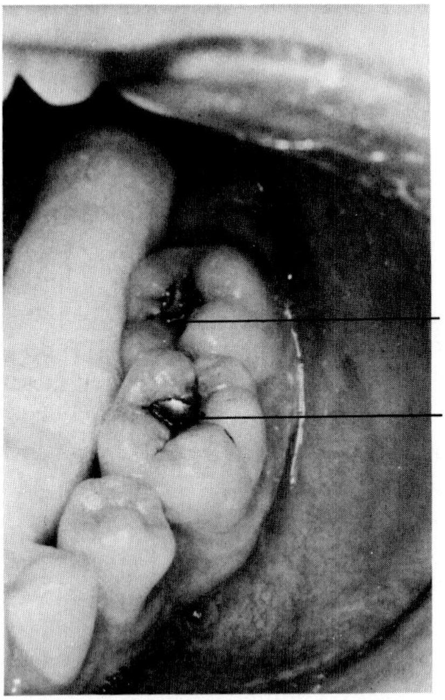

Fig. 6.9. The outline forms of these amalgam restorations cross several fissures. There is a danger that plaque will collect in these areas. Early secondary caries is present in one area, and 'ditching' of the restoration is seen. (By courtesy of *Dental Update*.)

the mechanism of marginal fracture is related to corrosion, so these newer alloys are likely to show improved marginal adaptation and clinical trials have confirmed this (Duperon *et al.* 1971).

In addition, ditching may be reduced by attention to detail in cavity preparation. As amalgam is a brittle material the amalgam-margin angle must exceed 70° as angles less than this are prone to fracture (Elderton 1984).

Although ditched margins predispose to plaque accumulation and therefore caries, restorations with ditched margins should not automatically be replaced. Research has shown that replacement restorations frequently contain the same in-built errors as their predecessors (Elderton 1977). Thus, where a margin is severely ditched, it may be more logical to repair that part of the restoration, concentrating efforts on improving it. Alternatively, ditched restorations may be accepted and put under review so that they may serve a little longer. This approach would seem particularly applicable in mouths which are not caries-prone.

Ditching is not the only discrepancy of fit than can hinder plaque control. Overhanging margins, which are particularly likely to occur gingivally, are very difficult to clean, encouraging both caries and periodontal diseases.

Every effort should be made to achieve a smooth junction between restoration and tooth by careful use of matrix bands and wedges, and by meticulous carving as soon as the band is removed. Despite all this care, ledges may still occur and may be obvious on bitewing radiographs. Such ledges should be removed by grinding with abrasive strips or with specially designed reciprocating handpieces and diamond-coated points or rotary instruments. Alternatively the restoration should be replaced.

Choice of restorative material in posterior teeth

Amalgam alloy is the material most commonly used in the restoration of posterior teeth. The freshly packed amalgam restoration has been shown to leak but cavity seal is improved when restorations have been in the mouth for some time (Nelson *et al.* 1952). This phenomenon has been attributed to the formation of corrosion products at the amalgam/dental tissue interface. Thus, corrosion of the alloy, a property long deplored by clinicians, may be responsible for its success in giving long clinical service (for review see Kidd 1976).

Many studies have shown that the initial leakage around an amalgam restoration may be minimized by applying a thin layer of cavity varnish to the walls and floor of the cavity before packing the amalgam (Going and Massler 1961; Phillips *et al.* 1961; Swartz and Phillips 1961). Little information is available on the duration of this beneficial effect, but it may prevent leakage around the freshly packed filling until corrosion products form and block the microspace between restoration and cavity wall. It would seem wise, therefore, to use a cavity varnish routinely in the caries-prone mouth.

From the point of view of their reduced corrosion resistance, the newer high copper-content alloys have posed a clinical dilemma. It is not known whether the reduced corrosion will have an effect on the long-term cavity sealing ability of the restorations. Logically, a cavity varnish should be used with such alloys but it is possible that this layer will eventually dissolve in the oral fluids leaving a channel along which leakage can occur.

Cast gold inlays are an alternative to amalgam for the restoration of posterior teeth. In any cast restoration the gap between restoration and tooth is filled by cement. It is thus obvious that the cavity sealing ability of a gold inlay is dependent on the seal of the cement lute. Unfortunately very little research work has been done on the cavity sealing ability of such cemented restorations, either in the laboratory or in the mouth. However, a limited comparison of zinc phosphate and glass ionomer cement using an *in vitro* artificial-caries system has shown that secondary caries-like lesions were formed adjacent to both materials. In addition, it is known that the commonly used luting agents are to some extent soluble in the oral fluids. For these reasons, current teaching is that cemented restorations are positively contra-indicated in the caries-prone mouth.

When composite resin materials first appeared on the market, it was hoped that their physical properties would make them suitable for posterior teeth. However, clinical trials showed that abrasion of the material led to a loss of anatomical form over the years. As far as recurrent caries was concerned, clinical trials carried out in dental hospitals were reassuring (for review see Barnes and Kidd 1980) but many practitioners reported a high incidence of recurrent caries around these restorations. It is interesting to speculate why clinical trials and general practitioner experience differed. It is possible that caries-susceptible patients were not used in the clinical trials. In addition there may have been differences in the way the two groups handled the materials.

With the advent of newer, more highly filled, composite materials, designed specifically for use in posterior teeth, the subject has come under discussion again. It appears that the wear resistance of the new materials is greatly improved but resistance to recurrent caries at the cervical margin of the Class II cavity may be poor, despite the fact that composites are bonded to enamel via the acid-etch technique and to dentine via bonding resins.

The problem is that these materials shrink as they set (Kidd 1985) and any adhesive material that shrinks in this way will move towards the stronger bond as it polymerizes. As the bond with the thick enamel of the axial wall is stronger than the bond with the thin enamel or dentine at the cervical margin, a gap is likely to form in this area. The fact that the materials are light-cured could exacerbate the problem because the surface nearest the light sets first and the material then shrinks towards the light, that is away from the cervical margin. To help to solve this problem light-reflectant wedges have been produced, and the polymerizing light is then applied buccally and reflected into the cervical area.

Another approach to the problem is to use a 2 mm thickness of a radiopaque glass ionomer cement at the base of the box. This material adheres to dentine, contains fluoride, which will exert a cariostatic effect (Kidd 1978), and can be etched to bond it physically to composite resin.

A novel concept in treatment of approximal caries has been to use an occlusal approach to the carious lesion which preserves the marginal ridge. This is called the internal cavity preparation (McLean and Gasser 1985). The cavity is restored with a glass ionomer cement or silver cement, which are injected through the occlusal access cavity. This is an ingenious idea because it preserves as much sound tooth as possible while restoring the lesion with a fluoride-releasing material. The material adheres to enamel and dentine and may thus support and strengthen the tissues. The results of clinical trials are awaited with interest.

Choice of restorative material in anterior teeth

When restoring intracoronal cavities in anterior teeth the clinician may choose to use composite resin, glass ionomer cement, or a combination of the two. With the composite materials acid-etching of the enamel, possibly combined with bevelling of the cavity wall, should improve marginal seal.

Glass ionomer cement contains available fluoride which will exert a cariostatic effect. This makes it the material of choice in a caries-prone mouth. The material also has the advantage of being chemically adhesive to enamel and dentine. Thus, where cavities are bounded by both enamel and dentine, it is possible to use glass ionomer cement to replace the missing dentine, then etch this material and the adjacent enamel before adding composite resin to complete the restoration (McLean *et al.* 1985).

Patient education and review

Although it may seem obvious, it must continually be borne in mind that the responsibility for patient care neither begins nor ends with the placement of a restoration. Unless patients are educated and motivated to prevent disease, time and money will be wasted. The experienced clinician will have learnt this by hard experience as, unless myopic or peripatetic, he will have seen his work fail over the years.

Having completed the restorative part of a treatment plan, every attempt must be made to ensure that the patient is able to clean perfectly around the restorations. This is particularly important where Class II restorations, crown, or bridges are present. Interdental cleaning is obligatory (see Chapter 9). Attempts should be made to find out whether the advice given on diet is being followed (see Chapter 2). Consideration must also be given to whether some form of topical fluoride therapy, such as mouth rinses should be continued (see Chapter 3). Finally, the dentist must decide when the patient should be seen again. The timing of the recall appointment will be based on the state of the mouth when the patient originally presented and the patient's response to preventive measures during treatment.

Problems in diagnosis of caries in restored teeth

One of the tasks of the dentist at the recall visit is to inspect restorations for any sign of new disease. This is so much a part of the everyday practice that the reader may consider the process is straightforward. However the problems are enormous and a search for their solution is probably one of the most pressing problems in preventive dentistry today.

A major problem in the diagnosis of caries in restored teeth is that the wall lesion cannot be seen until it is so advanced that the tooth tissue over it becomes grossly discoloured or the overlying tissue collapses to reveal a large hole (Plate 6.14). In many ways this is analogous to the problems in the diagnosis of fissure caries where histologically the white spot lesion forms on the walls of the fissure so that the fissure which looks clinically caries-free may histologically show signs of an early lesion.

Another problem is the filling with a defective margin, particularly the ditched amalgam restoration (Plate 6.15). There is a widely held view that recurrent caries is largely the result of marginal failure of restorations (Goldberg *et al.* 1981) and it has become common dental practice and teaching to replace defective restorations as a preventive procedure. Research work in extracted teeth

(Jorgensen and Wakumoto 1968) has shown that the larger the marginal defect, the more likely it is to show recurrent caries. This is hardly surprising as such defects are plaque traps. Again the situation is analagous to that of the fissure because both the marginal defect and the fissure are stagnation areas. However, just as not all fissures develop clinically detectable lesions, not all defective restorations will develop new caries. This is because the prerequisites for caries are a cariogenic plaque, i.e. specific micro-organisms, with a suitable dietary substrate. If either the substrate or the cariogenic plaque are not present, caries will not develop irrespective of tooth morphology.

The third problem to be considered in the diagnosis of caries in restored teeth is whether the dentist can distinguish new, recurrent caries around a restoration from residual caries that the dentist left during cavity preparation.

Recent work (Anderson and Charbeneau 1985; Anderson *et al.* 1985) has shown how commonly dentists leave residual caries in cavities. These investigators used a caries detector dye (Fusayama and Terachima 1972) in cavities passed as clinically satisfactory by teachers at a dental school. It is claimed that this red dye enhances the visual recognition of dentinal caries by staining the infected demineralized dentine which should be removed during cavity preparation (Plates 6.16, 6.17) but leaving unstained dentine which is only mildly demineralized, not infected, and capable of remineralization.

Their study showed that the enamel–dentine junction was stained red by the dye in 59 out of 100 teeth where cavities had been passed as clinically satisfactory using ordinary visual and tactile criteria. However, this is the very area where it is currently taught that the cavity should be made clinically caries-free because it is argued that residual caries in this area may flourish beneath a leaking restoration. It is thought-provoking that dentists cannot even diagnose caries within cavities when they can look directly at it and use probes!

Thus, to judge by this study the incidence of residual caries is very high indeed. Will all this residual caries progress? Logic suggests that the relevant factor is what happens in the plaque at the tooth surface because recurrent caries may be inevitable if a restoration leaks and a cariogenic plaque with a suitable dietary substrate remains.

One further problem in the diagnosis of caries within restored teeth is distinguishing active caries, which is likely to progress, from chronic, static lesions that are already arrested. Currently there are no clinical criteria on which to base this judgement.

Clinical methods to diagnose recurrent caries in restored teeth

As in the diagnosis of primary caries, the clinician needs good lighting, dry clean teeth, sharp eyes but 'blunt' probes, and good bitewing radiographs. Recurrent disease occurs more frequently at cervical and approximal margins so particular care must be taken in these areas (Mjor 1985).

A freshly cavitated lesion adjacent to a restoration will be obvious clinically (Plate 6.14) but sharp eyes may also pick up the pink, grey, or brown appearance of enamel undermined by caries, i.e. the wall lesion if it is assumed that this is new rather than residual disease (Plate 6.18).

Marginal staining of composite restorations produces considerable difficulty in diagnosis. Such staining represents marginal deterioration, but is this necessarily synonomous with caries?

The colour of corrosion products around amalgam restorations can also cause diagnostic problems as this grey or blue discoloration may also indicate caries (Plate 6.19). Judgement may be based partly on the size of the restoration and the size of the discoloured area. A large restoration may discolour the tooth *per se* without caries being present, whereas a smaller restoration with a large discoloured area around it is more likely to indicate caries.

Once again it is relevant to consider whether the discoloured area is new caries or residual disease. It is well known that arrested or slowly progressing dentine lesions are darkly staining (Miller and Massler 1962); such stain is probably picked up from exogenous dietary sources. If recurrent lesions pick up stain in a similar way it is possible that those lesions which are most obvious clinically because of their colour, may be the ones that are inactive, arrested, or slowly progressing!

Sharp probes should be used with as much care in the diagnosis of caries around restorations as in the diagnosis of primary disease. The probe may catch in a marginal discrepancy which is not carious or it may cause damage to the cavity margin or the filling. Despite these reservations, a curved probe is helpful cervically where evidence from bitewing radiographs is difficult to interpret. However the probe should be used with a light touch not a heavy hand.

Bitewing radiographs are very important in the diagnosis of caries within restored teeth although they usually reveal the caries once it is in dentine rather than showing the early lesion. Provided that the restorative material is radiopaque, the bitewing can be of value in detecting caries both proximally and occlusally.

The consequences of diagnostic difficulties

An experiment has been conducted where nine dentists were asked to examine in the laboratory specific areas of 228 extracted and filled teeth and indicate whether caries was present and the treatment that was required (Merrett and Elderton 1984). They found that caries was clearly considered to be a good reason for treatment in that these dentists proposed to treat 95 per cent of the teeth in which they diagnosed it. The teeth were then sectioned and the presence or absence of caries determined. Unfortunately there was a considerable lack of correspondence between the teeth in which caries was identified as present in the laboratory after sectioning and those in which it was assessed as present in the simulated clinical examinations.

One consequence of this depressing finding is that clinicians, and those who fund them, must currently accept that fillings may be done unnecessarily, or that caries may be missed and therefore the appropriate preventive and operative measures not taken. It is also currently inevitable that dentists will not agree in their diagnosis. This creates enormous problems for the practitioner who must continue to provide care in an incertain situation. The academic is privileged to be paid to address these problems and teachers should discuss them with students.

References

Anderson, M.H. and Charbeneau, G.T. (1985). A comparison of digital and optical criteria for detecting carious dentine. *J. prosth. Dent.* **53**, 643–6.

Anderson, M.H., Loesch, W.J., and Charbeneau, G.T. (1985). Bacteriologic study of a basic fuchsin caries-disclosing dye. *J. prosth. Dent.* **54**, 51–5.

Backer-Dirks, O. (1966). Post-eruptive changes in dental enamel. *J. dent. Res.* **45**, 503–11.

Barnes, I.E. and Kidd, E.A.M. (1980). Composite resin restorative materials—a review. *Dent Update* **7**, 273–83.

Black, G.V. (1895). An investigation of the physical characters of the human teeth in relation to their disease, and to practical dental operations, together with the physical characters of filling materials. *Dent. Cosmos* **37**, 553–71.

Black, G.V. (1908). *A work on operative dentistry. Vol. I The pathology of the hard tissues of the teeth.* Medico-Dental Publishing Company, Chicago.

Crabb, H.S.M. (1966). Enamel caries. Observations on the histology and patterns of progress of the approximal lesion. *Br. dent. J.* **121**, 115–29.

Dahl, J.E. and Eriksen, H.M. (1978). Reasons for replacement of amalgam restorations. *Scand. J. dent. Res.* **86**, 404–7.

Darling, A.I., Mortimer, K.V., Poole, D.F.G., and Ollis, W.D. (1961). Molecular sieve behaviour of normal and carious human dental enamel. *Archs. oral Biol.* **5**, 251–73.

Duperon, D.F., Neville, M.D., and Kasloff, Z. (1971). Clinical evaluation of corrosion resistance of conventional alloy, spherical-particle alloy and dispersion-phase alloys. *J. prosth. Dent.* **25**, 650–6.

Elderton, R.J. (1976). The prevalence of failure of restorations: a literature review. *J. Dent.* **4**, 207–10.

Elderton, R.J. (1977). The quality of amalgam restorations. In *Assessment of the quality of dental care*, (ed. H. Allred), pp. 45–81 London Hospital Medical College.

Elderton, R.J. and Nuttall, N.M. (1983). Variation among dentists in planning treatment. *Br. dent. J.* **154**, 201–6.

Elderton, R.J. (1984). Cavo-surface angles, amalgam-margin angles and occlusal cavity preparations. *Br. dent. J.* **156**, 319–24.

Elderton, R.J. (1987). Preventively-orientated restorations and restorative procedures. In Positive Dental Prevention, pp. 82–92 Heinemann, London.

Fusayama, T. and Terachima, S. (1972). Differentiation of two layers of carious dentine by staining. *J. dent. Res.* **51**, 866.

Goldberg, J., Tanzer, J., Munster, E., Amara, J., Thal, F., and Birkhead, D. (1981). Cross sectional clinical evaluation of recurrent enamel caries, restoration of marginal integrity and oral hygiene status. *J. Am. dent. Ass.* **102**, 635–41.

Going, R.E. and Massler, M. (1961). Influence of cavity liners under amalgam restorations on penetration by radioactive isotopes. *J. prosth. Dent.* **11**, 298–312.

Hallsworth, A.S., Robinson, C., and Weatherell, J.A. (1972). Mineral and magnesium distribution within the approximal carious lesion of dental enamel. *Caries Res.* **6**, 156–68.

Hals, E., Hoyer Andreassen, B., and Bie, T. (1974). Histopathology of natural caries around silver amalgam fillings. *Caries Res.* **8**, 343–58.

Hals, E. and Kvinnsland, I. (1974). Structure of experimental *in vitro* and *in vivo* lesions around composite fillings. *Scand. J. dent. Res.* **82**, 517–26.

Healey, H.J. and Phillips, R.W. (1949). A clinical study of amalgam failures. *J. dent. Res.* **28**, 439–46.

Holmen, L., Thylstrup, A., and Artun, J. (1987). Clinical and histological features observed during arrestment of active enamel carious lesions *in vivo*. *Caries Res.* **21**, 546–54.

Johnson, N.W. (1967*a*). Transmission electron microscopy of early carious enamel. *Caries Res.* **1**, 356–69.

Johnson, N.W. (1967*b*). Some aspects of the ultrastructure of early human enamel caries seen with the electron microscope. *Archs. oral Biol.* **12**, 1505–21.

Jorgensen, K.D. (1965). The mechanism of marginal fracture of amalgam fillings. *Acta odont. Scand.* **23**, 347–89.

Jorgensen, K.D. and Wakumoto, S. (1968). Occlusal amalgam fillings: marginal defects and secondary caries. *Odont. Tidskrift.* **76**, 43–53.

Kidd, E.A.M. (1976). Microleakage: a review. *J. Dent.* **4**, 199–206.

Kidd, E.A.M. (1978). Cavity sealing ability of composite and glass ionomer restorations. An assessment *in vitro*. *Br. dent. J.* **144**, 139–42.

Kidd, E.A.M. (1983). The histopathology of enamel caries in young and old permanent teeth. *Br. dent. J.* **155**, 196–8.

Kidd, E.A.M. (1985). Microleakage and shrinkage. In *Posterior composite resin dental materials*, (ed. G. Vanherle and D. Smith) pp. 263–8. 3M Co.

Kidd, E.A.M. and Joyston-Bechal, S. (1987). *Essentials of Dental Caries*, pp. 41–57. Wright, Bristol.

Kidd, E.A.M., Thylstrup, A., Fejerskou, O., and Silverstone, L.M. (1978). Histopathology of caries-like lesions created *in vitro* in fluorosed and sound enamel. *Caries Res.* **12**, 268–74.

Kostlan, J. (1962). Translucent zones in the central part of the carious lesion of enamel. *Br. dent. J.* **113**, 244–8.

Koulourides, T. (1966). Dynamics of tooth surface–oral fluid equilibrium. *Adv. oral Biol.* **2**, 149–71.

Koulourides, T., Keller, S.E., Manson-Hing, L., and Lilley, V. (1980). Enhancement of fluoride effectiveness by experimental cariogenic priming of human enamel. *Caries Res.* **14**, 32–9.

Krasse, B. (1985). *Caries risk. A practical guide for assessment and control.* Quintessence, Chicago.

Lavelle, C.L.B. (1976). A cross-sectional longitudinal survey into the durability of amalgam restorations. *J. Dent.* **4**, 139–43.

McLean, J.W. and Gasser, O. (1985). Glass-cermet cements. *Quint. Int.* **16**, 333–43.

McLean, J.W., Prosser, H.J., and Wilson, A.D. (1985). The use of glass-ionomer cements in bonding composite resins to dentine. *Br. dent. J.* **158**, 410–14.

Merrett, M.C.W. and Elderton, R.J. (1984). An *in vitro* study of restorative dental treatment decisions and dental caries. *Br. dent. J.* **157**, 128–33.

Mjor, I.A. (1981). Placement and replacement of restorations. *Oper. Dent.* **6**, 49–54.

Mjor, I.A. (1985). Frequency of secondary caries at various anatomical locations. *Oper. Dent.* **10**, 88–92.

Miller, W.A. and Massler, M. (1962). Permeability and staining of active and arrested lesions in dentine. *Br. dent. J.* **112**, 187–97.

Mitropoulos, C.M. (1985). A comparison of fibreoptic transillumination with bitewing radiographs. *Br. dent. J.* **159**, 21–3.

Mortimer, K.V. (1964). Some histological features of fissure caries in enamel. *Eur. Org. caries Res.* **2**, 85–94.

Nelson, R.J., Wolcott, R.B., and Paffenbarger, G.C. (1952). Fluid exchange at the margins of dental restorations. *J. Am. dent. Ass.* **44**, 288–95.

Phillips, R.W., Gilmore, H.W., Swartz, M.L., and Schenker, S.I. (1961). Adaptation of restorations *in vivo* as assessed by Ca^{45}. *J. Am. dent. Ass.* **62**, 9–20.

Pitts, N.B. (1984). Detection and measurement of approximal radiolucencies by computer-aided image analysis. *Oral. Surg.* **58**, 358–65.

Pitts, N.B. (1987). Temporary tooth separation with special reference to the diagnosis and management of equivocal approximal carious lesions. *Quint. Int.* **18**, 563–73.

Qvist, V., Thylstrup, A., and Mjor, I.A. (1986*a*). Restorative treatment pattern and longevity of amalgam restoration in Denmark. *Acta odont. Scand.* **44**, 343–9.

Qvist, V., Thylstrup, A., and Mjor, I.A. (1986*b*). Restorative treatment pattern and longevity of resin restorations in Denmark. *Acta. odont. Scand.* **44**, 351–6.

Richardson, A.S. and Boyd, M.A. (1973). Replacement of silver amalgam restorations by 50 dentists during 256 working days. *J. Can. dent. Ass.* **39**, 556–9.

Robinson, C., Weatherell, J.A., and Hallsworth, A.S. (1971). Variation in composition of dental enamel within thin ground sections. *Caries Res.* **5**, 44–57.

Rock, W.P. and Kidd, E.A.M. (1988). The electronic detection of demineralization in occlusal fissures. *Br. dent. J.* **164**, 243–7.

Sheiham, A. (1977). Is there a scientific basis for six-monthly dental examinations. *Lancet* **ii**, 442–4.

Silverstone, L.M. (1966). The primary translucent zone of enamel caries and of artificial caries-like lesions. *Br. dent. J.* **120**, 461–71.

Silverstone, L.M. (1968). The surface zone in caries and in caries-like lesions produced *in vitro*. *Br. dent. J.* **125**, 145–57.

Silverstone, L.M. (1970). The histopathology of early enamel caries in the enamel of primary teeth. *J. Dent. Child.* **37**, 17–27.

Silverstone, L.M. (1973). The structure of carious enamel, including the early lesion. In *Oral sciences reviews, No 4 Dental enamel.* (ed. A.H. Melcher and G. Zarb), pp. 100–60. Munksgaard, Copenhagen.

Simonsen, R.J. (1978). *Clinical applications of the acid-etch technique.* Quintessence, Chicago.

Swartz, M.L. and Phillips, R.W. (1961). *In vitro* studies on the marginal leakage of restorative materials. *J. Am. dent. Ass.* **62**, 141–51.

Thylstrup, A., and Fejerskov, O. (1981). Surface features of early carious enamel at various stages of activity. In *Proceedings of a workshop on tooth surface interactions and preventive dentistry*, (ed. G. Rolla, T. Sonju and G. Embery), pp. 193–205. IRL Press, London.

Thylstrup, A., and Fejerskov, O. (1986). *Textbook of cariology*, pp. 204–34. Munksgaard, Copenhagen.

von der Fehr, F.R. (1965). Maturation and remineralization of enamel. *Adv. Fluor. Res.* **3**, 83–95.
von der Fehr, F.R., Loe, H., and Theilade, E. (1970). Experimental caries in man. *Caries Res.* **4**, 131–48.

7

Prevention of caries: immunology and vaccination

W. M. EDGAR

Introduction

Mobilization or augmentation of the defence systems of the body is perhaps the most attractive approach to the prevention of infectious disease, as it involves working with natural functions, rather than cutting across them. The idea that caries might by prevented by such methods has a long history, but in the last two decades has stimulated increasing interest. There now exists a large body of research into the defence mechanisms of the mouth, and the possibility of preventing caries by stimulating these mechanisms.

The defences of the body are of two types, non-specific and specific. In the mouth, properties of saliva, such as its buffering power, its calcium and phosphate levels, and its lubricating and cleansing functions, may be thought of as non-specific defence mechanisms, but the term is normally reserved for antibacterial systems of saliva such as lysozyme, lactoperoxidase, and lactoferrin, which are active against many species of bacteria. However, no more will be said here of these non-specific antibacterial mechanisms as although they may be important in host resistance, ways of increasing their effectiveness are for the most part unknown.

Specificity of antibacterial action is the hallmark of the immune systems of the body. These systems have been exploited since the time of Jenner in controlling diseases that result from infection by a single, pathogenic strain or species of micro-organism, by vaccination. This process involves exposing the host to killed or attenuated forms of the organism (or to characteristic components or products) in order to instruct the host's immunological memory to mount an effective antibacterial response when the fully virulent organism is encountered.

To achieve the aim of mobilizing these specific immunological defences to prevent caries, we therefore need to understand the microbial aetiology of caries, the mechanisms involved in recognition of the aetiological agents by the immune system, and the ways in which the system might interfere with the pathological process leading to caries. With this knowledge, we can then sift the evidence relating caries and immunological responses in human populations and in animal experiments, with a view to arriving at a prognosis for successful and safe vaccination against caries in man.

Microbial specificity in caries

The search for a single organism as the cause of caries began shortly after the recognition of the role of bacteria in the aetiology of the disease. Clarke, in 1924, isolated an organism which he named *Streptococcus mutans* (because of its variable appearance on different culture media) in large numbers from human carious teeth, but the subsequent description of increased levels of lactobacilli in saliva from subjects with active caries led for many years to the widespread incrimination of that group of organisms as the major cause of caries.

Evidence from animal caries

It was not until the development of techniques whereby experimental animals could be bred and reared under germ-free conditions that the bacterial aetiology of caries could be proved. In the absence of bacteria, no caries developed in the teeth of susceptible animals fed a high-sugar, caries-conducive diet (Orland *et al.* 1955). When individual species were allowed to infect the mouths of these otherwise germ-free animals, variable levels of caries occurred depending upon the species introduced. Re-isolated from these animals, the organisms could be transferred to other germ-free animals who then also developed caries. Caries was induced in animals not normally susceptible by infecting them with faeces from animals having caries. All these observations indicated that (in animal experiments at least) caries was an infectious, transmissible disease (Fitzgerald and Keyes 1960).

Of the organisms studied (mostly isolated from human mouths) the evidence rapidly became overwhelming that one species, subsequently identified as the *Strep. mutans* of Clarke, was pre-eminent in causing caries in rats and hamsters both when introduced into germ-free animals (gnotobiotic experiments) and when inoculated in high numbers (superinfected) into the mouths of animals with their normal bacterial flora (Table 7.1). A few other species were also capable of producing caries, but usually less extensive and rapid, and not involving the smooth surface of the teeth.

This pre-eminence has led some workers to believe that *Strep. mutans* is specifically involved in caries in man. However, certain strains of other species (for example, lactobacilli and *Strep. milleri*) may give rise to almost as much caries under controlled test conditions as *Strep. mutans*. Furthermore, with most animal caries experiments, diets containing high levels of sugar (40–60 per cent) are usually administered in order to elicit rapid development of caries, and it has been argued that *Strep. mutans* is among the few organisms which can tolerate such high levels of sugar—much higher than in the mixed human diet. Experiments using a less severe dietary challenge have tended to suggest that animals whose oral flora included *Strep. mutans* were not markedly more caries-

Table 7.1. Cariogenicity of various microbial groups in rats with gnotobiotic and conventional floras. (Modified after Gibbons and van Houte (1975))

Organism	Caries		
	Smooth surfaces	Fissures	Root caries
Streptococci			
Strep. mutans	+ + +	+ + +	+
Strep. salivarius	−	−	− / + +
Strep. sanguis	−	− / +	−
Strep. milleri	− / +	+ / + +	−
Strep. mitis	−	− / +	−
Enterococci	−	− / +	−
Lactobacilli	−	+ / + +	−
Filaments	−	− / +	+ + +

References: Drucker and Green (1978); Fitzgerald (1968); Fitzgerald *et al.* (1960, 1980); Frank *et al.* (1972); Gibbons and van Houte (1975); Guggenheim (1968); Jordan and Hammond (1972); Keyes (1962, 1968); Krasse and Carlsson (1970); Orland *et al.* (1955); Rosen *et al.* (1968); Socransky (1970).

prone than those in which the organism was absent. In one experiment for example, with a group of rats fed a cariogenic diet for 21 days with a naturally acquired flora, only 67 out of 214 (31 per cent) of fissures with caries harboured the organisms, while in five out of 29 (17 per cent) of non-carious fissures the organism was nevertheless present (Huxley 1978). Thus caries could occur without detectable infection by *Strep. mutans*, and vice versa.

Virulence factors and *Strep. mutans*

The properties of an organism responsible for its pathogenicity are called virulence factors. With *Strep. mutans*, the most prominent features are its ability to form acid rapidly from dietary carbohydrates (in practice, mainly sucrose), its ability to tolerate acid conditions, and its ability to synthesize from sucrose an insoluble extracellular polysaccharide which is believed to help the organism to become attached to the teeth. This polysaccharide, a polymer of glucose (glucan) linked by $1 \rightarrow 3$ and $1 \rightarrow 6$ bonds, has been called 'mutan' to distinguish it from glucans synthesized by other species in which the $1 \rightarrow 6$ bond predominates.

The importance of these properties has been investigated by studying the amount of caries produced when a mutant form of the organism deficient in one of the properties is used to infect gnotobiotic animals. If, for example, mutan synthesis is an important virulence factor, than a mutant lacking this property should produce less caries than the parent strain. This was in fact the case (Tanzer and Freedman 1978; Mao and Rosen 1980), but only for caries of smooth surfaces and not for the pits and fissures. Conversely, a mutant synthesizing excessive mutan produces more rapid and extensive caries than the parent strain (Michalek *et al.* 1975). However, other organisms capable of producing extensive caries in animals do not synthesize mutan (Drucker and Greene 1978; Fitzgerald *et al.* 1980).

Mutants forming less acid than the parent strain gave greatly reduced caries, while those lacking the property of acid tolerance failed to become established on the animals teeth and did not produce any caries. Acid production from sugars by *Strep. mutans* has been found to be more rapid than other organisms from the mouth in test-tube experiments (e.g. Ranke and Ranke 1970; Minah and Loesche 1977), especially when the pH of the medium is low (Komiyama and Kleinberg 1974; Iwami and Yamada 1980). These properties are therefore probably the most important features of *Strep. mutans* giving rise to its virulence in animal experiments.

It is increasingly accepted that strains formerly designated as serotypes belonging to a single *Strep. mutans* species should more correctly be classified into five separate species on the basis of DNA homology and other studies. The two species predominant in man are *Strep. mutans* (formerly serotypes c, e, and f) and, less important, *Strep. sobrinus* (formerly serotypes d and g). *Strep. cricetus* (serotype a), *Strep. ferus* (serotype c), and *Strep. macacae* (serotype c) strains are rarely, if ever, isolated from the human mouth.

As defined above, *Strep. mutans* has been shown to produce more acid from sucrose and glucose than other members of the group and, in particular, to show enhanced acid production at pH 5 compared with pH 6.5. *Strep. mutans* and *Strep. sobrinus* are attached to pellicle by different receptors. Species differences such as these may contribute to variations in prevalence and virulence, although the relative cariogenicity of the various species is not well established.

Strep. mutans and caries in man

Numerous analyses of the microbial make-up of plaque in subjects of different caries experience have revealed a correlation between the presence of *Strep. mutans* and caries. Typically, subjects with high levels of caries harbour many *Strep. mutans*, but only occasionally caries is found in the absence of detectable numbers of *Strep. mutans*, and the organism may be found in the absence of disease.

Simple correlations of this kind do not of course prove that the organism causes the disease—it is equally possible that the acid conditions in a carious lesion favour the growth of the organism. To demonstrate a cause-and-effect relationship, it is necessary to carry out longitudinal studies observing microbial populations in plaque over a period of years during which caries develops in the underlying enamel. As such studies are laborious and expensive, only a few have been reported. In one, proportions of *Strep. mutans* (and *lactobacilli* rose *after* caries was diagnosed, suggesting that the carious lesion acted as a preferred ecological niche for these acid-tolerant organisms (Hardie *et al.* 1977). Another study found a significant rise in levels of *Strep. mutans* in the fissures of some children at the same time as caries was diagnosed, but not before diagnosis. In a minority of subjects, the appearance of caries was accompanied by an increase in lactobacilli, but not of *Strep. mutans* (Loesche and Straffon 1979). However, a further study by this group found that the proportion of *Strep. mutans* in molar fissures in caries-active children rose 6–24 months before diagnosis of caries in the fissures. Plaque in fissures in the same subjects which did not become carious, or in caries-inactive subjects, did not show the same rise in proportions of *Strep. mutans* (Loesche *et al.* 1984). Kristofferson *et al.* (1985) found that 83 per cent of approximal surfaces which never harboured *Strep. mutans* in 13-year-olds remained intact over 2 years, compared with only 35 per cent of surfaces from which the organism was regularly recovered. Caries incidence over 2 years was significantly associated with *Strep. mutans* counts in pre-school children (Alaluusua and Renkonen, 1983; Aaltonen *et al.* 1987). Overall, these studies show that *Strep. mutans* is an important factor in caries, but that it can not be regarded as the specific cause of the disease in man, as caries can occur in the absence of the organism.

Further evidence is given by studies of naturally occurring antibodies to oral organisms in subjects with varying levels of caries. Antibodies specific for *Strep. mutans* are present in higher concentrations in the sera of subjects with low levels of the disease, suggesting that they are exerting a protective effect. A similar relationship is not shown with antibodies to other species of organism, implying that they are not causally related to caries (Challacombe 1980). However, as we shall see later, the evidence relating naturally occurring antibodies and caries is confused, and as evidence for the specific role of *Strep. mutans* these findings must be viewed with caution.

Immunology of the oral cavity

Antigens of oral bacteria

The study of natural immune responses to a caries-producing organism, and the development of a vaccine, depend upon knowledge of the antigenic properties of the organism. The cell surface of *Strep. mutans* possesses very many antigens. The cell-wall enzyme glucosyltransferase (GTF) responsible for synthesis of insoluble extracellular mutan, has been extensively studied, as has the serotype-specific polysaccharide containing glucose, rhamnose, and sometimes galactose and galactosamine. In addition, the cell wall contains lipoteichoic acid, a polymer of glycerol and phosphate covalently linked to a glycolipid, which is found in virtually all Gram-positive organisms. This antigen may be responsible for some immunological cross-reactions between bacterial species, but specificity may be imparted by carbohydrate groups on the glycerol phosphate backbone. Glucans may be antigenic, but some reactions with glucans may have arisen from contamination with lipoteichoic acid or GTF.

A highly immunogenic antigen tightly bound to the cell wall of *Strep. mutans* gives antibodies in rabbits (Van de Rijn and Zabriski 1976) which cross-react with human heart tissue. Purification of antigens from cells of *Strep. mutans* has revealed at least two highly immunogenic proteins (Russell 1979). One, designated 'antigen A', is of low molecular weight (29 000 daltons) and the other, 'antigen B' (molecular weight 185 000 daltons) is similar to a protein having two antigenic determinants and called 'antigen 1/11' (Russell *et al.* 1980). It has been suggested that antigen B (and possibly 1/11) is responsible for cross-reactivity with heart tissue (Hughes *et al.* 1980; Russell 1979; Forester *et al.* 1983), although no evidence of heart damage has been reported in monkeys vaccinated for caries protection. Antigen 1/11 is present in all strains of *Strep. mutans* and *Strep. sobrinus*.

Most studies of natural immune responses in man and vaccination experiments in animals have used as the antigen whole bacterial cells, usually killed by heat or with formalin, but GTF preparations and ribosomal proteins have been employed as a vaccine in rats and monkeys, and purified cell-wall associated antigens (A, B, 1/11) have been used to vaccinate monkeys.

Antibodies in the mouth

Bacteria on the surface of the teeth may be affected by antibodies of two types—the secretory (salivary) antibodies of the isotype called s-IgA (Tomasi *et al.* 1965), and the serum antibodies (IgG, IgM, and IgA), which enter the mouth mainly via the gingival crevice (Challacombe *et al.* 1978).

s-IgA is present in external secretions such as tears, milk, sweat, and the products of glands of the respiratory and gastro-intestinal tracts, including saliva. In this secretory form it is dimeric, comprising two molecules of IgA united by a polypeptide 'secretory component' together with a shorter junctional peptide known as the 'J-chain'. Synthesis of monomeric IgA in response to antigenic stimulation occurs in the lymphoid tissue associated with the gastro-intestinal tract, both locally and in collections of lymphoid tissue such as the tonsils, mesenteric lymph nodes, and Peyers patches; addition of the secretory piece and dimer formation occurs during passage of the molecule through the epithelium of the gland. There is evidence that s-IgA antibodies formed by minor buccal and labial salivary glands may be elicited by penetration of antigen into the glands via the ducts (Krasse *et al.* 1978).

The functions of s-IgA are to bind with and aggregate foreign bodies and to inactivate antigens and toxins to prevent them adhering to surfaces and penetrating the epithelium. Formation of a s-IgA-antigen complex does not activate the complement mechanism, and s-IgA does not 'opsonize' bacteria to promote phagocytosis by polymorphonuclear leukocytes (PMNLs). IgA occurs in two subclasses: IgA1, which is susceptible to a proteolytic enzyme produced by certain oral bacteria including *Strep. sanguis*, and IgA2, which is more prevalent in secretions and is not cleaved by bacterial protease because it lacks a 13-peptide sequence where enzymic cleavage occurs.

Serum IgG is the major isotype in serum and is responsible for the humoral immune response, particularly the secondary or anamnaestic response where memory of a prior encounter with an antigen carried by primed lymphocytes leads to a brisk and sustained synthesis of antibody. The antigen is probably first bound and concentrated by macrophages and then 'presented' to the lymphocytes for more effective triggering of the cells to proliferate to antibody-secreting plasma cells. The B-lymphocytes involved in this humoral response are assisted in their function through the co-operative action of T-helper lymphocytes.

The principal functions of IgG are activation of complement, opsonization, and inhibition of antigens with biological activity, e.g. enzymes. In the activation of complement, antigen–antibody complexes stimulate a cascade-like sequence of changes in a group of nine serum factors ending up with release of a chemotactic factor which attracts phagocytic PMNLs, histamine release, and lysis of susceptible bacteria. Opsonization—coating of foreign particles such as bacteria with IgG molecules—results in increased phagocytosis by PMNLs, which have a binding site on their surfaces specific for parts of the bound IgG. Inhibition of GTF from *Strep. mutans* and of cell adhesion to surfaces may occur with sera from immunized animals (Ciardi *et al.* 1978; Hamada *et al.* 1979).

Cellular immune responses

Besides their helper function mentioned above, the principal function of T-lymphocytes is in the cell-mediated immune response. Antigens in the tissues, perhaps on the surface of a macrophage, are detected by specific receptors (not antibodies) on the surfaces of the T-cells, which are then stimulated to blastic transformation and proliferation. The blast cells form two populations, one of which (the killer T-cells) is cytotoxic to virally infected host cells or to cells bearing foreign histocompatability antigens—i.e. graft cells; the other subpopulation is responsible for release of soluble factors—the lymphokines—which have a large range of functions including chemotaxis and activation of macrophages, vascular permeability, and both stimulation and inhibition of other lymphocytes, perhaps related to T-cell helper and suppressor functions.

Cellular immune responses may be elicited in animals vaccinated with *Strep. mutans*, but it is unlikely that they play a direct part in the immunology of caries. However, they may modify a humoral immune response through (i) helper and suppressor actions of T-cells, and (ii) inflammation of the gingiva with accompanying increase in gingival fluid flow and hence access of IgG and PMNLs to the mouth.

Immunological microenvironments in the mouth

The plaque in the cervical region of the tooth and on root surfaces in older subjects is thus subjected to the influence both of salivary s-IgA and of serum immunoglobulins, complement factors, and PMNLs from the gingival crevice. IgA, IgG, IgM, and the third component of complement can be detected in plaque extracts, and in the free aqueous phase of plaque (plaque fluid) separated from the solid phase by centrifugation, but in view of the proteolytic activity of many plaque bacteria (including IgA protease) the proportion of these components present as functional antibodies is unknown.

Plaque in the fissures and more coronal parts of the smooth surfaces of the teeth is probably influenced only by salivary antibodies. PMNLs survive only for a very short time in human saliva, although in monkeys their survival may be more prolonged and in the gingival crevice they may persist for long periods.

Immunology and caries

Naturally induced immune responses to caries in man

Antibodies or oral bacteria including *Strep. mutans* can be detected in human serum and saliva. In order to see whether or not these antibodies might play a part in natural caries immunity, numerous comparisons of caries experience and levels of immunoglobulin or specific antibody have been carried out, but consistency in the results of such experiments is not apparent (Table 7.2). For example, IgA levels in saliva have been found to be higher, lower, or unchanged in subjects with little or no caries compared with subjects with high caries experience. Raised levels of serum antibodies to cariogenic bacteria have been found in caries-free or -inactive subjects and in those with active caries. Serum antibody against *Strep. mutans* fell in a group of subjects with high caries experience and active caries, during a 9-month period when their active lesions were treated, suggesting that a protective antibody response was no longer stimulated by the presence of antigen; in contrast salivary agglutinating activity rose during the same period. No similar changes in salivary or serum antibodies against *Strep. mutans* were observed. However, in view of the many conflicting reports noted above, the general applicability of such evidence remains in doubt.

Another approach has been to examine the caries experience of patients suffering from selective deficiencies in immunoglobulins of various classes. Such patients are rare, and numbers available for study have been small, but a trend emerges towards increased caries in patients with disturbances of salivary IgA secretion. However, these patients have often received antibiotic therapy for long periods, and caution is needed in making comparisons with normal age-matched controls.

Given these weak and uncertain correlations between antibody responses and caries, the apparent failure of naturally acquired immune mechanisms to prevent caries in the vast majority of people living in developed countries is not surprising. It seems likely that in communities where the dietary factors lead to weak cariogenic challenge, natural immune mechanisms might be effective in controlling caries, but that they fail in the face of the overwhelming challenge presented by the modern Western diet.

The aim of those attempting to develop a vaccine for human use is to stimulate an enhanced, prolonged response to cope with this increased dietary challenge. In other diseases effectively controlled by vaccination such as small pox, diphtheria, etc., natural immunity occurs, preventing re-infection or limiting the disease process, and the purpose of vaccination is to provide the lymphocytes with information allowing them to function optimally. Vaccination to prevent caries in man may therefore be more difficult to achieve as its purpose is to stimulate a response greater than that observed naturally.

Table 7.2. Immunoglobulins (Igs) and antibodies (abs) to *Strep. mutans* in serum and saliva related to caries experience in man

Reference	Saliva	Serum	Caries status
Geller and Rovelstad (1959)	high Igs	—	low
Kraus and Sinsinha (1962)	no corr Igs*	—	—
Toto *et al.* (1960)	no corr Igs	—	(Lactobacillus count)
Lehner *et al.* (1967)	low IgA, IgG	high IgG	low
Zengo *et al.* (1971)	high IgA†	—	caries free
Sims (1972)	no corr Igs	—	—
Serre *et al.* (1972)	no corr Igs	—	—
Everhart *et al.* (1972)	high IgA‡	—	low
Örstavik and Brandtzaeg (1975)	high IgA, parotid§	—	low
Stucel and Mandel (1978)	high IgA§	—	caries free
Arnold *et al.* (1978)	low s-IgA ± IgM‖	—	increased caries
Cole *et al.* (1978)	high IgS, IgG¶	—	low caries
Kennedy *et al.* (1968)	—	high abs	caries free
Challacombe *et al.* (1973)	low abs**	high abs**	low, treated
Lehner *et al.* (1978*a*)	no corr IgA, abs	low IgG:IgA, IgG:IgM abs	high (deciduous)
Huis in't Veld *et al.* (1978)	no corr IgA, abs	low IgG abs	caries free
McGhee *et al.* (1978)	rise in IgA abs	no abs elicited	oral vaccine
Gahnberg and Krasse (1983)	no rise IgA abs	—	oral vaccine
Cole *et al.* (1984)	no rise IgA abs	—	oral vaccine
Challacombe (1980)	rise in IgA abs	fall in IgG abs	treatment of caries
Weinmann (1936)	no corr PMNLs	—	—
Wright and Jenkins (1953)	no corr PMNLs	—	—
Friedman and Tonzetich (1968)	no corr PMNLs	—	—
Shklair *et al.* (1969)	high PMNLs	—	caries free
Lehner *et al.* (1976)	—	low SI††	high, treated
Ivanyi and Lehner (1978)	—	high SI†† mothers, neonates	active (mothers)
Aaltonen *et al.* (1985)	—	high IgG abs***	low (deciduous)
Aaltonen *et al.* (1987)	—	low IgG abs	high 2 yr increment (deciduous)

* No correlation between Ig levels and caries.
† In submandibular saliva.
‡ 20–29-year age group only.
§ Output/min.
‖ Subjects with deficiencies in various Ig classes.
¶ Subjects from communities with contrasting caries levels.
** abs to GTF.
†† Stimulation index; lymphoproliferative response to *Strep. mutans*.
*** Related to maternal transmission of *Strep. mutans* in saliva.

Caries vaccines in animals

Vaccination of rats and hamsters fed a cariogenic diet has given variable levels of protection using a range of antigens and routes of immunization (Table 7.3). In the past, the most popular type of vaccine was prepared from whole cells of *Strep. mutans*, usually killed by heat or by treatment with formalin, but increasingly, antigen preparations of varying purity derived from *Strep. mutans* are used as vaccines. Reductions in caries have usually been accompanied by a demonstrable antibody response in serum, saliva, or both.

Subcutaneous inoculation with formalin-killed cells of *Strep. mutans* in Freund's adjuvant in the vicinity of the salivary glands of rats whose mouths were subsequently infected with the same strain resulted in protection, but inoculation with similar antigens in sites remote from the salivary glands were less consistently successful. Both serum and salivary antibody responses were elicited by these subcutaneous injections close to the salivary glands. Injection of GTF preparations both from the same strain used for infection, and from different strains, have usually been effective, but in some cases increased levels of caries have been observed.

Oral vaccination elicits a s-IgA response in saliva and milk without detectable serum antibodies, and such vaccines have given protection. Passive immunization via antibodies in the milk of immunized dams has conferred protection in their pups, and rats fed with dried milk from cows immunized with *Strep. mutans* developed less caries than controls receiving conventional dried milk.

The evidence in rats and hamsters thus demonstrates the possibility of protection against caries, and that this protection may be afforded by s-IgA. The effect of the antibody seems to be to interfere with attachment of *Strep. mutans* to the tooth, either by inhibiting GTF activity, or blocking cell surface sites of attachment, or both. However, rodent teeth and saliva composition are very different from those of man, and experimental caries in rodents is known to differ in some respects from human caries, notably in the fact that only short-term experiments are possible owing to the animals' brief life-span. The immune response may last long enough to prevent caries over weeks or months, but not persist to confer protection over a number of years.

Caries in monkeys more closely resembles that in man, and their teeth, saliva, and immune systems are similar to the human pattern. For these reasons, vaccination experiments in monkeys can be expected to give more applicable findings. Reports of such experiments are fewer than with rodents owing to the expense of acquiring and maintaining the monkeys. However, protection against caries has been achieved by inoculation subcutaneously or submucosally with broken cells, cell walls, or heat-killed whole cells of *Strep. mutans* and by intravenous injection of live cells (Table 7.4). Vaccination with enzymes including GTF has given variable results; in some experiments protection was observed but in the experiments of Bowen *et al.* (1975) increased caries occurred in animals vaccinated with GTF. It is likely that some of the GTF preparations have been contaminated with other antigens. Vaccination with purified protein

Table 7.3. Vaccination with *Strep. mutans* against caries in rats and hamsters

Reference	C or G*	Vaccine	Route	Antibodies		Protection against caries (%)†
				Saliva	Serum	
Guggenheim *et al.* (1970)	C	live whole cells	i.v.	NR§	yes	−25 to −40
	G	live whole cells	i.v.	NR	yes	6 to 16
	C	GTF	i.v.	NR	yes	−15 to −27
	G	GTF	i.v.	NR	yes	−9 to 19
Hayashi *et al.* (1972)	C	GTF	i.p.	NR	yes	59
	GH‖	i.p.				28
Tanzer *et al.* (1973)	C	fk whole cells	s.c.	yes?	yes	0 to 69
Taubman and Smith (1974)	C	fk whole cells	s.c. (SGV)¶	yes	yes	15 to 58
McGhee *et al.* (1975)	G	fk whole cells	s.c. (SGV)	yes	yes	64
Gaffar (1976)	C**	fk whole cells	i.p.	NR	NR	−40
	C**	GTF	i.p.	yes	yes	−11 to 37
Taubman and Smith (1977)	C	crude GTF	s.c. (SGV)	yes	yes	34
	G	pure GTF	s.c. (SGV)	yes	yes	58
	C**	pure GTF	s.c. (SGV)	yes	yes	65
Michalek and McGhee (1977)	G	hk whole cells††	dams milk	yes	yes	45 (in pup)
	G	fk whole cells‡‡	dams milk	yes, in milk		51 (in pup)
Smith *et al.* (1978)	C**	GTF, various‖‖	s.c. (SGV)	yes	yes	36 to 69
Michalek *et al.* (1978)	G	fk whole cells	oral	yes	NR	21 to 68
	G	fk whole cells	cows' milk	NR	NR	56 to 88¶¶
Schöller *et al.* (1978)	G	GTF***	s.c. (SGV)	yes	yes	95†††
Hughes *et al.* (1983)	C	antigen A	s.c. (SGV)	NR	NR	72†††
Gregory *et al.* (1984)	G	ribosomes	s.c. (SGV)	IgA	IgG	18–94

* Conventional flora or gnotobiotic.
† Total caries, per cent reduction.
‡ formalin-killed.
§ Not recorded.
‖ In the vicinity of the salivary glands.
** Hamsters.
†† Injected i.v. in dam-elicited ab in milk.
‡‡ Injected s.c. in mammary gland region or orally via drinking water.
‖‖ GTF from one strain protective against caries on infecting with same or different strain.
¶¶ Milk from immunized cows fed to non-immunized rats.
*** From *Strep. sanguis*.
††† Smooth-surface lesions only.

Table 7.4. Vaccination with *Strep. mutans* against caries in monkeys

Reference	Vaccine	Route	Antibodies		N*	Protection against caries (%)
			Saliva	Serum		
Bowen (1969)	live cells	i.v.	NR	yes	3	80
Lehner *et al*. (1975)	hk† whole cells	s.c.	yes	yes	6	65‡
	hk† whole cells	s.m.§	yes	yes	6	51‡
Bowen *et al*. (1975)	live cells	i.v.	NR	yes	5	53
	broken cells	s.m.	NR	yes	4	100
	GTF	s.m.	yes	yes	11	increased caries
Evans *et al*. (1975)	fk‖ whole cells and GTF	CS (SGV)¶	no	yes		
		SGD**	yes	yes	4	NR††
Lehner *et al*. (1977)	hk or fk cells	s.c.	?yes	yes	6	69‡‡
Bahn *et al*. (1977)	GH§§	s.m.	NR	yes	10	23‖‖
	GTF	s.m.	NR	yes	5	69
	FTF¶¶	s.m.	NR	yes	5	62
	GH	s.m.	NR	yes	5	57
Schick *et al*. (1978)	cell walls***	s.m.	no	yes	6	33–50
	GTF	s.m.	no	yes	3	70
Lehner *et al*. (1978*b*)	passive†††	—	no	yes	3	80
Cohen *et al*. (1979)	fk whole cells	s.c.	NR	NR	8	55
	fk whole cells	s.m.	NR	NR	8	28‡‡‡
Lehner *et al*. (1980*a*)	antigen 1/11	s.c.	yes	yes	3	70
	fk whole cells	s.c.	yes	yes	3	73
Lehner *et al*. (1980*b*)	live cells	oral	?yes	no	6	34(NS)
Russell *et al*. (1982)	antigen A	s.c.	NR	yes	10	yes
	antigen B	s.c.	NR	yes	9	variable
Russell and Colman (1981)	GTF	s.c.	NR	yes	4	0
Lehner *et al*. (1985)	3800D fragment	s.c.	?yes	yes	6	100

* Number of animals per group.
† Heat killed.
‡ Fissures only, two years.
§ Submucosal injection.
‖ Formalin killed.
¶ Salivary gland vicinity.
** Instilled via salivary gland duct.
†† Reduced infection with *Strep. mutans*.
‡‡ First permanent molars only.
§§ Glycoside hydrolase enzyme.
‖‖ Short-term experiment.
¶¶ Fructosyl transferase enzyme.
*** Two strains.
††† Immune plasma injected; protection association with IgG fraction.
‡‡‡ Estimated from graph.

antigens from *Strep. mutans* have been successful in protecting against caries. It has been suggested that antigen A gives the most reliable protection, and that antigen B (perhaps the same as antigen 1/11) is less effective and may be responsible for cross-reactivity with heart tissue. Antigen A can be purified from the supernatants of cultures of *Strep. mutans* by passing the fluid through an immunosorbent affinity column prepared with monoclonal anti-antigen A antibody, followed by elution of the bound pure antigen.

The nature of the protective antibody response to vaccination in these experiments is not certain, but the present evidence suggests that IgG may play a more important part in monkeys than in rodents. Salivary IgA antibodies were elicited in monkeys using an oral vaccine (Challacombe and Lehner 1979), but the response was of short duration (Lehner *et al.* 1980*b*; Walker 1981). Protection against caries has been linked with increased phagocytosis (Scully and Lehner 1979), and passive immunization by injection of IgG (but not IgA) fractions separated from immune monkey plasma prevented caries in the recipients of the plasma, but no salivary antibodies were found in the animals receiving injections of the IgA fraction. It is possible that in monkeys, both serum and salivary antibodies are necessary to obtain maximum protection, with the former being more important in protecting the approximal and free smooth surfaces, and the latter having more effect in occlusal pits and fissures.

Towards a human caries vaccine

The protection against caries achieved in the animal experiments just described has general hopes for developing an effective vaccine for use in man. However, a number of major problems remain. First, in most of the experiments the caries in the control animals has been induced by infection with *Strep. mutans*, usually of the same strain as that used for vaccination. In gnotobiotic experiments, the plaque consists of a pure culture of the organism, while in animals with conventional flora, superinfection with *Strep. mutans* has been employed because of the need to achieve rapid caries in view of the prolonged vaccination period, after weaning and before administering the cariogenic diet. With monkeys, superinfection has also been employed. Thus the successful results of vaccination against caries associated with *Strep. mutans* may underestimate the difficulty of achieving success in man, where the association between the organism and caries is less clear, as discussed earlier.

Even if a vaccine were successful in giving a response which eliminated the target organism, other organisms might step in to fill the gap. A vaccine against the most prevalent of the serotypes of *Strep. mutans* (serotype c) that acted specifically to eliminate this serotype might simply lead to a shift towards other members of the *Strep. mutans* group without reducing the level of cariogenic challenge. A less specific vaccine giving rise to antibodies reacting with *Strep. sobrinus* as well as *Strep. mutans* would avoid this problem. This type of cross-protection has been observed when caries resulting from infection with one strain of *Strep. mutans* was prevented by immunizing with GTF from a different strain (Table 7.3). However elimination of all strains of *Strep. mutans* may not necessarily lead to reduced caries, as other species may take over the role of the target species.

The evidence at present does not allow us to decide confidently the nature of the antibody action or actions which is likely to confer maximum protection. Inhibition of bacterial attachment, perhaps including inhibition of GTF activity, may be important in the action of salivary IgA antibodies, while the action of IgG antibodies derived from the serum may involve opsonization and subsequent phagocytosis by crevicular PMNLs as well as complement-mediated lysis. We have seen that the two classes of antibody may be involved in protecting different tooth surfaces, but IgA may also inhibit the functions of IgG and so the proportion of the two isotypes elicited by vaccination, as well as their concentrations, may be important.

Recent work using purified cell wall protein antigens for *Strep. mutans* as vaccines has established their effectiveness, and after more extensive investigation of their relationship with the cell-wall antigen responsible for reaction with human heart tissue the development of a vaccine for human testing is under way. However, the immunization schedules used must be readily acceptable for human use, and further elucidation of the mechanisms involved in conferring protection might reveal more acceptable antigens, adjuvants, and routes.

GTF preparations are attractive possible vaccines, as they may constitute an important target of the antibacterial mechanism of the immune response, have the advantage of not eliciting heart-reactive antibodies, and have been shown in rats to offer cross-protection between different strains of *Strep. mutans*. However, these antigens have been less successful in conferring protection both in rats and monkeys.

In some animal studies, oral vaccination with whole-cell or cell-wall vaccines stimulated a secretory IgA response but did not elicit serum antibodies, including any possible heart-reactive antibody. If it could be shown that a salivary s-IgA response confers adequate protection, the oral route offers hope of a safe and acceptable method. However, later studies in man and monkeys (Table 7.2, 7.4) did not support such a hope. Even safer, passive immunization (e.g. through the consumption of immune cows' milk) could confer protection while by-passing the need for active immunization of children.

A programme of vaccination against caries could probably be easily implemented alongside other vaccination procedures in childhood. It is uncertain however if it would be widely accepted in the present climate of public opinion which is cautious about vaccination against disease that are not life-threatening. With falling levels of caries in children in most developed countries, it may be that vaccination would be most valuable for high-risk groups, or perhaps for developing countries where other caries control methods are less applicable.

It should be clear from the foregoing that formidable obstacles must be overcome before safety and effectiveness could be guaranteed. Furthermore, in view of the complex bacterial aetiology of caries in man, it seems likely that even the most effective vaccination programme targeted against a single cariogenic species could only provide partial protection. The potential benefits of vaccination (alongside other preventive measures including treatments and diet control) in the elimination of caries from the community may, if they can be achieved, prove sufficient to warrant the effort and expense of development. However even if the effort is successful, vaccination will not remove the need for continued fluoride therapy, or allow young patients to consume limitless cariogenic foods with impunity.

Recommended reading

Roit, I.M. and Lehner, T. (1980). *Immunology of oral diseases*. Blackwell, Oxford.

Secretory immunity and infection ((1978). (ed. J.R. McGhee, J. Mestecky, and J.L. Babb). In *Advances in Experimental Medicine and Biology*, Vol. 107. Plenum Press, New York.

Hamada, S. and Slade, H.D. (980). Biology, immunology and cariogenicity of *Streptococcus mutans*. *Microbiol. Rev.* **44**, 331–44.

McGhee, J.R. and Michalek, S.M. (1981). Immunobiology of dental caries. *A. Rev. Microbiol.* **35**, 595–638.

Molecular microbiology and immunology of Streptococcus mutans (1986). (ed. S. Hamada, S.M. Michalek, H. Kiyona, L. Menaker and J.R. McGhee). Elsevier, Amsterdam.

Russell, R.R.B. and Johnson, N.W. (1987). The prospects for vaccination against dental caries. *BR. dent. J.* **162**, 29–34.

Krasse, B., Emilson, C-G., and Gahnberg, L. (1987). An anticaries vaccine: report on the status of research. *Caries Res.* **21**, 225–76.

References

Aaltonen, A.S., Tenovuo, J., Lehtonen, O-P., Saksala, R., and Meurman, O. (1985). Serum antibodies against oral *Streptococcus mutans* in young children in relation to dental caries and maternal close-contacts. *Archs. oral Biol.* **30**, 331–35.

Aaltonen, A.S., Tenovuo, J., and Lehtonen, O-P (1987). Increased dental caries activity in preschool children with low baseline levels of serum IgG antibodies against the bacterial species *Streptococcus mutans*. *Archs. oral Biol.* **32**, 55–60.

Alaluusua, S. and Renkonen, O-V. (1983). *Streptococcus mutans* establishment and dental caries experience in children from 2 to 4 years old. *Scand. J. dent. Res.* **91**, 453–7.

Arnold, R.R., Prince, S.J., Mestecky, J., Lynch, D., Lynch, M., and McGhee, J.R. (1978). In *Secretory immunity and infection*, (ed. J.R. McGhee, J. Mestecky and J.L. Babb), pp. 401–10. Plenum Press, New York.

Bahn, A.N., Shklair, I.L., and Hayashi, J.A. (1977). Immunization with dextransucrases, Levansucrases and glysocidic hydrolases from oral streptococci. *J. dent. Res.* **56**, 1586–98.

Bowen, W.H. (1969). A vaccine against dental caries. A pilot experiment in monkeys (*Macaca irus*). *Br. dent. J.* **126**, 159–60.

Bowen, W.H., Cohen, B., Cole, M.F., and Colman, G. (1975. Immunization against dental caries. *Br. dent. J.* **139**, 45–58.

Challacombe, S.J. (1980). Serum and salivary antibodies to *Streptococcus mutans* relation to the development and treatment of human dental caries. *Archs oral Biol.* **25**, 495–502.

Challacombe, S.J. and Lehner, T. (1979). Salivary antibody responses in Rhesus monkeys immunised with *Streptococcus mutans* by the oral, submucosal or subcutaneous routes. *Archs. oral Biol.* **24**, 917–25.

Challacombe, S.J., Guggenheim, B., and Lehner, T. (1973). Antibodies to an extract of *Streptococcus mutans*, containing glycosyltransferase activity, related to dental caries in man. *Archs. oral Biol.* **18**, 657–68.

Challacombe, S.J., Russell, M.W., Hawkes, J.E., Bergmeier, L., and Lehner, T. (1978). Passage of immunoglobulins from plasma to the oral cavity in Rhesus monkeys. *Immunology* **35**, 923–31.

Ciardi, J.E., Bowen, W.H., Reilly, T.A., Hsu, S.D., Gomez, I., Kuzmiak-Jones, H., and Cole, M.F. (1978). Antigens of *Streptococcus mutans* implicated in virulence-production of antibodies. In *Secretory immunity and infection*, (ed. J.R. McGhee, J. Mestecky and J.L. Babb), pp. 281–92. Plenum Press, New York.

Clarke, J.K. (1924). On the bacterial factor in aetiology of dental caries. *J. exp. Pathol.* **5**, 141–7.

Cohen, B., Colman, G., and Russell, R.R.B. (1979). Immunisation against dental caries: further studies. *Br. dent. J.* **147**, 9–14.

Cole, M.F. *et al.* (1978). Immunoglobulins and antibodies in plaque fluid and saliva in two populations with contrasting levels of caries. In *Secretory immunity and infection*, (ed. J.R. McGhee, J. Mestecky and J.L. Babb), pp. 383–92. Plenum Press, New York.

Cole, M.F., Emilson, C-G., Hsu, S.D., Li, S-H., and Bowen, W.H. (1984). Effects of peroral immunization of humans with *Streptococcus mutans* on induction of salivary and serum antibodies and inhibition of experimental infection. *Infec. Immunity* **46**, 703–9.

Drucker, D.B. and Green, R.M. (1978) The relative cariogenicities of *Streptococcus milleri* and other viridans group streptococci in gnotobiotic hooded rats. *Archs. oral Biol.* **23**, 183–7.

Evans, R.T., Emmings, F.G., and Genco, R.J. (1975). Prevention of *Streptococcus mutans* infection of tooth surfaces by salivary antibodies in Irus monkeys (*Macaca fascicularis*). *Infec. Immunity* **12**, 293–302.

Everhart, D.L., Grisby, W.R., and Carter, W.H. (1972). Evaluation of dental caries experience and salivary immunoglobulins in whole saliva. *J. dent. Res.* **51**, 1487–91.

Fitzgerald, R.J. (1968). Dental caries research in gnotobiotic animals. *Caries Red.* **2**, 139–46.

Fitzgerald, R.J. and Keys, P.H. (1960). Demonstration of the etiologic role of streptococci in experimental caries in the hamster. *J. Am. dent. ss.* **61**, 9–19.

Fitzgerald, R.J., Jordan, H.V., and Stanley, H.R. (1960). Experimental caries and gingival pathologic changes in the gnotobiotic rat. *J. dent. Res.* **39**, 923–35.

Fitzgerald, R.J., Fitzgerald, D.B., Adams, B.O., and Duany, L.F. (1980). Cariogenicity of human oral lactobacilli in hamsters. *J. dent. Res.* **59**, 832–7.

Forester, H., Hunter, N., and Knox, K.W. (1983). Characteristics of a high molecular weight extracellular protein of *Streptococcus mutans*. *J. gen. Microbiol.* **129**, 2779–88.

Frank, R.M., Guillo, B., and Llory H. (1972). Caries dentaires chez le rat gnotobiote inoculé avec *Actinomyces viscosus* et *Actinomyces naeslundii*, *Archs. oral Biol.* **17**, 1249–53.

Friedman, S.D. and Tonzetich, J. (1968). A study of human oral leucocytes in relation to caries incidence. *Archs. oral Biol.* **13**, 647–59.

Gaffar, A. (1976). Effects of specific immunization on dental caries in hamsters. *J. dent. Res.* **55**, C221–3.

Gahnberg, L. and Krasse, B. (1983). Salivary immunoglobulin A antibodies and recovery from challenge of *Streptococcus mutans* after oral administration of *Streptococcus mutans* vaccine in humans. *Infec. Immunity* **39**, 514–19.

Geller, J.H. and Rovelstad, G.H. (1959). Electrophoresis of saliva: relationship of protein components to dental caries. *J. dent. Res.* **38**, 1060–5.

Gibbons, R.J. and van Houte, J. (1975). Dental caries. *A. Rev. Med.* **26**, 121–36.

Gregory, R.L., Michalek, S.M., Schechmeister, I.L., and McGhee, J.R. (1984). Effective immunity to dental caries: protection of gnotobiotic rats by a local immunisation with a ribosomal preparation from *Streptococcus mutans. Microbiol. Immunol.* **27**, 787–800.

Guggenheim, B. (1968). Streptococci of dental plaques. *Caries Res.* **2**, 147–64.

Guggenheim, B., Mühlemann, H.R., Regolati, B., and Schmid, R. (1970). The effect of immunization against streptococci or glucosyltransferases on plaque formation and dental caries in rats. In *Dental plaque*, (ed. W.D. McHugh), pp. 287–96. Livingstone, Edinburgh.

Hamada, S., Tai, S., and Slade, H.D. (1979). Serotype-dependent inhibition of glucan synthesis and cell adherence of *Streptococcus mutans* by antibody against glucosyltransferase of serotype e *S. mutans. Microbiol. Immunol.* **23**, 61–70.

Hardie, J.M. *et al.* (1977). A longitudinal epidemiological study on dental plaque and the development of dental caries—interim results after two years. *J. dent. Res.* **56**, C90–8.

Hayashi, J.A., Shlair, I.L., and Bain, A.N. (1972). Immunization with dextransucrases and glycosidic hydrolases. *J. dent. Res.* **51**, 436–42.

Huis in't Veld, J., Bannet, D., van Palenstein Helderman, W., Sampaio Camargo, P., and Backer Dirks. O. (1978). Antibodies against *Streptococcus mutans* and glucosyltransferases in caries-free and caries-activity military recruits. In *Secretory immunity and infection*, (ed. J.R. McGhee, J. Mestecky and J.L. Babb). Plenum Press, New York.

Hughes, M., MacHardy, S.M., Sheppard, A.J., and Woods, N.C. (1980). Evidence for an immunological relationship between *Streptococcus mutans* and human cardiac tissue. *Infec. Immunity* **27**, 576–88.

Hughes, M., MacHardy, S.M., and Sheppard, A.J. (1983). Manufacture and control of a dental caries vaccine for parenteral administration to man. In *Glycosyltransferases, glucans, sucrose and dental caries*, (ed. R.J. Doyle and J.E. Ciardi), pp. 259–68. IRL Press, Washington, D.C.

Huxley, H.G. (1978). *Streptococcus mutans* and dental caries in Long-Evans rats with a naturally-acquired oral flora. *Archs. oral Biol.* **23**, 703–7.

Iwami, Y. and Yamada, T. (1980). Rate-limiting steps of the glycolytic pathway in the oral bacteria *Streptococcus mutans* and *Strep. sanguis* and the influence of acidic pH on the glucose metabolism. *Archs. oral Biol.* **25**, 163–9.

Ivanyi, L. and Lehner, T. (1978). The relationship between caries index and stimulation of lymphocytes by *Strep. mutans* in mothers and their neonates. *Archs. oral Biol.* **23**, 851–6.

Jordan, H.V. and Hammond, B.F. (1972). Filamentous bacteria isolated from human root surface caries. *Archs. oral Biol.* **17**, 1333–42.

Kennedy, A.E., Shklair, I.L., Hayashi, J.A., and Bahn, A.N. (1968). Antibodies to cariogenic streptococci in humans. *Archs. oral Biol.* **13**, 1275–9.

Keyes, P.H. (1962). Recent advances in dental caries research. Bacteriology. *Int. dent. J.* **12**, 443–64.

Keyes, P.H. (1968). Research in dental caries. *J. Am. dent. Ass.* **76**, 1357–73.

Komiyama, K. and Kleinberg, I. (1974). Comparison of glucose utilization and acid formation by *Strep. mutans* and *Strep. sanguis* at different pH. *J. dent. Res.* **53** (spec. issue), 241.

Krasse, B. and Carlsson, J. (1970). various types of streptococci and experimental caries in hamsters. *Archs. oral Biol.* **15**, 25–32.

Krasse, B., Gahnberg, L., and Bratthall, D. (1978). Antibodies reacting with *Strep. mutans* in secretions from minor salivary glands in humans. In *Secretory immunity and infection*, (ed. J.R. McGhee, J. Mestecky, and J.L. Babb), pp. 349–54. Plenum Press, New York.

Krause, F.W. and Sirisinha, S. (1961). Gamma-globulin in saliva. *Archs. oral Biol.* **7**, 221–33.

Kristoffersson, K., Grondahl, H-G., and Bratthall, D. (1985). The more *Streptococcus mutans*, the ore caries on approximal surfaces. *J. dent. Res.* **64**, 58–61.

Lehner, T., Caldwell, J., and Clarry, E.D. (1967). Immunoglobulins in saliva and serum in dental caries. *Lancet* **i**, 1294–6.

Lehner, T., Challacombe, S.J., and Caldwell, J. (1975). An immunological investigation into the prevention of caries in deciduous teeth of Rhesus monkeys. *Archs. oral Biol.* **20**, 305–10.

Lehner, T., Challacombe, S.J., Wilton, J.M.A., and Ivanyi, L. (1976). Immunopotentiation by dental microbial plaque and its relationship to oral disease in man. *Archs. oral Biol.* **21**, 749–53.

Lehner, T., Caldwell, J. and Challacombe, S.J. (1977). Effects of immunization on dental caries in the first permanent molars in Rhesus monkeys. *Archs. oral Biol.* **22**, 393–7.

Lehner, T., Murray, J.J., Winter, G.B., and Caldwell, J. (1978*a*). Antibodies to *Strep. mutans* and immunoglobulin levels in children with dental caries. *Archs. oral Biol.* **23**, 1061–7.

Lehner, T., Russell, M.W., Wilton, M.M.A., Challacombe, S.J., Scully, C.M., and Hawkes, J.E. (1978*b*). Passive immunization with antisera to *Streptococcus mutans* in the prevention of caries in Rhesus monkeys. In *Secretory immunity and infection*, (ed. J.R. McGhee, J. Mestecky, and J.L. Babb), pp. 303–16. Plenum Press, New York.

Lehner, T., Russell, M.W., and Caldwell, J. (1980*a*). Immunization with a purified protein from *Streptococcus mutans* against dental caries in rhesus monkeys. *Lancet* **i**, 995–6.

Lehner, T., Challacombe, S.J., and Caldwell, J. (1980*b*). Oral immunisation with *Streptococcus mutans* in rhesus monkeys and the development of immune responses and dental caries. *Immunol.* **41**, 857–64.

Lehner, T., Caldwell, J., and Giasuddin, A.S.M. (1985). Comparative immunogenicity and protective effect against dental caries of a low (3800) and high (18 000) molecular weight protein in rhesus monkeys. (*Macaca mulatta*). *Archs. oral Biol.* **30**, 207–12.

Loesche, W.J. and Straffon, L.H. (1979). Longitudinal investigation of the role of *Streptococcus mutans* in human fissure decay. *Infec. Immunity* **26**, 498–507.

Loesche, W.J., Eklund, S., Earnest, R., and Burt, B. (1984). Longitudinal investigation of bacteriology of human fissure decay: epidemiological studies in molars shortly after eruption. *Infec. Immunity* **46**, 765–72.

McGhee, J.R., Michalek, S.M., Webb., J., Navia, J.M., Rahman, A.F.R., and Legler, D.W. (1975). Effective immunity to dental caries: protection of gnotobiotic rats by local immunization with *Streptococcus mutans*. *J. Immunol.* **114**, 300–5.

McGhee, J.R., Mestecky, J., Arnold, R.R., Michalek, S.M., Prince, S.J., and Babb, J.L. (1978). Induction of secretory antibodies in humans following ingestion of *Streptococcus mutans*. In *Secretory immunity and infection*, (ed. J.R. McGhee, J. Mestecky and J.L. Babb), pp. 177–84. Plenum Press, New York.

Mao, M.W.H. and Rosen, S. (1980). Cariogenicity of Mutans of *Strep. mutans*. *J. dent. Res.* **59**, 1620–6.

Michalek, S.M. and McGhee J.R. (1977). Effective immunity to dental caries: passive transfer to rats of antibodies to *Strep. mutans* elicits protection. *Infec. Immunity* **17**, 644.

Michalek, S.M., Shiota, T., Ikeda, T., Navia, J.M., and McGhee, J.R. (1975). Virulence of *Streptococcus mutans:* biochemical and pathogenic characteristics of mutant isolates. *Proc. Soc. exp. Biol. Med.* **150**, 498–502.

Michalek, S.M., McGhee, J.R., Arnold, R.R., and Mestecky, J. (1978). Effective immunity to dental caries: selective induction of secretory immunity by oral administration of *Streptococcus mutans* in rodents. In *Secretory immunity and infection*, (ed. J.R. McGhee, J. Mestecky and J.L. Babb), pp. 261–70. Plenum Press, New York.

Minah, G.E. and Loesche, W.J. (1977). Sucrose metabolism by prominent members of the flora isolated from cariogenic and non-cariogenic dental plaques. *Infec. Immunity* **17**, 55–61.

Orland, F.J., Blayney, J.R., Harrison, R.W., Reyniers, J.A., Trexler, P.C., Ervin, R.F., Gordon, H.A., and Wagner, M. (1955). Experimental caries in germfree rats inoculated with enterococci. *J. Am. dent. Ass.* **50**, 259–72.

Örstavik, D. and Brandtzaeg, P. (1975). Secretion of parotid IgA in relation to gingival inflammation and dental caries experience in man. *Archs. oral Biol.* **20**, 701–4.

Ranke, E. and Ranke, B. (1970). Zur bedeutung verschiedener Plaque-Streptokokken fur die Karies. *Deut. zahnartl. Z.* **25**, 270–3.

Rosen, S. Lenny, W.S., and O'Malley, J.E. (1968). Dental caries in gnotobiotic rats inoculated with *Lactobacillus casei*. *J. dent. Red.* **47**, 358–63.

Russell, M.W., Bergmeier, L.A., Zanders, E.D., and Lehner, T. (1982). Protein antigens of *Streptococcus mutans:* purification and properties of a double antigen and its protease-resistant component. *Infec. Immunity* **28**, 486–93.

Russell, R.R.B. (1979). Wall-associated protein antigens of *Streptococcus mutans*. *J. gen. Microbiol.* **114**, 109–15.

Russell, R.R.B., Beighton, D., and Cohen, B. (1980). Immunization of monkeys (*Macaca fascicularis*) with antigens purified from *Streptococcus mutans*. *Br. dent. J.* **152**, 81–4.

Russell, R.R.B. and Colman, G. (1981). Immunization of monkeys. (*Macaca fascicularis*) with purified *Streptococcus mutans* glucosyltransferase. *Archs. oral Biol.* **26**, 23–6.

Schick, H.J., Klimek, F.J., Weimann, E., and Zwisler, O. (1978). Preliminary results in the immunization of Irus monkeys against dental caries. In *Secretory immunity and infection*, (ed. J.R. McGhee, J. Mestecky and J.L. Babb), pp. 703–12. Plenum Press, New York.

Schöller, M., Klein, J.P., and Frank, R.M. (1978). Dental caries in gnotobiotic rats immunized with purified glycosyltransferase from *Strep. sanguis*. *Archs. oral Biol.* **23**, 501–4.

Scully, C.M. and Lehner, T. (1979). Opsonization, phagocytosis and killing of *Strep. mutans* by polymorphonuclear leucocytes, in relation to dental caries in the Rhesus monkey (*Macaca mulatta*). *Archs. oral Biol.* **24**, 307–12.

Serre, A., Benfredi, G., and Levey, D. (1972). Les immunoglobulines A salivaires, Etude des correlations avec les indices de carie et de quelques facteurs de variabilité de resultats. *Revue Immunol., Paris* **36**, 47–54.

Shklair, I.L., Rovelstad, G.H., and Lamberts, B.L. (1969). Study of some factors influencing phagocytosis of cariogenic streptococci by caries-free and caries-active individuals. *J. dent. Res.* **48**, 842–5.

Sims, W. (1972). The concept of immunity in dental caries. II. Specific responses. *Oral Surg.* **34**, 69–86.

Smith, D.J., Taubman, M.A., and Ebersole, J.L. (1978). Effects of local immunization with glucosyltransferase fractions from *Streptococcus mutans* on dental caries in hamsters caused by homologous and heterologous serotypes of *Streptococcus mutans*. *Infec. Immunity* **21**, 843–51.

Socransky, S.S. (1970). Relationship of bacteria to the etiology of periodontal disease. *J. dent. Res.* **49**, 203–22.

Stuchel, R.N. and Mandel, I.D. (1978). Studies of secretory IgA in caries-resistant and caries-susceptible adults. In *Secretory immunity and infection*, (ed. J.R. McGhee, J. Mestecky and J.L. Babb), pp. 341–8. Plenum Press, New York.

Tanzer, J.M. and Freedman, M.L. (1978). Genetic alteration of *Streptococcus mutans* virulence. In *Secretory immunity and infection*, (ed. J.R. McGhee, J. Mestecky and J.L. Babb), pp. 661–72. Plenum Press, New York.

Tanzer, J.M., Hageage, G.L., and Larson, R.H. (1973). Variable experiences in immunization of rats against *Streptococcus mutans*—associated dental caries. *Archs. oral Biol.* **18**, 1425–40.

Taubman, MA. and Smith, D.J. (1974). Effects of local immunization with *Streptococcus mutans* on induction of salivary immunoglobulun A antibody and experimental dental caries in rats. *Infec. Immunity* **9**, 1079–91.

Taubman, M.A. and Smith, D.J. (1977). Effect of local immunization with glucosyltransferase fractions from *Streptococcus mutans* in dental caries in rats and hamsters. *J. Immunol.* **118**, 710–20.

Tomasi, T.B., Tan, E.M., Solomon, A., and Prendergast, R.A. (1965). Characteristics of an immune system common to certain external secretions. *J. exp. Med.* **121**, 101–24.

Toto, P.D., Grisamore, T., Rapp, G.W., Delow, R., and Hammond, H. (1960. The correlation of *Lactobacillus* count and gamma globulin level of human saliva. *J. dent. Res.* **39**, 285–8.

Van de Rijn, I. and Zabriskie, J.B. (1976). Immunological relationship between *Streptococcus mutans* and human myocardium. In *Immunological aspects of dental caries*, (ed. W.H. Bowen, R.J. Genco and T.C. O'Brien), pp. 187–94. Information Retrieval Inc., Washington, DC.

Walker, J. (1981). Antibody responses of monkeys to oral and local immunization with *Streptococcus mutans*. *Infec. Immunity* **31**, 61–70.

Weinmann, J. (1936). Role of leukocytes in saliva. *J. dent. Res.* **15**, 360.

Wright, D.E. and Jenkins, G.N. (1953). Leukocytes in the saliva of caries-free and caries-active subjects. *J. dent. Res.* **32**, 511–23.

Zengo, A.N., Mandel, I.D., Goldman, R., and Khurana, H.J. (1971). Salivary studies in human caries resistance. *Archs. oral Biol.* **16**, 557–60.

8

Dental caries—a genetic disease?

J. J. MURRAY

MANDEL and Zenco (1973) summarized our present knowledge concerning genetic and chemical aspects of caries resistance in the following way:

> Despite many years of intensive investigation, a number of aspects of caries aetiology remains ill defined. Caries researchers prefer to attribute this lack of definition to the complexity of the problem rather than the simplicity of the investigators. Indeed, the prevailing view is that caries is a multifactorial disease, divisible in a general way into the holy trinity of bacterial factors, dietary factors and host susceptibility. (See Fig. 8.1)

It is widely accepted that environmental factors appear to play a commanding role in caries susceptibility and the first two sections of this book have been concerned with the evidence regarding diet and fluorides in the prevention of caries. Hereditary aspects have generally been relegated in the dental literature to a relatively minor position, although the general public do seem to feel that 'bad teeth run in families'. A survey on public attitudes towards dental health carried

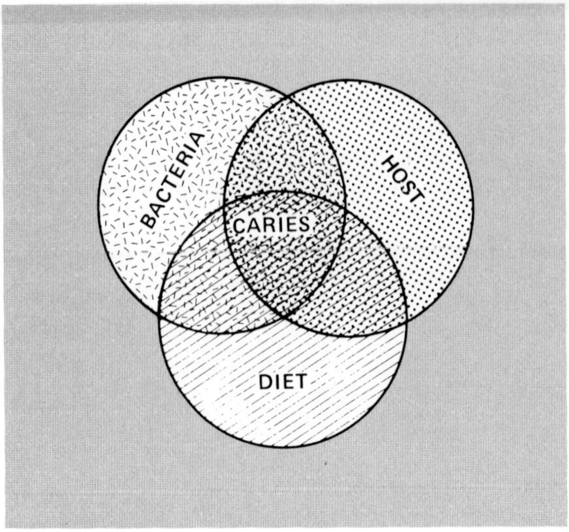

Fig. 8.1. The relationship between bacteria, host, and diet in the initiation of caries. (After Mandel and Zenco (1973).)

out for the National Dental Health Action Campaign (1977) found that although most people believe in the effectiveness of brushing teeth, a sizeable minority believe that healthy teeth are inherited rather than the result of proper dental hygiene and that brushing one's teeth makes them feel better but does not stop decay. The idea that heredity plays some part in the aetiology of dental caries has a long history. Jobson, in his book *Outlines of the Anatomy and Physiology of the Teeth* (1934), says:

> Although caries of the teeth does not appear to arise from causes which affect the general health, many persons of robust constitution being observed to be exceedingly prone to this disease, and others, although of a more delicate frame, are almost wholly free from it, yet it is undoubtedly materially influenced by predisposing causes. The first of these, perhaps, is hereditary predisposition; for it will generally be remarked that, if the patients have bad teeth, the malformation will, in all probability, be reproduced in their offspring; and it is by no means uncommon to find the teeth of different individuals of a family decaying in exactly the same way at corresponding periods of life.

In animals the very precise studies by Hunt *et al.* (1962) and by Shaw *et al.* (1962) have demonstrated that genetically caries-susceptible strains of rats can be developed as a result of selective breeding. Evidence concerning the possibility of an hereditary factor in human dental caries comes from twin and family history studies.

Human twin and family history studies

The great problem in human studies relating to caries experience is to try to differentiate between possible inherited or genetic factors influencing caries and 'familial' factors due to different members of a family sharing a similar environment with respect to diet and oral hygiene practices. Parent–child similarities in dental caries rates have been reported (Garn *et al.* 1976) but a correlation between caries experience in husbands and wives (genetically unrelated individuals living together and sharing a common diet), has also been shown (Garn *et al.* 1977). In order to try and clarify the position a number of investigators have concentrated on caries experience in monozygotic and dizygotic twins.

At least nine studies involving almost 1200 pairs of twins have been reported in the literature over the last 50 years (Table 8.1). In the main they have concluded that although environmental factors clearly have greater influence, genetic factors also contribute to the causation of dental caries. These 'genetic factors' may influence aspects of the oral cavity such as enamel structure, tooth and arch shape, and buffering power of saliva.

Many epidemiological studies have shown that when a large number of people, all within a narrow age group, are examined for dental caries, the resulting frequency distribution is one-peaked, has a large range, and approximates to a normal distribution (Fig. 8.2). Some studies on caries susceptibility have focused on the extremes of the distribution, either the most vulnerable individuals or the most resistant. Klein and Palmer (1940) carried out the first large-

Table 8.1. Summary of studies concerned with dental caries in twins

Reference	No. monozygotic	No. dizygotic pairs	No. unrelated pairs	Age in years	Findings
Bachrack and Young (1927)	130	171		3–14	Identical twins more alike in total caries experience, but the differences between the two twin types were not statistically significant.
Dahlberg and Dahlberg (1942)	37	89		7–14	No differences in caries between identical and like-sexed fraternal twins.
Horowitz *et al.* (1958)	30	19		18–65	Measurable genetic component of susceptibility to dental caries.
Goodman *et al.* (1959)	19	19		19	Intra-pair variance of dizygotic twins exceeded that of monozygotic twins.
Mansbridge (1959)	96	128		5–17	Resemblance in caries experience greater between identical twins than between fraternal twins, but difference was not statistically significant.
Finn and Caldwell (1963)	35	31	25	7–15	Greater variation in caries prevalence in the dizygotes than among the monozygotes.
Fairpo (1968)	83	95		5–15	Using site for site comparison, statistically significant differences were found between monozygotic and dizygotic twins.
Karwan *et al.* (1970)	73	124			Greater agreement on caries incidence and distribution on monozygotes than dizygotes.
Bordoni *et al.* (1973)	17		17	4–8	Concluded that their data had established a genetic component related to caries experience.
TOTAL	520	676			

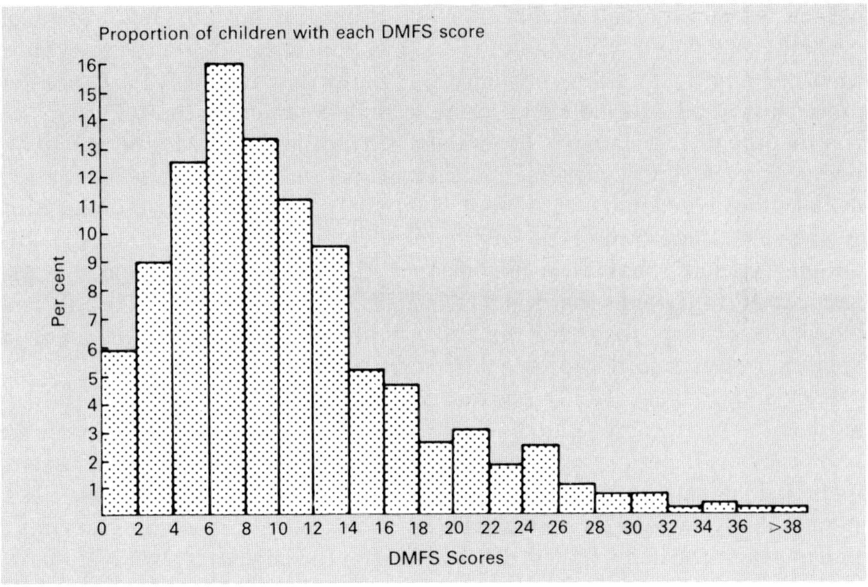

Fig. 8.2. The base line values of 1452 children, aged 11–13 years, who participated in a fluoride toothpaste trial, showing the proportion of children with each DMFS score. The histogram is one-peaked and is rather skewed to the left, but shows many of the characteristics of a normal distribution. (Murray and Shaw, unpublished data.)

scale family study concerned with the caries experience of siblings; 4416 school children were examined and their caries status recorded by means of the DMF index. Caries-resistant children were defined as those who showed no evidence of clinical caries when examined with mirror and probe. Caries-susceptible children were defined as those with six or more cavities at 10 years age, with one additional cavity included for each additional year of age. The 306 siblings of the 148 caries resistant children had a much lower mean DMF than the 182 siblings of the 117 susceptible children. In a later study of 5400 persons from 1150 families of Japanese ancestry residing in the United States, Klein (1946) found among the siblings a definite reflection of the caries score of their parents. although these reports suggest that caries 'runs in families' this may well be a reflection of the dietary habits of the families rather than evidence of inherited factors.

The dental records of every Swedish conscript enrolling for military training during the period 1944–47 were examined by Böök and Grahnén (1953). Swedish males, aged 20 years, who were caries free on clinical and radiological examination at the time of entering into military training, were selected as propositi for their study. An attempt was made to trace each propositus, or index case, together with the parents and siblings. Of the 55 caries-free index cases, 40 could be located and examined; in addition 30 fathers, 33 mothers, 43 brothers, and 56 sisters were seen, a total of 202 individuals. The control propositi were defined as follows: a male individual, 20 years of age, who at the registration for compulsory military training in 1944–1947 inclusive had the registration number immediately below or above the registration number of a caries-free propositus. In all 114 individuals were examined to form a control group: 23 control propositi, 20 fathers, 23 mothers, 27 brothers, and 21 sisters. Parents and siblings of adult caries-free individuals had, on average, significantly less dental decay as compared with properly selected control individuals (Table 8.2). After due consideration of the environment conditions of the two groups, the authors concluded that the group difference could hardly be determined by differences in living conditions, oral hygiene, dieting habits, or general health conditions, and they suggested that the variability in caries experience is appreciably determined by polygenic factors.

Böök and Grahnén (1953) provide an appendix to their paper giving the caries data for each examined individual arranged by family groups. During the years between the initial examination for military training and te survey examination some carious lesions had occurred in 21 out of the 40 index cases. Almost all of them had a very low DMF of 1, 2, or 3. Only two index cases had a DMF of 6 and one had a DMF of 10. The data for the families of their index cases showed that 14 out of the 162 relations had a DMF of 6 or less. In comparison only one person in the control group had a DMF of 6 or less.

Horowitz *et al.* (1965) carried out a similar study in the United States and confirmed the Böök and Grahnén findings (Table 8.2). Dental records of two large insurance companies showed that the number of adults who were completely caries free was only 0.07–0.08 per cent. By screening medical, dental, and college students, hospital personnel, and dental clinic patients, these workers obtained a list of 100 people aged 17 years or over, residing in the New York City area, who were caries free on clinical radiographic examination. From this group, 33 index cases were selected for a family history study by mean of a personal interview. Information was obtained regarding the presumed caries status of 126 other members of their immediate families. Ten of the 33 index cases reported that they thought at least one other adult member of the immediate family was completely free of caries. Seven of these relations were contacted and in five families the report regarding caries immunity was found to be correct on clinical and rediographic examination. Thus there were five confirmed caries immune people out of the 126 immediate relatives of the 33 selected index cases, a proportion about 30 times greater than that occurring in the general population.

Although the studies involving twins and families have suggested a genetic factor or influence associated with caries experience, the mechanism whereby this genetic influence may be exerting its effect has never been isolated. Have those 'caries-resistant' individuals inherited a set of genes which result in more perfect enamel or dentine being formed? Are the shapes of their teeth slightly different, in particular are their teeth more widely spaced or are the pits and fissures shallower or more rounded than other people? Do the differences lie in the

Table 8.2. Family studies of caries immunity

Reference	No. of index cases	No. of index cases examined	No. of immediate family examined	No. of adults caries resistant		Proportion of caries immunity in the adult general population
				No.	Percentage	
Böök and Grahnén (1953)	55	40	162	14*	9	0.1
Horowitz *et al.* (1965)	100	33	126	5**	4	0.08

* Caries immunity if DMF $\leqslant 6$
** caries immunity in DMF = 0.

calcium and phosphate levels in saliva, or in differences in salivary flow rate, or in the buffering capacity of saliva? These factors, and many others, have been considered by dental researchers, but either because of the 'complexity of the problem' or the 'simplicity of the investigators' a number of aspects of caries aetiology remain ill-defined.

Dental caries—an auto-immune disease?

In 1966 a revolutionary concept of dental caries aetiology, involving precise mathematical calculations, was put forward by Burch and Jackson who stated that

> Specific random events appear to be implicated in the initiation of dental caries. We shall argue that these initiating events are possibly somatic mutations and that they give rise to the growth of 'forbidden clones' of cells producing auto-antibodies. That is to say, spontaneous disturbed tolerance auto-immune factors may be involved in the pathogenesis of dental caries.

Burch (1968*a*) substituted the term 'auto-aggressive' for 'auto-immune' and stated that the emergence of an auto-aggressive condition in a genetically predisposed person can be divided into two phases: *Initiation*, which is a purely stochastic phenomenon, normally involving spontaneous mutations; and *progression*, which is in part a sequential phenomenon, although accidental environmental factors may accelerate this phase and therapeutic measures may retard it. The interval between the initiation of a disease and its symptomatic or clinical onset is termed the *latent period.*

In relation to dental caries, Jackson *et al.* (1967) have postulated that the target cells are odontoblasts and that the random event is a special form of gene mutation in a central growth-control stem cell. An interval or latent period elapses between the random initiating event and the clinical manifestation of dental caries. They suggested that the forbidden clone propagated by the mutant stem cell synthesizes primary 'auto-antibodies' (mutant MCPs) that attack odontblasts and disturb their metabolism. Presumably this destroys the integrity of the protein matrix extending from the odontoblast, through the dentine, to the enamel. Exogenous factors such as acids and/or chelating agents complete the degenerative change to produce the lesions diagnosed as dental caries. As Edgar (1974) remarked, 'Clearly, if confirmed, their conclusions would cast doubt on the validity of much of the theoretical basis of current caries research, and would throw into question the present conventional approaches to preventive dentistry.

Objections to the Burch–Jackson hypothesis

A number of important objections can be made to the Burch–Jackson hypothesis so far expounded. They concern the method for selecting the clinical material on which the calculations were based, the idea of latent period, the original concept of the 'forbidden-clone' theory as expounded by Burnet, patterns of caries in incisor teeth, and the lack of any histological evidence to support their hypothesis.

Clinical material

The initial data on which this hypothesis rests are based on a fairly small sample of 1441 adults, aged 15–64 years. The method of applying correction factors to the missing (M) fraction of the DMF index can only be an estimate of caries experience. As people get older an increasing proportion of caries-free teeth are extracted for periodontal and prosthetic reasons. However, Jackson (1961) used only one figure for the proportion of extracted tooth types which were carious or filled. Thus the estimated DMF rates, particularly in the older age groups, were an over-estimate of caries experience. Yet it is these data that were used to calculate the stochastic equations and to draw the graphs which show how closely their data fits theoretical calculations.

Latent period

The idea of 'latent period' is especially relevant because of the effect of fluoride on dental caries. According to the Burch–Jackson hypothesis a tooth is genetically susceptible to an attack or it is completely resistant. Once a 'forbidden clone' of cells have been formed as a result of a mutation, a carious lesion may develop. The interval between the mutation and the observation of a clinically carious lesion is known as the latent period. The latent period for premolars is given as 7.5 years (Burch and Jackson 1966) (Fig. 8.3). They postulated that preventive measures may merely lengthen the duration of the latent period. Burch (1968) prophesized that this was how water fluoridation worked—by lengthening the latent period— and that by adjusting this value alone, the curves for caries in tooth types in fluoride and low-fluoride areas would be identical. However, it is not possible to fit the data of caries experience in adults from the natural fluoride area of Hartlepool to that from the low-fluoride area of York merely by lengthening the length of the latent period (Figs. 8.4 and 8.5).

Burnet's forbidden clone theory

According to Burnet (1959): 'If the form of age incidence of a disease is reproducibly similar in different environments, this must be regarded as one of its characteristics and therefore calls for interpretation. Since it can be expressed graphically as a define curve, it is susceptible to mathematical treatment and may therefore be relevant as evidence to test this or that hypothesis of aetiology.' The crucial words in my view are 'reproducibly similar in different environments'. In a later paper Jackson and Burch say: 'For a given environment we find that the data for caries fit our hypotheses', but when one examines these words they show an important difference from Burnet. For a given environment

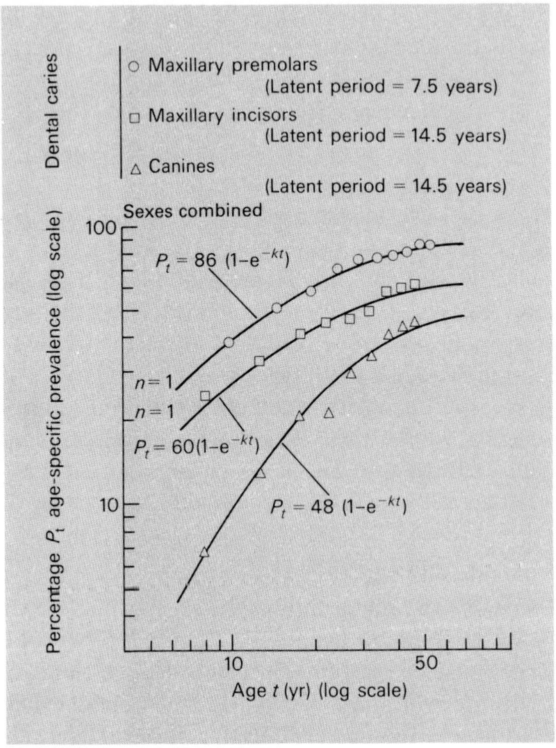

Fig. 8.3. Age-specific prevalence of dental caries, corrected for latent period, according to Burch and Jackson (1966); for maxillary premolars, latent period correction is 7.5 years. (By courtesy of the Editor, *British Dental Journal*.)

we could all make our predictions concerning caries experience—no plaque, no caries—lots of plaque and sucrose, caries. Burnet's point was that a disease involving mutations should appear irrespective of the local environment.

Approximal incisor caries patterns in children

A most important part of the evidence that Burch and Jackson present is the anatomical site distribution of caries in incisor teeth. Their suggestion that genetic factors have an overriding influence on the siting and timing of caries attack is based on data collected from many sources and the subject of a number of publications (Jackson 1968; Jackson and Burch 1968; Jackson and Burch 1970; Jackson *et al.* 1967, 1972, 1973*a*, *b*, 1975).

They argue an initial attack of caries on maxillary incisors is quickly associated with a definite anatomical distribution of lesions which persists as long as the incisors remain in the mouth. A surface is either attacked or spared, and if it is spared it remains free from further attack. An 'all-or-none' response to a cariogenic attack is inexplicable in conventional terms. In their view the traditional acidogenic theory offers no plausible explanation for this phenomenon. Instead they conclude that: 'The distinction between the susceptibility and resistance to dental caries is qualitative in character. A site on a tooth is either at risk with re-

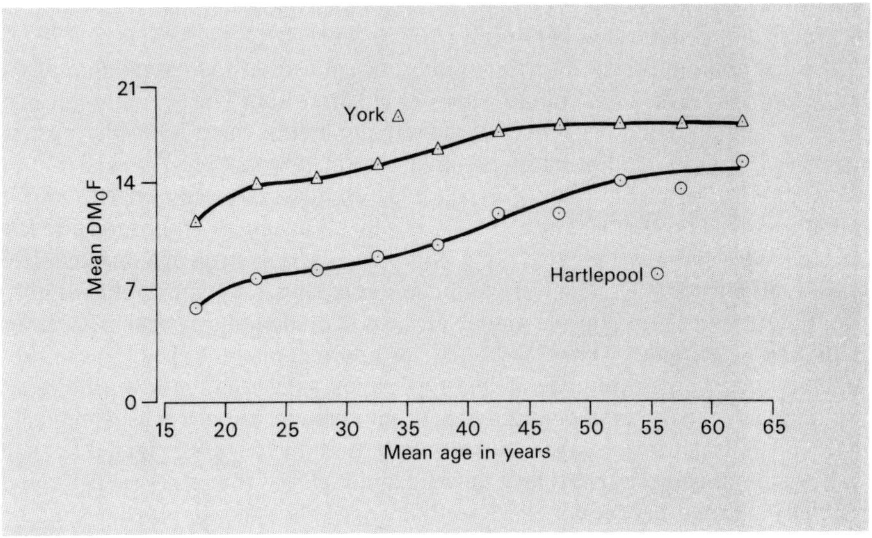

Fig. 8.4. Observed DMF values of 3902 dentate adults from Hartlepool, a natural fluoride area, and York, a low fluoride area.

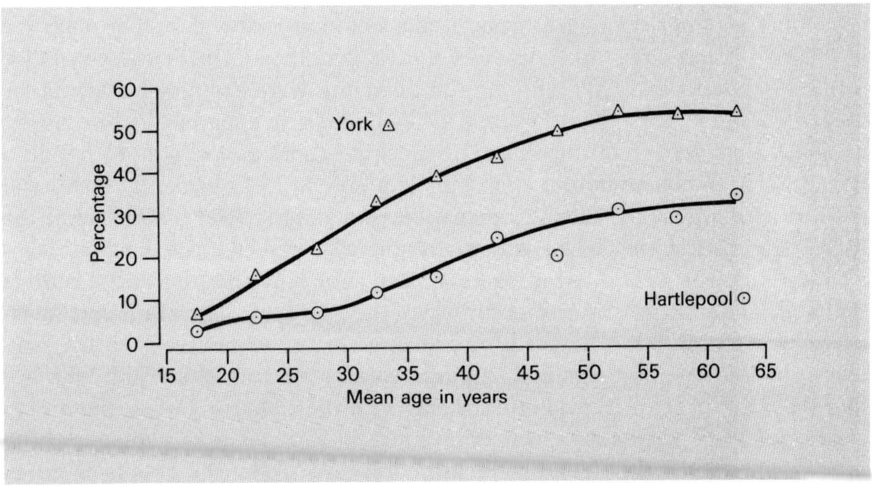

Fig. 8.5. The percentage DMF of maxillary canines from Hartlepool and York. Figures 4 and 5 show that the shape of the curves from Hartlepool, for all tooth types or for an individual tooth type, is not the same as that found in York.

spect to dental caries or it is completely resistant. This qualitative distinction is determined by genetic factors' (Burch 1968; Jackson 1968; Jackson *et al.* 1967).

The first anatomical site data to be published concerned approximal mandibular incisor caries in 2437 11–12-year-old children from Leeds, a low-fluoride area; 101 children (4.1 per cent) had mandibular incisor caries. Considering first the mesial surfaces of adjacent mandibular central incisors they observed that in 13 children a carious lesion occurred on the right surface only, in 14 cases a lesion occurred on the left surface only, but in 27 instances both right and left surfaces were carious. This gives an R only : R + L : L only ratio of almost exactly 1 : 2 : 1. Similar simple ratios were found for other sites: for example the number of carious lesions found on the mesial surfaces of mandibular lateral incisors for R only : R + L : L only, were 25 : 22 : 20, or approximately 1 : 1 : 1. These preliminary analyses, yielding Mendelian-type ratios, suggested to the authors that the anatomical pattern of dental caries in mandibular incisors was genetically determined. In a further paper, Jackson and Burch (1968) investigated the site distribution of caries in maxillary incisors and reported that the specificity and regularities in the distribution of DF teeth are most conspicuous. Considering the mesial surface of maxillary central incisors, 75 lesions occurred on the right only; in 110 cases both right and left mesial surfaces were affected, and in 65 cases only the left surface was carious. This means that there were more single attacks (140) than double attacks, giving a single/double ratio of 1.3 : 1. The corresponding figures for the mesial surface of lateral incisors were R only 175, R + L 157, L only 138, giving a single/double ratio of 313 : 157 or 2 : 0.

Few studies have been published to substantiate or refute the initial patterns of incisor caries reported by Jackson *et al.* (1967). Yet if the Burch–Jackson theory that dental caries is primarily a genetic disease is correct, then the Mendelian-type ratios for single : double attacks at adjacent incisor sites should be observed in different populations. In order to test their hypothesis, the dental charts for 1432 11–12-year-old children living in Berkshire were examined in detail for incisor caries (Murray *et al.* 1976): 197 had clinically apparent incisor caries; 175 (12.2 per cent) had maxillary incisor approximal caries; and 41 children (2.0 per cent) had mandibular approximal incisor caries. Considering the mesial surfaces of mandibular central incisors, Jackson *et al.* (1967) reported that the ratio of right surfaces affected only: right and left surfaces affected: left surfaces affected only was 1 : 2 : 1, whereas in the Berkshire study we reported a ratio of 3 : 15 : 2. The ratio for the mesial surface of the maxillary central incisors given by Jackson and Burch (1968) was approximately 2 : 3 : 2, whereas in the Berkshire children the corresponding figures were 1 : 4 : 1.7. Thus, although we found a number of attacks on one surface, with the adjacent surface remaining caries free, there were many more double attacks reported in our study for each approximal site tha that found by Jackson and co-workers. Our results do not of themselves disprove Jackson's hypothesis; it may well be that our own findings are in error. Nevertheless, is a simple genetic basis has an overriding influence on dental caries—at least in incisor teeth—one would have thought that the pattern should be evident in a sample of 1400 children of similar age. So far no other studies have been reported which substantiate or refute the pattern of caries in incisor teeth of children referred to in this section.

Approximal incisor caries patterns in adults

Jackson and co-workers extended their work by examining the chartings made by dental practitioners for many thousands of patients aged 15–60+ years. He stated (Jackson 1968) that as each member of a pair of mesial surfaces of central incisors shares a common environment, it would be reasonable to expect that if caries occurred on one mesial surface, it would be accompanied by an attack on the other surface either immediately or after a short interval of time. Accordingly the single/double ratio might be fairly high in the youngest age groups, but it would fall with age and approach zero in the highest age groups. However, he reported that, taking a sample of people with at least one carious incisor, and ignoring any charts with missing or crowned incisors, the single/double ratio 'freezes' from about 18 years onwards to a level of approximately 0.8 : 1. This means that when an attack occurs on one mesial surface of a maxillary central incisor it is unlikely to be accompanied by an attack on the remaining surface in more than approximately 45 per cent of instances. Similar findings were reported for other adjacent maxillary incisor sites.

However, as Edgar (1974) remarked, Jackson's findings depend wholly upon the assumption that successive age groups reflect the pattern of attack in the lifetime of an individual. This assumption may or may not be valid, depending upon whether or not successive age groups are unbiased samples from the general population and have had identical histories. The selection of subjects for inclusion in the surveys of Jackson and associates was not random, being based upon a sub-population of subjects with at least one carious maxillary incisor. Subjects from the general population may be 'recruited' into this sub-population at any rate by experiencing caries attacks in hitherto caries-free teeth; conversely they may be lost from the sub-population by extraction of one or all of their maxillary incisors. These population changes could, in theory, explain the findings of Jackson *et al.* without implying the existence of an all-or-none aetiological factor. Jackson observed different people of different ages passing through the same stage of caries development, while Edgar observed the same people passing through different stages of caries development through their middle-life.

By a 15-year retrospective study of the records of 150 patients, Edgar showed that when the records were considered longitudinally, the single/double ratio fell with increasing age, in contrast to the results from Jackson's cross-section survey. He concluded that 'whatever properties of teeth and environment may be involved in governing the distributions of caries observed, and these may include a proportion of inherited properties, it seems unnecessary to postulate the existence of an all-or-none genetic component. Furthermore, clear evidence of continuous, if declining, increments of caries occurring over 15 years even in the oldest subjects casts grave doubt upon the existence of absolutely caries-free sites.' There is obviously a need for further longitudinal studies to elucidate this point.

Histological evidence

According to the Burch–Jackson hypothesis, after a mutation in a stem cell a forbidden clone of cells synthesizes primary auto-antibodies that attack odontoblasts and disturb their metabolism, destroying the integrity of the protein matrix extending from the odontoblast, through the dentine, to the enamel. As far as I am aware, no histological evidence is available to support this suggestion.

Family history study of caries resistance and caries susceptibility

Nevertheless, in spite of modern diet, with its high carbohydrate consumption, and the fact that very few people are so meticulous in their oral hygiene regimes that their mouths are always free from dental plaque (two of the factors mentioned by Mandel and Zenco) the fact remains that the majority of teeth surfaces do maintain their integrity, at least macroscopically. Eighty per cent of the tooth surfaces present in York adults, even at the age of 45 years and over, remained caries free; and in the natural fluoride area of Hartlepool 90 per cent of sites present in the mouth were sound clinically. For many years innumerable dental research workers have asked the question 'Why does a tooth become carious?' and yet the number of people who have asked the converse—'Why does a tooth *not* decay?'—have been very few indeed. There has been one symposium on this topic, under the auspices of the Ciba Foundation, in London in 1964, resulting in the book *Caries-resistant teeth* (1965), which recorded the papers and discussion occurring at the symposium. It was asking the question 'Why do some tooth surfaces not decay?' that led Jackson to examine the dental charts of so many children and to the realization that, in spite of the ubiquitous nature of dental plaque, only a minority had maxillary incisor caries and only a very small proportion had mandibular incisor caries. Just because I have criticized some aspects of the 'auto-immune' hypothesis does not mean that I reject that dental caries might have a genetic component.

It is for this reason that we looked in detail at the examination charts of children who participated in a recent toothpaste trial (Murray and Shaw 1980). Why is it that out of 1431 children, aged 13–15 years, only 39 have mandibular incisor caries and only 44 children are caries free? Is there a big difference in their diet—or their standard of oral hygiene? Is the prevalence of dental caries in their families different—do the parents of children with mandibular incisor caries also have a high caries experience and are the parents of caries-free children also relatively immune from this disease?

In order to try and answer some of these questions, a letter was sent to the families of the 83 children who were defined as caries resistant and caries susceptible (Shaw and Murray 1980), requesting their consent to the completion of a questionnaire in their homes and a dental examination. Only two of the families, both with children in the caries-susceptible group, refused to co-operate. Questionnaires and clinical examinations were completed for 147 of their parents and 132 siblings in their own homes. Although the mean age of the parents of the two groups was similar (43.8 years and 43.9 years) only 8 per cent of parents of the caries-resistant children were edentulous compared with 37 per cent of parents of caries-susceptible children. The mean DMFS for dentate parents of caries-resistant children was 43.6 compared with a mean DMFS of 64.2 for dentate parents of caries-susceptible children. The ages of the siblings of the caries-resistant and caries-susceptible children were also similar (13.5 years and 14.5 years) but, like the parents, a large difference in caries experience was observed. The mean DMFS value was three times higher in siblings of the caries-susceptible group compared with siblings of the caries-resistant group (21.3 as against 7.6). These differences do not necessarily show a genetic component but could, in fact, be due to better oral hygiene and dietary habits being followed in the families of the 'caries-resistant' group than in the household containing the 'caries-susceptible' children. However, the results of the questionnaire showed that the intake of refined sugars did not vary widely between the groups, although the parents and siblings of the caries-susceptible group did consume slightly more snacks than their caries-resistant counterparts. There were no differences between the groups in dental attendance and tooth-brushing habits.

One drawback of this type of enquiry is that it is unrealistic to relate to lifetime caries experience with a single assessment of food intake. However, attempts were made in this questionnaire to determine long-term dietary habits rather than give a quantitative estimate of consumption within the preceding 24 hours, as has been used in many dietary histories. It is difficult to escape the conclusion that good and bad teeth were 'running in the families' of these two groups of children, as mentioned by Jobson in 1834, and that perhaps genetic factors or other environmental factors not assessed in this particular study may play a significant role on the caries process.

Saliva and plaque in caries-resistant and caries-susceptible individuals

One other factor, which might have a genetic component, is the composition of saliva and plaque. Conflicting results have been obtained from investigation of calcium and phosphorus content of saliva and plaque, and their relationship to dental caries. Some workers (Maijer and Klassen 1972; Turtola 1978) have observed a rise in salivary calcium concentration with increasing caries activity whilst others (Ahrens 1961; Ashley 1971; Shannon and Feller 1979) have noted a trend to higher calcium levels in lower caries groups. In the toothpaste trial referred to in the previous section, an attempt was made to collect saliva and plaque samples from the caries-resistant and caries-susceptible children, and to carry out calcium and phosphorus analyses. Results showed that the plaque collected from posterior teeth of the caries-resistant children had significantly higher values of calcium and phosphorus than that found in plaque from the caries-susceptible group. Similar trends were also evident for the calcium and phosphorus analyses of saliva (Shaw *et al.* 1983).

Conclusion

Böök and Grahnén (1953) pointed out that to distinguish a genetic trait in a population depends, among other things, on the frequency of that trait. The more common a genetic trait, the more difficult it will be to demonstrate its genetic character. The extremely high prevalence of dental caries in western populations will tend to make the genetic analysis rather inefficient, even if dental caries were very strongly genetically determined. The evidence gathered together in this chapter suggests that the assertion by Jackson and co-workers that genetic factors have an overriding influence on the siting and timing of caries attacks has not been sustained. The effect of diet, fluoride supplements, and the presence and composition of dental plaque are of overwhelming importance in the causation of dental caries, and the methods now available for changing the environment of the tooth provide us with the opportunity of preventing dental caries. Nevertheless, some 'host component' remains, although still ill-defined.

References

Ahrens, G. (1961). Beziehungen zwischen dem phosphatgehalt des speichels und karies. *Arch. oral Biol.* **6**, 241–8.

Ashley, F.P. (1971). Relationship between dietary sugar intake, parotid saliva, plaque calcium and phosphorus concentrations and caries. *J. dent. Res.* **50**, 1212.

Bachrack, F.H. and Young, M. (1927). A comparison of the degree of resemblance in dental characters shown in pairs of twins of identical and fraternal types. *Br. dent. J.* **48**, 1293–304.

Böök, J.A. and Grahnén, H. (1953). Clinical and genetical studies of dental caries. II. Parents and siblings of adult highly resistant (caries-free) propositi. *Odont. Rev.* **4**, 1–53.

Bordoni, N., Dono, R., Manfredi, C., and Allegrotti, I. (1973). Prevalence of dental caries in twins. *J. Dent. Child.* **40**, 440–3.

Burch, P.R.J. (1968*a*). Of growth and disease. *New Scient.* **40**, 484–6.

Burch, P.R.J. (1968*b*). *An enquiry concerning growth, disease and ageing.* Oliver and Boyd, Edinburgh.

Burch, P.R.J. and Jackson. D. (1966). Periodontal disease and dental caries. Some new aetiological consideration. *Br. dent. J.* **120**, 127–34.

Burnet, F.M. (1959). *The clonal selection theory of acquired immunity.* Cambridge University Press, London.

CIBA Foundation (1965). *Caries-resistant teeth*, (ed. G.E.W. Wolstenholme and M. O'Connor). Churchill, London.

Dahlberg, G. and Dahlberg, B. (1964). Über Karies und andere Zahnveränderungen bei Zwillingen. *Uppsala Läk-Förh.* **47**, 395–416.

Edgar, W.M. (1974). A 15-year retrospective survey of the distributions of clinical caries attacks in human permanent maxillary incisors. *Archs. oral Biol.* **19**, 1203–9.

Fairpo, C.G. (1968). Comparison of dental caries experienced in identical and like-sexed fraternal twins. *J. dent. Res.* **47**, 971.

Finn, S.B. and Caldwell, (1963). Dental caries in twins—1. A comparison of the caries experience of monozygotic twins and unrelated children. *Archs. oral Biol.* **8**, 571–85.

Garn, S.M. and Clark, D.C. (1977). Husband-wife similarities in dental caries experience. *J. dent. Res.* **56**, 186.

Garn, S.M., Rowe, N.H., and Cole, P.E. (1976). Parent-child similarities in dental caries rates. *J. dent. Res.* **55**, 1129.

Goodman, H.O., Luke, J.E., Rosen, S., and Hackel, E. (1959). Heritability of dental caries and some related salivary components. (Abstr.) *J. dent. Res.* **38**, 662.

Horowitz, S.L., Osborne, R.H., and George, F.V. (1958). Caries experience in twins. *Science, NY* **128**, 300–1.

Horowitz, S.L., Zengo, A.N., and Mandel, I.D. (1965). Studies in dental caries immunity. *NY St. dent. J.* **31**, 49–53.

Hunt, H.R., Hoppert, C.A., and Rosen, S. (1962). The inheritance factor in dental caries in rats (*Rattus norvegicus*). In *Genetic and dental health*, (ed. C.J. Witkop). McGraw-Hill, New York.

Jackson, D. (1961). An epidemiological study of dental caries prevalence in adults. *Archs. oral Biol.* **6**, 80–93.

Jackson, D. (1968). Genes and dental caries. *Proc. R. Soc. Med.* **61**, 265–9.

Jackson, D. and Burch, P.R.J. (1968). The anatomical site distribution of clinical dental caries in the maxillary incisor teeth of 11- and 12-year-old children. *Archs. oral Biol.* **13**, 809–17.

Jackson, D. and Burch, P.R.J. (1970). Dental caries: distribution by age-group, between homologous (right-left) mesial and distal surfaces of human permanent maxillary incisors. *Archs. oral Biol.* **15**, 1059–67.

Jackson, D., Sutcliffe, P., and Burch, P.R.J. (1967). The anatomical site distribution of clinical dental caries in the mandibular incisor teeth of 11- and 12-year-old children. Aetiological implications. *Archs. oral Biol.* **12**, 1343–53.

Jackson, D., Burch, P.R.J., and Fairpo, C.G. (1972). Dental caries: distribution, by age-group, between the mesial and distal surfaces of human permanent mandibular incisors. *Archs. oral Biol.* **17**, 1343–50.

Jackson, D., Fairpo, C.G., and Burch, P.R.J. (1973*a*). Human lingual pit caries: distribution between right and left maxillary incisors. *Archs. oral Biol.* **18**, 181–7.

Jackson, D., Fairpo, G.G., and Burch, P.R.J. (1973*b*). Distribution of symmetric and asymmetric patterns of caries attack in human permanent maxillary incisor teeth: genetic implications. *Archs. oral Biol.* **18**, 189–95.

Jackson, D., Fairpo, G.G., and Burch, P.R.J. (1975). Distribution of symmetric and asymmetric patterns in caries attack in human permanent mandibular incisor teeth: genetic implications. *Archs. oral Biol.* **20**, 11–16.

Jobson, D.W. (1834). *Outlines of the anatomy and the physiology of the teeth. Their diseases and treatment with practical observations on artificial teeth.* William Tait, Edinburgh.

Klein, H. (1946). The family and dental disease: iv dental disease (DMF) experience in parents and offspring. *J. Am. dent. Ass.* **33**, 735–43.

Klein, H. and Palmer, C.E. (1940). Dental caries in brothers and sisters of immune and susceptible children. *Milbank Mem. Fund. Q.* **18**, 67–82.

Maijer, R. and Klassen, G.A. (1972). Ionized calcium concentration in saliva and its relationship to dental disease. *J. Can. dent. Ass.* **38**, 333–6.

Mandel, I.D. and Zenco, A.N. (1973). In *Genetic and chemical aspects in caries resistance in comparative immunology of the oral cavity*, (ed. S.E. Mergenhagen and H.W. Scherp). DHGW Publ. No. (NIH) 73–438. US Government Printing Office, Washington DC.

Mansbridge, J.N. (1959). Heredity and dental caries. *J. dent. Res.* **38**, 337–47.

Murray, J.J. and Shaw, J.H. (1980). Classification and prevalence of enamel opacities in the human deciduous and permanent dentitions. *Archs. oral Biol.* **24**, 7–13.

Murray, J.J., Shaw, J.H., and Campbell, G.A. (1976). Distribution of incisor caries in 11- and 12-year-old English children. *Archs. oral Biol.* **21**, 187–93.

National Dental Health Action Campaign (1977). (Public survey.) *Public attitudes towards dental health.* carried out by Market and Opinion Research International, MORI).

Shannon, I.L. and Feller, R.P. (1979). Paratid saliva glow rate, calcium, phosphorous and magnesium concentrations in relation to dental caries experience in children. *Paediat. Dent.* **1**, 16–20.

Shaw, J.H. and Murray, J.J. (1980). A family history study of caries-resistance and caries-susceptibility. *Br. dent. J.* **148**, 231–5.

Shaw, J.H., Griffiths, D., and Wollman, D.H. (1962). Comparison of dental caries activity in strains of laboratory rats. *J. dent. Res.* **41**, 1312–21.

Shaw, L., Murray, J.J., Burchell, C.K., and Best, J.S. (1983). Calcium and phosphorus content of plaque and saliva in relation to dental caries. *Caries Res.* **17**, 543–8.

Turtola, L. (1978). Dental caries and its prevention. *Proc. Finn. dent. Soc.* **74**, 36–7.

9

Prevention in the ageing dentition

A. W. G. WALLS

IT is well established that the structure of the population within the United Kingdom is changing. This is a result of an improvement in economic status, health care, and social environment during the last century, which has produced a dramatic increase in average life expectancy. In 1911, the average life expectancy at birth was 49 years for men and 52 years for women, compared with 70 and 76 years respectively in the 1970s. This is a product of a reduction in mortality in infancy, childhood, and young adulthood: for those aged 65, life expectancy has only risen 1 year for men and 4 years for women during the same period.

This alteration in life pattern means that more people are surviving into their 'old age', producing a major change to health and social services. As we age, our bodies undergo a number of alterations or 'age changes'. These changes effect all parts of the body, including the oral environment.

An age change can be defined as:

> An alteration in form or function to a tissue or organ, as a result of biological activity associated with minor disturbances of normal cellular turnover.

As such, there is a limited number of age changes that affect the mouth, most of which have no bearing upon the dentition. These changes are confined to alterations in the oral mucosa and connective tissue, including the periodontium. They comprise thinning of the mucous membrane, and increased collagen density with a decreased rate of collagen turnover. There are significant changes in the structure of all of the salivary glands with increasing age. These changes are greatest in the submandibular and minor salivary glands and least in the parotid gland (Scott 1986). Studies on the alteration of salivary flow with age are complicated by the involvement of the salivary glands in systemic disease, and the influence of a wide variety of medications upon salivary function (Baker and Ettinger 1985). A number of investigations into salivary function with age, in which the medical history of the participants has been carefully controlled, have been reported recently. It would appear that there is little alteration in functional capacity of the parotid gland with increasing age, either in terms of stimulated or resting flow rates (Ben-Aryeh *et al.* 1984; Heft and Baum 1984; Baum 1986).

There is, however, some diminution in flow from minor salivary glands (Gandara *et al.* 1985) and the submandibular gland (Pedersen *et al.* 1985) with increasing age. It would appear that these functional changes are manifest in the predominantly mucous secreting glands, where the acinar structure deteriorates with age. The lack of any perceived age-related alteration in parotid flow may be a reflection of a considerable 'functional reserve' within this gland, or of the very wide variation in 'normal' flow rates from the parotid irrespective of the age of the individual.

If an age change is a cellular phenomenon by definition, then there can be no 'age changes' to enamel—there is a continued surface maturation of enamel with increased crystal growth and altered orientation, but this is a product of exposure in the oral environment, and not an age change. Conversely, both dentine and the pulp undergo some age-dependent alteration in structure. There is an increase in peritubular dentine formation and in secondary dentine deposition with ageing, giving a more highly mineralized tissue. This is associated with a reduced number of odontoblasts. The vascularity of the pulp is reduced, with an increase in pulpal fibrous tissue, and areas of ectopic calcification within the pulp are not uncommon.

There are two problems, root surface caries and tooth wear, which increase in prevalence with increasing age, but cannot be regarded as age changes. They are more properly regarded as age-related, or age-associated phenomena. As such they can be regarded in the same light as atherosclerotic vascular disease where there is an increased prevalence with ageing, but the disease process is not a *sine qua non* of ageing. It is to these two clinical problems that the remainder of this chapter will be devoted.

Root surface caries

Caries on the root surface (Fig. 9.1) has been defined as:

> A cavitation or softened area in the root surface which might, or might not, involve adjacent enamel or existing restorations (Hix and O'Leary 1976).

Epidemiology

There is wide variation in the prevalence of root surface caries, from as low as 7.3 per cent (Burt *et al.* 1986), amongst individuals living in a community with high levels of natural water fluoridation, to 100 per cent (Fejerskov *et al.* 1985) in patients over the age of 60 attending a gerontology clinic. The prevalence of root surface caries increases with increasing age of the population. This increase is independent of the population studied (Fig. 9.2). Whilst these figures give us an estimate of the total number of the population that have one or more root carious lesion, they do not give an indication of the magnitude of the problem within any given individual. The mean number of lesions per person affected has been reported by a number of workers: it varies, depending upon the age and

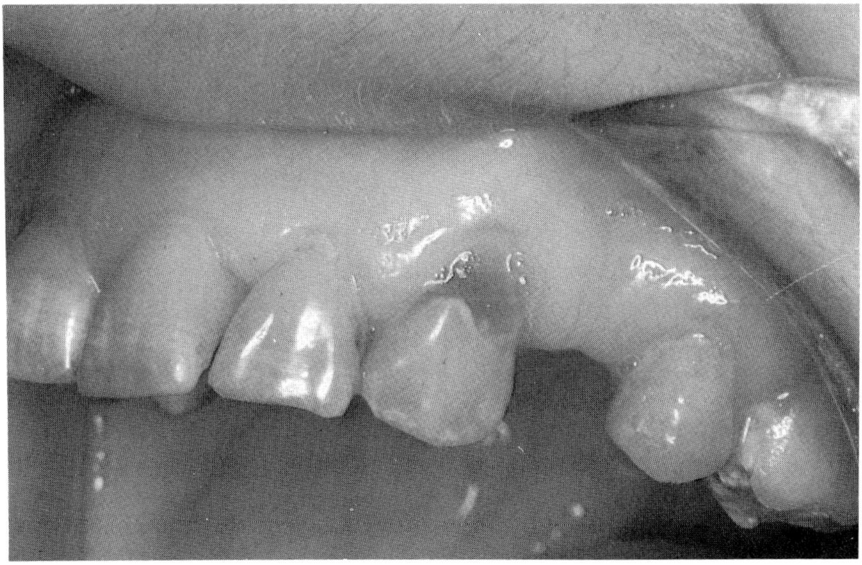

Fig. 9.1. An extensive active root surface caries lesion at the buccal cervical margin of an upper canine.

nature of the population studied, from 0.2 for 28–29-year olds from a non-fluoridated western community (Katz *et al.* 1982) to 6.4 in primitive tribesmen 30 or more years old (Schamschula *et al.* 1974) (Fig. 9.3.)

Once again these figures are useful, but they do not give any idea of the likelihood that any given individual will develop root caries. It goes without saying that for a tooth to develop root caries, the root will be exposed in the mouth. A true 'attack rate' for root caries should relate the incidence of no lesions to the number of surfaces at risk, i.e. exposed root surfaces. The root caries index (RCI) proposed by Katz (1985) computes a true attack rate for root caries. There is some conflict concerning the effect of age upon the RCI. In an early study (Katz *et al.* 1982) the RCI increased with increasing age of the population sampled (1.1 per cent at 20–29 years to 22.9 per cent at 50–59 years); however, the sample size was relatively small (n = 473). In a more recent study using a much larger sample (n = 3361), the RCI rates varied between 11 and 18 per cent, with 'no discernible pattern associated with age' (Katz *et al.* 1985). It would seem likely that between 10 and 20 per cent of exposed root surfaces will develop root caries, and that the increase in incidence of root caries with age is a manifestation of gingival recession, rather than ageing. Miller *et al.* (1987) reported that over 50 per cent of their sample exhibited at least one site with gingival recession. The prevalence of gingival recession increased with increasing age of the individual (11 per cent of 18–19-year-olds exhibited one site with recession compared to 88 per cent of those 80 or more years old).

When assessing these data concerning the prevalence of root surface caries, it

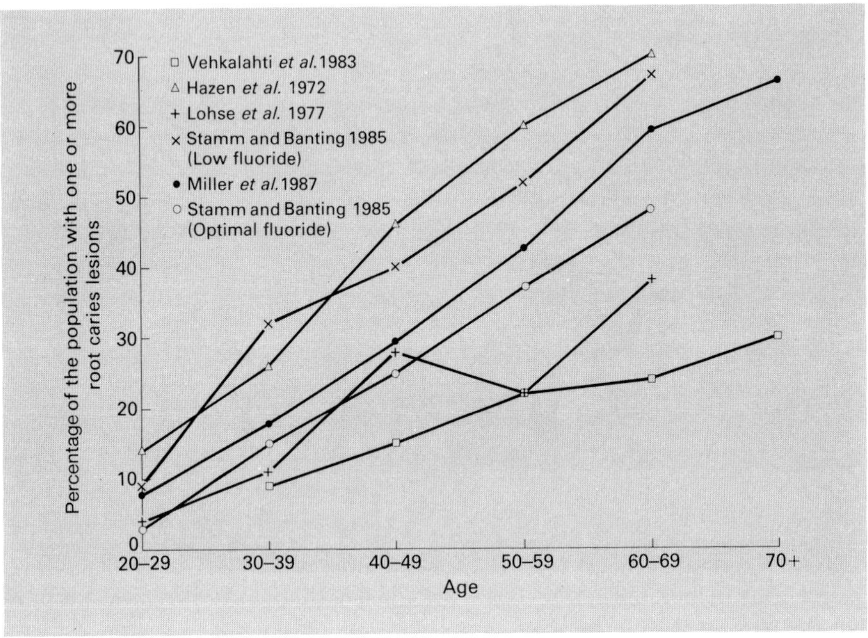

Fig. 9.2. A graphical presentation of the data from a number of studies demonstrating the increasing prevalence of root surface caries with age. This increase is independent of the nature of the population studied.

must be borne in mind that the examiners were looking for decayed or restored root surfaces. In 'western' countries some of these restorations will have been placed to repair 'cervical abrasion' lesions and not root caries. Such lesions rarely become carious in their own right, and inclusion of these restorations would increase the prevalence figures for root surface decay. There are three possible solutions which have been adopted to counter this problem: firstly, a restored surface can be discounted as far as caries revalence is concerned (Vehkalahti *et al.* 1983); secondly, some allowance can be made for the problem, e.g. areas of restored tooth structure that appeared to be related to tooth-brush abrasion were not recorded as restored root caries (Hix and O'Leary 1976); or finally, all carious and restored surfaces can be included as 'root caries' (Beck *et al.* 1985). Each solution brings with it further difficulties in terms of under or overestimation of the prevalence of root caries.

Distribution within the mouth

There is a characteristic distribution for root caries lesions within the oral cavity (Katz *et al.* 1982; Fejerskov *et al.* 1985; Katz *et al.* 1985), with an increased prevalence in mandibular molar teeth, followed by maxillary anterior teeth, and maxillary posteriors. Manibular anteriors seem to be least susceptible to root car-

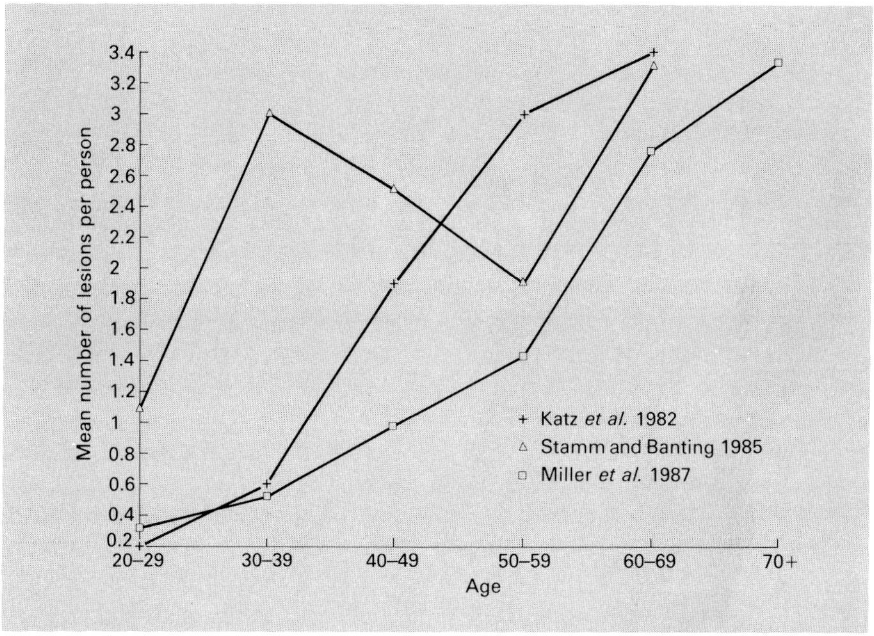

Fig. 9.3. A graphical presentation of the data from a number of studies illustrating the increase in the number of root carious lesions per person with increasing age. This trend is independent of the population studied.

ies. In addition, the buccal and interproximal surfaces are more susceptible to attack than the palatal or lingual aspects of affected teeth.

This perceived pattern of attack may be distorted by two factors. Firstly, the pattern of tooth loss amongst the elderly will influence the perceived pattern of root caries. There is a well-established pattern of tooth loss with increasing age (Fig. 9.4) (van Wyk *et al.* 1977). It may be that those teeth lost would be the most susceptible to root caries, and those retained would have relatively low susceptibility yet are seen as carious in numbers out of proportion to their 'true susceptibility' as they are the only teeth present.

Secondly, the high prevalence rates on buccal tooth surfaces may be a reflection of their susceptibility to cervical abrasion, which is subsequently restored.

Risk factors

The increasing prevalence of root surface caries with increasing age is probably a reflection of increased root exposure in the mouth rather than ageing. As would be expected, subjects with periodontal disease have an increased level of root surface caries; however, the attack rate is greater for those with untreated periodontal disease than after periodontal care (Hix and O'Leary, 1976). It is important to realize that root surface exposure does not automatically lead to root

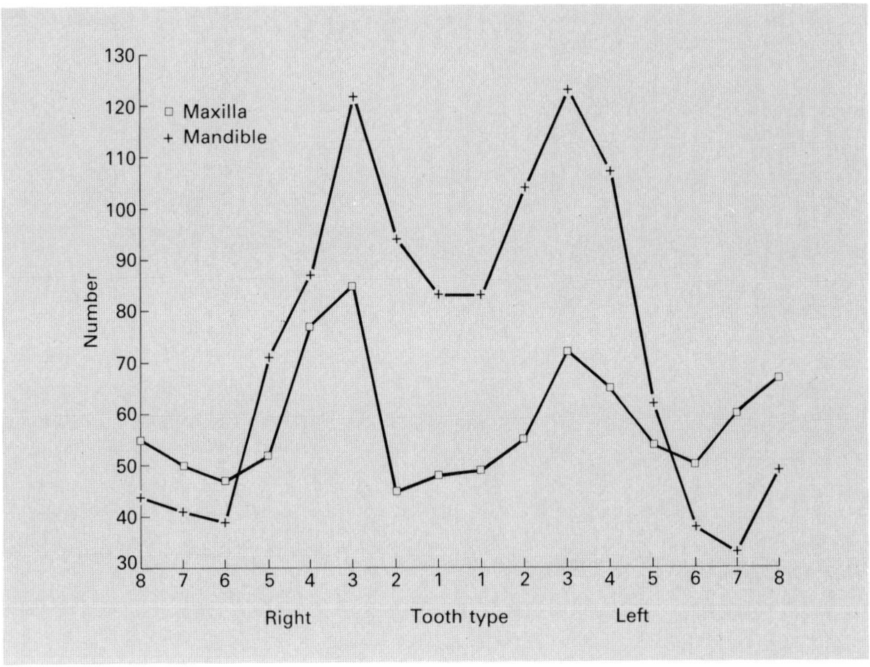

Fig. 9.4. The pattern of tooth retention in an ageing population. (After van Wyk *et al.* 1977.)

caries. Indeed, one report from a developing country whose inhabitants exhibit extensive gingival recession with age found virtually no root caries (Muya *et al.*in Fejerskov and Nyvad 1986), whereas a second report from a primitive culture found very high levels of root surface caries, which correlated well with the high levels of periodontal destruction (Schamschula *et al.* 1974). It may be that the root surface within a periodontal pocket, or protected from the oral environment as a result of periodontal architecture, is at greater risk than when it is fully exposed.

High levels of root surface caries have also been reported in chronically ill, institutionalized, older adults (Banting *et al.* 1980), drug addicts (Hecht and Friedman 1949), and in individuals with altered salivary function, either as a result of a disease process or radiation-induced damage to the salivary glands (Fig. 9.5) (Wescott *et al.* 1975).

The prevalence of root surface caries has been correlated with the number of 'fermentable carbohydrate assaults' (Hix and O'Leary, 1976), and there may be a relationship between coronal caries experience and root caries experience. The majority of workers who have related root caries to coronal caries have found that the individuals with decayed or filled root surfaces had greater experience of decayed or restored coronal surfaces (Banting *et al.* 1980; Beck *et al.* 1985; Burt

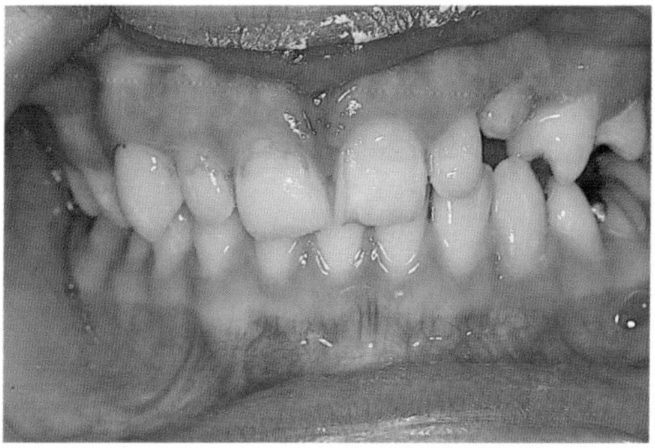

Plate 9.1. Extensive buccal tooth surface loss on the upper central and upper left lateral incisors. This subject chewed lemons as part of a 'diet'. The extensive wear occurred over a 2-year period.

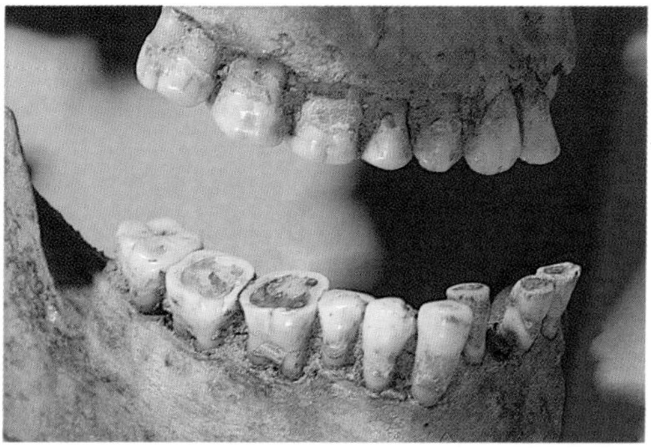

Plate 9.2. The characteristic flat occlusal table and broad contact areas of a 'primitive man'. This pattern of tooth wear is thought to be associated with a coarse, abrasive diet. (Illustration courtesy of Dr A. D. G. Beynon).

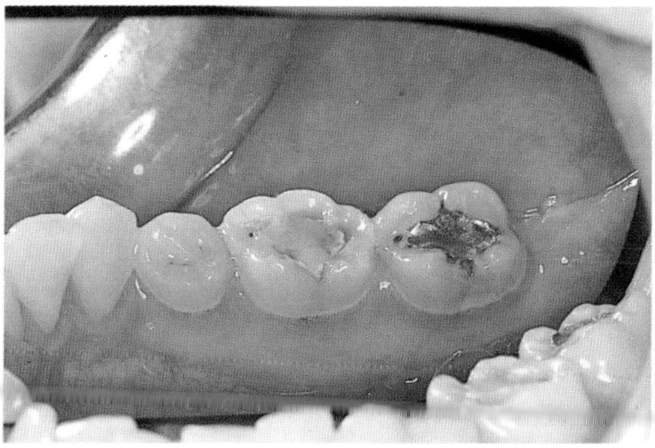

Plate 9.3. Extensive tooth wear of the lower right first molar in a 23-year-old man. There is also faceting of the lower first premolar and anterior teeth. This subject gave a history of recurrent regurgitation of stomach contents between the ages of 9 and 14 years, and admitted a clenching/grinding habit.

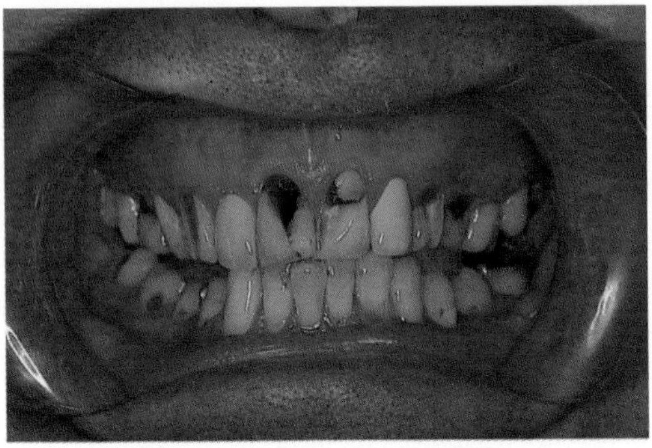

Plate 9.4. Marked tooth wear of the buccal surfaces of the upper anterior teeth. The two upper lateral incisors had been restored with porcelain bonded to metal crowns. Note the caries occurring in the exposed coronal dentine. This subject worked in a brick works and had not worn the protective mask provided by his employer. The abrasive dust laden atmosphere probably contributed to the buccal tissue loss. Eighteen months prior to this picture being taken, he had transferred to office work. This change in local environment allowed the carious lesions to develop on the exposed dentine surfaces.

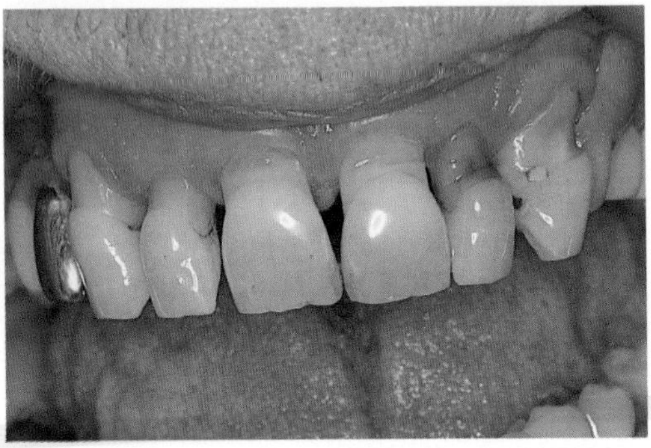

Plate 9.5. V- or U-shaped notching at the exposed cervical root surface, beneath the cement–enamel junction. This pattern of tooth wear may be associated with an improper oral hygiene technique.

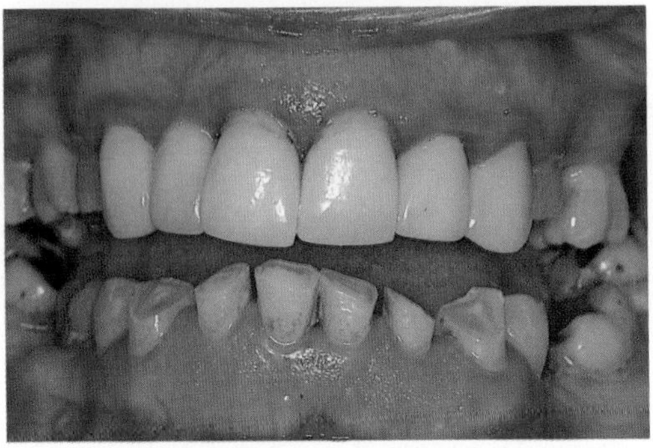

Plate 9.6. Gross destruction of the lower anterior teeth associated with rough, over-contoured, palatal surfaces on the porcelain bonded to metal restorations in the upper arch. The upper restorations had been in place for between 6 and 10 years.

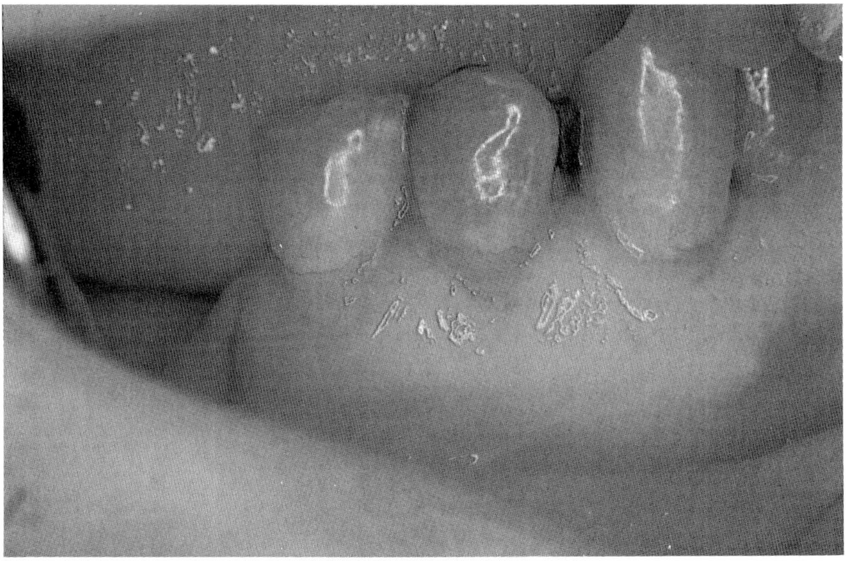

Fig. 9.5. Extensive and rapidly developing root surface caries lesions in an individual with radiation-induced xerostomia. This patient had a pharyngeal carcinoma; both parotid and submandibular glands were involved in the irradiated field.

et al. 1986 (in an optimally fluoridated community); Vehkalahti 1987), or previous root caries experience (Banting *et al.* 1985). However, other workers (Sumney *et al.* 1973; Banting *et al.* 1985) have not been able to demonstrate a correlation with coronal caries experience. Two large studies have demonstrated slightly higher prevalence rates for males than females (Vehkalahti *et al.* 1983; Katz *et al.* 1985).

The various 'at risk' groups have relatively little in common, except perhaps the chronically ill/drug addict/impaired salivary flow group, who may all suffer from a combination of impaired oral hygiene and altered salivary protection at the root surface.

Microbiology and histology

It is well established that coronal decay is a disease process of microbial origin. There is no doubt that bacteria have a similar part to play in the aetiology of root surface caries. There is, however, some debate concerning the species of bacteria that are responsible for root surface lesions in man. *Streptococcus mutans* is of prime importance in initiating coronal caries, although other species may be of greater significance in extension of the carious lesion into dentine. The bacterial species most commonly associated with root surface caries are *Actinomyces viscosus/naeslundii*, *Strep. mutans* and lactobacilli.

A. viscosus is one of the dominant species, and has been reported as constituting up to 40 per cent of the cultivable flora of root surface caries plaque (Syed *et al.* 1975). Animal studies have also demonstrated that *A. viscosus* can cause both periodontal destruction and root surface caries in rodents (Socransky *et al.* 1970, Jordan *et al.* 1972). However, it has been demonstrated that, although Actinomyces species can frequently be isolated from root surface plaque, there is *no difference* in the prevalence or proportion of isolation of Actinomyces species between carious and caries-free root surfaces (Bryan *et al.* 1985; Ellen *et al.* 1985*a*). This may be a reflection of the predominance of *A. viscosus* in mature root-surface plaque (Kmet *et al.* 1985).

Strep. mutans and lactobacilli can also be isolated from root-surface caries plaque in varying proportions (Brown *et al.* 1983; Ellen *et al.* 1984, 1985*b*). Ellen *et al.* (1984, 1985*b*)have correlated the detection of *Strep. mutans* and lactobacilli, even at very low levels, with the development of root surface caries within that individual. This pattern held true for the mouth as a whole, but was not site-specific—i.e. if *Strep. mutans* and/or lactobacilli were encountered then it was more likely that that individual would develop root caries somewhere in their mouths, although not necessarily at the site of sampling. The development of root surface caries, in periodontally involved subjects, has also been correlated with the frequency of ingestion of fermentable carbohydrates (Hix and O'Leary 1976), and with high salivary lactobacillus counts (Ravald and Hamp 1981).

The macroscopic and microscopic appearance of root surface lesions will depend upon the stage of progression of the disease. A root surface that is exposed in the mouth will take up mineral from oral fluids forming a hypermineralized surface layer. This phenomenon occurs whether the root surface is dentine or cementum (Selvig 1969; Westbrook *et al.* 1974; Hals and Selvig 1977). The hypermineralized layer is not present on root surfaces that have not been exposed in the mouth (Hals and Selvig 1977). The early root caries lesion is characterized by demineralization beneath this hypermineralized surface. Demineralization is accompanied by dissolution of apatite crystals and splitting of the collagen bundles within the dentine matrix (Furseth 1970; Furseth and Johansen 1971). Clinically detectable softening of the root surface occurs at a relatively early stage of the lesion, with surface breakdown at a number of discrete, localized sites (Ferjerskov and Nyvad 1986). Bacterial penetration into the demineralized surface occurs rather quickly after the onset of decay, but the rate of progression of the lesion is slow, resulting in a clinical picture of extensive, but shallow, carious lesions on the root surface.

Prevention

In addition to its role in reducing coronal caries prevalence, long-term exposure to a water supply containing optimum levels (1 p.p.m. or *pro rata* for the climatic conditions) of fluoride has a beneficial effect in reducing the prevalence of root surface caries (Stamm and Banting 1978, 1980; Brustman 1986). However, the reduction in caries prevalence is not as great as that for coronal lesions. The preventive effect may be 'dose-related', as it has been reported that the attack rate

Table 9.1. Composition of a 'remineralizing mouthwash' (Johansen *et al.* (1987))

Calcium	5 mM
Phosphate	3 mM
Fluoride	0.25 mM (5 p.p.m.)
Stabilized with Sodium Chloride at pH 7.0	

amongst citizens in a population with 3.5 mg/l fluoride in their water supply is significantly less than that for subjects exposed to 0.7 mg/l (both populations had a natural fluoridated water supply in New Mexico, where 0.7 mg/l was deemed optimal). The RCI figures for the two populations were 1.22 and 6.68 per cent respectively (Burt *et al.* 1986).

Subjects who have suffered the ravages of periodontal disease are 'at risk' of root surface caries. However, it has been demonstrated that the development of new carious lesions can be prevented, during the maintenance phase of treatment, by vigorous and regular individual and professional tooth cleaning (Lindhe and Nyman 1975). It is debatable whether this level of motivation and professional support could be made available on a wide scale. In addition, such vigorous oral hygiene may lead to iatrogenic problems of its own (*vide infra*). Current stratagems during the maintenance phase of periodontal care include the use of sodium or stannous fluoride mouth-rinses, fluoride-containing prophylaxis pastes, and topical use of acidulated phosphate fluoride (APF) gels. This latter medicament is apparently useful in preventing dentine sensitivity as well as radicular decay (Ramfjord 1987).

A variety of regimens have been described for the prevention and remineralization of root surface caries in individuals with reduced salivary flow, either as a result of radiation or gland dysfunction. All of these include the use of topical fluorides, either as a mouth rinse (Davis *et al.* 1985), or in gel form. 0.4 per cent stannous fluoride (Wescott *et al.* 1975). 1.1 per cent neutral sodium fluoride (Daly *et al.* 1972; Dreizen *et al.* 1977), and 1.23 per cent APF (Johansen and Olsen 1979) gels have been advocated. Stannous fluoride and neutral sodium fluoride gels were proposed for daily use in custom-fitted polyvinyl guards. Johansen and Olsen (1979) took a different approach, with an initial phase of daily application of APF gel for 4 weeks and a 'remineralizing mouthwash' (Table 9.1), followed by a 'maintenance phase' using the mineralizing mouthwash alone (in conjunction with a fluoride-containing dentifrice and salivary stimulation with sugar-free chewing-gum) for the duration of the study. This approach was modified to exchange neutral sodium fluoride for the APF gel in a later study (Johansen *et al.* 1987). All of these treatments are of benefit in the xerostomic patient, giving a reduction in caries prevalence. Johansen *et al.* (1987) claim a high level of remineralization of root surface lesions with their intensive regimen. In addition to a sodium fluoride rinse, Davis *et al.* (1985) used a combined sodium fluoride and chlorhexidine gluconate rinse, and found it to have similar benefit to the sodium fluoride preparation. It may be that, in addition to their remineralizing role, many of these treatments act by reducing the *Strep. mutans* colonization of the root surface (Brown *et al.* 1983; Keene *et al.* 1984).

The second aspect of management for individuals with reduced salivary flow is salivary substitution with some form of oral lubricant. A number of 'salivary substitutes' attempt to increase salivary flow with an acid stimulus. These substances can cause demineralization of tooth tissue in their own right, and should not be used in partially dentate individuals (Kidd and Joyston-Bechal 1984). There are a number of commercially available salivary substitutes; the effects of these agents upon enamel *in vitro* have been reported by Joyston-Bechal and Kidd (1987). They found that two commercial products (Luborant and Saliva Orthana) contained 2 p.p.m. fluoride with a pH in the region of 6.7. These agents proved to be very acceptable remineralizing media for enamel *in vitro*.

There has been some debate as to whether topical fluoride treatments would have similar benefits in caries-susceptible individuals with 'normal' salivary function because of enhanced clearance of the topical agent from the mouth. Johansen *et al.* (1987) reported on the use of the sodium fluoride remineralizing solution/fluoride dentifrice/chewing-gum regimen in 30 subjects in a dental practice and 90 subjects in a dental school. All subjects exhibited high caries activity in both coronal and radicular sites. None of the carious lesions were restored at the outset of the trial. Their results after up to 6 years of follow-up demonstrate 'remineralization' of 50–60 per cent of radicular and 50 per cent of coronal carious lesions, and virtually no new lesions amongst the treatment group. There was a trend for the results in 'healthy' individuals to be better than in those who were 'ill'.

Management of root surface caries

Root surface caries can provide the restorative dentist with a severe clinical problem, especially if the decay extends subgingivally or into the furcation region of periodontally involved molar teeth.

There are three possible treatment modalities;

1. Prevention/remineralization, using fluoride gels and/or mouth rinses, with or without a 'remineralizing' mouth rinses and/or chlorhexidine gluconate mouth rinse.

There is little doubt that remineralization of a carious root surface lesion is practicable, using a combination of a supersaturated, fluoride-containing calcium phosphate solution and/or some form of long-term topical fluoride therapy (Mellberg 1986). One drawback of this approach is that the remineralized tissue takes on the appearance of an arrested carious lesion. The surface is dark brown or black with a leathery texture intially, and will eventually harden to give a polished highly mineralized layer. Some patients may not be prepared to tolerate this discoloration of the root surface.

2. Surface recontouring

It has been suggested that the earliest form of interceptive management for root caries should simply comprise removal of the softened dentine, followed by recontouring of the root architecture to give a smooth, cleansable surface. The freshly exposed dentine is treated with topical fluoride agents to stimulate the formation of a hypermineralized surface layer (Banting and Ellen 1976). This technique is attractive, in that it corrects the problems without a restoration but does not have the potential complication of aesthetic impairment of the root surface. It does, however, result in the removal of tooth tissue, which must produce some 'waisting' of the root surface contour. In addition, it has been demonstrated that the carious process extends beyond the junction with 'clinically sound dentine' in the majority of cases (Billings *et al.* 1982). The significance of this finding in terms of progression of the disease process is unclear.

This approach is only applicable for shallow lesions, where excellent results have been reported (Billings *et al.* 1985).

3. Restoration of the defect

Once the carious lesion has become well established, repair using an appropriate restorative material will become necessary. A wide variety of materials—amalgam, gold, composite resin, and glass polyalkenoate (ionomer) cements—have been used for restoration of the root surface. Silver amalgam and gold have the disadvantage that they require finite cavity form, and the cavity design must provide some form of mechanical retention. These two requirements inevitably result in destruction of sound tooth tissue beyond the margins of, and deep to, the lesion. In addition, neither material is tooth-coloured and thus they may not be acceptable to the patient when placed in the front of the mouth.

There are two 'aesthetic' restorative materials that are commonly used in this situation, composite resin and glass ionomer cements. Until recently, it was necessary to provide mechanical retention for composite material. However, a number of commercially available 'dentine bonding agents' are now available to provide a chemical bond between either the organic or the inorganic phase of dentine and the resin phase of a composite. The long-term durability of these systems has not been proven as yet, because they have not been available for sufficient time. It is likely that their success will be greatest in relatively shallow cavities where a large surface area of dentine is available for bonding and there is low bulk within the composite material. These criteria are met when restoring root surface caries.

Glass ionomer cements are also adhesive materials, which bind to the mineral component of dentine and enamel. Their physical properties are inferior to those of the composite resins, but are more than adequate for restoration of root surface caries (Walls 1986). The majority of the clinical trials of glass polyalkenoate cements have concerned their usage in restoration of cervical deficiencies in tooth substance (these have been summarized by Knibbs 1988). The results of the early clinical trials were mixed, with some problems of retention of material in non-undercut cavities, and of colour match with the adjacent tooth structure. More recent results are somewhat better, with very good retention and much better aesthetics. These improvements have been brought about as a result of modifications to the material, and greater awareness on behalf of clinicians of the techniques required for successful use of an adhesive restorative material. One major advantage of these cements is that they leach fluoride into the local environment, which has been shown to exhibit a caries-inhibitory effect upon adjacent tooth substance *in vitro* (Kidd 1978; Wesenberg and Hals 1980; Hicks 1986).

If the aesthetics of a glass polyalkenoate cement restoration prove unacceptable, then it is possible to use the cement as an adhesive lining material by removing a surface layer, etching the cement surface, and replacing the surface with a composite resin (McLean *et al.* 1985).

Tooth wear

Tooth wear can be defined as:

> The loss of mineralized tooth substance from the surface of the teeth, as a result of physical and/or chemical attack. The chemical assault must not be of bacterial origin.

It will occur as a natural phenomenon on all functional or contacting surfaces of the dentition with use in the oral environment. Consequently it would be expected that the quantity of occlusal, interproximal and, to a certain extent, buccal and lingual wear will increase with increasing age of the individual concerned. In certain individuals, wear in excess of this physiological norm will occur; under these circumstances the wear becomes pathological.

There is very little published information concerning the prevalence of tooth wear within the community, or indeed the levels of wear that are 'normal' and/or acceptable for any age group. A number of indices have been described to attempt to quantify the severity of tissue damage. The majority of these focus upon one particular 'type' of wear, i.e. cervical wear, and are only applicable for that specific pattern of tissue loss. One recently proposed index (Smith and Knight 1984*a*) attempted to overcome this problem by subjectively scoring every visible surface of a tooth for wear. A set of approximate 'population norms' were established by examining a small group of patients within three dental hospitals (100 subjects in all). The same authors have described the use of this index as an adjunct during the diagnostic phase, for subjects with a worn dentition, in an endeavour to clarify any aetiological factors from the pattern of wear within an individual compared to the 'population norm' (Smith and Knight 1984*b*).

There are some epidemiological data concerning the prevalence of cervical wear within the community. Sognnaes *et al.* (1972) examined nearly 11 000 extracted teeth, 18 per cent of which 'had typical patterns of erosion-like lesions'. They were unable to give an age-related breakdown of their results. Xhonga and Valdmanis (1983) found that approximately 25 per cent of their sample of adults exhibited tooth cervical damage. This figure increases to 56 per cent amongst an elderly population (Hand *et al.* 1986). Premolars are the most frequently involved teeth, followed by incisors in all age groups (Xhonga and Valdmanis 1983; Hand *et al.* 1986). In subjects with cervical tooth wear, the lesions progress at between 1 and 2 μm per day (Nordhe and Skogedal 1982; Xhonga *et al.* 1972).

Aetiology

Physiological wear

There are three mechanisms for tooth wear:

Erosion The progressive loss of hard tooth substance by chemical dissolution, not involving bacterial action.

Attrition The progressive loss of hard tooth substance caused by mastication, or contact between occluding or approximal surfaces.

Abrasion The progressive loss of hard tooth substance caused by mechanical factors other than mastication or tooth to tooth contacts.

Tooth wear, as a result of normal function, will be a product of all three of these mechanisms. Attrition or abrasion will occur, to a limited extent, with sound tooth tissue. These two mechanical effects will potentiate the damage caused by an erosive component, as the softened surface produced after acid attack will be more readily removed by mechanical trauma. Whilst the definition of erosion precludes damage caused by bacterial acid production, it may be that this is of significance during wear of exposed root surfaces. The dentine of an exposed root surface is relatively soft and consequently prone to mechanical damage; any further softening, via an erosive element which may include plaque acids, will only potentiate this.

Pathological wear

Pathological wear is normally the product of an exacerbation of one of the mechanisms responsible for 'physiological wear'. This tends to result in a pattern of tooth tissue loss that may be of use in determining the cause of wear in a particular clinical situation (Table 9.2). A variety of aetiological factors have been implicated for wear with a preponderance of erosion or attrition or abrasion.

Erosion. Sognnaes (1963) has postulated three linked 'mechanisms of hard tissue destruction' which may occur during erosion:

(1) absence or loss of a protective salivary organic coating on a tooth;

(2) loss of mineral from the tooth surface with a decalcifying agent (either extrinsic or intrinsic);

(3) destruction of decalcified tooth tissue with biochemical and/or biophysical and/or mechanical action.

Table 9.2. Pattern of tooth loss with different aetiological agents

Erosion	The worn surface will be smooth with a dull surface finish. Acid-resistant restorations will stand proud the surrounding tooth tissue.
Dietary	The pattern of loss will depend upon the dietary habit. e.g. An individual who chews citrus fruits will lose tissue from the incisal and labial aspects of the upper incisors (Plate 9.6).
Medicinal	Tissue loss from the occlusal surfaces of the lower molars and the occlusal and palatal surfaces of the uppers.
Gastric Reflux	Tissue loss from the occlusal surfaces of the molars and the palatal aspects of the upper anteriors and premolars.
Occupational	Tissue loss from the surfaces exposed to acid attack, classically the buccal surfaces of the upper and lower anterior teeth.
Attrition	Smooth polished surfaces with multiple facets that are mirror images of each other. Pitting of the worn surface will occur when there is a significant element of erosion allied to the attrition (Plate 9.8).
Abrasion	Smooth polished defects in the mineralized surfaces of the teeth. The pattern of tissue loss will correspond to the abrasive stimulus.
Industrial	Loss of buccal contour from the surfaces exposed to environmental polution. The appearance will be similar to that for erosive industrial damage.
Iatrogenic	Damage to tooth substance as a result of improper use of oral hygiene aids giving notching or waisting at the gingival margin. Use of abrasive dentifrices can cause marked damage to the buccal enamel of upper anterior teeth, giving dish-shaped wear facets.

Whilst it is probable that loss of the protective function of saliva (both buffering and as an organic coating) would result in exacerbated erosion, this is not borne out by clinical data from individuals with impaired salivary function. However, the pattern of dental decay in these individuals, if left untreated, is so extensive and rapidly progressing that any underlying tendency for increased erosion would be very difficult to detect. Equally, treatment regimes for the xerostomic patient may have some benefit in helping to overcome erosive tooth damage.

A number of sources of extrinsic or intrinsic acids or chelating agents have been described in the literature (Table 9.3) which may be responsible for tooth loss (Plate 9.1). The pattern of tissue loss is not the same for all sources of decalcifying agent, indeed it can be almost pathognomonic of the particular form of damage (Table 9.2).

Attrition. Wear as a result of tooth to tooth contact will cause an increase in the area of teeth in contact, and may result in increased masticatory efficiency (Woda *et al.* 1987). The extent of attrition will depend upon the use to which an individual (or race) puts their teeth. It is well documented that attrition is increased in populations where the teeth are used as a tool (i.e. Eskimos, etc.) and in primitive tribal groups or early man, where the diet has a greater abrasive component (Plate 9.2) (Lavelle 1973; Murphy 1959; Begg 1954). Lavelle (1973) also reported a marked decrease in attrition amongst the population of Britain when comparing Romano-British skulls to those of the nineteenth century.

Table 9.3. Possible demineralizing agents that have been implicated in the aetiology of erosive tooth wear. (Adapted from Giunta 1983)

Dietary
Fruits
(lemons, oranges, bananas, etc.)
Fruit juices
Carbonated beverages
(both 'Diet' and 'normal')
Vinegar
Vitamin C
Medicinal
HCl replacement
Vitamin C
Aspirin
Regurgitation
Hiatus hernia
Chronic alcoholism
(recurrent vomiting)
Anorexia nervosa
Occupational
Industrial acid
Idiopathic
'Acid saliva'

Parafunctional clenching or grinding habits will produce abnormal patterns of wear (Pavone 1985), indeed Xhonga (1977) has reported a four-fold increase in the rate of loss of tooth tissue in bruxists compared to non-bruxist controls. The aetiology of such habits is a complex mixture of psychological, emotional, dental, systemic, occupational, and idiopathic factors (see Pavone 1985). The systemic problems include abnormal jaw movements associated with tardive dyskinesias, which are more common in an elderly population (Karmen 1975). There may be an erosive component contributing to the magnitude of tooth tissue loss in a bruxist. If this is the case, any exposed dentine surfaces will be worn away more rapidly than the enamel, producing 'cupping' of the contact surfaces, with contact between the enamel margins of the defect alone (Plate 9.3).

Abrasion. There are two forms of attack which may be responsible for generalized abrasive wear of the dentition. Firstly, individuals who work in an environment polluted by abrasive dust particles (i.e. coal mine, brick works), and who fail to wear a protective mask, may suffer abrasive wear on any tooth surfaces exposed during speech (Plate 9.4). In addition, such individuals may have a pattern of wear similar to that of a bruxist or a primitive tribesman because of the presence of an abrasive paste in their mouths during normal function.

Secondly, the use and abuse of dental scaling instruments and/or oral hygiene aids (Epstein 1976; Bevenius *et al.* 1988). All of the 'normal' oral hygiene aids—tooth-brushes, dental floss, 'bottle brushes'—can produce abrasive wear. The most common site of damage is the exposed root surface, where the softer dentine is easily damaged during oral hygiene procedures. The classical picture is that of a V- or U-shaped defect immediately apical to the cemento-enamel junction of an exposed tooth surface (Plate 9.5). This is usually attributed to improper use of a tooth brush; a horizontal scrubbing action, the use of excessive force, hard brush bristles, increased brushing frequency, and the use of an excessively abrasive dentifrice, are factors in the severity or rapidity of damage.

Other patterns of damage may be associated with the over-zealous or improper use of dental floss and interdental 'bottle brushes', where grooving or waisting of the root surface is a problem. This form of destruction is a complication during the maintenance phase of management in patients with periodontally involved teeth and extensive root surface exposure.

There is some correlation between clinical signs of clenching or grinding habits (notably occlusal faceting) and the presence of cervical 'erosions' in the same patient (Xhonga 1977; Pavone 1985). It remains unclear whether this is a cause-and-effect relationship, or whether those individuals whose personalities predispose to their developing a clenching or grinding habit are also those who would use an improper oral hygiene technique.

Enamel will also be lost as a result of tooth brush/dentifrice abrasion. This results in blurring of the surface anatomy of the tooth, but is unlikely to cause clinically significant damage unless a very abrasive dentifrice is used. Dentifrices designed to remove stain associated with tobacco smoking or those which 'whiten the teeth' are sufficiently abrasive to cause marked enamel damage. Their use should be discouraged.

Localized abrasive wear is usually the result of some form of habit. An example of this would be notching of the incisal edges of teeth as a product of holding pins or tacks between the teeth at work. Equally, grooving of a small segment of the dentition by a pipe-stem would fall into this category. It has been suggested that an active partial denture clasp may cause cervical abrasion if it rests on a dentine surface.

One final group of individuals for whom abrasive wear may be a problem are the quadraplegics, who often use their teeth as a tool, either for communication or artistic purposes. Great care must be taken to design any necessary appliances to minimize damage to tooth tissue.

Prevention and management

The management of a patient presenting with a worn dentition falls into three areas: firstly, diagnosis, treatment planning, and the elimination of any aetiological factors (if possible); secondly, the restorative reconstruction of the worn dentition; and finally, a maintenance phase, where the patient is taught how to care for their reconstructed mouth without causing further iatrogenic wear. The complexities of treatment planning and restorative reconstruction are beyond the scope of this chapter.

There are few measures, beyond instruction in 'correct' use of oral hygiene aids, which can be regarded as preventing tooth wear, especially when a degree of wear is to be expected with increasing age. However, there are a number of steps that can be taken, once diagnosis of pathological wear has been made, to prevent the condition from getting any worse. These procedures are all designed to negate the aetiological factor which has become dominant in the wear process.

Erosion

It is obvious that removal of the decalcifying agents in erosive wear will help to arrest its progress. It should be relatively easy to perform dietary counselling for a subject whose erosion is of dietary origin. This should arrest the rapid progress of the tissue loss, if the dietary advice is followed.

Achlorhydria is a distressing condition where gastric acids secretion is either markedly diminshed, or fails. One treatment for this is oral ingestion of dilute hydrochloride acid, which can cause marked erosive damage. If this form of treatment is to be followed, then the acid should be sucked through a straw, to minimize contact with tooth surfaces. Two preparations are now available in tablet form. Unfortunately, the tablets of betaine hydrochloride must be dissolved in water prior to use. This solution is also markedly acidic and must be sucked through a straw.

A number of medications with low pH have been reported as producing erosive damage (aspirin, chewable vitamin C, 'iron tonic') (Giunta 1983). The ports have usually concerned excessive or abnormal use of these agents, and the erosion can be controlled by modifying the habitual pattern of use, or changing the form of medication, e.g. by using vitamin C tablets rather than the chewable form.

Erosion as a result of gastric regurgitation may present a more complex problem. Any preventitive measures should begin with eliminating the cause if at all possible. Subjects who are suspected as suffering from anorexia nervosa with bulimia, or chronic alcoholism with vomiting, should be referred to a physician or phychiatrist for medical help. There are a number of medicaments which may cause nausea or vomiting as a side-effect. The patient's physician could be consulted to see if an alternative therapeutic agent is available. Regurgitation as a result of incompetence of the cardiac sphincter at the base of the oesophagus can cause severe erosion, because reflux is more common when the patient is supine but salivary secretion (and hence protection) is at its lowest at night. Once again medical/surgical advice should be sought.

If there is an obvious time during which reflux/regurgitation occurs, then it may be possible to protect the dentition using a soft splint. This should extend well onto the palatal mucosa in the upper arch, and it may be of benefit to place a fluoride gel or antacid preparation inside the splint before use. (Kleier *et al.* 1984).

It has been demonstrated that a fissure-sealed enamel surface would be more resistant to acid attack than a non-sealed surface (Silverstone 1975). As a result it has been suggested that resin impregnation of the surface of a crown (after etching) may help to prevent erosive wear. Whilst this is attractive, and may be of benefit on non-functional surfaces, it has been shown that a resin-impregnated surface is considerably softer than an intact enamel surface (Davidson and Bekke-Hoekstra 1980). Consequently the 'sealed' surface would probably be lost rather rapidly as a result of attrition, which would then expose the fresh enamel surface to further erosion. This process would negate the benefits of sealing the surface in the first place.

If the acidic attack is of industrial origin, then appropriate measures should be taken to protect the mouth from acid vapour.

There is some evidence that topical fluoride therapy is of benefit in the control of erosive tooth tissue loss (Davis and Winter 1977). Indeed, a management regimen similar to that for patients with profound xerostomia (*vide supra*) may be of benefit during the care of patients in whom an aetiological factor cannot be eliminated.

Definitive reconstruction, utilizing full coronal restorations, should be delayed in a case of erosive wear, until the aetiological factors involved have been identified and controlled. The marginal gaps around full coronal restorations would be highly susceptible to acid attack, leading to rapidly progressing decay beneath the restoration, if reconstruction should be done whilst the erosive challenge exists.

Attrition

Wear as a result of normal masticatory function cannot be eliminated—indeed, current thinking that an increase in dietary fibre is beneficial may result, in time, in an increase in occlusal and interproximal wear. The pattern of wear would be similar to that seen in 'primitive man', although the severity should not be as great. The most difficult problem to be surmounted in the care of a subject with attrition is deciding when the perceived wear is in excess of the physiological 'norm' and thus requiring treatment.

The management of a subject with a bruxing habit is a complex subject, depending upon the aetiology of the condition. Management regimens can include occlusal splint therapy, either hard or soft and with or without occlusal adjustment, psychotropic medication, and psychological counselling. There is no evidence concerning the effect of any of these treatment modalities upon wear *per se*. However, on an empirical basis, the provision of some form of occlusal splint should be of benefit. Such splints are made from either a flexible material or an acrylic resin and would act as a buffer, preventing tooth to tooth contact. Any wear would be most likely to occur upon the splint itself, rather than the teeth.

It is important to recognize a bruxing habit in subjects who are undergoing restorative care, especially if full coronal restorations are contemplated. Porcelain is a very hard material, and can have an abrasive surface if poorly glazed or if it has been adjusted and not glazed. Regular contact with opposing natural tooth tissue will result in very rapid wear of the natural tooth, producing a complicated management problem (Plate 9.6). It is always desirable to produce tooth-to-artificial crown contacts on a metallic surface, or, if this is not practicable for aesthetic reasons, on a highly glazed porcelain surface.

Abrasion

Prevention should again be aimed at removing the cause of the damage. Consequently, the use of an appropriate mask in a dust-laden environment, teaching correct oral hygiene techniques, and an alteration in the habitual use of the teeth as a 'third hand' may all be of benefit in preventing the progression of abrasive wear.

Conclusions

Both root surface caries and tooth wear pose problems in the ageing population, especially amongst certain 'at risk' groups.

The management of carious lesions on the root surface can present many difficulties, especially when the lesion occurs in situations that are relatively inaccessible to the restorative dentist. We know it is possible to prevent root surface caries with rigorous personal, and professional, oral hygiene. However, it is impracticable to provide the level of care required to produce this benefit on a national basis, and, in addition, the probabilility of iatrogenic tooth wear to the root surface is very high. It has been demonstrated that topical fluorides are of benefit in helping to prevent root surface decay and, when used in conjunction with a remineralizing solution, may be able to arrest early lesions. The use of these preventive regimens must be extended to include those in the 'at risk' categories for root surface caries, and should be considered for individuals who have high coronal caries experience, and/or exhibit a high prevalence of early root surface lesions.

Tooth wear is a normal functional phenomenon. It can be expected to increase in magnitude with increasing age of the individual concerned. Physiological wear is a product of *mild* conditions of the following.

Erosion—decalcification of surface mineral from dietary acids.

Attrition—as a result of normal tooth to tooth contact during mastication and deglutition, and from abrasive food substances. This will primarily occur on the occlusal and interproximal tooth surfaces.

Abrasion—routine use of a tooth-brush and dentifrice will cause some loss of mineralized tissue.

When one or more of these mechanisms becomes abnormal in its expression, pathological wear occurs; in this case the wear is greater than the physiological norm.

A large number of aetiological factors can be identified as contributing to pathological wear. The perceived pattern of wear often gives a reasonable indication of the aetiological factors in any one individual. As a degree of wear is normal, the prevention of wear is impracticable. However, once the wear is diagnosed as being pathological, progression can be prevented by eliminating, or counteracting, the aetiological factor(s) concerned. Restorative reconstruction of the damaged dentition can then be undertaken, if this is deemed appropriate.

References

Baker, K.A. and Ettinger, R.L. (1985). Intra-oral effects of drugs in elderly persons. *Gerodontics* **1**, 111–16.

Banting, D.W. and Ellen, R.P. (1976). Carious lesions on the roots of teeth: a review for the general practitioner. *J. Can. dent. Ass.* **42**, 496–502.

Banting, D.W., Ellen, R.P., and Fillery, E.D. (1980). Prevalence of root surface caries among institutionalised older persons. *Commun. Dent. oral Epidemiol.* **8**, 84–8.

Banting, D.W., Ellen, R.P. and Fillery, E.D. (1985). A longitudinal study of root caries: baseline and incidence data. *J. dent. Res.* **64**, 141–4.

Baum, B.J. (1986). Salivary gland function during ageing. *Gerodontics.* **2**, 61–4.

Beck, J.D., Hand, J.S., Hunt, R.J., and Field, M.M. (1985). Prevalence of root and coronal caries in a noninstitutionalized older population. *J. Am. dent. Ass.* **111**, 964–7.

Begg, P.R. (1954). Stone age man's dentition. *Am. J. Orthodont.* **40**, 298–312.

Ben-Aryeh, H., Miron, D., Szargel, R., and Gutman, D. (1984). Whole saliva secretion rates in old and young healthy subjects. *J. dent. Res.* **63**, 1147–8.

Bevenius, J., Angmar-Mansson, B., and Thesander, M. (1988). An elderly patient with iatrogenic damage from repeated scaling. *Gerodotics.* **3**, 181–2.

Billings, R.J., Brown, L.R., and Kaster, A.G. (1985). Contemporary treatment stategies for root surface dental caries. *Gerodontics* **1**, 20–7.

Billings, R.S., Brown L.R., Simmons, F.F., Braden, J.C., and Cadena, L.M. (1982). *In vitro* studies on treatment of incipient root caries. *J. dent. Res.* **61**, 210. (Abstr. 285).

Brown, L.P., Billings, R.J., O'Niell, P.A. Wheatcroft, M.G., and Kater A.G. (1983). Microbiological comparisons of carious and non-carious root and enamel tooth surfaces. *J. dent. Res.* **62**, (spec. iss.), 295. (Abstr. 1137).

Brustman, B.A. (1986). Impact of exposure to fluoride-adequate water on root surface caries in the elderly. *Gerodontics.* **2**, 203–7.

Bryan, A.R., Reynolds, H.S., and Zambon, J.J. (1985). Prevalence of *Actinomyces* species in human root surface caries. *J. dent. Res.* **64**, (spec. iss.), 192 (Abstr. 162).

Burt, B.A., Ismail, A.I., and Eklund, S.A. (1986). Root caries in an optimally fluoridated and a high-fluoride community. *J. dent. Res.* **65**, 1154–8.

Daly, T.E., Drane, J.B., and MacComb, W.S. (1972). Management of the problems of the teeth and jaws in patients undergoing irradiation. *Am. J. Surg.* **124**, 539–42.

Davidson, C.L. and Bekke-Hoekstra, I.A. (1988). The resistance of superficially sealed enamel to wear and carious attack *in vitro*. *J. oral Rehab.* **7**, 299–305.

Davis, B. and Winter, P.J. (1977). Dietary erosion of adult dentine and enamel. Protection with a fluoride toothpaste. *Br. dent. J.* **143**, 116–19.

Davis, J., Harper, D.S., and Hurst, P.S. (1985). NaF and chlorhexidine for prevention of post-irradiation oral disease. *J. dent. Res.* **64**, 206. (Abstr. 287).

Dreizen, S., Brown, L.R., Daly, T.E., and Drane, J.B. (1977). Prevention of xerostomia-related dental caries in irradiated cancer patients. *J. dent. Res.* **56**, 99–104.

Ellen, R.P., Banting, D.W., and Fillery, E.D. (1984). Microbiological assessment of root caries risk in a chronically hospitalized population. *J. dent. Res.* **63**, (spec. iss.), 218. (Abstr. 430).

Ellen, R.P., Banting, D.W., and Fillery, E.D. (1985*a*). Longitudinal microbiological investigation of a hospitalized population of older adults with a high root surface caries risk. *J. dent. Res.* **64**, 1377–87.

Ellen, R.P., Banting, D.W., and Fillery, E.D. (1985*b*). *Streptococcus mutans* and lactobacillus detection in the assessment of dental root surface caries risk. *J. dent. Res.* **64**, 1245–9.

Epstein, J. (1976). Cervical erosion and abrasion. *IADS Newsletter* **4**, 29–43.

Fejerskov, O. *et al.* (1985). Root surface caries in a population of elderly Danes. *J. dent. Res.* **64**, 187. (Abstr. 116).

Fejerskov, O. and Nyvad, B. (1986). Pathology and treatment of dental caries in the aging individual. In *Geriatric dentistry*, (eds. P. Holm-Pedersen and H. Loe), pp. 238–62. Munksgaard, Copenhagen.

Furseth, R. (1970). Further observations on the fine structure of orally exposed and carious human dental cementum. *Archs. oral Biol.* **16**, 71–7.

Furseth, R. and Johansen, E. (1971). The minimal phase of sound and carious human dental cementum studied by electron microscopy. *Acta odont. Scand.* **28**, 305–13.

Gandara, B.K., Izutsu, K.T., Truelove, E.L. Ensign, W.Y., and Sommers, E.E. (1985). Age-related salivary flow rate changes in controls and patients with oral lichen planus. *J. dent. Res.* **64**, 1149–51.

Giunta, J.L. (1983). Dental erosion resulting from chewable vitamin C tablets. *J. Am. dent. Ass.* **107**, 253–6.

Hals, E. and Selvig, K.A. (1977). Correlated electron probe microanalysis and microradiography of carious and normal dental cementum. *Caries Res.* **11**, 62–75.

Hand, J.S., Hunt, R.J., and Reinhardt, J.W. (1986). The prevalence and treatment implications of cervical abrasion in the elderly. *Gerodontics.* **2**, 167–70.

Hazen, S.P., Chilton, N.W., and Mumma, R.D. (1972). The problem of root caries: 3. a clinical study. *J. dent. Res.* **51** (suppl.), 219.

Hecht, S.S. and Friedman, J. (1949). The high incidence of cervical caries among drug addicts. *Oral Surg.* **2**, 1428–42.

Heft, M.W. and Baum, B.J. (1984). Unstimulated and stimulated parotid salivary flow rate in individuals of different ages. *J. dent. Res.* **63**, 1182–5.

Hicks, M.J. (1986). Artificial lesion formation around glass-ionomer restorations in root surfaces: a histological study. *Gerodontics.* **2**, 108–14.

Hix, J.O. and O'Leary, T.J. (1976). The relationship between cemental caries, oral hygiene status and fermentable carbohydrate intake. *J. Perio.* **47**, 394–404.

Johansen, E. and Olsen, T. (1979). Topical fluoride in the prevention and arrest of dental caries. In *Continuing evaluation of the use of fluorides*, AAS Selected Symposium 11. (eds. E. Johansen, D.R. Taves, and T. Olsen). West View Press, Boulder, Colorado.

Johansen, E., Papas, A., Fong, W., and Olson, T.O. (1987). Remineralization of carious lesions in elderly patients. *Gerdontics.* **3**, 47–50.

Jordan, H.V. and Hammond, T.H. (1972). Filamentous bacteria isolated from human root surface caries. *Archs. oral Biol.* **17**, 1333–42.

Joyston-Bechal, S. and Kidd, E.A.M. (1987). The effect of three commercially available saliva substitutes on enamel *in vitro*. *Br. dent. J.* **163**, 187–90.

Karmen, S. (1975). Tardive dyskinesia. A significant syndrome for geriatric dentistry. *Oral Surg.* **39**, 52–7.

Katz, R.V. (1985). Development of an index for the prevalence of root caries. *J. dent. Res.* **63**, 814–18.

Katz, R.V., Hazen, S.P., Chilton, N.W. and Mumma, R.D. (1982). Prevalence and intra-oral distribution of root surface caries in an adult population. *Caries Res.* **16**, 265–71.

Katz, R.V., Newitter, D.A., and Clive, J.M. (1985). Root caries prevalence in adult dental patients. *J. dent. Res.* **64**, 293 (Abstr. 1069).

Keene, H.J., Fleming, J., Brown, L.R., and Dreizen, S. (1984). *Lactobacilli* and *S. mutans* in cancer patients using fluoride gels. *J. dent. Res.* **63** (spec. iss.), 218. (Abstr. 429).

Kidd, E.A.M. (1978). Cavity sealing ability of composite and glass ionomer cement restorations. *Br. dent. J.* **144**, 139–42.

Kidd, E.A.M. and Joyston-Bechal, S. (1984). Mouth lubricants and saliva substitutes. *Caries Res.* **18**, 155. (Abstr. 6).

Kleier, D.J., Aragon, S.B. and Averbach, R.E. (1984). Dental management of the chronic vomiting patient. *J. Am. dent. Ass.* **108**, 618–21.

Kmet, P., Boyar, R., and Bowden, G.L. (1985). Microbial colonization of exposed root surfaces and enamel. *J. dent. Res.* **64** (spec. iss.), 331. (Abstr. 1411).

Knibbs, P.J. (1988). Glass ionomer cement: 10 years of clinical use. *J. oral Rehab.* **14**, 103–15.

Lavelle, C. (1973). Alveolar bone loss and tooth attrition in skulls from different population samples. *J. perio. Res.* **8**, 395–9.

Lindhe, J. and Nyman, S. (1975). The effect of plaque control and surgical pocket elimination on the establishment and maintenance of periodontal health. A longitudinal study of periodontal therapy in cases of advanced disease. *J. clin. Perio.* **2**, 67–79.

Lohse, W.G., Carter, H.G., and Brunelle, J.A. (1977). The prevalence of root surface caries in a military population. *Milit. Med.* **141**, 700–3.

McLean, J.W. Wilson, A.D., Powis, D.R. (1985). The use of glass ionomer cements in bonding composite resins to dentine. *Br. dent. J.* **158**, 410–14.

Mellberg, J.R. (1986) Demineralization and remineralization of root surface caries. *Gerodontal.* **5**, 25–31.

Miller, A.J. *et al.* (1987). *Oral health of United States adults*, United States Department of Health and Human Services. National Institute of Health Publications No. 87–2868.

Murphy, T.R. (1959). The changing pattern of dentine exposure in human tooth attrition. *Am. J. phys. Anthrop.* **17**, 167–78.

Muya, R.J. *et al. Changing and developing dental health services in Tanzania* 1980–2000. Reported in Fejerskov and Nyvad (1986) (*vide supra*).

Norde, H. and Skogedal, O. (1982). The rate of cervical abrasion in dental students. *Acta odont. Scand.* **40**, 45–7.

Pavone, B.W. (1985) Bruxism and its effect on the natural teeth. *J. prosth. Dent.* **53**, 692–6.

Pedersen, W., Schubert M., Izutsu, K., Mersai, T., and Truelove, E. (1985). Age-dependent decreases in human submandibular gland flow rates as measured under resting and post-stimulation conditions. *J. dent. Res.* **64**, 822–5.

Ramfjord, S.P. (1987). Maintenance care for treated periodontitis patients. *J. clin. Perio.* **14**, 433–7.

Ravald, N. and Hamp, S.E. (1981). Prediction of root surface caries in patients treated for advanced periodontal disease. *J. clin. Perio.* **8**, 400–14.

Schamschula, R.G., Barmes, D.E., Keyes, P.H., and Gulbinat, W. (1974). Prevalence and inter-relationships of root surface caries in Lufa, Papua New Guinea. *Commun. Dent. oral Epidemiol.* **2**, 295–304.

Scott, J. (1986). Structure and function in aging salivary glands. *Gerodontics.* **5**, 149–58.

Selvig, K.A. (1969). Biological changes at the tooth–saliva interface in periodontal disease. *J. dent. Res.* **48**, 846–55.

Silverstone, L.M. (1975). The adic etch technique: *in vitro* studies with special reference to the enamel surface and the enamel–resin interface. In *Proceedings of the International Symposium on the acid etch technique*, (ed. L.M. Silverstone and I.L. Dogon) pp. 13–39. North Carolina Publishing Co., St Pauls, Minnesota.

Smith, B.G.N. and Knight, J.K. (1984*a*). An index for measuring the wear of teeth. *Bri. dent. J.* **156**, 435–8.

Smith, B.G.N. and Knight, J.K. (1984*b*). A comparison of patterns of tooth wear with aetiological factors. *Bri. dent. J.* **157**, 16–19.

Socransky, S.S., Hubersak, C., and Propas, D. (1970). Induction of periodontal destruction in gnotobiotic rats by a human oral strain of *Actinomyces naeslundii*. *Archs oral Biol.* **15**, 993–5.

Sognnaes, R.F. (1963). Dental hard tissue destruction with special reference to idiopathic erosion. In *Mechanisms of hard tissue destruction*, p. 91. American Association for the Advancement of Science, Washington DC.

Sognnaes, R.F., Wolcott, R.B., and Xhonga, F.A. (1972). Dental erosion. 1. Erosion-like patterns occurring in association with other dental conditions. *J. Am. dent. Ass.* **84**, 571–6.

Stamm, J.W. and Banting, D.W., (1978). The occurrence of root caries in adults with a life-long history of fluoridated water consumption. *J. dent. Res.* **57** spec. iss., 149. (Abstr. 298).

Stamm, J.W. and Banting, D.W. (1980). Comparison of root caries prevalence in adults with life-long residence in fluoridated and non-fluoridated communities. *J. dent. Res.* **59** spec. iss., 405. (Abstr. 552).

Stamm, J.W., and Banting, D.W. (1985). Reported in Banting, D.W. (1985). Dental caries. In *Oral health and aging*, (ed. A.F. Tryon) pp. 247–86. PSG Publishing Co., Massachusetts, USA.

Sumney, D.L., Jordan, H.V., and Englander, H.R. (1973). The prevalence of root surface caries in selected populations. *J. Periodontol.* **44**, 500–4.

Syed, S.A., Loesche, W.J., Pape, H.L. jun., and Grenier, E. (1975). Predominant cultivable flora from human root surface carious lesions. *Infect. Immun.* **11**, 727–31.

van Wyk, C.W., Farman, A.C., and Staz, J. (1977). Tooth survival in institutionalised elderly cape coloreds from the Cape Peninsula of South Africa. *Commun. Dent. oral Epidemiol.* **5**, 185–9.

Vehkalahti, M.M. (1987). Relationship between root caries and coronal decay. *J. dent. Res.* **66**, 1608–10.

Vehkalahti, M.M., Rajala, M., Tuomien, R., and Paunio, I. (1983). Prevalence of root caries in an adult Finnish population. *Commun. Dent. oral Epidemiol.* **11**, 188–90.

Walls, A.W.G. (1986) Glass polyalkenoate (glass-ionomer) cements: a review. *J. Dent.* **14**, 231–46.

Wescott, W.B., Starche, E.N., and Shannon, I.L. (1975). Chemical protection against post-irradiation dental caries. *Oral Surg.* **40**, 709–19.

Wesenberg, G. and Hals, E. (1980). The *in vitro* effect of a glass ionomer cement on dentine and enamel walls. *J. oral Rehab.* **7**, 35–42.

Westbrooke, J.L., Miller, A.S., Chilton, N.W., Williams, F.L., and Mumma, R.D.J. (1974). Root surface caries: a clinical, histopathological and microradiographic examination. *Caries Res.* **8**, 249–55.

Woda, A., Gourdon, A.M., and Faraj, M. (1987). Occlusal contacts and tooth wear. *J. pros. Dent.* **57**, 85–93.

Xhonga, F.A. (1977). Bruxism and its effect on the teeth. *J. oral Rehab.* **4**, 65–76.

Xhonga, F.A. and Valdmanis, S. (1983). Geographic comparisons of the increase of dental erosion: a two centre study. *J. oral Rehab.* **10**, 269–77.

Xhonga, F., Wolcott, R.B., and Sognnaes, R.F. (1972). Dental Erosion. II. Clinical measurements of dental erosion progress. *J. Am. dent. Ass.* **84**, 577–82.

10

The prevention and control of chronic periodontal disease

W. M. M. Jenkins

Introduction

'Periodontal disease' is a term which includes all pathological conditions of the periodontium, viz, the gingiva and supporting structures (cementum, periodontal membrane, and alveolar bone). It is, however, commonly used in reference to those diseases—gingivitis and periodontitis—which are plaque-induced and which affect the marginal periodontium.

Gingivitis is an inflammatory response of the gingiva without destruction of the supporting tissues. The commonest form of gingival disease is chronic gingivitis caused by bacterial plaque. In chronic gingivitis, loss of gingival resistance to probing and gingival enlargement occur; these result in a gingival pocket.

Periodontitis is an inflammatory lesion of the supporting structures, the commonest form of which is described as chronic periodontitis. It results from an apical extension of the inflammatory process, initiated in the gingiva. Destruction of the periodontal membrane results in a periodontal pocket.

The pathogenesis of periodontal disease

The appearance of normal healthy periodontium is illustrated diagrammatically in Fig. 10.1a. The oral epithelium is keratinized but the crevicular (sulcular) epithelium and the junctional epithelium are not. The junctional epithelium is attached to the enamel surface and underlying connective tissue by a basal lamina and hemi-desmosomes, and its free surface (from which desquamation takes place) lines the bottom of the histological crevice. The depth of the histological crevice—the distance from the crest of the free gingiva to the coronal extent of the junctional epithelium—measures only 0.5 mm. Clinically, however, the crevice depth is considered to be the distance to which a blunt probe will penetrate and, because it will readily penetrate the fragile junctional epithelium, the clinical crevice depth is more in the order of 2 mm. If gingival recession occurs the junctional epithelium will form an attachment to cementum.

The pathogenesis of gingivitis and of periodontitis are described in detail by

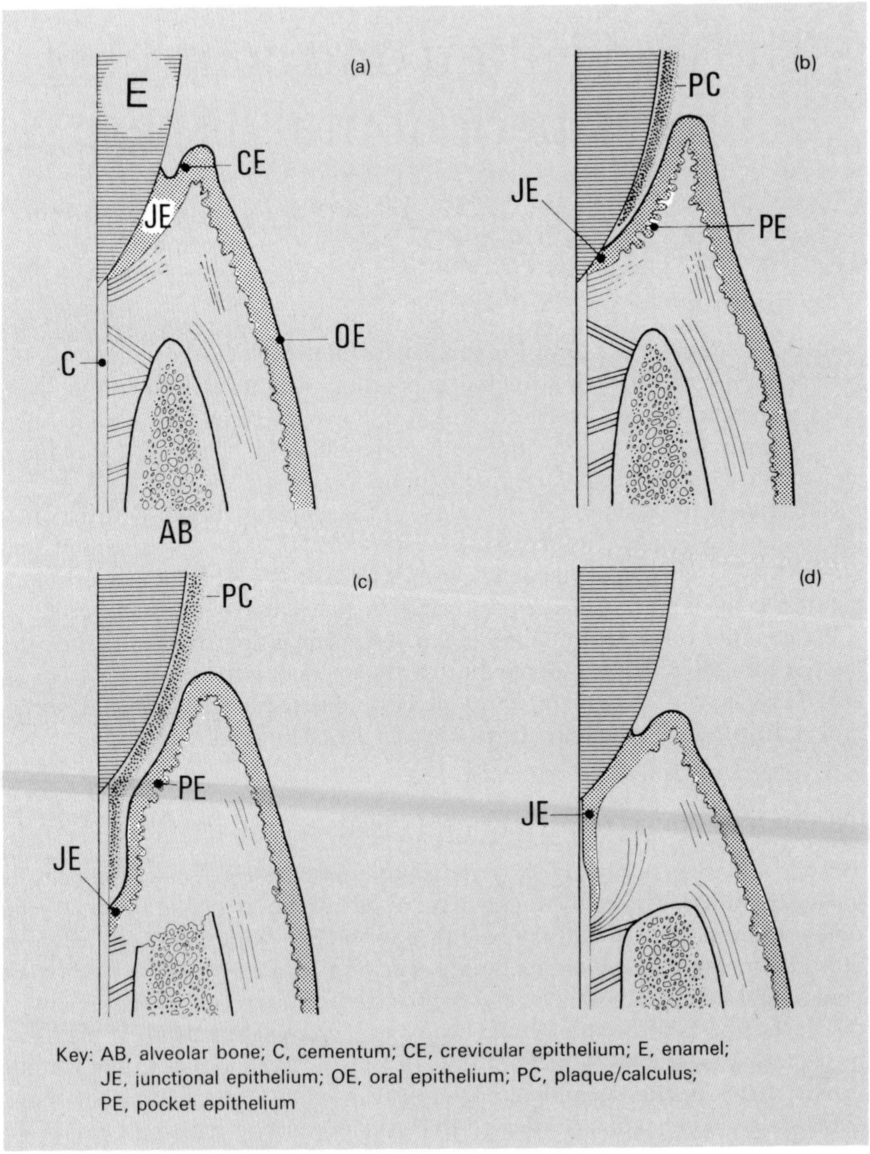

Key: AB, alveolar bone; C, cementum; CE, crevicular epithelium; E, enamel; JE, junctional epithelium; OE, oral epithelium; PC, plaque/calculus; PE, pocket epithelium

Fig. 10.1. (a) Periodontal health. (b) Chronic gingivitis (late phase). (c) Chronic periodontitis. (d) Repair following debridement.

Page (1986) and Listgarten (1986) respectively. When plaque is allowed to accumulate freely there is an acute exudative inflammatory response within 2–4 days in the connective tissue underlying the coronal portion of junctional epithelium. This occurs without clinically detectable changes. After 10–21 days of persistent plaque accumulation, collagen destruction in this zone is marked and a dense infiltrate of chronic inflammatory cells is found. The clinical changes of chronic gingivitis can now be detected: redness, swelling, reduced resistance to probing, and an increased tendency of the gingiva to bleed on probing or when the teeth are brushed.

Bacterial deposits do not extend below the gingival margin in the subclinical stages of developing gingivitis. Gingival enlargement, however, helps to create a subgingival flora as supragingival deposits become located within the gingival pocket. Apical advancement of subgingival plaque occurs at a later stage (Fig. 10.1(b)) as the junctional epithelium separates from the tooth surface and becomes 'pocket epithelium', characterized by the formation and lateral extension of rete pegs, and by areas of micro-ulceration.

After the development of chronic gingivitis, an equilibrium is usually established between the increased mass of bacteria and the host defences, maintaining a state of chronic gingivitis indefinitely. If and when periodontitis does supervene, it is thought to be precipitated either by a proportional increase in pathogenic micro-organisms within the subgingival bacterial flora, by impaired host resistance, or by both factors in combination.

As soon as the destructive process extends apically to affect the alveolar bone and fibre attachment of the root surface, periodontitis is said to have developed (Fig. 10.1(c)). Thus, periodontitis is characterized by loss of (connective tissue) attachment. Junctional epithelium proliferates apically to maintain an epithelial barrier at the base of the deepening pocket, and the denuded cementum becomes contaminated by micro-organisms and their products. Periodontitis is detected most readily with a probe, a blood-stained or purulent exudate being elicited by probing to the base of the pocket beyond the amelo-cemental junction.

Chronic gingivitis is a condition which can be largely reversed by plaque control. Furthermore, the removal of existing plaque and calculus deposits together with pathologically altered cementum, accompanied by daily plaque control, forms the basis of treatment in the early stages of chronic periodontitis. Although loss of fibre attachment is irreversible, repair processes may take place following treatment in which the junctional epithelium is re-established by involution of pocket epithelium and a gingival fibre structure regenerates (Fig. 10.1(d)). More advanced lesions may not respond to treatment without surgical intervention.

Implications for prevention

As gingivitis is caused by supragingival plaque accumulation and as gingivitis is a prerequisite for the development of periodontitis, both diseases can be prevented by an adequate standard of plaque control.

Although there is great variation in individual susceptibility to periodontitis in particular, there are no predictive tests which would single out, for priority preventive care, individuals at high risk of developing rapidly destructive forms of periodontitis. Regular and frequent dental visits are, therefore, indicated to establish and maintain good oral hygiene and to identify inflammatory changes at an early and reversible stage.

Epidemiology

Unlike caries, periodontal disease has existed since ancient times (Ruffer 1921).

Factors affecting the prevalence and severity of periodontal disease

Most of the early population studies of periodontal disease were carried out using the Periodontal Index (PI) (Russell 1956). This is based on a non-linear scale of 0–8 treating gingivitis and periodontitis as different stages in one disease process. The scoring criteria were designed to permit rapid evaluation of every tooth in the dentition and to yield a mean severity score for the mouth or the population group. Studies with the PI were instrumental in establishing that periodontal disease is more common and more severe in males, certain racial groups, individuals of low economic and educational status, older age groups, and groups with inadequate oral hygiene practices. For any particular age group, however, the association between oral hygiene and periodontal disease is so strong as to leave little variation in PI scores to be accounted for by any factor independent of age or oral hygiene. Analysis of the difference in PI scores for males v. females, negroids v. caucasians, high income groups v. low income groups, etc., show that these differences tend to disappear when comparison is limited to groups of the same age with the same standard of oral hygiene. Whether the increase in periodontal disease with advancing age simply reflects the duration of exposure to aetiological agents, rather than the result of the ageing process itself, is not known. This literature is reviewed by Scherp (1964) and Waerhaug (1971).

It should not be overlooked that there is significant variation in periodontal disease experience among different individuals of the same age and standard of oral hygiene; preventive measures, applied randomly to a large group, may not be appropriate for all individuals in that group.

Limitations of the PI

Early epidemiological studies using mean severity scores such as the PI gave rise to the concept of linear progression of periodontal disease from gingivitis, through the early stages of periodontitis, to advanced destruction and tooth loss. This, however, is true only on a population level when the population group is large enough to mask the effect of variation between individuals and between single teeth in the same mouth. It is now known that gingivitis does not necessarily progress to periodontitis and that most periodontitis lesions progress very slowly, if at all. Further criticism of the PI arises from the subjective nature of the scoring criteria, which lead to examiner variability, and from the tendency to underestimate the magnitude of the disease. Recent epidemiological surveys, therefore, have used more stringent criteria, and gingivitis statistics are usually reported separately from periodontitis data. Nevertheless, at present, there are no universally agreed diagnostic criteria, and so comparison of data on the occurrence and distribution of periodontal disease, particularly with respect to periodontitis, reveals enormous variation between surveys (Jenkins and Mason 1984).

Prevalence and severity of gingivitis

In general, the prevalence of gingivitis increases with increasing age, beginning in the deciduous dentition and reaching a peak at puberty. A slight decline during adolescence is then followed by a gradual rise throughout adult life. The age of onset is around 3–5 years (Parfitt 1957; Moller 1963). By puberty almost all children have gingivitis, e.g. 99.4 per cent of 13-year-old children in Scotland (McHugh *et al.* 1964). The severity of gingivitis, like the prevalence rate in children, increases until puberty after which the decline in severity is rather greater than the decline in prevalence (Parfitt 1957). There is a further increase in severity during the third decade to accompany the rising prevalence (Marshall-Day *et al.* 1955). The hormonal changes associated with puberty may be responsible for the peak which is recognized in this age group (Sutcliffe 1972). Alternatively, the rising prevalence before puberty may be attributed to an increase in gingival sites at risk as the permanent dentition develops (Murray 1974). Furthermore, the temporary decline in prevalence and severity after puberty may reflect an increased social awareness and resulting improved oral hygiene (Greene 1963).

In a review of the epidemiology of gingivitis, Stamm (1986) has demonstrated the existence of large variations in the reported prevalence of gingivitis in the deciduous and mixed dentitions. These variations are attributed to the difficulty of applying suitable diagnostic criteria and standards in this age group.

Prevalence and severity of periodontitis

The absolute criterion of periodontitis is the demonstration of inflammation apical to the amelo-cemental junction by the occurrence of bleeding on probing. Such painstaking examination, however, is inappropriate for large epidemiological surveys. Instead, rough estimates of the occurrence of periodontitis have been obtained by enumerating pockets in excess of 3 mm or by measuring loss of attachment or loss of marginal bone on radiographs. None of these methods gives a precise diagnosis. Pockets in excess of 3 mm may occur due to gingival swelling without loss of attachment, while loss of attachment may be accompanied by gingival recession without significant pocketing. Loss of attachment and reduction in alveolar bone height is evidence of previous destruction, not of existing disease. Furthermore, attachment loss may occur due to trauma from oral hygiene devices. The data which follow, therefore, must be interpreted with caution.

Periodontitis in prepubertal children is uncommon. However, loss of attachment affected between 11 and 47 per cent of adolescents in the 12–16-year age range (Lennon and Davies 1974; Hoover *et al.* 1981; Mann *et al.* 1981). In youths, 17 to 26 years of age, and in adults of all ages, loss of attachment was virtually universal (Ismail *et al.* 1987).

The number of teeth affected by loss of attachment increased with increasing age from 30 per cent of teeth at risk in 17–26-year-olds to 67 per cent in 27–46-year-olds (Ismail *et al.* 1987). Although a majority of teeth in 27–46-year-olds were affected, only 10 per cent of teeth at risk had loss of attachment in excess of 3 mm and only 1.5 per cent in excess of 6 mm. Thus, only a small proportion of teeth affected by periodontitis progressed to an advanced stage of the disease by 27 to 46 years of age.

In a 47–74-year-old population at least 34 per cent of individuals had at least one tooth with attachment loss in excess of 6 mm (Ismail *et al.* 1987). Advanced loss of attachment, therefore, appears to be common in older age groups.

In recent years it has become apparent that teeth affected by severe loss of attachment are unevenly distributed within populations, and that in any population there will exist a group at 'high risk' of losing many teeth due to periodontal disease. Drawing on his own research findings and on evidence from recent epidemiological literature, Schaub (1984) concluded: '. . . that 10–15 per cent of adult populations with natural teeth will lose teeth because of progressive periodontal disease and that approximately half of them will lose most of their teeth'.

Periodontal treatment needs

The epidemiological data summarized above yields important information on the prevalence and severity of periodontal disease at different ages and in various populations. However, they cannot easily be converted to give a reliable estimate of treatment needs or, therefore, to plan and develop preventive or curative services. This deficiency has recently been overcome by introduction of the Community Periodontal Index of Treatment Needs (CPITN) designed by the World Health Organization and the International Dental Federation (Ainamo *et al.* 1982).

Examination is carried out with a specially designed probe; colour-coded for pocket depth measurement and with a ball tip for calculus detection. A score is given to each sextant according to the worst finding in all teeth of that sextant as follows:

Pocket of 6 mm depth or more	Code 4
Pocket of 4 or 5 mm depth	Code 3
Supra- or subgingival calculus	Code 2
Bleeding on probing	Code 1
No disease	Code 0

Using the CPITN, Cushing and Sheiham (1985) examined a random sample of 448 dentate individuals, aged 20 to 60 years, in the north-west of England and assessed their treatment needs. Only 2 per cent (Code 0) did not require any treatment. Seven per cent (Code 1) required oral hygiene instruction only. Eighty-four per cent (Codes 2 and 3) required oral hygiene instruction and scaling, while 7 per cent (Code 4) required complex treatment. By combining these data with the number of sextants requiring treatment, the manpower resource requirements were estimated at 1 week of work for a dental surgeon and 6 months of work for a dental hygienist. These estimates did not include time taken for intitial examination, treatment planning, and monitoring and maintenance care, which would increase the dentist-time required.

Intra-oral distribution of periodontal disease

The tooth surface most often coated in plaque and affected by gingivitis or periodontitis is the approximal surface (Hugoson and Koch 1979). The teeth most severely affected by gingivitis are the molars and lower anteriors (Suomi and Barbano 1968). The first teeth to be affected by periodontitis are usually the first molars (Hugoson and Rylander 1982).

In a 40- to 44-year-old age group, where periodontal destruction had progressed sufficiently to be easily scored but before a significant number of teeth had been removed from the calculation by extraction, Bossert and Marks (1956) reported the following pattern of periodontitis: lower incisors and upper molars were most severely affected; lower canines and molars, upper incisors, and premolars were moderately affected; those least affected were the lower premolars and upper canines.

Although studies of large populations, such as that quoted above, suggest that certain teeth are preferentially affected by periodontitis, this pattern is frequently not detectable in single subjects where attachment loss may appear to follow a random distribution throughout the dentition. At present, there is no satisfactory explanation for differences in susceptibility to periodontitis among teeth or individual tooth surfaces.

Tooth mortality

There is great variation in tooth mortality statistics in different parts of the world depending on oral hygiene, caries susceptibility, and the availability and effectiveness of dental services. The dentist's and patient's attitude, together with technical difficulties associated with provision of treatment, may also be significant factors determining the timing of extractions which obscure the significance of caries and periodontal disease. This must be borne in mind when interpreting tooth mortality statistics.

In recent years, there has been reasonably good agreement that, in developed countries, periodontal disease accounts for about 20–30 per cent of all extractions (Curilovic 1979; Ainamo *et al.* 1984; Kay and Blinkhorn 1986), and that over 35 to 40 years of age, more teeth are extracted because of periodontal disease than because of caries (Curilovic 1979; Kay and Blinkhorn 1986). By contrast in India, where caries experience was low, 66 per cent of all extractions were related to periodontal disease and, after the age of 30, the figure rose to 80 per cent (Mehta *et al.* 1958).

The first teeth to be extracted because of periodontal disease are molars, while canines are least frequently extracted for periodontal reasons (Bossert and Marks 1956).

The rate of periodontal destruction

In discussing the rate of progress of periodontitis, it is essential to consider the behaviour of single lesions, differences between individuals, and the pattern which emerges from looking at population averages.

With regard to individual lesions, perhaps affecting only one tooth surface, recent observations suggest that progression may be episodic in some cases, acute episodes being interspersed with periods of repair (Goodson *et al.* 1982). At sites of active disease, attachment loss of up to 4–5 mm per year has been observed (Goodson *et al.* 1982). In some patients, especially those with early-onset aggressive periodontitis, the disease process may arrest spontaneously and, thereafter, progress at a slow rate, if at all.

The difference in rate of progress between individuals has been highlighted by Löe *et al.* (1986), who reported on a 15-year longitudinal study of Sri Lankan tea labourers, aged initially 14 to 31 years. All were, therefore, in a similar age range and all displayed gross accumulation of plaque and calculus, and widespread gingivitis. Nevertheless, three distinct sub-populations were identified, based on proximal-surface loss of attachment and tooth mortality rates. Eight per cent of the total population exhibitied rapidly progressive periodontitis and had a peak annual rate of proximal-surface attachment loss of 1 mm per year. Eighty-one per cent exhibited moderately progressive periodontitis with a peak annual rate of destruction of 0.5 mm per year. Eleven per cent exhibited essentially no progression beyond gingivitis. Thus, the rate of periodontal destruction may vary at different stages of the disease, between single tooth surfaces and between individuals.

It has already been noted that the amount of periodontal disease in a large population is strongly correlated to age and oral hygiene. Thus, Löe *et al.* (1978), in a comparative longitudinal study, showed that the average rate of buccal- and mesial-surface attachment loss in a young adult population with reasonably good oral hygiene was almost 0.1 mm per year, compared with 0.3 mm per year for young adults with poor oral hygiene. Furthermore, Axelsson and Lindhe (1978) showed that among individuals not receiving periodontal care, young adults exhibited 0.17 mm of attachment loss per year, compared with 0.3 mm per year for the over 50-year-olds.

While these population averages are well accepted, there is no satisfactory evidence that individual lesions, once initiated, progress faster in older individuals or when plaque control is poor (Haffajee *et al.* 1983). This apparent contradiction is explained by the occurrence in these population groups of a larger number of periodontitis-affected sites so that, if measurements are taken from several teeth and several points around each tooth, higher mean rates of attachment loss will be observed.

Periodontal disease trends

Evidence is accumulating of an improvement in gingivitis in children and adults during the last 25 years. This evidence has been obtained by repeating cross-sectional studies of the same age range after an interval of several years using the same survey criteria. Thus, Anderson (1981) reported a decline in gingivitis and improvement in dental cleanliness over a 15-year period among 12-year-old English children from two schools. Cuttress (1986) reported a decline in gingivitis prevalence over a 6-year period in the 15 to 19 year age group in New Zealand, from 98 per cent of subjects and 51 per cent of teeth to 79 per cent of subjects and 34 per cent of teeth.

Improvements in gingivitis and oral hygiene among adults as well as children have been reported in the U.S.A. over a 12-year period (Douglass *et al.* 1985), and in Sweden over a 10-year period (Hugoson *et al.* 1986). In the Swedish study, the improvement in gingivitis and plaque control was most noticeable on buccal and lingual surfaces and was less marked interproximally (Hugoson *et al.* 1986).

From this evidence of a decline in gingivitis prevalence, a future decline in periodontitis might be anticipated. However, more teeth are being placed at risk because more teeth are being retained and the proportion of the population in older age groups is increasing. Periodontal disease, therefore, is likely to remain an important problem for the foreseeable future.

Aetiology of periodontal disease

It is well established that periodontal disease is initiated by bacterial plaque. It is, however, recognized that other aetiological factors exist—those which predispose to plaque accumulation and those which modify the inflammatory response.

Plaque and other acquired tooth deposits

'*Plaque*' is the soft, non-mineralized, bacterial deposits which form on teeth that are not adequately cleaned' (Löe 1969). It accumulates on tooth surfaces not exposed to friction from cheeks, lips, tongue and food, and its composition varies according to its location. Plaque is the subject of a number of detailed reviews (Bowen 1976; Newman 1980; Theilade 1986).

The earliest deposit to form on a cleaned tooth surface is the 'acquired pellicle'. It is a structureless film of glycoproteins selectively adsorbed to the surface of hydroxyapatite crystals from saliva, and is visible within minutes following a polish with pumice. The formation of pellicle is accompanied by bacterial colonization as micro-organisms in saliva adsorb to the pellicle. After three or four hours colonies of Gram-positive and Gram-negative cocci will be established. After seven days, Gram-positive cocci constitute about 50 per cent of plaque bacteria and, at this stage, Gram-positive and Gram-negative rods, filaments, fusobacteria, and spirilla are found. As the plaque matures further, spirochaetes and vibrios appear, and filamentous bacteria, especially *Actinomyces* may become predominant.

There appear to be many mechanisms for bacterial adherence: some organisms interact with salivary constituents which serve as the binding material; the occurrence in plaque of *Streptococcus mutans* is dependent on sucrose from which it synthesizes extracellular polysaccharides to mediate its attachment. The synthesis of surface polymers may also account for the ability of bacteria of one species to bind to one another or to bacteria of a different species. 'Corn-cob' structures, i.e. filamentous bacteria coated with cocci, represent one example of such interspecies binding. In addition to extracellular polysaccharides, plaque contains intracellular polysaccharides in the form of storage granules synthesized from dietary sugars.

Micro-organisms constitute at least 70 per cent of the bulk of plaque and the intermicrobial matrix comprises a protein and carbohydrate substrate derived partly from endogenous sources, viz, saliva, epithelial cells and crevicular exudate, and partly from the diet. The exact structural, bacteriological, and biochemical composition of plaque is subject to great variation depending on: the concentration of bacteria in saliva; the site and duration of plaque formation; the nature of competitive resident flora; oxygen and nutrient availability; the composition of the diet; and the presence of periodontal disease.

Recent bacteriological studies of plaque during development of gingivitis suggest that there are more than 200 different species in mature plaque. Gingivitis is believed to result from quantitative changes in plaque rather than the overgrowth of specific micro-organisms.

Periodontitis is caused by subgingival downgrowth of those bacteria best able to evade host defences and survive in a low oxygen environment. Thus, the composition of subgingival plaque differs from plaque on the adjacent visible tooth surface. For example, in subgingival plaque, Gram-positive bacteria are found in lower proportions and Gram-negative bacteria in higher proportions than in supragingival plaque. The subgingival flora comprises a layer of tooth-attached plaque as well as a loosely adherent component in direct association with the pocket epithelium. The tooth-attached plaque consists mainly of Gram-positive rods and cocci, while the unattached plaque contains a predominance of Gram-negative organisms including motile forms. Many different bacterial species are thought to be of aetiological significance in periodontitis. The reader is referred to a recent review by Theilade (1986).

Mineralization within plaque results in calculus formation. Its inorganic content (70–90 per cent) is mostly crystalline and amorphous calcium phosphate.

The organic component includes protein, carbohydrates, lipid, and various non-vital micro-organisms, predominantly filamentous ones. The rate of calculus formation between individuals is very variable, and children form less calculus than adults. Calcification may commence in 1-day-old plaque but the mechanism for calculus formation is not known. In supragingival locations, however, it is thought to result from interactions between saliva, tooth surfaces and plaque, while in subgingival locations gingival exudate from periodontal pockets is the fluid medium involved. Subgingival calculus forms more slowly and is usually more difficult to remove by virtue of the intimate relationship which it forms with the rougher root surface. Calculus is always covered by soft plaque and retains toxic bacterial products. Mandell and Gaffar (1986) have recently reviewed the aetiological significance of calculus.

Materia alba is a disorganized white debris probably comprising the outer layers of mature plaque.

Stains are caused by food substances such as tea and coffee, by tobacco, by the products of chromogenic bacteria, or by metallic particles. These pigments become absorbed by plaque or pellicle.

Factors predisposing to plaque accumulation

Tooth malalignment

The relationship between tooth alignment and plaque accumulation is disputed. While some studies (e.g. Buckley 1980) have demonstrated a low but statistically significant correlation between malalignment and plaque accumulation, others (e.g. Ingervall *et al.* 1977) have shown that tooth crowding does not favour plaque accumulation. A further alternative conclusion, reached by Ainamo (1972), is that the relationship between crowding and periodontal disease becomes evident only when cleanliness is moderate. When oral hygiene is very good this relationship will not be apparent and when it is very poor it will be masked by generalized severe periodontal disease.

Restorations

Bacteria accumulate more readily on restoration surfaces (Glantz 1969), with the possible exception of porcelain (Newcomb 1974), than on tooth enamel. Furthermore, the surface finish of a restorative material may influence the degree of plaque accumulation. A highly polished surface should be more amenable to cleansing procedures than a rough surface. However, no standards of acceptable surface roughness have been established.

Restorations with overhanging or otherwise defective cervical margins form retention sites for plaque and may have a profound effect on periodontal health (Björn *et al.* 1969, 1970). Subgingival restoration margins produce more plaque accumulation and result in poorer gingival health than margins which are level with the gingival crest or in a supragingival position (Silness 1980). Excessive axial crown contours tend to enhance plaque accumulation and gingival inflammation (Yuodelis *et al.* 1973).

Removable partial dentures

It has been observed (Addy and Bates 1979) that patients provided with partial dentures accumulate more plaque on abutment teeth. The fitting surfaces of the dentures themselves become coated with plaque, and plaque accumulation both on abutment teeth and denture is increased by day and night wear. These factors help to account for the common observation of gingivitis around abutment teeth. Moreover, El Ghamrawy (1979) has shown that the microbial composition of plaque in denture subjects changes more rapidly, resembling the 4- to 9-day-old plaque of non-denture wearers as early as the second day.

Calculus

The surface texture of calculus promotes plaque accumulation and retention of irritant bacterial deposits. There is no evidence, however, that calculus itself is capable of initiating periodontal disease.

Factors modifying the inflammatory response

Host defence mechanisms appear to be both protective and destructive, and in most cases the tissue damage sustained is minor relative to the protection provided. An intact and normal functioning host response would appear to be compatible with, at worst, slowly progressive periodontal disease. However, changes in the capacity of various components of the host response to deal with the bacterial challenge may cause an increased susceptibility to periodontal disease. In addition, a number of systemic abnormalities are thought to affect the host response to local irritants, increasing the severity of periodontal disease. These factors are reviewed by Pennel and Keagle (1977), and include various endocrinopathies, stress, blood dyscrasias, certain genetic disorders, and alteration in the levels of circulating sex hormones during puberty, pregnancy or medication with oral contraceptives.

Rationale for prevention and management of periodontal disease

Professional care

Dental health education

The objective of oral hygiene education is to produce a change in behaviour which will result in a reduction of plaque accumulation sufficient, if possible, to prevent the initiation and progression of dental caries and periodontal disease, and to make the patient as independent as possible of professional support.

Health education for the prevention of periodontal disease is usually given to individual patients in a dental surgery and involves oral hygiene instruction. A successful outcome will depend not only on mastery of plaque control techniques but also on a change of behaviour and compliance with the suggested plaque control regime. Kegeles (1963) has suggested various steps which must be taken before a recommended health action is adopted:

(1) belief in susceptibility to the disease;

(2) belief that the disease is undesirable;

(3) belief that prevention is possible;

(4) belief that prevention is desirable.

Clearly, therefore, the clinician must use an educative approach aimed at changing the patient's attitude to periodontal disease and dental care (Blinkhorn *et al.* 1983). Furthermore, plaque control skills must be taught using proper educational principles such as step-size advancement, self-pacing, repeated feedback, and reinforcement as well as active participation by the patient.

Dental health education and instruction in oral hygiene is traditionally carried out by dental personnel at the chairside, but this process is labour-intensive and, with repetition, is likely to affect the mood of the instructor and, thereby, the effect of the instruction. In recent years, however, the need for oral hygiene instruction to be given at the chairside has been questioned. Glavind *et al.* (1985) have shown that a self-educational programme, comprising self-examination and instruction manuals, was as effective as chairside instruction by dental personnel in changing oral hygiene habits.

The dental surgery has frightening overtones for many people, who then find it difficult to concentrate on advice being given (Blinkhorn *et al.* 1983). This fact alone might explain the success of self-education manuals—the lack of personal contact being compensated for by the freedom to assimilate information in a better environment.

Regardless of the means employed, it is well known that oral hygiene instruction usually has no long-term effect unless periodically reinforced. Gjermo (1967), for example, found that the initial improvement observed 1 month after individual instruction of schoolchildren was not maintained at the second examination 7 months later. Thus, initial incentives for behavioural change appear to fade after the target behaviour has been achieved. According to the Committee on Oral Health Care for the Prevention and Control of Periodontal Disease (Committee Report 1966*a*): 'Probably the most important and difficult problem that remains to be solved before much progress can be made in the prevention of periodontal disease is how to motivate the individual to follow a prescribed effective oral health-care programme throughout his life.'

Improved oral hygiene alone has no effect on the gingival condition, pocket depth, or subgingival flora of deep periodontal lesions (Beltrami *et al.* 1987). In patients with existing periodontal disease, therefore, dental health education must be supported by attention to the subgingival environment.

Scaling

Although calculus does not seem to behave as a mechanical irritant it may act as a reservoir for toxic microbial and tissue breakdown products by virtue of its permeable structure (Baumhammers and Rohrbaugh 1970). Furthermore, the irregular calculus surface is always covered in plaque (Committee Report 1966b) which may be difficult to remove by standard tooth cleaning methods (Baumhammers *et al.* 1973). The removal of calculus deposits is therefore of paramount importance in the prevention and treatment of periodontal disease. The beneficial effect of calculus removal upon gingival health has been emphasized in numerous clinical and histological studies (see Lövdal *et al.* 1961; O'Bannon 1964).

Ideally, subgingival scaling should result in a plaque-free environment allowing renewal of junctional epithelium and the epithelial attachment. Failure to achieve complete plaque and calculus removal will allow recolonization of the root surface to take place. There is some evidence, however, that periodontopathic micro-organisms do not reappear in the pocket flora for at least 6 months after scaling (Listgarten *et al.* 1978).

Root planing

Scaling alone is sufficient to remove completely plaque and calculus from enamel leaving a smooth clean surface. Root surfaces, however, whether supra- or subgingival, may have deposits of calculus embedded in cemental irregularities (Zander 1953; Moskow 1969). A portion of cementum must, therefore, be removed to eliminate these deposits. Furthermore, plaque accumulation results in contamination of cementum by toxic substances, notably endotoxins (Hatfield and Baumhammers 1971; Aleo *et al.* 1974, 1975). Evidence suggests that this cementum is biologically unacceptable to adjacent gingival tissue and should be removed by root planing, a procedure which may result in exposure of dentine. While this is not the aim of treatment, it may be unavoidable (Van Volkinburg *et al.* 1976). There is little evidence that the degree of root smoothing *per se* is of biological importance (Garrett 1977) although it gives the best clinical indication that calculus and altered cementum have been completely removed.

Polishing

Polishing enamel results in reorientation of surface crystals to create a smoother surface (Boyde 1971). It appears from experimental studies that polishing to a high gloss may inhibit pellicle (Muhler *et al.* 1964), plaque (Swartz and Philips 1957), and calculus (Barnes *et al.* 1971) formation.

Surgical pocket therapy

Recent evidence suggests that there is no certain magnitude of initial probing depth beyond which non-surgical instrumentation is ineffective, provided sufficient skill and perseverance are applied (Badersten *et al.* 1984). Non-surgical scaling and root planing, however, as a definitive procedure in deep pockets, is very time consuming, and surgical intervention may be required to provide the operator with better access to the plaque-infected root surface for pockets of more than approximately 5 mm depth (Waerhaug 1978*a*, *b*).

Correction of other factors predisposing to plaque accumulation

An individual's prospects of achieving an adequate standard of oral hygiene may depend on the existence of an environment where there is optimum access to plaque deposits. The importance of removing calculus and altered cementum, which harbour toxic substances, has already been discussed. The dentist must also determine whether to institute orthodontic treatment for correction of tooth malalignment, and should practise high standards of restorative dentistry to avoid creating reservoirs of plaque.

Reinforcement of host defence mechanisms

Systemic factors which undermine the normal host response, some of which may be amenable to medical attention, have already been listed. It has also been suggested that the host response to injurious agents might be altered by immunization. Although there is much speculation that specific organisms or groups of organisms are responsible for periodontal disease, research has not advanced to the stage where immunization procedures could be remotely contemplated (Socransky and Crawford 1977).

Home care

The manual tooth-brush

Design characteristics. Design variations include dimensions of the head, the length, diameter, and modulus of elasticity of the filaments and their number, distribution, and angulation. Operating efficiency may further depend on the moisture content, temperature of the water used, and brushing technique. These variables confound comparison of the many investigations carried out to determine optimum tooth-brush characteristics. Although current opinion favours a soft-textured nylon multitufted brush with a short head, there is no clear-cut evidence that one particular type of tooth-brush is superior to others with respect to plaque removal and prevention of gingivitis (Bergenholtz 1972). Furthermore, concern that hard-textured brushes might abrade the tooth surface appears to be unfounded as tooth-brushes alone have no abrasive action on the tooth surface (Sangnes 1976). Certain tooth-brush filaments may, however, traumatize the gingiva (Breitenmoser *et al.* 1979).

Tooth-brushing methods. Greene (1966) grouped tooth-brushing methods into the following categories based on the direction of the brushing stroke: (i) vertical; (ii) horizontal; (iii) roll technique; (iv) vibrating techniques (Charters, Stillman, Bass); (v) circular technique; (vi) physiological technique; (vii) scrub brush method. Comparative studies of these different methods have yielded conflicting results and each technique has its own protagonists. In a sample of 800 individuals, Wade (1971) showed that more than one-third used no definite brushing stroke but, of those who employed an identifiable stroke, almost half used the roll method. This, however, may be one of the least efficient methods according to several studies (Rodda 1968; Frandsen *et al.* 1970; Hansen and Gjermo 1971; Gibson and Wade 1977) and the advice of the Health Education Council (1979). Current opinion now favours the Bass method (Gibson and Wade 1977) or a modification of it.

The automatic tooth-brush

Automatic tooth-brushes have found a place in the home care of physically or mentally handicapped individuals (Kelner 1963; Smith and Blankenship 1964). Well-informed individuals with reasonable digital skill, however, use the manual brush just as effectively (McKendrick *et al.* 1968). Fears that the automatic brush may damage the tissues have not been realized (Chasens and Marcus 1968).

Interdental cleaning

It is well established that periodontal conditions are worst in interdental areas where standard tooth-brushes are ineffective at removing approximal plaque (Hansen and Gjermo 1971). Furthermore, bacterial deposits remaining after brushing will promote the regrowth of fresh plaque (De La Rosa *et al.* 1979). The importance of total plaque removal is emphasized by Brecx *et al.* (1980) in a study of early plaque formation. Using light and electron microscopy, they concluded that the establishment of a complex and presumably pathogenic flora on cleaned tooth surfaces may be accelerated when plaque remains on other tooth surfaces. The need for effective interdental cleaning has led to the manufacture of various devices. They should be recommended in accordance with individual dexterity and interdental anatomy.

Woodpoints (toothpicks). The woodpoint is effective only where sufficient interdental space is available to accommodate it. Bergenholtz *et al.* (1974), in a study of open interdental spaces, demonstrated that triangular woodpoints are superior to round or rectangular ones, which are ineffective on lingual aspects of proximal surfaces. Triangular woodpoints in this study were more effective overall than dental floss. In a more recent study, testing various characteristics both *in vitro* and *in vivo*, Bergenholtz *et al.* (1980) concluded that triangular woodpoints with low surface hardness and high strength values are preferable.

Dental floss. There is little apparent difference in the cleaning ability of waxed and unwaxed floss (Keller and Manson-Hing 1969; Gjermo and Flötra 1970; Hill *et al.* 1973; Bergenholtz and Brithon 1980). Nor is there much evidence that dental floss is wholly effective. Wolffe (1976) reported that subjects using dental floss removed only 50 per cent of proximal plaque. Furthermore, some clinical trials have shown that floss is no more effective at removing approximal plaque than a woodpoint, interspace brush, or a standard tooth-brush (Wolffe 1976; Schmid *et al.* 1976). On the other hand, Bergenholtz *et al.* (1974) showed that, when tooth-brushing was accompanied by flossing, more plaque was removed from the approximal surfaces than by tooth-brushing alone while Gjermo and Flötra (1970) and Bergenholtz and Brithon (1980) demonstrated that floss was superior to woodpoints especially in removing plaque from the lingual aspect of proximal surfaces. Although flossing requires more digital skill and is almost twice as time-consuming as the use of woodpoints (Gjermo and Flötra 1970), there appears to be no alternative method of cleaning approximal surfaces when a normal papilla fills the interdental space.

Interspace brush (single-tufted tooth-brush). This device was introduced to improve access to certain tooth surfaces. Wolffe (1976) showed that its effectiveness at plaque removal was equal to woodpoints or dental floss while Gjermo and Flötra (1970) demonstrated that the combined use of the interspace brush and woodpoints compensated for the lack of effectiveness of woodpoints alone.

The interdental brush (bottle brush). Large interdental spaces are cleaned most thoroughly by the interdental brush (Gjermo and Flötra 1970), which is manufactured in different sizes. The larger type is held by its wire handle while smaller versions, of which the Proxabrush® is an example, are attachable to a metal or plastic handle. Studies comparing the interdental brush with a rubber cone stimulator (Nayak and Wade 1977) and with dental floss (Bergenholtz and Olsson 1984) have shown it to be superior in cleaning large interdental spaces. Waerhaug (1976) showed that individuals who used the interdental brush habitually were able not only to maintain supragingival approximal surfaces free of plaque, but could also remove subgingival plaque to a depth of 2–2.5 mm below the gingival margin.

Irrigation devices

These provide a steady or pulsating stream of water escaping through a nozzle under pressure and have been extensively studied in clinical trials. Only surface layers of soft plaque are removed (Lobene 1969; Fine and Baumhammers 1970; Hugoson 1978) and the reduction in gingivitis is correspondingly modest when used as an adjunct to brushing by subjects uninstructed in use of the tooth-brush (Lobene 1969; Lainson *et al.* 1970; Gupta *et al.* 1973).

Studies have also been made of individuals with healthy gingiva, practising prescribed tooth-brushing and interdental cleaning regimes, who employed an irrigating device as well. Conflicting results have been reported. Hoover and Robinson (1971), for example, found that the additional use of an irrigating device resulted in significantly less plaque, calculus, and gingivitis. Hugoson (1978), on the other hand, found that an irrigator conferred no additional benefit in subjects with healthy gingiva who used the tooth-brush and woodpoints as their only other hygiene aids.

Water irrigating devices should clearly not be used as a substitute for tooth-brushing and may be of negligible adjunctive value in prevention of periodontal disease, especially as they are time consuming and messy to use (Lainson *et al.* 1972). They may yet have a role in the delivery of chemical agents to the oral cavity (Lobene *et al.* 1972; Cumming and Löe 1973*a*; Agerbaek *et al.* 1975; Lang and Räber 1981; Lang and Ramseier-Grossman 1981).

Toothpaste

Toothpaste contains detergents, abrasives, and additives such as fluoride. Little is known of its contribution to plaque removal *per se* although one study demonstrated that, during the 24-hour period after brushing, the rate of plaque regrowth in the group using toothpaste was 27 per cent lower than in the group brushing without toothpaste (De La Rosa *et al.* 1979). This effect may possibly be attributed to its fluoride content rather than its physical cleansing action. Although the degree of abrasivity does not influence the amount of plaque removal achieved, the abrasive property of toothpaste keeps the pellicle layer thin and prevents the accumulation of surface stains (Bergenholtz 1972). Paste with a high dentine abrasion value may cause destructive lesions in the cervical tooth region but the optimum degree of abrasivity which will reduce surface pellicle without damaging tooth structure has not been determined.

Frequency of tooth cleaning

Plaque forms continuously and tooth surfaces cannot be maintained in a plaque-free state by conventional mechanical means. The object of plaque control in prevention of periodontal disease is, therefore, the periodic removal of accumulated plaque at intervals which are sufficiently frequent to prevent pathological effects arising from recurrent plaque formation. Accordingly, individuals with healthy gingiva and no history of periodontal disease can prevent gingivitis by *complete* mechanical plaque removal every 48 hours (Lang *et al.* 1973). On the other hand, if inflammation is already present, colonization of the cleaned tooth surface occurs much sooner (Saxton 1973), plaque grows more rapidly (Lang *et al.* 1973; Goldman *et al.* 1974; Hillam and Hull 1977; Goh *et al.* 1986), and matures faster (Brecx *et al.* 1980). To control gingivitis, rather than prevent its onset, therefore, more frequent plaque removal may be necessary. Furthermore, individual susceptibility to gingivitis and periodontitis (Van der Velden *et al.* 1985) may be an important factor to consider in selecting a suitable frequency of tooth cleaning. In their experimental gingivitis model, Löe *et al.* (1965) showed that, following the first clinical signs of inflammatory change, the introduction of oral hygiene measures, twice daily, achieved resolution of gingivitis within a few days. This was true even of the more susceptible individuals who had developed gingivitis at an early stage of plaque accumulation.

Accordingly, to achieve gingival health, the interval between tooth cleaning sessions need be no less than 12 hours and no greater than 48 hours, depending on prevailing gingival conditions and individual susceptibility to periodontal disease.

Duration and technique of tooth cleaning

Questionnaire surveys in Scandinavian countries (e.g. Frandsen 1985) have revealed a frequency of tooth-brushing of once or twice daily in a majority of individuals, although the reported use of floss was negligible. When gingivitis occurs, therefore, it is important not to jump to the convenient, but probably erroneous conclusion that tooth-brushing has been too infrequent. Cumming and Löe (1973*b*) have shown that, among individuals who brush at least twice daily, the same surfaces consistently remain cleaned or not cleaned at each tooth cleaning session. Thoroughness of technique, therefore, is an important factor in prevention of gingivitis. Furthermore, in a study to analyse the effect of habitual tooth-brushing in 13-year-old children, the duration of brushing was found to have a greater influence on plaque removal than either its frequency or pattern (Honkala *et al.* 1986). Studies of tooth-brushing duration in uninstructed children (MacGregor *et al.* 1986) and uninstructed adults (MacGregor and Rugg-Gunn 1985) revealed brushing times of only 51 and 33 s respectively.

Diet and natural cleansing

It has been shown by tube-feeding experiments in dogs (Egelberg 1965) and monkeys (Bowen 1974) that plaque formation is not dependent on the presence of food in the mouth.

The effect of diet on plaque accumulation is reviewed by Theilade and Theilade (1976). They conclude that the effect of dietary sugars on plaque quantity in man is generally far less pronounced than could be anticipated from theoretical considerations. They further state that there is great individual variation in the amount of plaque formation and its response to different dietary regimes. Although diet may influence the quantitative proportions of plaque micro-organisms, the clinical significance of such changes with respect to the initiation and progress of periodontal disease is not known.

It has been shown conclusively in a number of studies that the traditional concept of natural cleansing by detersive foodstuffs is not valid. This concept is cited by the Health Education Council (1979) as an example of a dental health message, popular in the past, which has little or no evidence to support it. Cervical tooth regions are not subject to physical stress from food particles during mastication (Wilcox and Everett 1963) and excessive chewing of raw vegetables and fruit has no effect on the quantity of plaque accumulating there (Bergenholtz *et al.* 1967; Lindhe and Wicén 1969).

It is clear, therefore, that dietary advice, although important in caries prevention, is not beneficial with respect to periodontal disease.

Prolonged preventive programmes based on plaque control

The components of an effective preventive programme based on plaque control are dental health education, oral hygiene instruction, and professional tooth cleaning. The relative importance of each component has been assessed in a number of studies. These have measured various parameters of oral cleanliness and periodontal health, viz, plaque and calculus accumulation, gingival inflammation, gingival bleeding, pocket depths, attachment levels, and bone resorption. This work has been carried out both in children and adults. Due to partial eruption and immature tooth-contact relationships, the pattern of plaque accumulation in children may differ from adults. Children, moreover, form less calculus, the reason for which is unknown. In childhood, there is a marked age-related predisposition to gingivitis (Matsson and Goldberg 1985). Young children (3–5 years) are much less susceptible to gingivitis than adults when plaque is allowed to accumulate freely (Mackler and Crawford 1973; Matsson 1978; Matsson and Goldberg 1985) while, at puberty, gingivitis reaches a peak (Parfitt 1957), which may be partly attributable to hormonal factors. With regard to preventive procedures, manual dexterity in young children is limited and so is their response to any form of activity which does not produce immediate benefits. It is appropriate, for all these reasons, that preventive programmes in child and adult populations should be given separate consideration.

Preventive programmes in children

It is generally assumed that good oral hygiene practices are best acquired in childhood when they may be integrated with other developing health habits. Preventive programmes in schools provide continual opportunities for peer influence and the stimulating effect of daily personal interaction.

Evidence for the effectiveness of dental health education programmes in schools is equivocal (for review see Flanders 1987). Although there may be significant improvements in knowledge and attitudes, changes in behaviour, as measured by reduction in plaque and gingivitis, are usually short-lived. Craft (1984) reported the effect of the 'Natural Nashers' health education programme in the United Kingdom. This was a very large trial involving 6700 13–14-year-olds who received a teacher-mediated dental health education programme comprising three 70–80 minute sessions, at weekly intervals. The programme employed active learning principles and included a slide presentation, experimental work, and use of work sheets. Improvement in plaque and gingivitis levels, while statistically significant, was small and faded considerably between the 5- and 28-week observation periods. Nevertheless, the exposure to such a dental health programme might conceivably improve the uptake of subsequent practice-based preventive care.

Supervised tooth-brushing in schools is an alternative approach which has been evaluated in several studies. Lindhe and Koch (1966), for example, in a study of 12- to 13-year-old school children, showed that a 3-year supervised daily brushing regimen in the last year of the study *reduced* gingivitis in 56 per cent of all tooth areas examined, whereas the control group showed a 75 per cent *increase* in gingivitis, typical for this stage of childhood.

Tooth-brushing, professionally supervised on a *daily* basis, is labour-intensive and may be unnecessary in younger children less predisposed to develop gingival inflammation. Thus, Bennie *et al.* (1978) reported significant reductions in plaque and gingivitis compared with controls among a group of children who, from the age 6–11 years, participated in a *fortnightly* supervised tooth-brushing regime.

Although supervised tooth-brushing may produce an overall improvement in gingival health, the reduction of gingivitis is unevenly distributed within the dentition. Lindhe *et al.* (1966) found that their test group had 80 per cent less gingivitis than controls in the upper anterior region but only 13 per cent less in the lower molar regions. Furthermore, Lindhe and Koch (1966) noted that gingivitis scores were somewhat higher for approximal surfaces than for buccal and lingual surfaces. Another major criticism of this type of preventive programme is the lack of any prolonged effect after it is withdrawn. Lindhe and Koch (1967) showed a substantial increase in gingivitis one year after the end of their 3-year supervised tooth-brushing programme in children who at follow-up were 16 to 17 years of age. Likewise, Horowitz *et al.* (1977), observing the effect of a 2-year supervised daily brushing and flossing regime in schoolchildren, initially 10- to 13-years-old, noted that the benefits virtually disappeared during the summer vacation. These limitations, inherent in a tooth-brushing regimen, have to some extent been overcome in later studies in which dental personnel have introduced various other preventive strategies to children on an individual basis.

In 1974, Axelsson and Lindhe reported the effect of a rigorous preventive programme in school children aged initially 7 to 14 years. The test groups received fortnightly professional tooth cleaning, oral hygiene instruction and motivation, and topical fluoride applications. Parental involvement was obtained at the beginning of the study and after 1 year. The experimental group after 2 years demonstrated low plaque scores and negligible signs of gingivitis. The control group children, on the other hand, had much higher plaque and gingivitis scores. In the test groups there were no significant differences between gingivitis scores of approximal and buccal/lingual areas. Thus it appears that careful fortnightly interproximal cleaning with floss or polishing tips prevents gingivitis in those areas in children. Furthermore the plaque control programme was equally effective for molars and incisors.

This study was continued for two further years. During the third year the interval between prophylactic sessions was prolonged to 4 weeks in the younger age groups and to 8 weeks in the oldest age group (Lindhe *et al.* 1975). During the fourth year all children were recalled every 8 weeks (Axelsson and Lindhe 1977). The excellent standard of oral hygiene was maintained during the third and fourth years and there was no significant change in gingival condition. Significant differences, however, were once again observed between test and control groups. This introductory 2-year programme of fortnightly prophylactic and oral hygiene sessions, followed by recall at intervals of one or two months during the third and fourth years, practically eliminated all signs of gingivitis in schoolchildren.

An alternative and less ambitious prophylactic programme was described by Badersten *et al.* (1975) who carried out professional tooth cleaning including interdental cleaning, oral hygiene instruction, and fluoride rinsing at monthly intervals in 113 schoolchildren, 10–12-years old. After 1 year the gingivitis frequency in the experimental group was significantly less than in the control group where no reduction occurred. However, the frequency of inflamed gingival units in the trial group fell only from 76 per cent to 60 per cent, a reduction in gingivitis which, although statistically significant, was clearly inferior to the result achieved by Axelsson and Lindhe (1974). This was attributed to the lesser effect of monthly prophylactic sessions and the lack of parental support within a lower socio-economic group.

A further trial with a similar design was carried out by Hamp *et al.* (1978) primarily to assess the effect of preventive measures in a large group (1100) of school children between the ages of 7 and 17 years. Specially trained dental nurses administered oral hygiene instruction and professional tooth cleaning, and applied topical fluoride every third week. Over the 3-year trial period, the frequency of plaque infected surfaces in the experimental group fell from 64.1 per cent to 29.2 per cent and the frequency of inflamed gingival units from 41.1 per cent to 18.8 per cent. Differences between test and control groups were highly significant at re-examination.

Further studies were designed to ascertain the separate effect of each component of the prophylactic regimen.

Poulsen *et al.* (1976) attempted to determine the benefits that might be obtained by professional tooth cleaning alone in 78 7-year-old children. Thus the experimental group received thorough mechanical cleaning every 2 weeks while a control group were given no professional tooth cleaning. Both groups received fortnightly supervised fluoride rinsing. Throughout the study, home-care standards were not intentionally influenced. After 1 year, there was a statistically significant difference in plaque accumulation between the groups and an improvement in gingivitis in the test group. This study was continued for one further year during which the interval between professional tooth-cleaning sessions was increased to 3 weeks. Results were reported by Agerbaek *et al.* (1978). Plaque and gingivitis scores increased in the experimental group but remained significantly lower than in the control group where there was no appreciable change in oral cleanliness or gingival health. These studies (Poulsen *et al.* 1976; Agerbaek *et al.* 1978) demonstrate that the frequency of professional tooth cleaning is of major importance when it is the only plaque control measure used, although it is difficult to assess the value of tooth cleaning *per se* because the involvement of the children itself may have motivated them to practice better home care. This view is supported by Lindhe *et al.* (1966) in whose tooth-brushing study a control group, receiving a fortnightly rinsing programme only, demonstrated a significant improvement in plaque control and gingival health.

Axelsson *et al.* (1976) carried out a 2-year trial involving 164 children, age 13–14 years, in which they attempted to judge the significance of oral hygiene instruction and professional cleaning in a crossover study: Children who received detailed oral hygiene instruction once every 3 months failed to demonstrate a reduction in plaque scores and gingivitis. Those children, however, who were placed on a fortnightly plaque-control programme, including professional cleaning (Axelsson and Lindhe 1974), demonstrated low levels of plaque and gingivitis which showed no significant increase when professional tooth cleaning was withdrawn during the second year of the trial and only fortnightly oral hygiene instruction was given.

The benefits of fortnightly professional tooth-cleaning cannot be attributed entirely to the repeated removal of 2-week old plaque. This has been demonstrated in a study by Axelsson and Lindhe (1981) involving 13–14-year-old children who received fortnightly professional tooth cleaning in a split-mouth design. The children were divided into two groups only one of which received oral hygiene instruction at 2-week intervals. There was an equal reduction in plaque and gingivitis in the untreated quadrants of both groups of children showing that the subjective impression of tooth cleanliness, as identified in the cleaned jaw quadrants of the group not receiving oral hygiene instruction, was sufficient to motivate the children towards a standard of home care which was equal to that achieved by the group who did receive oral hygiene instruction.

The fortnightly programme of Axelsson and Lindhe (1974), which has produced the most impressive reductions not only of gingivitis but also of caries, required about 160 min/child per year (Lindhe and Axelsson 1973). Traditional dental treatment, for children not participating in the trial, required about 140 min/child per year and cost over twice as much as the preventive programme. Furthermore, the trial participants achieved a much better standard of dental health—gingivitis was negligible and practically no caries developed. Attempts by others to match these results have, however, been unsuccessful. Although other trials (Ashley and Sainsbury 1981) have achieved similar reductions in plaque and gingivitis, their effect on caries has not been sufficiently large to make such programmes cost effective.

Preventive programmes in adults

From a practical standpoint, it is more important to prevent the progression of periodontitis, which is widespread in adults, than to abolish gingivitis. However, as gingivitis either precedes or accompanies destructive periodontal disease and plaque is the common aetiological agent, those measures which effect a reduction of gingivitis in children are pertinent also for adults. On the other hand, in adults periodontal as well as gingival pockets are common, and these contain a microflora which perpetuates the disease. Pocket therapy, i.e. the complete removal of subgingival irritants, is therefore an integral part of all types of periodontal care which may be achieved by surgical or non-surgical means in suitably selected cases. The discussion which follows concerns non-surgical methods of periodontal care which are aimed indiscriminately, not only at inhibition of gingivitis but also at elimination of early destructive lesions (Fig. 10.1(d)) and control of advanced ones.

The success of a preventive regimen depends largely on the extent to which it will preserve attachment levels. In children, attachment loss occurs infrequently, and the consequences of plaque accumulation can be measured only by its effect on the gingiva. Preventive regimens in adults, however, may be assessed by comparing changes in attachment level with untreated control values.

Adams and Stanmeyer (1960) subjected 103 men, living in an Antarctic base, to monthly individual oral hygiene instruction and after $1\frac{1}{2}$ years were able to demonstrate a substantial improvement in oral cleanliness, in sharp contrast to the poor results achieved from a preliminary phase of group instruction.

It was later shown by Brandtzaeg and Jamison (1964) that, 35 days after oral hygiene instruction, Norwegian army recruits had greater oral cleanliness and better periodontal health, compared with non-participating controls. These observations were confirmed by Fay (1964), who found a significant difference in gingivitis compared with controls as much as 4 months after oral hygiene instruction, and by Tan and Saxton (1978) who found a small improvement in gingivitis lasting 3 months after oral hygiene instruction.

Chawla *et al.* (1975), in a 2-year study of 14–28-year-old Indians united by a total lack of dental awareness, showed that plaque and gingivitis could be reduced for a prolonged period by oral hygiene instruction alone, repeated at 6-month intervals. A greater improvement in gingivitis with less attachment loss was achieved by professional cleaning without oral hygiene instruction at 6-month intervals, although plaque scores in this group were significantly higher. Moreover, those individuals for whom oral hygiene instruction was combined with professional cleaning every 6 months showed no further improvement in gingivitis compared with the group who received scaling and polishing alone. The value of scaling and root-planing procedures at 6-month intervals, in the total absence of day-to-day plaque control, has been confirmed in a 3-year study of attachment loss in dogs (Morrison *et al.* 1979). These findings may have important implications in the preventive care of certain groups such as the physically or mentally handicapped. The ability of periodic scaling to reduce gingivitis and retard attachment loss suggests that the removal of subgingival deposits may allow renewal of the epithelial attachment protecting the underlying tissue from toxic plaque products. There may, furthermore, be a significant delay before periodontopathic organisms are re-established within the periodontal pocket, following scaling (Listgarten *et al.* 1978).

By contrast, Suomi *et al.* (1973*b*) found that when scaling and polishing was carried out, unsupported by oral hygiene instruction, the participants showed progressive gingivitis and attachment loss regardless of whether the procedure was repeated annually, six monthly or three monthly. This study, however, was carried out in 17–22-year-olds with comparatively good dental health who might not be expected to require much calculus removal or to benefit substantially from it.

Other studies tend to support the view that, in young individuals in a dentally conscious society, the gingival tissues will show a greater response to improved personal oral hygiene than to professional cleaning (Tan and Saxton 1978), and, when oral hygiene instruction is included with a scaling regime, the results are better than those achieved by scaling alone (Lightner *et al.* 1968; 1971; Tan and Saxton 1978).

The converse is also true that oral hygiene instruction accompanied by professional cleaning, will have a greater effect on gingival health than oral hygiene instruction alone (Fay 1964; Tan and Saxton 1978). The need for scaling will clearly depend to a large extent on the rate of calculus formation and the presence of pathological pockets which harbour subgingival deposits of plaque and calculus.

The optimum time interval between preventive appointments was the subject of an investigation by Lightner *et al.* (1971). In a 4-year study they showed that the preventive regime which involved the greatest amount of professional care, i.e. oral hygiene instruction with scaling and polishing in one 40 minute appointment every 3 months, produced the greatest decrease in gingivitis. Nevertheless, it was found that one course of treatment per year, administered in two 40-minute appointments, 5–11 days apart, was more economical and almost as effective.

These findings lend support to the earlier work of Lövdal *et al.* (1961), who carried out the first long-term study to evaluate the combined effect of oral hygiene instruction and scaling on the incidence of gingivitis. Their study group, originally comprising 1428 men and women, was followed for a period of 5 years, during which time prophylactic visits were arranged at 3- or 6-month intervals according to the severity of individual cases. After 5 years, there was a reduction in gingivitis of between one-eighth and one-half, depending on whether the participants started the study with good or poor oral hygiene respectively. The improvement was limited, however, to those areas where pocket depths did not exceed 5 mm and which, therefore, were reasonably accessible to scaling instruments.

The effect of such a prophylactic regimen, not only on gingival health but also on attachment levels, was later observed by Suomi *et al.* (1971*a*), who carried out a 3-year study in which they subjected their test group to dental health education, oral hygiene instruction, and professional tooth cleaning at 2–4 month intervals. They showed that a matched control group, who were not recruited to the oral hygiene programme, had substantially greater plaque scores, more gingivitis, and their rate of attachment loss, at 0.1 mm/year, was more than $3\frac{1}{2}$ times greater than their experimental counterparts. Furthermore, Suomi *et al.* (1971*b*) showed that, during the 3-year trial period, the experimental group showed almost no radiographic evidence of bone loss in the region studied—the lower right posterior teeth—whereas the controls exhibited 0.19 mm of marginal bone destruction. Two and a half years after the experiment had been discontinued and the preventive regimen disbanded, Suomi *et al.* (1973*a*) showed that the former experimental group continued to demonstrate cleaner teeth and better periodontal health than the former control group. Nevertheless, the difference between groups with respect to oral hygiene and gingivitis had diminished.

A similar 3-year study was carried out by Axelsson and Lindhe (1978) to include an investigation on caries increment. Their experimental group of 375 adults received scaling, root planing, and oral hygiene instruction at 2-month intervals for the first 2 years and three-monthly during the third year. One hundred and eighty matched controls received only traditional dental care at yearly intervals and, during this period, demonstrated persistent gingivitis and progressive loss of periodontal attachment. The experimental group, on the other hand, showed negligible signs of gingivitis and no loss of periodontal support.

The deficiencies of traditional dental care were further highlighted by Björn (1974) who carried out a 6-year longitudinal study of dental health in 653 individuals. Those attending regularly for traditional dental care during the 6-year period suffered the same loss of periodontal support as those who attended sporadically.

Söderholm (1979) described a longitudinal study of 454 Swedish shipyard workers who, for 9 years between 1965 and 1974, received traditional dental care. Then, for 4 years between 1974 and 1978, they were enrolled instead on a treatment programme with a strong preventive emphasis which included scaling and oral hygiene instruction at 3-month intervals. The preventive programme reduced the proportion of tooth surfaces coated in plaque from 60 per cent to 20 per cent approximately, and the rate of periodontal bone loss from about 0.1 mm per year to zero; the rate of tooth loss was halved, at 0.1 teeth per individual per year. A cost–benefit analysis was reported by Björn (1982). Thus, traditional care was estimated at 2 h of 'dentist time' and 16 min of 'dental auxillary time' per year, while the preventive programme required 54 minutes of 'dentist time' and 1 h 54 min of 'dental auxillary time' per year. Although the participants spent 32 min more per year in the dental chair during the preventive programme, their dental care cost 10–20 per cent less, because the greater proportion of dental care was performed by an auxilliary. Furthermore, during the 4 years of prevention the participants enjoyed a much better standard of periodontal health and an improved periodontal prognosis.

Chemoprophylaxis

Plaque control by mechanical debridement is highly labour-intensive, whether professionally administered or practised personally. Satisfactory home care further demands a measure of manual dexterity and a high degree of motivation which many individuals do not possess. Not surprisingly, therefore, a large number of chemical agents have been tested for their ability to reduce plaque accumulation.

In spite of the wide range of antimicrobial substances of proven effectiveness in the treatment of many different infections, the nature of dental plaque infection limits the usefulness of chemical agents. Of major significance are the apparent non-specific nature of chronic gingivitis and the proliferative capacity of oral bacteria. Streptococci, for example, have a generation time of 30 min and a reduction in their numbers of, say, 75 per cent by a single short exposure to a bactericidal mouthwash would be followed by a gradual increase to the original numbers within 1 h. Even after a 99.9 per cent reduction in their numbers a normal bacterial count would be restored within 5 h. This rough calculation has been confirmed by *in vivo* experiment (Strålfors 1962). Effective suppression of oral bacteria can, therefore, only be achieved by frequent topical application, by the topical use of a drug which is retained for long periods within the mouth, or by continual systemic administration where the dosage is adjusted such that the lowest level in the saliva is above the minimal inhibitory concentrations for plaque bacteria.

This review is limited to a consideration of drugs which have been tested as preventive agents for their effects on *supragingival* plaque accumulation. These include various antibiotics and antiseptics. Therapeutic agents directed against *subgingival* plaque lie outwith the scope of this discussion.

Antibiotics

Several antibiotics (see reviews by Parsons 1974; Loesche 1976) have been shown to suppress plaque formation and gingivitis to various degrees, whether used topically or systemically. These include broad-spectrum antibiotics, such as tetracycline and kanamycin; those with a narrower spectrum, such as penicillin, erythromycin and spiramycin; those specifically antagonistic towards Gram-positive organisms, such as vancomycin and niddamycin (CC10232); and those with a purely Gram-negative spectrum, such as polymyxin. However, the dangers of indiscriminate use of antibiotics, whether applied topically or administered systemically, are well documented—selection of resistant strains, promotion of hypersensitivity, and superinfection. None of the presently available antibiotics, therefore, can be recommended for routine control of supragingival plaque.

Bisbiguanide antiseptics

Various antiseptic mouthwashes can achieve a temporary reduction in the number of bacteria in saliva (Slanetz and Brown 1949) or plaque (Strålfors 1962). However, only those agents that remain active in the mouth, to exert a prolonged effect after administration, are capable of significant plaque inhibition. Thus, Gjermo *et al.* (1970) demonstrated that the cationic bisbiguanide, chlorhexidine, was a much more effective plaque-inhibitor *in vivo* than other antiseptics with equal or better *in vitro* activity. Of the cationic bisbiguanides, chlorhexidine has received by far the greatest attention. Other members of this group have been shown to possess similar potential as plaque inhibitors but they share side effects in common with chlorhexidine (Gjermo *et al.* 1973; Baker *et al.* 1979), and have, therefore, not been promoted to any significant extent.

Chlorhexidine

As chlorhexidine is currently the most extensively tested and most effective chemical anti-plaque and anti-gingivitis agent, its properties are described in more detail below.

Mode of action. Chlorhexidine is a cationic bisbiguanide with a broad spectrum of bactericidal activity against Gram-positive and Gram-negative organisms (Davies *et al.* 1954). It was marketed by ICI (Macclesfield, England) in 1953 as a general disinfectant for skin and mucous membranes. It is used principally in the form of chlorhexidine gluconate.

The positively-charged chlorhexidine binds to bacteria cell walls and to various oral surfaces including the hydroxyapatite of tooth enamel, the organic pellicle covering the tooth surface, mucous membrane and salivary protein (Rölla *et al.* 1970; 1971). Besides acting immediately on oral bacteria it is slowly desorbed from these sites to exert a prolonged bactericidal effect, and subsequently, as its concentration falls, a bacteriostatic effect for several hours (Bonesvoll 1977). It interacts with bacteria, damaging permeability barriers and precipitating cytoplasm. The pharmacodynamics of chlorhexidine in the mouth indicate that the frequency of application should not be less than twice daily. A 0.2 per cent aqueous mouth rinse twice daily has been shown to reduce the salivary bacterial count by 85–95 per cent over a 22-day period (Schiött *et al.* 1970), and essentially to prevent plaque accumulation and gingivitis development in subjects whose habitual mechanical cleaning is suspended (Löe and Schiött 1970*a*). Suppression of the salivary flora, however, does not appear to play a major part in dental plaque inhibition, which is primarily a result of the local antibacterial activity of chlorhexidine that has become bound to tooth surface components (Davies *et al.* 1970).

Method of application. Chlorhexidine may be administered as a mouth rinse, as a toothpaste or gel, in an oral irrigator, or as a spray. It is generally accepted that 10 ml of 0.2 per cent chlorhexidine, used for 1 min twice daily, is a convenient and satisfactory mouthwash regimen which will produce absolute plaque control in all individuals (Löe and Schiött 1970*a*). However, there is some scope for variation of the concentration, volume, duration of exposure, and number of doses per day. Thus, gingivitis may be prevented to a significant extent with reduced dosage and frequency of use, viz. 15 ml of 0.2 per cent chlorhexidine once daily (Lang *et al.* 1982); 10 ml of 0.1 per cent chlorhexidine twice daily (Flötra *et al.* 1972; Axelsson and Lindhe 1987); 15 ml of 0.1 per cent chlorhexidine once daily (Lang *et al.* 1982); and 15 ml of 0.12 per cent chlorhexidine twice daily (Grossman *et al.* 1986; Segreto *et al.* 1986; Siegrist *et al.* 1986). In theory, side-effects should be less when using reduced concentrations of the drug, thereby leading to better compliance for long-term usage. However, a mouthwash concentration of 0.1 per cent must be close to the threshold of effectiveness for chlorhexidine. It is reported that 30 ml of 0.1 per cent chlorhexidine once daily failed to prevent plaque and gingivitis (Lang and Räber 1981), and several investigators have found interindividual variation in the effectiveness of 10 ml of 0.1 per cent chlorhexidine twice daily (Schroeder 1969; Gjermo *et al.* 1970; Flötra *et al.* 1972). An 'all or none' response occurs so that plaque inhibition will be optimal in some subjects but completely absent in others. Therefore, when prolonged use is planned, the minimum concentration necessary should be individually assessed. For short-term use, 10 ml of 0.2 per cent chlorhexidine remains the mouthwash regimen of choice.

A more intensive programme of mouth rinsing has been shown to allow resolution of a superficial gingivitis produced by 17 days of uninterrupted plaque accumulation (Löe and Schiött 1970b). This regimen comprised six one-minute rinses with 10 ml of 0.2 per cent chlorhexidine in the space of one hour followed by twice daily rinsing with the same solution. After 6 days the teeth were virtually plaque free.

It was further shown by Flötra *et al.* (1972) that twice daily 0.2 per cent chlorhexidine mouthwashes, accompanied by customary personal oral hygiene regimens, although producing a large reduction in supragingival plaque, had a less dramatic effect on established gingivitis where subgingival plaque had formed. Following subgingival scaling, the experimental group receiving chlorhexidine showed substantial improvement in gingival health in those areas where pocket depths did not exceed 3 mm. However, even after subgingival scaling, the continued use of chlorhexidine had no therapeutic effect where pocket depths exceeded 3 mm. Presumably, therefore, chlorhexidine mouthwash is unable to eliminate subgingival plaque or to prevent recolonization of deep pathological pockets from subgingival deposits of bacteria not removed by scaling.

As an alternative to the mouthwash, the use of a toothpaste or gel containing 0.5 to 1.0 per cent chlorhexidine gluconate has not produced consistently good results. Johansen *et al.* (1975) and Emilson and Fornell (1976) found no significant effects on either plaque or gingival health. Lennon and Davies (1975), Hansen *et al.* (1975), Hoyos *et al.* (1977), and Bain and Strahan (1978) obtained small but significant reductions in plaque deposition only; Bassiouny and Grant (1975), Russell and Bay (1975), Saxton *et al.* (1976), and Joyston-Bechal *et al.* (1979) obtained significant reductions both in plaque accumulation and gingival inflammation.

The high reactivity of the chlorhexidine molecule and its incompatibility with many standard toothpaste constituents could account for these conflicting reports. Alternatively, there may be considerable variation in the ability of different individuals to apply chlorhexidine toothpaste/gel to all tooth surfaces effectively with a tooth-brush. Differences in study design and sample characteristics also tend to invalidate strict comparison of these reports. Nevertheless, analysis of these accumulated data points to the tentative conclusion that chlorhexidine gel is of little adjunctive value in individuals with moderate or good oral hygiene, while it will have its greatest therapeutic effect among those with high plaque levels and frank gingivitis. This conclusion is supported by the work of Flötra (1973) and Usher (1975), who demonstrated significant reductions in plaque, debris and gingivitis when chlorhexidine gel was applied in trays to the teeth of severely handicapped individuals for whom conventional cleaning methods were unacceptable. The efficacy of gel application in trays has recently been confirmed by Francis *et al.* (1987*a*) in a study of handicapped children, but unfortunately most of the parents and house parents found the technique awkward and felt they would not be willing to continue the regimen for long periods (Francis *et al.* 1987*b*).

Although early studies have testified to the value of a 0.2 per cent mouthwash used twice daily in 10 ml doses for one minute, it has been shown that if larger volumes are used, much lower concentrations are necessary and, therefore, local side-effects such as staining of teeth and fillings are reduced. Fifty millilitres of a 0.1 per cent solution or 100 ml of a 0.075 per cent solution achieved better plaque control than 20 ml of 0.2 per cent solution once daily (Cumming and Löe 1973*a*). In this study, it was further shown that the distribution of chlorhexidine to the more inaccessible areas of the dentition may be improved with the use of an oral irrigator. Optimal results were obtained using 700 ml of 0.05 per cent chlorhexidine once daily. This essentially prevented plaque formation. In a more recent study on the use of chlorhexidine with an oral irrigator, Lang and Ramseier-Grossman (1981) established that 400 ml of a 0.02 per cent solution of chlorhexidine once daily was the lowest concentration and dose to achieve complete plaque inhibition. Reducing the concentration further did not achieve complete plaque control even when the dose was increased.

Dever (1979) tested the effect of chlorhexidine applied in a spray (5 ml of 0.2 per cent solution) to the dentition of handicapped children, and found it to be moderately successful in preventing plaque accumulation and gingivitis. In a similar study, (Francis *et al.* 1987*b*) showed that the spray method of chlorhexidine application was considerably more popular among the parents and house parents of handicapped children than the mouthwash or gel application in trays. In this study, however, the spray delivered a lower dose of chlorhexidine (1.5–2 ml of 0.2 per cent solution) and consequently the effect on plaque and gingivitis was minimal (Francis *et al.* 1987*a*). Nevertheless, the comparative simplicity of this mode of delivery for handicapped children would seem to merit further research.

Safety and side effects. Bacteriological studies conducted after long-term use of chlorhexidine mouthwash have shown that, although the number of salivary and plaque organisms were reduced, there was no detectable shift in microbial populations, no residual effects on salivary or plaque bacteria after cessation of rinsing (Schiött *et al.* 1976a; Briner *et al.* 1986*a*) and little evidence of bacterial mutation or selection of resistant strains (Schiött *et al.* 1976*b*; Briner *et al.* 1986*b*). Furthermore, after a 22-day period of twice daily mouth rinsing with 0.2 per cent chlorhexidine the total salivary bacterial count increased to the control level within 48 h (Schiött *et al.* 1970), and plaque formed at normal rates after 24 h (Löe and Schiött 1970*a*).

Data accumulated over a period of 20 years concerning the safety of chlorhexidine in animal (Case 1977) and human (Rushton 1977) studies have been reviewed. It is known to have low irritancy and is most unlikely to produce sensitization. Absorption after oral ingestion is very low and long-term use has produced no changes in haematological or biochemical parameters. Prolonged application has failed to show carcinogenic or teratogenic effects.

The majority of side-effects are of a local nature. It has an unpleasant taste and produces disturbances in taste sensation which may last for several hours. Brown discoloration of teeth and fillings is common, both with mouthwash and gel preparations of chlorhexidine, a side-effect which is shared with other cationic antiseptics. Brown staining of the dorsum of the tongue occurs with the mouthwash but not with the toothpaste/gel. There is an interaction between locally adsorbed chlorhexidine and factors derived from diet such as the tannin-like substances in red wine, tea and coffee (Jensen 1977; Addy *et al.* 1979; Praynito *et al.* 1979). This interaction is responsible for the characteristic stain.

Desquamative lesions of the oral mucosa occur in a small number of individuals, perhaps due to precipitation of acidic mucins and proteins that cover and protect mucous membranes (Flötra *et al.* 1971). A few cases of unilateral or bilateral parotid gland swelling have been reported after use of chlorhexidine mouth rinses. The clinical features are suggestive of mechanical obstruction of the parotid duct (Rushton 1977).

There is a tendency for more supragingival calculus to be formed (Löe *et al.* 1976; Grossman *et al.* 1986; Segreto *et al.* 1986) which counteracts the benefits of chlorhexidine.

On the whole, these local side-effects appear to diminish if the drug concentration is reduced and probably occur to a lesser extent with the toothpaste/gel than with the mouthwash.

Clinical applications. Although the side-effects are minor, their existence has placed limitations on the application of chlorhexidine to clinical practice. Nevertheless, chlorhexidine has been shown to serve a useful function in the following circumstances.

1. The post-operative management of periodontal wounds: this literature has been reviewed by Davies (1977). Chlorhexidine may be used as an alternative to periodontal dressing or after its removal, when it permits a rapid resolution of post-operative gingival inflammation due to its ability to prevent new plaque formation. Although rinsing with chlorhexidine while a periodontal dressing is *in situ* has no siginficant effect on the wound, incorporation of chlorhexidine acetate powder into a methacrylic-gel dressing will promote healing.

2. The management of desquamative forms of gingivitis: individuals with painful gingival lesions may be placed on a chlorhexidine mouthwash regimen instead of tooth-brushing.

3. Plaque control during intermaxillary fixation: patients with jaw fractures, which have been treated by intermaxillary fixation, will be unable to perform mechanical cleansing procedures on lingual tooth areas, and may benefit from a chlorhexidine mouthwash.

4. Long-term plaque control in handicapped patients: a large variety of disabling conditions may prevent the practice of effective mechanical plaque control. Other individuals may have serious diseases for which absolute dental plaque control is essential to avoid the hazards of tooth extraction. These include haemophiliacs, patients with acute leukaemia, and those who have received radiotherapy in the region of the jaws.

Beneficial effects have been obtained from the continued use of chlorhexidine mouthwash, toothpaste, or gel application on a long-term basis. In this respect, it should be noted that no serious side-effects have been reported after two years continuous use of chlorhexidine in humans (Löe *et al.* 1975).

Unfortunately, the success of chlorhexidine in these specific situations is not equalled by its effect on established periodontal disease. As previously noted, the standard mouthwash regimen will not remove existing supragingival plaque or penetrate below the gingival margin to remove subgingival plaque. Furthermore, if chlorhexidine mouthwash is used during the initial phase of hygiene therapy, it will mask the effects of personal mechanical plaque control upon which successful long-term treatment of periodontal disease is dependent, and make proper evaluation of the patient's efforts impossible. Chlorhexidine, therefore, should be reserved for prevention of plaque accumulation only where mechanical plaque removal is impracticable.

Other antiseptics

While it is generally recognized that chlorhexidine is currently superior to all other plaque-inhibiting drugs, numerous other antiseptics have been tested in the hope of finding a chemical agent as safe and as effective as chlorhexidine but with less significant local side-effects (for review see Addy 1986).

A number of mouthwashes are commercially available and have been tested using chlorhexidine as a positive control. On the whole, their ability to prevent plaque formation and gingivitis is modest although further research work is proceeding to find optimal regimens and to confirm their safety.

Quaternary ammonium compounds. Like chlorhexidine, quaternary ammonium compounds are cationic surface-active agents. Cetylpyridinium chloride (Cetrimide®) and benzalkonium chloride are the most studied, and are almost as effective as chlorhexidine in plaque control if they are used in a mouthwash four times daily instead of twice daily (Bonesvoll and Gjermo 1978). This study suggested that, although quaternary ammonium compounds are adsorbed in greater amounts, they are also desorbed from binding surfaces much faster than chlorhexidine.

Phenolic compounds. Listerine® mouthwash, a well-established commercial preparation of phenolic compounds, is shown in comparative studies to be less effective in plaque inhibition than chlorhexidine mouthwash (Lang and Brecx 1986; Axelsson and Lindhe 1987) but possibly more effective in preventing gingivitis (Axelsson and Lindhe 1987), perhaps due to prostaglandin synthetase inhibitor activity (Dewhirst 1980).

Sanguinarine. Veadent® mouthwash contains zinc chloride and sanguinaria, a plant extract. Recent studies have found that it substantially reduces the amount of plaque and gingivitis relative to a placebo mouthwash (Wennström and Lindhe 1986). However, studies by Lang and Brecx (1986), Wennström and Lindhe (1986), and Etemadzadeh and Ainamo (1987), showed that the plaque-inhibiting effect of sanguinarine mouthwash was inferior to that of chlorhexidine.

Hexetidine. Bergenholtz and Hanström (1974) showed that the anti-plaque activity of hexetidine (Oraldene®) was small compared to that of chlorhexidine, and that increasing its concentration led to painful mucosal erosions.

Stannous fluoride. Mouthwashes of stannous fluoride have been shown in several studies to possess an antibacterial effect. This is attributed mainly to the stannous ion, a divalent cation whose positive charge interferes with bacterial adhesion (Skjörland *et al.* 1978). Svatun *et al.* (1977) showed that 0.2 or 0.3 per cent stannous fluoride mouthwash has a plaque-inhibiting potential significantly greater than the placebo mouthwash but inferior to chlorhexidine.

Not only are the above antiseptics inferior to chlorhexidine with respect to plaque inhibition, but none are without side-effects. Thus cetylpyridinium chloride, Listerine® and sanguinarine are all reported to cause brown staining of teeth (Lang and Brecx 1986), while stannous fluoride has a metallic taste, stains teeth, increases calculus formation, and may cause desquamative lesions (Svatun *et al.* 1977).

Concluding remarks

Periodontal disease is caused by bacterial plaque. It is a worldwide problem but one which is more acute in underdeveloped countries where standards of personal hygiene are low. In modern countries, ritual, if not entirely efficient, oral hygiene practices have reduced the rate of attachment loss to approximately 0.1 mm/year. This figure, however, is a population mean, which includes measurements taken at stable healthy sites and at sites of rapid destruction where attachment loss may proceed at a much faster rate. Thus, it is estimated that periodontal disease accounts for about 20–30 per cent of all extractions.

In spite of the almost universal prevalence of periodontitis, it progresses to tooth loss in only 10–15 per cent of the population (Schaub 1984). Prevention is labour-intensive and because the means do not exist at present to discriminate between high-risk and low-risk individuals, it could be argued that preventive programmes are wasteful. This might be true if the only objective of a preventive strategy was to prevent tooth loss. Less aggressive forms of periodontal disease, however, while posing no threat to tooth survival, may nonetheless be unacceptable to the victim: bleeding gingiva and bad taste may be distressing; red swollen gingiva, exposed roots and migrated teeth may be unaesthetic; and halitosis is socially undesirable. Freedom from periodontal symptoms and a sense of personal well-being must, therefore, be an important objective of preventive periodontal care. As living standards improve and health expectations rise, an increasing number of individuals may be unwilling to accept mere tooth survival as a suitable yardstick of dental fitness.

Increasing the availability and utilization of present systems of restorative dental care is no answer. Indeed, it has been shown that periodontal disease may progress at the same rate in those receiving regular traditional reparative dental care as in those who attend sporadically (Björn 1974). Adequate dental health education and a greater measure of professional preventive care are needed to achieve satisfactory control of periodontal disease.

Numerous programmes in schools and among adults have been evaluated. The large body of information on the merits and limitations of preventive strategies, which these studies make available, may be used in the planning and implementation of dental health programmes both at a population level and in dental practices, where the specific needs of each patient can be met.

Preventive efforts directed towards groups of children are, in some ways, more acceptable and make less demand on resources than similar schemes in adults. In children, calculus deposits are less common, the disease is largely reversible and indoctrination may be more successful. Daily group-instruction in toothbrushing, however, is of questionable value. Doubts have been expressed regarding its cost-effectiveness. Furthermore, this measure has little effect approximally and in molar areas, and the habit is not automatically maintained when supervision is withdrawn. On the other hand, regular professional tooth cleaning, with individual oral hygiene instruction and motivation by enthusiastic dental personnel, may have a significant preventive effect on both periodontal disease and caries in children or adults. The precise nature of this form of preventive care and the interval between preventive visits should take account of individual variation in the rate of plaque and calculus accumulation, in susceptibility to gingivitis and destructive periodontal disease, and in the response to preventive procedures. It should also be remembered that deep pockets, not accessible to adequate personal or professional cleaning, may require surgical intervention.

In a dentally conscious society, emphasis should be placed on further improvement in personal oral hygiene while, in individuals unable, through handicap or lack of motivation, to maintain adequate standards of cleanliness, attachment loss may be slightly retarded by periodic scaling and root planing.

Destructive changes are common by adolescence, accompanying gingivitis in individuals who harbour plaque deposits on their teeth. Although it is understood that periodontitis represents the apical extension of a lesion which was initiated in the gingiva, it is by no means certain that the onset of destructive changes is dependent on the duration or severity of pre-existing gingivitis. It is quite possible that periodontitis might develop at any time in response to the emergence of certain specific plaque micro-organisms and alterations in the immune response. Should this latter hypothesis be correct, then a prolonged phase of plaque control during childhood would not exempt an individual from the destructive effects of plaque accumulation in adolescence. The need for periodontal preventive care to continue throughout adolescence and into adult life would then assume greater importance.

With regard to the practical aspects of plaque control, oral hygiene aids should be prescribed to suit individual needs and capabilities. A few individuals may be able to maintain periodontal health by tooth-brushing alone without further effort. For others whose brushing technique fails to remove approximal plaque, interdental cleaning is necessary. Where gingival tissue fills the interdental space, dental floss is the only suitable agent. Where a little gingival recession has occurred, a triangular woodpoint will gain access and may be more acceptable to the patient. Large interdental spaces are best cleaned by an interdental brush.

Chemical anti-plaque agents are now available, their development promoted by a lack of public enthusiasm for mechanical methods of plaque control. The broad-spectrum antiseptic, chlorhexidine, has been exhaustively tested and remains the agent of choice in chemical control of supragingival plaque. It is a valuable means of prophylaxis for selected patients but has not achieved the status of a universal panacea for the prevention of dental plaque infections. Indeed, Löe (1979), who pioneered the early studies on the dental uses of chlorhexidine, has stated: 'I am somewhat concerned about the indiscriminate use of this and other agents . . . I strongly believe that at this point in time the use of chlorhexidine should be based on firm diagnostic criteria, should be appropriately monitored and frequency of application prescribed on the basis of disease characteristics'.

Clearly, for the majority of individuals with a positive attitude towards oral health, the means already exist to maintain reasonably good periodontal conditions throughout life, using comparatively simple forms of personal and professional care. There remains, however, a minority of individuals who are highly susceptible to the destructive effects of plaque accumulation. Current research is aimed at finding methods to identify these individuals at an early stage of the disease so that more intensive preventive care can be made available to them.

References

Adams, R. and Stanmeyer, W. (1960). The effects of a closely supervised oral hygiene program upon oral cleanliness. *J. Perio.* **31**, 242.

Addy, M. (1986) Chlorhexidine compared with other locally delivered antimicrobials. A short review. *J. clin. Perio.* **13**, 957.

Addy, M. and Bates, J.F. (1979). Plaque accumulation following the wearing of different types of removable partial dentures. *J. oral. Rehab.* **6**, 111.

Addy, M., Praynito, S.W., Taylor, L., and Cadogan, S. (1979). An *in vitro* study of the role of dietary factors in the aetiology of tooth staining associated with the use of chlorhexidine. *J. perio. Res.* **14**, 403.

Agerbaek, N., Melsen, B., and Rölla, G. (1975). Application of chlorhexidine by oral irrigation systems. *Scand. J. dent. Res.* **83**, 284.

Agerbaek, N., Poulsen, S., Melsen, B., and Glavind, L. (1978). Effect of professional toothcleansing every third week on gingivitis and dental caries in children. *Commun. Dent. oral Epidemiol.* **6**, 40.

Ainamo, J. (1972). Relationship between malalignment of the teeth and periodontal disease. *Scand. J. dent. Res.* **80**, 104.

Ainamo, J., Barmes, D., Beagrie, G., Cutress, T., Martin, J., and Sardo-Infirri, J. (1982). Development of the World Health Organisation (WHO) community periodontal index of treatment needs (CPITN). *Int. dent. J.* **32**, 281.

Ainamo, J., Sarkki, L., Kuhalampi, M.L., Palolampi, L., and Piirto, O. (1984). The frequency of periodontal extractions in Finland. *Commun. dent. Hlth.* **1**, 165.

Aleo, J., De Renzis, F, and Farber, P. (1975). *In vitro* attachment of human gingival fibroblasts to root surfaces. *J. Perio.* **46**, 639.

Aleo, J., De Renzis, F., Farber, P., and Varbonceur, A. (1974). The presence and biological activity of cementum bound endotoxin. *J. Perio.* **45**, 672.

Anderson, R.J. (1981). The changes in the dental health of 12-year-old schoolchildren in two Somerset schools. A review after an interval of 15 years. *Br. dent. J.* **150**, 218.

Ashley, F.P. and Sainsbury, R.H. (1981). The effect of a school-based plaque control programme on caries and gingivitis. *Br. dent. J.* **150**, 41.

Axelsson, P. and Lindhe, J. (1974). The effect of a preventive programme on dental plaque, gingivitis and caries in schoolchildren. *J. clin. Perio.* **1**, 126.

Axelsson, P. and Lindhe, J. (1977). The effect of a plaque control programme on gingivitis and dental caries in schoolchildren. *J. dent. Res.* **56** (spec. iss. C), 142.

Axelsson, P. and Lindhe, J. (1978). Effect of controlled oral hygiene procedures on caries and periodontal disease in adults. *J. clin. Perio.* **5**, 133.

Axelsson, P. and Lindhe, J. (1981). Effect of oral hygiene instruction and professional toothcleaning on caries and gingivitis in schoolchildren. *Commun. Dent. oral Epidemiol.* **9**, 251.

Axelsson, P. and Lindhe, J.(1987). Efficacy of mouthrinses in inhibiting dental plaque and gingivitis in man. *J. clin. Perio.* **14**, 205.

Axelsson, P., Lindhe, J., and Wäseby, J. (1976). The effect of various plaque control measures on gingivitis and caries in schoolchildren. *Commun. Dent. oral Epidemiol.* **4**, 232.

Badersten, A., Egelberg, J., and Koch, G. (1975). Effect of monthly prophylaxis on caries and gingivitis in schoolchildren. *Commun. Dent. oral Epidemiol.* **3**, 1.

Badersten, A., Nilveus, R., and Egelberg, J. (1984). Effects of non-surgical periodontal therapy. II Severely advanced periodontitis. *J. clin. Perio.*. **11**, 63.

Bain, M.J. and Strahan, J.D. (1978). The effect of a 1% chlorhexidine gel in the initial therapy of chronic periodontal disease. *J. Perio.* **49**, 469.

Baker, P.J., Coburn, R.A., Genco, R.J., and Evans, R.T. (1979). Alkyl-bisbiguanides as *in vitro* inhibitors of bacterial growth and dental plaque formation. *J. perio. Res.* **14**, 352.

Barnes, G.P., Stookey, G.K., and Muhler, J.C. (1971). *In vitro* studies of the calculus-inhibiting properties of tooth surface polishing agents and chelating agents. *J. dent. Res.* **50**, 966.

Bassiouny, M.-A. and Grant, A.A. (1975). The toothbrush application of chlorhexidine. *Br. dent. J.* **139**, 323.

Baumhammers, A. and Rohrbaugh, E. (1970). Permeability of human and rat dental calculus. *J. Perio.* **41**, 39.

Baumhammers, A., Conway, J.C., Saltzberg, D., and Matta, R.K. (1973). Scanning electron microscopy of supragingival calculus. *J. Perio.* **44**, 92.

Beltrami, M., Bickel, M., and Baehni, P.C. (1987). The effect of supragingival plaque control on the composition of the subgigival microflora in human periodontitis. *J. clin. Perio.* **3**, 161.

Bennie, A.M., Tullis, J.I., Stephen, K.W., and MacFadyen, E.E. (1978). Five years of community preventive dentistry and health education in the County of Sutherland. *Commun. Dent. oral Epidemiol.* **6**, 1.

Bergenholtz, A. (1972). Mechanical cleaning in oral hygiene. In *Oral hygiene*, (ed. A. Frandsen), p. 27. Munksgaard, Copenhagen.

Bergenholtz, A. and Brithon, J. (1980). Plaque removal by dental floss or toothpicks. An intra-individual comparative study. *J. clin. Perio.* **7**, 516.

Bergenholtz, A. and Hanström, L. (1974). The plaque inhibiting effect of hexetidine (Oraldene®) mouthwash compared to that of chlorhexidine. *Commun. Dent. oral Epidemiol.* **2**, 70.

Bergenholtz, A. and Olsson, A. (1984). Efficacy of plaque-removal using interdental brushes and waxed dental floss. *Scand. J. dent. Res.* **92**, 198.

Bergenholtz, A., Hugoson, A., and Sohlberg, F. (1967). The plaque-removing property of some oral hygiene aids. *Svensk, tandläkare Tidskrift* **60**, 447.

Bergenholtz, A., Bjorne, A., and Vikström, B. (1974). The plaque-removing ability of some common interdental aids. An intra-individual study. *J. clin. Perio.* **1**, 160.

Bergenholtz, A., Bjorne, A., Glantz, P.-O., and Vikström. B. (1980). Plaque removal by various triangular toothpicks. *J. clin. Perio.* **7**, 121.

Björn, A.-L. (1974). Dental health in relation to age and dental care. *Odont. revy* **27** (suppl.) 29.

Björn, A.-L. (1982). Economy aspects of preventive dentistry. In *Dental health care in Scandinavia*, (ed. A. Frandsen), p. 217. Quintessence, Chicago.

Björn, A.-L., Björn, H., and Grkovic, B. (1969). Marginal fit of restorations and its relation to periodontal bone level. Part I Metal fillings. *Odont. Revy* **20**, 311.

Björn, A.-L., Björn, H., and Grkovic, B. (1970). Marginal fit of restorations and its relation to periodontal bone level. Part II Crowns. *Odont. Revy* **21**, 337.

Blinkhorn, A.S., Fox, B., and Holloway, P.J. (1983). *Notes on Dental Health Education*. Scottish Health Education Group, Edinburgh, and Health Education Authority, London.

Bonesvoll, P. (1977). Oral pharmacology of chlorhexidine, *J. clin. Perio.* **4**, 49.

Bonesvoll, P. and Gjermo, P. (1978). A comparison between chlorhexidine and some quarternary ammonium compounds with regard to retention, salivary concentration and plaque-inhibiting effect in the human mouth after mouth rinses. *Archs. oral Biol.* **23**, 289.

Bossert, W.A. and Marks, H.H. (1956). Prevalence and characteristics of periodontal disease of 12 800 persons under periodic dental observation. *J. Am. dent. Ass.* **52**, 429.

Bowen, W.H. (1974). Effect of restricting oral intake to invert sugar or casein on the microbiology of plaque in *Macaca fascicularis (irus)*. *Archs. oral Biol.* **19**, 231.

Bowen, W.H. (1976). The nature of plaque. *Oral Sci. Rev.* **9**, 3.

Boyde, A. (1971). The tooth surface. In *The prevention of periodontal disease*, (ed. J.E. Eastoe, D.C.A. Picton and A.G. Alexander). Kimpton, London.

Brandtzaeg, P. and Jamieson, H.C. (1964). The effect of controlled cleansing of the teeth on periodontal health and oral hygiene in Norwegian army recruits. *J. Perio.* **35**, 308.

Brecx, M., Theilade, J., and Attström, R. (1980). Influence of optimal and excluded oral hygiene on early formation of dental plaque on plastic films. A quantitative and descriptive light and electron microscopic study. *J. clin. Perio.* **7**, 361.

Breitenmoser, J., Mormann, W., and Mühlemann, H.R. (1979). Damaging effects of toothbrush bristle end form on gingiva. *J. Perio.* **50**, 212.

Briner, W.W. *et al.* (1986*a*). Effect of chlorhexidine gluconate mouthrinse on plaque bacteria. *J. perio. Res.* **21** (suppl. 16), 44.

Briner, W.W. *et al.* (1986*b*). Assessment of susceptibility of plaque bacteria to chlorhexidine after six months oral use. *J. perio. Res.* **21** (suppl. 16), 53.

Buckley, L.A. (1980). The relationship between irregular teeth, plaque, calculus and gingival disease. *Br. dent. J.* **148**, 67.

Case, D.E. (1977) Safety of Hibitane I. Laboratory experiments. *J. clin. Perio* **4**, 66.

Chasens, A.I. and Marcus, R.W. (1968). An evaluation of the comparative efficiency of manual and automatic toothbrushes in maintaining the periodontal patient. *J. Perio* **39**, 156.

Chawla, T.N., Nanda, R.S., and Kapoor, K.K. (1975). Dental prophylaxis procedures in control of periodontal disease in Lucknow (rural India). *J. Perio.* **46**, 498.

Committee Report (1966*a*). Oral health care for the prevention and control of periodontal disease. In *World workshop in periodontics*, (ed. S.P. Ramfjord, D.A. Kerr and M.M. Ash), p. 444. University of Michigan Press, Ann Arbor.

Committee Report (1966*b*). The etiology of periodontal disease. In *World workshop in periodontics*, (ed. S.P. Ramfjord, D.A. Kerr and M.M. Ash), p. 167. University of Michigan Press, Ann Arbor.

Craft. M.H. (1984). Dental health education and periodontal disease: health policies, disease trends, target groups and strategies. In *Public health aspects of periodontal disease*, (ed. A. Frandsen), p. 149. Quintessence, Chicago.

Cumming, B.R. and Löe, H. (1973*a*). Optimal dosage and method of delivering chlorhexidine solutions for the inhibition of dental plaque. *J. perio. Res.* **8**, 57.

Cumming, B.R. and Löe, H. (1973*b*). Consistency of plaque distribution in individuals without special home care instruction. *J. perio. Res.* **8**, 94.

Curilovic, Z. (1979). Die ursachen des zahnverlustes in der Schweitz. Resultate einer umfrage bei privatzahnarzten. *S.S.O.* **89**, 727.

Cushing, A.M. and Sheiham, A. (1985). Assessing periodontal treatment needs and periodontal status in a study of adults in north-west England. *Commun. dent. Hlth.* **2**, 187.

Cutress, T.W. (1986). Periodontal health and periodontal disease in young people: global epidemiology. *Int. dent. J.* **36** 146.

Davies, G.E., Fransis, J., Martin, A.R., Rose, F.L., and Swain, G. (1954). 1:6 di-4 chlorophenyldiguanidohexane (Hibitane). Laboratory investigation of a new antibacterial agent of high potency. *Br. J. Pharmacol.* **9**, 192.

Davies, R.M. (1977). Use of Hibitane following periodontal surgery. *J. clin. Perio.* **4**, 129.

Davies, R.M., Jensen, S.B., Schiött, C.R., and Löe, H. (1970). The effect of topical application of chlorhexidine on the bacterial colonization of the teeth and gingiva. *J. perio. Res.* **5**, 96.

De La Rosa, M.R., Guerra, J.Z., Johnston, D.A., and Radike, A.W. (1979). Plaque growth and removal with daily toothbrushing. *J. Perio.* **50**, 661.

Dever, J.G. (1979). Oral hygiene in mentally handicapped children. A clinical trial using a chlorhexidine spray. *Australia dent. J.* **24**, 301.

Dewhirst, F.F. (1980). Structure-activity relationships for inhibition of prostaglandin cyclooxygenase by phenolic compounds. *Prostaglandins* **20**, 209.

Douglass, C.W., Gammon, M.D., and Orr, R.B. (1985). Oral health status in the United States: prevalence of inflammatory periodontal diseases. *J. dent. Educ.* **49**, 365.

Egelberg, J. (1965). Local effect of diet on plaque formation and development of gingivitis in dogs. III. Effect of frequency of meals and tube feeding. *Odont. Revy* **16**, 50.

El Ghamrawy, R. (1979). Qualitative changes in dental plaque formation related to removable partial dentures. *J. oral Rehab.* **6**, 183.

Emilson, C.G. and Fornell, J. (1976). The effect of toothbrushing with chlorhexidine gel on salivary microflora, oral hygiene and caries. *Scand. J. dent. Res.* **84**, 308.

Etemadzadeh, H. and Ainamo, J. (1987). Lacking anti-plaque efficacy of 2 sanguinarine mouth rinses. *J. clin. Perio.* **14**, 176.

Fay, H. (1964). Effect of prophylaxis and dental health education on periodontal status. *Dent. Abstr.* **9**, 248.

Fine, D.H. and Baumhammers, A. (1970). Effect of water pressure irrigation on stainable material on the teeth. *J. Perio.* **41**, 468.

Flanders, R.A. (1987). Effectiveness of dental health educational programs in schools. *J. Am. dent. Ass.* **14**, 239.

Flötra, L. (1973). Different modes of chlorhexidine application and related local side effects. *J. perio. Res.* **8** (suppl. 12), 41.

Flötra, L., Gjermo, P., Rölla, G., and Waerhaug, J. (1971). Side effects of chlorhexidine mouthwashes. *Scand. J. dent. Res.* **79**, 119.

Flötra, L., Gjermo, P., Rölla, G., and Waerhaug, J. (1972). A 4-month study on the effect of chlorhexidine mouthwashes on 50 soldiers. *Scand. J. dent. Res.* **80**, 10.

Francis, J.R., Hunter, B., and Addy, M. (1987*a*). A comparison of three delivery methods of chlorhexidine in handicapped children. I Effects on plaque, gingivitis and tooth staining. *J. Perio.* **58**, 451.

Francis, J.R., Addy, M., and Hunter, B. (1987*b*). A comparison of three delivery methods of chlorhexidine in handicapped children. II Parent and house-parent preferences. *J. Perio.* **58**, 456.

Frandsen, A. (1985). Changing patterns of attitudes and oral health behaviour. *Int. dent. J.* **35**, 284.

Frandsen, A.M., Barbano, J.P., Suomi, J.D., Chang, J.J., and Burke, A.D. (1970). The effectiveness of the Charters', scrub and roll methods of toothbrushing by professionals in removing plaque. *Scand. J. dent. Res.* **78**, 459.

Garrett, J.S. (1977). Root planing: a perspective. *J. Perio.* **48**, 553.

Gibson, J.A. and Wade, A.B. (1977). Plaque removal by the Bass and roll brushing techniques. *J. Perio.* **48**, 456.

Gjermo, P.E. (1967). Effect of combined audiovisual motivation and individual instruction in oral hygiene. *J. perio. Res.* **2**, 248.

Gjermo, P. and Flötra, L. (1970). The effect of different methods of interdental cleaning. *J. Perio. Res.* **5**, 230.

Gjermo, P., Baastad, K.L., and Rölla. A. (1970). The plaque-inhibiting capacity of 11 antibacterial compounds. *J. perio. Res.* **5**, 102.

Gjermo, P., Rölla, G., and Arskaug, L. (1973). Effect on dental plaque formation and some *in vitro* properties of 12 bis-biguanides. *J. perio. Res.* **8** (suppl. 12), 81.

Glantz. P.-O. (1969). On wettability and adhesiveness. *Odont. Revy* **20** (suppl. 17),

Glavind, L., Christensen, H., Pedersen, E., Rosendahl, H., and Attstrom, R. (1985). Oral hygiene instruction in general dental practice by means of self-teaching manuals. *J. clin. Perio.* **12**, 27.

Goh, C.J.W., Waite, I.M., Groves, B.J., and Cornick, D.E.R. (1986). The influence of gingival inflammation and pocketing on the rate of plaque formation during non-surgical periodontal treatment. *Br. dent. J.* **161**, 165.

Goldman, R.S., Abelson, D.C., Mandel, I.D., and Chilton, N.W. (1974). The effect of various disclosants on plaque accumulation in human subjects. *J. perio. Res.* **9**, 381.

Goodson, J.M., Tanner, A.C.R., Haffajee, A.D., Sornberger, G.C., and Socransky, S.S. (1982). Patterns of progression and regression of advanced destructive periodontal disease. *J. clin. Perio.* **9**, 472.

Greene, J.C. (1963). Oral hygiene and periodontal disease. *Am. J. publ. Hlth.* **53**, 913.

Greene, J.C. (1966). Oral health care for prevention and control of periodontal disease. In *World workshop in periodontics*, (ed. S.P. Ramfjord, D.A. Kerr and M.M. Ash), p. 399. University of Michigan Press, Ann Arbor.

Grossman, E. *et al.* (1986). Six-month study of the effects of a chlorhexidine mouthrinse on gingivitis in adults. *J. perio. Res.* **21** (suppl. 16), 33.

Gupta, O.P., O'Toole, E.T., and Hammermeister, R.O. (1973). Effects of a water pressure device on oral hygiene and gingival inflammation. *J. Perio.* **44**, 294.

Haffajee, A.D., Socransky, S.S., and Goodson, J.M. (1983). Clinical parameters as predictors of destructive periodontal disease activity. *J. clin. Perio.* **10**, 257.

Hamp, S.-E., Lindhe, J., Fornell, J., Johansson, L.Å., and Karlsson, E. (1978). Effect of a field program based on systematic plaque control on caries and gingivitis in schoolchildren after 3 years. *Commun. Dent. oral Epidemiol.* **6**, 17.

Hansen, F. and Gjermo, P. (1971). The plaque-removing effect of four toothbrushing methods. *Scand. J. dent. Res.* **79**, 502.

Hansen, F., Gjermo, P., and Eriksen, H.M. (1975). The effect of a chlorhexidine-containing gel on oral cleanliness and gingival health in young adults. *J. clin. Perio.* 2, 153.

Hatfield, C.G. and Baumhammers, A. (1971). Cytotoxic effects of periodontally involved surfaces of human teeth. *Archs. oral. Biol.* **16**, 465.

Health Education Council (1979). *The scientific basis of dental health education. A policy document*. London.

Hill, H.C., Levi, F.A., and Glickman, I. (1973). The effects of waxed and unwaxed dental floss on interdental plaque accumulation and interdental gingival health. *J. Perio.* **44**, 411.

Hillam, D.G. and Hull, P.S (1977). The influence of experimental gingivitis on plaque formation. *J. clin. Perio.* **4**, 56.

Honkala, E., Nyyssonen, V., Knuuttila, M., and Markkanen, H. (1986). Effectiveness of children's habitual toothbrushing. *J. clin. Perio.* **13**, 81.

Hoover, D.R. and Robinson, H.B.G. (1971). The comparative effectiveness of a pulsating oral irrigator as an adjunct in maintaining oral health. *J. Perio.* **42**, 37.

Hoover, J.N., Ellegaard, B., and Attström. R. (1981). Periodontal status of 14–16-year-old Danish schoolchildren. *Scand. J. dent. Res.* **89**, 175.

Horowitz, A.M., Suomi, J.D., Peterson, J.K., and Lyman, B.A. (1977). Effects of supervised daily dental plaque removal by children: 24 months' results. *J. publ. Hlth. Dent.* **37**, 180.

Hoyos, D.F., Murray, J.J., and Shaw, L. (1977). The effect of chlorhexidine gel on plaque and gingivitis in children. *Br. dent. J.* **142**, 366.

Hugoson, A. (1978). Effect of the Water Pik® device on plaque accumulation and development of gingivitis. *J. clin. Perio.* **5**, 95.

Hugoson, A. and Koch, G. (1979). Oral health in 1000 individuals aged 3–70 years in the community of Jonkoping, Sweden. *Swed. dent. J.* **3**, 69.

Hugoson, A. and Rylander, H. (1982). Longitudinal study of periodontal status in individuals aged 15 years in 1973 and 20 years in 1978 in Jonkoping, Sweden. *Commun. Dent. oral. Epidemiol.* **10**, 37.

Hugoson, A. *et al.* (1986). Oral health of individuals aged 3–80 years in Jonkoping, Sweden, in 1973 and 1983. II A review of clinical and radiographic findings. *Swed. dent. J.* **10**, 175.

Ingervall, B., Jacobsen, U., and Nyman, S. (1977). A clinical study of the relationship between crowding of teeth, plaque and gingival condition. *J. clin. Perio.* **4**, 214.

Ismail, A.I., Eklund, S.A., Striffler, D.F., and Szpunar, S.M. (1987). The prevalence of advanced loss of periodontal attachment in two New Mexico populations. *J. perio. Res.* **22**, 119.

Jenkins, W.M.M. and Mason, W.N. (1984). Periodontitis in the United Kingdom. *Br. dent.J.* **156**, 43.

Jensen, J.E. (1977). Binding of dyes to chlorhexidine treated hydroxyapatite. *Scand. J. dent. Res.* **85**, 334.

Johansen, J.R., Gjermo, P., and Eriksen, H.M. (1975). Effect of 2 years use of chlorhexidine-containing dentifrices on plaque, gingivitis and caries. *Scand. J. dent. Res.* **83**, 288.

Joyston-Bechal, S., Smales, F.C., and Duckworth, R. (1979). The use of a chlorhexidine-containing gel in a plaque control programme. *Br. dent. J.* **146**, 105.

Kay, E.J. and Blinkhorn, A.S. (1986). The reasons underlying the extraction of teeth in Scotland. *Br. dent. J.* **160**, 287.

Kegeles, S.S. (1963). Why people seek dental care: The test of conceptual formulation. *J. Hlth. hum Behav.* **4**, 166.

Keller, S.E. and Manson-Hing, L.R. (1969). Clearance studies of proximal tooth surfaces. Part III and IV: *in vivo* removal of interproximal plaque. *Ala, J. med. Sci.* **6**, 399.

Kelner, M. (1963). Comparative analysis of the effect of automatic and conventional toothbrushing in mental retardates. *Penn. dent. J.* **30**, 102.

Lainson, P.A., Berquist, J.J., and Fraleigh, C.M. (1970). Clinical evaluation of Pulsar®. A new pulsating water pressure cleansing device. *J. Perio.* **41**, 401.

Lainson, P.A., Berquist, J.J., and Fraleigh, C.M. (1972). A longitudinal study of pulsating water pressure cleansing devices. *J. Perio.* **43**, 444.

Lang, N.P. and Brecx, M.C. (1986). Chlorhexidine digluconate—an agent for chemical plaque control and prevention of gingival inflammation. *J. perio. Res.* **21** (suppl. 16), 74.

Lang, N.P. and Räber, K. (1981). Use of oral irrigators as vehicle for the application of antimicrobial agents in chemical plaque control. *J. clin. Perio.* **8**, 177.

Lang, N.P. and Ramseier-Grossman, K. (1981). Optimal dosage of chlorhexidine digluconate in chemical plaque control when applied by the oral irrigator. *J. clin. Perio.* **8**, 189.

Lang, N.P., Cumming, B.R., and Löe, H. (1973). Toothbrushing frequency as it relates to plaque development and gingival health. *J. Perio.* **44**, 396.

Lang, N.P., Hotz, P., Graff, H., Geering, A.H., and Saxer, U.P. (1982). Effects of supervised chlorhexidine mouthrinses in children. A longitudinal clinical trial. *J. perio. Res.* **17**, 101.

Lennon, M.A. and Davies, R.M. (1974). Prevalence and distribution of alveolar bone loss in a population of 15-year-old schoolchildren. *J. clin. Perio.* **1**, 175.

Lennon, M.A. and Davies, R.M. (1975). A short-term evaluation of a chlorhexidine gel on plaque deposits and gingival status. *Pharmacol. Ther. Dent.* **2**, 13.

Lightner, L.M., O'Leary, T.J., Jividen, G.J., Crump, P.P., and Drake, R.B. (1968). Preventive periodontic treatment procedures: results after one year. *J. Am. dent. Ass.* **76**, 1043.

Lightner, L.M., O'Leary, T.J., Drake, R.B., Crump, P.P., and Allen, M.F. (1971). Preventive periodontic treatment procedures: results over 46 months. *J. Perio.* **42**, 555.

Lindhe, J. and Axelsson, P. (1973). The effect of controlled oral hygiene and topical fluoride application on caries and gingivitis in Swedish schoolchildren. *Commun. Dent. oral Epidemiol.* **1**, 9.

Lindhe, J. and Koch, G. (1966). The effect of supervised oral hygiene on the gingivae of children. Progression and inhibition of gingivitis. *J. perio. Res.* **1**, 260.

Lindhe, J. and Koch, G. (1967). The effect of supervised oral hygiene on the gingivae of children. Lack of prolonged effect of supervision. *J. perio. Res.* **2**, 215.

Lindhe, J. and Wicén, P.-O. (1969). The effects on the gingivae of chewing fibrous foods. *J. perio. Res.* **4**, 193.

Lindhe, J., Koch, G., and Månsson, J. (1966). The effect of supervised oral hygiene on the gingiva of children. *J. perio. Res.* **1**, 268.

Lindhe, J., Axelsson, P., and Tollskog, G. (1975). Effect of proper oral hygiene on gingivitis and dental caries in Swedish schoolchildren. *Commun. Dent. oral Epidemiol.* **3**, 150.

Listgarten, M.A. (1986). Pathogenesis of periodontitis. *J. clin. Perio.* **13**, 418.

Listgarten, M.A., Lindhe, J., and Hellden, L. (1978). Effect of tetracycline and/or scaling on human periodontal disease. Clinical, microbiological and histological observations. *J. clin. Perio.* **5**, 246.

Lobene, R.R. (1969). The effect of a pulsed water pressure cleansing device on oral health. *J. Perio.* **40**, 667.

Lobene, R.R., Soparkar, P.M., Hein, J.W., and Quigley, G.A. (1972). A study of the effects of antiseptic agents and a pulsating irrigating device on plaque and gingivitis. *J. Perio.* **43**, 564.

Löe, H. (1969). Present day status and direction for future research on the etiology and prevention of periodontal disease. *J. Perio.* **40**, 678.

Löe, H. (1979). Mechanical and chemical control of dental plaque. *J. clin. Perio.* **6**, 32.

Löe, H. and Schiött, C.R. (1970*a*). The effect of mouthrinses and topical application of chlorhexidine on the development of dental plaque and gingivitis in man. *J. perio. Res.* **5**, 79.

Löe, H. and Schiött, C.R. (1970*b*). The effect of suppression of the oral microflora upon the development of dental plaque and gingivitis. In *Dental plaque*, (ed. W.D. McHugh), p. 247. Livingstone, Edinburgh.

Löe, H., Theilade, E., and Jensen, S.B. (1965). Experimental gingivitis in man. *J. Perio.* **36**, 177.

Löe, H., Schiött, C.R., Glavind, L., and Karring, T. (1975). Effects and side effects during two years use of chlorhexidine in humans. *J. dent. Res.* **54** (spec. iss. A), 123.

Löe, H., Schiött, C.R., Glavind, L., and Karring, T. (1976). Two years oral use of chlorhexidine in man. I General design and clinical effects. *J. perio. Res.* **11**, 135.

Löe, H., Anerud, A., Boysen, H., and Smith, M.R. (1978). The natural history of periodontal disease in man. *J. Perio.* **49**, 607.

Löe, H., Anerud, A., Boysen, H., and Morrison, E. (1986). Natural history of periodontal disease in man. Rapid, moderate and no loss of attachment in Sri Lankan laborers 14 to 46 years of age. *J. clin. Perio.* **3**, 431.

Loesche, W.J. (1976). Chemotherapy of dental plaque infections. *Oral Sci. Rev.* **9**, 65.

Lövdal, A., Arno, A., Schei, O., and Waerhaug, J. (1961). Combined effect of subgingival scaling and controlled oral hygiene on the incidence of gingivitis. *Acta odont. Scand.* **19**, 537.

MacGregor, I.D.M. and Rugg-Gunn, A.J. (1985). Toothbrushing duration in 60 uninstructed young adults. *Commun. Dent. oral Epidemiol.* **13**, 121.

MacGregor, I.D.M., Rugg-Gunn, A.J., and Gordon, P.H. (1986). Plaque levels in relation to the number of toothbrushing strokes in uninstructed English schoolchildren. *J. perio. Res.* **21**, 577.

McHugh, W.D., McEwan, J.D., and Hitchin, A.D. (1964). Dental disease and related factors in 13-year-old children in Dundee. *Br. dent. J.* **117**, 246.

McKendrick, A.J.W., Barbenel, L.M.H., and McHugh, W.D. (1968). A two year comparison of hand and electric toothbrushes. *J. perio. Res.* **3**, 224.

Mackler, S.B. and Crawford, J.J. (1973). Plaque development and gingivitis in the primary dentition. *J. Perio.* **44**, 18.

Mandell, I.D. and Gaffar, A. (1986). Calculus revisited. A review. *J. clin. Perio.* **13**, 249.

Mann, J., Cormier, P.P., Green, P., Ram, C.A., Miller, M.F., and Ship, I.I. (1981). Loss of periodontal attachment in adolescents. *Commun. Dent. oral Epidemiol.* **9**, 135.

Marshall-Day, C.D., Stephens, R.G., and Quigley, L.F. (1955). Periodontal disease: prevalence and incidence. *J. Perio.* **26**, 185.

Matsson, L. (1978). Development of gingivitis in pre-school children and young adults. *J. clin. Perio.* **5**, 24.

Matsson, L. and Goldberg, P. (1985). Gingival inflammatory reaction in children at different ages. *J. clin. Perio.* **12**, 98.

Mehta, F.S., Sanjana, M.K., Shroff, B.C., and Doctor, R.H. (1958). Relative importance of the various causes of tooth loss. *J. All India dent. Ass.* **30**, 211.

Moller, P. (1963). Oral health survey of preschool children in Iceland. *Acta odont. Scand.* **21**, 47.

Morrison, E.C., Lang, N.P., Löe, H., and Ramfjord, S.P. (1979). Effects of repeated scaling and root planing and/or controlled oral hygiene on the periodontal attachment level and pocket depth in beagle dogs. I. Clinical findings. *J. perio. Res.* **14**, 428.

Moskow, B.S. (1969). Calculus attachment in cemental separations. *J. Perio.* **40**, 125.

Muhler. J.C., Dudding, N.J., and Stookey, G.K. (1964). Clinical effectiveness of a particular particle size distribution of zirconium silicate for use as a cleaning and polishing agent for oral hard tissues. *J. Perio.* **35**, 481.

Murray, J.J. (1974). The prevalence of gingivitis in children continuously resident in a high fluoride area. *J. Dent. Child.* **41**, 133.

Nayak, R.P. and Wade, A.B. (1977). The relative effectiveness of plaque removal by the Proxabrush® and rubber cone stimulator. *J. clin. Perio.* **4**, 128.

Newcomb, G.M. (1974). The relationship between the location of subgingival crown margins and gingival inflammation. *J. Perio.* **45**, 151.

Newman, H.N. (1980). Update on plaque and periodontal disease. *J. clin. Perio.* **7**, 251.

O'Bannon, J.Y. (1964). The gingival tissues before and after scaling the teeth. *J. Perio.* **35**, 69.

Page, R.C. (1986). Gingivitis. *J. clin. Perio.* **13**, 345.

Parfitt, G.J. (1957). A five year longitudinal study of the gingival condition of a group of children in England. *J. Perio.* **28**, 26.

Parsons, J.C. (1974). Chemotherapy of dental plaque. A review. *J. Perio.* **45**, 177.

Pennel, B.M. and Keagle, J.G. (1977). Predisposing factors in the etiology of chronic inflammatory periodontal disease. *J. Perio.* **48**, 517.

Poulsen, S., Agerbaek, N., Melsen, B., Korts, D.C., Glavind, L., and Rölla, G. (1976). The effect of professional tooth cleansing on gingivitis and dental caries in children after 1 year. *Commun. Dent. oral Epidemiol.* **4**, 195.

Praynito, S., Taylor,L., Cadogan, S., and Addy, M. (1979). An *in vivo* study of dietary factors in the aetiology of tooth staining associated with the use of chlorhexidine. *J. perio. Res.* **14**, 411.

Rodda, J.C. (1968). A comparison of four methods of toothbrushing. *NZ dent. J.* **64**, 162.

Rölla, G., Löe, H., and Schiött, C.R. (1970). The affinity of chlorhexidine for hydroxyapatite and salivary mucins. *J. perio. Res.* **5**, 90.

Rölla, G., Löe, H., and Schiött, C.R. (1971). Retention of chlorhexidine in the human oral cavity. *Archs. oral Biol.* **16**, 1109.

Ruffer, M.A. (1921). *Studies in the palaeopathology of Egypt*. University of Chicago Press.

Rushton, A. (1977). Safety of Hibitane II. Human experience. *J. clin. Perio.* **4**, 73.

Russell, A.L. (1956). A system of classification and scoring for prevalence surveys of periodontal disease. *J. dent. Res.* **35**, 350.

Russell, B. and Bay. L. (1975). The effect of toothbrushing with chlorhexidine gluconate toothpaste on epileptic children. *J. dent. Res.* **54** (spec. iss. A), L114.

Sangnes, G. (1976). Traumatization of teeth and gingiva related to habitual tooth cleaning procedures. *J. clin. Perio.* **3**, 94.

Saxton, C.A. (1973). Scanning electron microscope study of the formation of dental plaque. *Caries Res.* **7**, 102.

Saxton, C.A., Cowell, C.R., Sheiham, A., and Wagg, B.J. (1976). Testing therapeutic measures for controlling chronic gingivitis in man: the results of two studies. *J. clin. Perio.* **3**, 220.

Schaub, R.M.H. (1984). Barriers to effective periodontal care. Unpublished thesis. University of Groningen.

Scherp, H.W. (1964). Current concepts in periodontal disease research: epidemiological contributions. *J. Am. dent. Ass.* **68**, 667.

Schiött, C.R., Löe, H., Jensen, S.B., Kilian, M., Davies, R.M., and Glavind, K. (1970). The effect of chlorhexidine mouthrinses on the human oral flora. *J. perio. Res.* **5**, 84.

Schiött, C.R., Briner, W.W., and Löe, H. (1976*a*). Two years use of chlorhexidine in man II. The effect on the salivary bacterial flora. *J. perio. Res.* **11**, 145.

Schiött, C.R., Briner, W.W., Kirkland, J.J., and Löe, H. (1976*b*). Two years oral use of chlorhexidine in man. III Changes in sensitivity of the salivary flora. *J. perio. Res.* **11**, 153.

Schmid, M.O., Balmelli, O.P., and Saxen, U.P. (1976). Plaque-removing effect of a toothbrush, dental floss and a toothpick. *J. clin. Perio*, **3**, 157.

Schroeder, H.E. (1969). *Formation and inhibition of dental calculus*. Hans Huber, Stuttgart.

Segretto, V.A. *et al.* (1986). A comparison of mouthrinses containing two concentrations of clorhexidine. *J. perio. Res.* **21** (suppl. 16), 23.

Siegrist, B.E., Gusberti, F.A., Brecx, M.C., Weber, H.P., and Lang, N.P. (1986). Efficacy of supervised rinsing with chlorhexidine digluconate in comparison to phenolic and plant alkaloid compounds. *J. perio. Res.* **21** (suppl. 16), 60.

Silness, J. (1980). Fixed prosthodontics and periodontal health. *Dent. Clinics N. Am.* **24**, 317.

Skjörland, K., Gjermo, P., and Rölla, G. (1978). Effect of some polyvalent cations on plaque formation *in vivo*. *Scand. J. dent. Res.* **86**, 103.

Slanetz, L.W. and Brown, E.A. (1949). Studies on the number of bacteria in the mouth and their reduction by the use of oral antiseptics. *J. dent. Res.* **28**, 313.

Smith, J.F. and Blankenship. J. (1964). Improving oral hygiene in handicapped children by the use of an electric toothbrush. *J. Dent. Child.* **31**, 198.

Socransky, S.S. and Crawford, A.C.R. (1977). Recent advances in the microbiology of periodontal disease. In *Current therapy in dentistry*, (5th edn.), p. 3. Mosby, St. Louis.

Söderholm, G. (1979). Effect of a dental care program on dental health conditions. A study of employees of a Swedish shipyard. Unpublished thesis. University of Lund, Sweden.

Stamm, J.W. (1986). Epidemiology of gingivitis. *J. clin. Perio.* **13**, 360.

Strålfors, A. (1962). Disinfection of dental plaques in man. *Odont. Tidskr.* **70**, 183.

Suomi, J.D. and Barbano, J.P. (1968). Patterns of gingivitis. *J. Perio.* **39**, 71.

Suomi, J.D., Green, J.C., Vermillion, J.R., Doyle, J., Chang, J.J., and Leatherwood, E.C. (1971*a*). The effect of controlled oral hygiene procedures on the progression of periodontal disease in adults: results after third and final year. *J. Perio.* **42**, 152.

Suomi, J.D., West, T.D., Chang, J.J., and McClendon, B.J. (1971*b*). The effect of controlled oral hygiene procedures on the progression of periodontal disease in adults: radiographic findings. *J. Perio.* **42**, 562.

Suomi, J.D., Leatherwood, E.C., and Chang, J.J. (1973*a*). A follow-up study of former participants in a controlled oral hygiene study. *J. Perio.* **44**, 662.

Suomi, J.D., Smith, L.W., Chang, J.J., and Barbano, J.P. (1973*b*). Study of the effect of different prophylaxis frequencies on the periodontium of young adult males. *J. Perio.* **44**, 406.

Sutcliffe, P. (1972). A longitudinal study of gingivitis and puberty. *J. perio. Res.* **7**, 52.

Svatun, B., Gjermo, P., Eriksen, H.M., and Rölla, G. (1977). A comparison of the plaque-inhibiting effect of stannous fluoride and chlorhexidine. *Acta odont. Scand.* **35**, 247.

Swartz, M.L. and Philips, R.W. (1957). Comparison of bacterial accumulation on rough and smooth enamel surfaces. *J. Perio.* **27**, 304.

Tan, H.H. and Saxton, C.A. (1978). Effect of a single dental health care instruction and prophylaxis on gingivitis. *Commun. Dent. oral Epidemiol.* **6**, 172.

Theilade, E. (1986). The non-specific theory in microbial etiology of inflammatory periodontal diseases. *J. clin. Perio.* **13**, 905.

Theilade, E. and Theilade, J. (1976). Role of plaque in the etiology of periodontal disease and caries. *Oral Sci. Rev.* **9**, 23.

Usher, P.J. (1975) Oral hygiene in mentally handicapped children. *Br. dent. J.* **138**, 217.

Van der Velden, U., Abbas, F., and Hart, A.A.M. (1985). Experimental gingivitis in relation to susceptibility to periodontal disease. I Clinical observations. *J. clin. Perio.* **12**, 61.

Van Volkinburg, J., Green, E., and Armitage, G. (1976). The nature of root surfaces after curette, cavitron and alphasonic instrumentation. *J. perio. Res.* **11**, 374.

Wade, A.B. (1971). Brushing practices of a group with periodontal disease. In *The prevention of periodontal disease*, (ed. J.E. Eastoe, D.C.A. Picton and A.G. Alexander), p. 218. Kimpton, London.

Waerhaug, J. (1971). Epidemiology of periodontal disease. In *The prevention of periodontal disease*, (ed. J.E. Eastoe, D.C.A. Picton and A.G. Alexander). Kimpton, London.

Waerhaug, J. (1976). The interdental brush and its place in operative and crown and bridge dentistry. *J. oral Rehab.* **3**, 107.

Waerhaug, J. (1978*a*). Healing of the dento-epithelial junction following subgingival plaque control I. As observed in human biopsy material. *J. Perio.* **49**, 1.

Waerhaug, J. (1978*b*). Healing of the dento-epithelial junction following subgingival plaque control II. As observed on extracted teeth. *J. Perio.* **49**, 119.

Wennström, J. and Lindhe, J. (1986). The effect of mouthrinses on parameters characterising human periodontal disease. *J. clin. Perio.* **13**, 86.

Wilcox, C.E. and Everett, F.G. (1963). Friction on the teeth and the gingiva during mastication. *J. Am. dent. Ass.* **66**, 513.

Wolffe, G.N. (1976). An evaluation of proximal surface cleansing agents. *J. Clin. Perio.* **3**, 148.

Yuodelis, R.A., Weaver, J.D., and Sapkos. S. (1973). Facial and lingual contours of artificial complete crown restorations and their effects on the periodontium. *J. prosth. Dent.* **29**, 61.

Zander, H.A. (1953). The attachment of calculus to root surfaces. *J. Perio.* **24**, 16.

11

Social factors and preventive dentistry

JOHN F. BEAL

These things one ought to consider most attentively . . . the mode in which the inhabitants live, and what are their pursuits, whether they are fond of drinking and eating to excess, and given to indolence, or are fond of exercise and labour, and not given to excess in eating and drinking (Hippocrates c. 400 BC)

ONE of the most common criticisms that teachers at dental schools make of their students is that the students treat the individual tooth rather than the mouth as a whole. In reality that comment only goes half way. It is essential that we recognize that we are responsible not just to a mouth but to a patient. We are, therefore, required to consider what makes that patient 'tick'. What are his or her attitudes to their teeth? How were those attitudes formed, can they be changed, and if so how? Often it is necessary to go a step further. For example, if we consider water fluoridation we are concerned not for the dental health of an individual patient, but for that of a community which may include more than one million people. Again we must know something about that community. We must learn how public opinion is formed, how it can be measured, why some people are against fluoridation and how we can influence the decision-making process in order to promote the fluoridation of the water supply.

It can be seen, therefore, that preventive dentistry is not a mechanistic matter based purely on a knowledge of clinical techniques. It requires an understanding of the society in which we live. We need to know what social factors are relevant, how individuals are influenced by their upbringing, how we can best communicate with different groups and so on. This chapter examines the relationship between such social factors and dental health, and tries to suggest ways in which traditional approaches in preventive dentistry might be modified in the light of this extra dimension.

Social class

Before looking at the relationship between social status and dental health, it is necessary to examine the concept of social stratification. In all societies members are divided into various social strata or layers. Some are recognized as 'superior'

Table 11.1. The Registrar General's Social Class

Social Class	Description	Examples
I	'Professional' and top managerial occupations	Doctor, dentist, university lecturer, company secretary
II	'Intermediate' occupations, i.e. minor professions and lower managerial	Teacher, nurse, chiropodist, supermarket manager
III	'Skilled' occupations:	
	—non-manual	Draughtsman, clerk, policeman
	—manual	Plumber, tool-maker, coalminer
IV	'Semi-skilled' occupations	Gardener, storekeeper, postman
V	'Unskilled' occupations	Labourer, kitchen hand, office cleaner

and others as 'inferior'. Each person, therefore, has a social *status* which is the position he or she occupies within the social system. This determines the amount of *prestige* or social importance which will be given to that person. There are, broadly speaking, two types of status, *ascribed* and *achieved*. An ascribed status is one which is determined at birth such as sex or caste. An achieved status on the other hand is gained during the lifetime of the person and may, for instance, be based upon the occupation of the individual. A status group may be either *open* or *closed*. An open form of stratification is found in the Australian aborigines where status is related to age and where each man becomes successively a hunter, a warrior, and eventually reaches the heights of elderhood. Every man passes through each social position. The caste system, conversely, is an example of a closed status grouping. It is a permanent rank and determines one's whole lifestyle including what type of occupation one can have, who one can mix with, and even who one can marry. Contact between those of different castes is limited and governed by predetermined rules, and movement from one caste to another is not allowed.

In western society, social status is based upon the class system. This is a relatively open system in which mobility from one group to another is not necessary, as with the aborigines, but it is permitted and can be made with comparative ease. There are numerous systems of dividing the population in to social classes, ranging from the early classifications of Marx and Weber to the more generally used one of the Registrar General's Social Class (Office of Population Censuses and Surveys 1980). This system is based upon the occupation of an individual and divides the population into five groups or classes. Table 11.1 shows the type of occupation allocated to each social class together with examples for each class. One of the disadvantages of this particular classification is that about a half of the population falls into Class III. This class is, therefore, frequently subdivided into non-manual and manual categories.

The advantage of this type of classification is that it enables us to make generalizations about the lifestyles, behaviour and attitudes of others, based upon the pattern for that group as a whole. Of course not everyone from a social class will share the same lifestyle. However, the differences between those from the various classes are often great enough to identify patterns and trends. A number of these differences between the social classes have an important bearing on preventive dentistry. Mention will be made later of various other sociological factors which are themselves associated with social class. However, two of these factors are fundamental in understanding the relationship between social status and health. The first factor is income, where those in the higher social classes in general receive a higher income. The other factor is education. Most of those in Social Class I have a university or college education. At the other end of the scale the majority of subjects in Social Class V left full time education at the minimum school leaving age and went straight into a job or at least started looking for work.

Even though social class is a status which is achieved during the lifetime of an individual, it also has an ascribed component as a minor takes the social class of his or her father. In fact, the whole family is recognized as a unit of social class, a married woman being classified according to the social class of her husband.

In many cases there is a social gradient from those in Social Class I to those in Social Class V. However, it is often simpler to divide the population into just two groups in order to make broad statements about social differences. For the sake of convenience, Classes I, II and sometimes Class III non-manual are combined under the title of 'middle class' whilst Classes III manual, IV, and V form the 'working class'.

Social class and disease

It has long been recognized that there are a number of health inequalities related to social class. Susser and Watson (1971) point out that Edwin Chadwick in 1842 published a series of tables illustrating the connection between mortality and social class. This pattern is still found today. The infant mortality statistics in England and Wales (Office of Population Censuses and Surveys (1986*a*) show that babies whose fathers had unskilled jobs run twice the risk of stillbirth and death under one year than babies whose fathers worked in the professions. Exactly the same relationship is found in the mortality rates of men aged 16–64 years in England and Wales (Office of Population Censuses and Surveys 1986*b*).

Further, The Black report (Report of a Research Working Group 1980) states that 'an extraordinary variety of causes of death such as cancer, heart and respiratory disease differentiate between classes'. Brotherston (1976) and Blaxter (1976) have indicated that in spite of the widely held expectation that the social gradient would reduce following the formation of the National Health Service, the differences not only remain, but the gap has, in fact, widened. Indeed the gap is still widening (Whitehead 1987).

It is not only in death that inequalities exist between the rich and the poor. The pattern of morbidity is also related to social class. Some diseases are more associated with those from the working classes whilst a few are found more commonly in the middle classes. Examples of diseases in which the incidence is higher in the lower social classes are bronchitis, pneumonia, tuberculosis, rheumatic heart disease, ulcer, and cancer of the stomach (Susser and Watson 1971). Blaxter has shown how, although overall rates for the infectious respiratory diseases have fallen, the differences between the classes have widened over the past 50 years. Conversely, a number of the diseases of affluence, formerly associated with those from the higher social groups, are now found to show no differences between classes, or even a reverse trend with the incidence being higher in the lower social groups (Blaxter 1976).

In 65 of the 78 disease categories used for men (Office of Population Censuses and Surveys 1986*a*; Townsend *et al.* 1987) social classes IV and V had a higher mortality than either class I or class II. Only one cause, malignant melonoma, showed the reverse trend. In women a similar social gradient was found in 62 of the 82 categories, with only 4 categories more common in social classes I and II. The rest are neutral. Clearly so-called 'diseases of affluence' have all but disappeared and what is left is a general health disadvantage of the poor (Whitehead 1987).

A knowledge of the social distribution of disease can be important, for example, in refuting allegations by anti-fluoridationists when they claim that fluoridation causes some particular disease. It was suggested at one time, for example, that as the incidence of cancer of the stomach was higher in Slough, where the natural level of fluoride was one part per million, compared with nearby fluoride-free Gerrards Cross, that the cause of this difference must be the fluoride. In fact, Slough is a large industrial town, whereas Gerrards Cross is a London commuter community with a much higher social-class composition. As cancer of the stomach is found more frequently in those from the lower social classes it would be expected that Slough would have a higher incidence of the disease. The only way of accurately making comparisons of disease levels in different communities is to use the process of *standardization*, a statistical technique which can be used to eliminate the effect of differences in the age, racial and social composition of the populations concerned.

Social class and dental disease

As with many other diseases, social class differences exist in the prevalence of dental disease. Until about a century ago, dental caries was confined largely to the better off sections of the community. In the second half of the nineteenth century, however, dental caries increased considerably (Corbett and Moore 1976) following the 400 per cent increase in sugar consumption during the reign of Queen Victoria. Refined sugar was no longer the privilege of the rich but became cheap and available to all (James 1981).

A number of studies have demonstrated the present relationship between social status and dental caries. One of the largest dental surveys was the national study of child dental health carried out in England and Wales in 1973 (Todd 1975). Table 11.2 shows that those from the higher social classes were more likely to have no experience of dental decay and less likely to have widespread

Table 11.2. Decay experience of 5-year-old children according to Social Class (Todd 1975)

Social Class	Percentage of children with no deciduous decay experience	Five or more deciduous teeth involved
I, II, and III non-manual	38	30
III manual	24	41
IV and V	23	43

Table 11.3. Percentage of adults in Darlington with good, fair, and poor gingival health according to Social Class (Bulman *et al.* 1968)

Social Class	Gingival health		
	Good	Fair	Poor
I, II, and III non-manual	30	16	54
III manual, IV and V	8	12	80

Table 11.4. An indication of the need for full and partial dentures according to Social Class. (Based on Gray *et al.* 1970)

Social Class	Percentage edentulous	Mean number of missing and unrestorable teeth
I, II, and III non-manual	27	9.6
III manual	34	10.6
IV and V	46	11.8

decay. Children from Social Classes IV and V were more likely to have had toothache than those from the higher groups.

In a subsequent survey in 1983 Todd and Dodd (1985) showed that a similar pattern continues to exist. Five-year-olds from social classes IV and V had twice as many teeth with decay experience as their counterparts from professional households. Thus in both the prevention of decay and the control of it, children of parents from the top social class group do significantly better than the others. Bulman *et al.* (1968) showed that a similar pattern is found with regard to gingival disease in adults (Table 11.3) as have Cushing and Sheiham (1985). Thus the need for treatment for both dental caries and periodontal disease is greater in the lower social classes. A measure of the total met and unmet need for full dentures is indicated by the proportion of the population who are edentulous. In the case of partial dentures, an approximation of the relative need between groups may be ascertained from the mean number of missing teeth plus the mean number of unrestorable teeth. Table 11.4 shows that for both of these

Table 11.5. Percentage of adults in Salisbury with different dental attendance patterns according to Social Class (Bulman *et al.* 1968)

Social Class	Frequency of dental visits in last five years				
	Regular	Occasional	Rarely (pain)	Rarely (dentures)	No visits
I and II	33	23	10	15	19
III non-manual	28	20	18	3	30
III manual	14	17	15	11	43
IV	6	8	23	11	53
V	—	9	18	9	64

indicators, the lowest social classes have the greatest need for treatment (Gray *et al.* 1970).

Social class and medical treatment

In 1969, Titmuss drew attention to differences in the use of health services and concluded that middle-class members of the community were more efficient in the use of the National Health Service and were receiving greater benefits from it. Although in general the lower social classes make less use of medical services there are differences in the utilization of the various parts of the service. For instance, the crude rate of visits to general medical practitioners by middle-aged adults is higher in the working-class groups. However, if this is adjusted to take into account the differences in chronic morbidity, then those from the higher social classes are found to visit their general practitioner more than twice as much as those from Social Classes IV and V. An even greater disparity of utilization in relation to actual need is found in the hospital outpatient consultation rates (Blaxter 1976). Conversely, Brotherston (1976) points out that hospital inpatient services in Scotland have a higher utilization by the lower social groups. Preventive services generally are used much more by the middle classes (Blaxter 1984). These include early attendance for antenatal care, child welfare clinics, and immunization and vaccination services (Brotherston 1976). Bergner and Yerby (1976) show similar social differences in health-service utilization in the United States.

Social class and dental treatment

All of the indicators already described showed that those from the lower social classes have more dental disease and thus need more dental treatment than those from the higher social classes. In view of this, it might be expected that those from the lower social classes would visit the dentist more frequently in order to obtain this greater amount of treatment. Bulman *et al.* (1968) investigated the frequency of dental visits according to social class. Table 11.5 shows that, in contrast to their respective dental needs, one in three from the highest social group had been attending the dentist on a regular basis, whereas none of

Table 11.6. Percentage of mother's choosing different types of treatment for 5-year-old children with decayed primary and permanent teeth according to Social Class (Beal and Dickson 1974*a*)

Social Class	Primary teeth		Permanent teeth	
	Fill	Extract	Fill	Extract
I and II	54	46	90	10
III	40	60	58	42
IV and V	24	76	46	54

the subjects from Social Class V had visited regularly. Less than one in five from Social Classes I and II had not seen a dentist for 5 years compared with nearly two in every three from Class V. A similar trend was found by Todd (1975) and Todd and Dodd (1985), who reported that not only were mothers from the highest social groups more regular in their own dental attendance, but also that they took their children to the dentist at an earlier age. This social differential in the pattern of regular dental visits is consistent with the pattern already described for the usage of preventive health services generally. Even the choice of dental service is found to differ between the social groups. Middle-class mothers take their children to their own general dental practitioner who is a 'family dentist'. In contrast many more working-class mothers, who are less likely to go to a dentist themselves, send their children to the School Dental Service (now part of the Community Dental Service) after receiving a note informing them that a school screening inspection has indicated a need for treatment (Todd 1975).

Such social class differences are found not only with attendance patterns for routine dentistry but also with referrals for specialist treatment such as orthodontics. Jenkins *et al.* (1984*a,b*) reported more referrals for orthodontic advice and treatment from the higher social groups, who were also more likely to seek treatment for minor malocclusions.

Not only are attendance patterns different, but the mother's attitude and choice of treatment for her child differs from one social class to another. It has been shown (Beal and Dickson 1974*b*) that in the West Midlands those from Social Classes I and II are more than twice as likely to favour the restoration of carious primary teeth than the mothers from the lower social classes. Table 11.6, however, shows that even amongst mothers in the higher social groups only just over a half of the sample wanted primary teeth filled. In contrast, the treatment preference for decayed permanent teeth is, from the dentist's point of view, much more favourable. Nine out of ten mothers from Classes I and II favoured fillings. Even so, as many as 54 per cent of Social Class IV and V mothers wanted the teeth extracted. Todd and Dodd (1985) found a rather higher overall percentage (88 per cent) of mothers of 5 year-old children who wanted decayed permanent teeth to be filled. The social gradient rose from 78 per cent in social classes IV and V to 95 per cent in classes I and II.

Attendance at the dentist brings differences in the dental treatment actually

Table 11.7. Percentage of 5-year-old children who have been to the dentist and who have different treatment experience according to Social Class (Todd 1975; Todd and Dodd 1985)

Social Class	No fillings No extractions		Had fillings		Had extractions	
	1973	1983	1973	1983	1973	1983
I, II, and III non-manual	38	61	38	26	17	7
III manual	20	49	35	29	28	12
IV and V	23	37	22	39	23	15

received by different social groups. Table 11.7 shows that, in both studies, of those 5-year-old children who have visited the dentist, a greater proportion of those from the highest social group had never had to have any treatment. This social group were also found to have been less likely to have had teeth extracted.

The situation with regard to fillings is, however, changing. In 1973 those from the highest social group were more likely to have had fillings whereas in 1983 they were less likely to have received restorative treatment. In a study into the dental health of adults, Sheiham and Hobdell (1969) showed that, in the younger age groups, those in Social Class I had on average three times as many teeth filled as those in Class V, whilst the latter had four times as many teeth both extracted and decayed as the former.

Cooper (1975) stated that the most important determinant of demand for medical services is the availability of resources. This has been suggested as an important reason for social class differences in the use of dental services (Lennon 1976). O'Mullane and Robinson (1977) compared the uptake of dental services in two towns, one where the dentist to population ratio was favourable and the other where it was unfavourable. They found that in the unfavourable area there was considerably greater utilization by the higher social classes, whilst in the favourable area there was a more similar pattern of usage throughout the social scale with only a slight bias in favour of the higher social groups. The net effect of having a greater availability of dentists seemed to be that only slightly more Social Class I and II individuals sought treatment whereas the percentage of patients from Social Class IV and V greatly increased. These results suggest that an increase in the availability of dental resources does not lead to an even greater utilization by the middle classes, but to an equalization between the classes. If this is true then one way of reducing the inequalities in the use of dental services may be to encourage dentists to practise in areas of greatest need by offering financial or other incentives (Dental Strategy Review Group 1981).

Taylor and Carmichael (1980) have shown, in Newcastle, that general dental practitioners are more numerous in areas of high social class. The Community Dental Service, which should be complementary to the General Dental Services, does not always have clinics located in the dentally deprived areas. One way of providing dental services to these communities in lower social class areas is by

Table 11.8. Percentage of 5-year-old children exhibiting various patterns of behaviour related to dental health shown according to Social Class (Beal and Dickson 1974*a*)

Social Class	Child brushes at least once a day	Child was given sugared dummy	More than 25p weekly spent on child's sweets
I and II	92	17	2
III	74	29	15
IV and V	64	30	13

the use of mobile dental caravans by the community service. As with medical services, the supply would then create its own demand (Carmichael 1981).

In summary, then, it can be seen that those from the higher social classes have less dental disease but are more regular attenders at the dentist, they are also less likely to have had any dental treatment. Conversely, those in the lower social groups have more dental disease but visit the dentist less frequently. They are more likely to have teeth extracted and, until recently, were less likely to have fillings although this situation is changing.

Social class and dental knowledge, attitudes, and behaviour

Although a number of studies investigating social differences in knowledge, attitudes, and behaviour have been carried out in the United States, fewer British studies have been conducted.

It is, however, possible to identify differences between those from various socio-economic backgrounds in their level of knowledge, dental attitudes, and behaviour patterns.

In general, as might be expected, those from the higher social classes, who have a higher level of education, are more knowledgeable about dentally related matters. In a study into the level of knowledge in Bristol mothers, it was found that 83 per cent of those from Social Classes I and II were aware of the importance of frequency of sugar consumption in the aetiology of caries compared to 59 per cent from Classes IV and V (J. F. Beal, unpublished data).

Another demonstration of the different levels of knowledge is related to awareness that blackcurrant juice can be harmful to the teeth of young children. In a study of the mothers of 5-year-old children in West Midlands, it was shown (Beal and Dickson 1974*a*) that twice as many mothers from Social Classes I and II knew that blackcurrant juice could be harmful to the teeth compared with the number from Classes IV and V. The importance of this can be seen from the fact that the level of knowledge was closely related to reported behaviour. It was found that those who knew about the harmful potential were twice as likely to not give blackcurrant juice to their children, or if they did provide it, then it was given much less frequently.

It is also possible to identify a number of other types of behaviour which are related to dental health and in which social gradients have been demonstrated. Table 11.8 shows three such behaviour patterns. It can be seen that children from the higher social classes are more likely to brush their teeth regularly, but less likely to be given a sugared dummy in infancy, or to have relatively large amounts of money spent on their sweets (more than 25p per week at 1971 prices).

There are a number of respects in which the general cultural patterns differ between the middle-class and working-class sections of the community. A number of these differences affect attitudes towards dentistry and the prevention of dental disease. It is most important that these should be understood by the dental practitioner in order for him to help the patient to improve his or her dental health.

The life orientation associated with the working classes is one of *immediate gratification*, whereas that more commonly found in middle-class individuals is of *deferred gratification*. This means that the middle-class person sees value in foregoing the pleasures of today in order to gain greater benefit in the future. Those from this group place great emphasis on education and training. They encourage their children to spend their evenings doing homework and studying for examinations, with the expectation that this will result in a 'better job'. They also save and invest their money in order to purchase what they want in the future or perhaps provide a pension after retirement. Those from the lower social groups, however, tend to be less interested in education. They do not buy so many books for their young children, and make fewer visits to the public lending library. Their children are not given the same encouragement to do their homework, or stay on at school in order to take examinations leading to attendance at college or university. Indeed, the working-class boy or girl with a father in a unskilled or semi-skilled occupation may find great difficulties in studying at home. Not only are they less likely to receive parental support, especially if a girl, but the facilities at home may not be particularly conducive to study, and she or he may have to work in the room in which siblings and parents are watching television. In addition, the working-class child is often subjected to a conflict of cultures between the school and home environments. Whilst the child will have been socialized into a working-class culture, the teachers communicate using the speech and ideas appropriate to their own middle-class background and experience. In addition, the whole school pattern is based upon competition and individual achievement, values which are associated with the middle classes (Bernstein 1961, 1965). This factor is one of the most important impediments to mobility up the social scale for children from such families. Although a quarter of students at British universities come from working-class homes, only 2 per cent of them have fathers who are semi-skilled or unskilled manual workers (Worsley *et al.* 1970).

Saving is also less common in working-class families, partly because they tend to have a lower income, and expensive items have to be bought on hire purchase. Their children, although they receive more pocket money than middle-class children, are not encouraged to save a proportion of it, but are allowed to spend it all without making any conditions as to its 'sensible use' (Newson and Newson 1976). This results in more money being available for the purchase of snacks and sweets, and it has been shown that working-class children and their parents spend more on sweets than middle-class children (Beal and Dickson 1974*b*).

The patient's occupation and circumstances relating to his or her employment are factors which should be borne in mind by every dentist preparing a treatment plan whether or not it includes preventive therapy. Many middle-class employees are paid a salary. When they are absent from work to visit the dentist they suffer no loss of income. The working-class person, however, is often paid an hourly wage or 'piece work', whereby remuneration depends upon productivity. Absence from work will, therefore, result in financial loss. Especially during times of economic recession and high unemployment some patients may be reluctant to undergo long courses of treatment involving many visits to the dentist for fear of losing their job. This may well influence the treatment plan in such a way as to require the minimum number of visits. On the other hand, it may also serve as an incentive for the patient to practice the self-help aspects of preventive dentistry in order to reduce the future need for dental treatment.

Dentists have been granted a protected monopoly in the provision of dental treatment and this privilege carries with it the responsibility of ensuring that an appropriate service is offered to the community. This should include making the service available when it is reasonable for patients to attend. Rogers *et al.* (1984) found that pre-school children whose parents worked were less likely to visit the dentist, especially if the parents would lose money if absent from work. They suggest that there is a need for practitioners to consider evening or Saturday sessions when it would be possible for parents to bring their children for treatment.

Whilst there remain items of preventive treatment, such as the application of topical fluorides and fissure sealants, which are not provided to all children who need them free of charge within the General Dental Services, ability to pay will continue to be an important factor in the uptake of preventive services. Although some groups of skilled manual workers have narrowed the gap in recent years there remains a differential in the income of middle-class and working-class persons. There is also a difference in the income curve of the two classes. Those in the working classes can expect, after any initial training, to get the set rate for the job which will, apart from cost-of-living rises, remain the same until retirement. Many middle-class persons earn nothing during training, which is often carried out full-time at places of higher education. After qualification they frequently enter posts in which they become *spiralists*, that is they are graded at the bottom of a hierarchical ladder. They can, however, espect annual increments as well as the cost-of-living rises. In addition, they seek promotion up the hierachy, usually involving further training and qualifications, and will earn a higher salary with each successive step up the ladder. It is frequently not before they are well into middle age, or even older, that they earn their maximum income. It is interesting to note that dentists in the General Dental Services of the National Health Service have more in common with the working class in this respect, for they are not eligible for promotion within the service, do not get annual increments, and they cannot, because of the set fee per item of treatment, charge more because of greater experience as can professional groups like barristers or their own counterparts in wholely private dental practice.

One of the problems associated with using a classification of social class based upon the occupation of an individual is that this relates only to present achieved status and provides no information about social origin. It has, however, already been stated that social class is a relatively open system, that is, movement from one status group to another can be achieved during a person's lifetime. *Social mobility* may be either horizontal or vertical. Horizontal mobility takes place when someone changes from one occupation to another within the same social class. Vertical mobility is exhibited by a person who changes from an occupation classified in one social class to another which falls in a different social class.

The results of studies in other fields have indicated that those who have shown vertical social mobility have attitudes and behaviour which are different from their socially static contemporaries (Rosser and Harris 1965). As a group they fit neither into the cultural pattern of the social class into which they were born and brought up, nor into that into which they have moved. Goldthorpe *et al.* (1968) have described the conflict between their past and their present, and between their background and their aspirations that is found in these individuals. Blau (1956) describes this 'pattern of acculturation' in the following way: 'Both groups exert some influence over mobile individuals since they have, or have had, social contacts with members of both, being placed by economic circumstances amidst the one while having been socialized among the other. Hence their behaviour is expected to be intermediate between that of the two non-mobile classes.' This coincides with findings in the sphere of dental health (Beal and Dickson 1975*a*). As a group, the pattern of preference for restoring or extracting decayed teeth, of mothers' dental attendance, of a child's first dental attendance, of the child's tooth-brushing regularity, and of the amount spent on sweets, fall mid-way between the social group they had left and the one they had joined. Whether girls born into those working-class families with 'middle-class attitudes' are more likely to marry a middle-class husband, or whether a working-class girl who marries into the middle class changes her own attitudes to conform to those of her husband's social peers, and vice versa for downward mobility, is uncertain. The work of Goldthorpe *et al.* (1968, 1969) suggests that it is the former.

Some sociologists have suggested that with increasing affluence of the working class they will begin to adopt the cultural patterns which are traditionally associated with the middle classes, a process developed as the thesis of the *embourgeoisement* of the working class. Goldthorpe *et al.* (1969) have examined this in a study of automobile workers at Luton. They concluded that the differences they found in some subgroups of car workers were much more likely to be due to factors such as social mobility than to the process of embourgeoisement. Although increasing affluence and education of the working class may well eventually lead to changes in dental attitudes and behaviour, it is essential that any dentist responsible for providing treatment to a working-class community is constantly aware, albeit subconsciously, of the different cultural background of many of his or her patients.

Other social factors related to dental health

In this chapter so far the Registrar General's Social Class has been the only indicator of status that has been examined in relation to dental health. There are, however, many other factors associated with the concept of class by various social scientists. These include income, education, type of housing, and voting behaviour. All are found to be related to Social Class and they have each shown a social gradient in dental attitudes (Beal and Dickson 1974*b*). However, dental behaviour was found to be much more strongly related to area of residence than to any of the individual social variables. In fact, the area of residence was the only factor to be consistently associated with each of the attitudes and behaviour patterns investigated. It may be that the area differences reflect a combination of the other differences. It was found that mothers in one area tended to be from the higher social classes, have a higher income, longer full-time education, and live in their own house, whilst in another area there was a tendency for the mothers to be nearer to the lower end of all the social scales. Alternatively it may reflect a form of group learning, a process whereby members of the community are influenced in their attitudes and behaviours by others who live near to them even if they are not in the same social class. Certainly many of the factors associated with their environment are shared. For example, in the area with more mothers from the higher social groups there are more dentists. It would, therefore, be easier even for working-class mothers in that area, to go to the dentist for regular check-ups and to have children's teeth filled, whilst in other areas the mothers tend to wait until emergency extractions are necessary.

A summary of some differences in beliefs and values in working-class and middle-class persons are presented in Table 11.9. The dentally related beliefs and values have been added to general ones which are based on the work of Goldthorpe *et al.* (1969).

One of the unfortunate results of the social difference described is that those children who most need the dental services are the very ones who are least often taken to the dentist. The less educated and less well-off are not only least likely to take steps to prevent dental disease from occuring, but when it does occur, they do not take steps to seek dental treatment until it is too late to treat them conservatively. Hence they regard the dentists as providing an emergency service only, and they have decayed teeth extracted and eventually replaced by dentures.

It is, therefore, this group who most need and in the past have obtained the greatest benefit from water fluoridation. Prior to the widespread use of fluoride in toothpaste the prevalance of dental caries was perhaps the only social or health indicator in which children from fluoridated inner city areas such as Birmingham were as well-off or even better than nearby children in high class but

Table 11.9. Social class and dental health. A summary of differences in beliefs and values in working-class and middle-class persons. (Adapted from Goldthorpe *et al.* (1969))

	Working-class perspective	**Middle-class perspective**
General beliefs	The social order is divided into 'us' and 'them'; those who do not have authority and those who do	The social order is a hierarchy of differentially rewarded positions; a ladder containing many rungs
	The division between 'us' and 'them' is virtually fixed, at least from the point of view of one man's life chances	It is possible for individuals to move from one level of the hierarchy to another
	What happens to you depends a lot on luck; otherwise you have to learn to put up with things	Those who have ability and initiative can overcome obstacles and create their own opportunities. Where a man ends up depends on what he makes of himself
Dental beliefs	Tooth decay is inevitable. If you are born with weak teeth they will rot whatever you do	Tooth decay and loss of teeth signifies failure to look after them properly
	By the time you are in your 30s or 40s they will fall out or have to be pulled out anyway	It is up to each one of us to care for his teeth and get regular treatment. If you look after them they will last into old age
General values	'We' ought to stick together and get what we can as a group. You may as well enjoy yourself while you can instead of trying to make yourself 'a cut above the rest'	Every man ought to make the most of his own capabilities and be responsible for his own welfare. You cannot expect to get anywhere in the world if you squander your time and money. 'Getting on' means making sacrifices
Dental values	I don't like going to the dentist so I won't go until I have pain, then I will have them out. I am not interested in prevention	It is worth the time, money, and discomfort of going for regular check-ups and treatment—and for having preventive treatment
	The children enjoy their sweets—it is cruel to stop them	It is important to control the children's sweets so they don't get a lot of decay
	They can spend their pocket money on sweets if they like	I control how they spend their pocket money, so they won't buy lots of sweets

unfluoridated residential areas (Beal and James 1970, 1971). However, there is some doubt about whether this is still the case (French *et al.* 1984; Bradnock *et al.* 1984). The general improvement in dental health (see Chapter 15) has been found in all social groups, and there is evidence that even with the additional benefit of water fluoridation, children in the lower social groups may have more dental decay than those from the higher social groups living in non-fluoridated communities. The fact remains, however, that even if fluoridation does not totally obviate the influences of social background, it is the deprived sections of the community which gain the greatest improvement in absolute terms, especially in the reduction of the proportion of children with a high caries experience.

In addition to those factors associated with social status, there are others which are related to dental health. Obviously the prevalence and severity of both dental caries and periodontal disease is related to age. The relationship between sex and oral health, especially periodontal health, has been demonstrated on numerous occasions. Amongst children, girls are found to have cleaner teeth and less gingivitis (Todd 1975). In adults, females are also shown to have better oral cleanliness (Sheiham 1969), less calculus, and less periodontal disease (Gray *et al.* 1970). This latter study and its follow-up 10 years later (Todd and Walker 1980) also found that females make more regular visits to the dentist, have more teeth filled but fewer teeth which were sound and untreated, and fewer teeth with active decay. Women also become edentulous at an earlier age. Todd (1975) did not demonstrate any significant difference between boys and girls in the caries experience in primary teeth. In the permanent teeth, however, she showed that girls had a higher mean DMF which was due mainly to their higher mean number of fillings.

Ethnic origin is another factor for which not only dental health but also attitudes and behaviour are found to vary from group to group. Studies conducted in Britain in the late 1960s and early 1970s found that negroid children tended to have less caries experience than other ethnic groups (Downer 1970; Varley and Goose 1971; Beal 1973).

The position with Asian children was more confused with studies giving conflicting results, although in general they seemed to have a similar caries experience to white children. More recent studies have shown changes in the relative caries status of those from different ethnic groups. Paul and Bradnock (1986) found that Asian children of 4 and 5 years had more caries than white children, a finding confirmed by Perkins and Sweetman (1986), who also reported that Afro-Caribbean children had a similar total caries experience to the white group. A similar pattern has been found in 5-year-olds (J. F. Beal, unpublished data) but the situation in 14-year-olds is quite different. In this age group the Asian children had less caries than the white sample. Such findings could be related to different patterns of sugar consumption in Asian children at different ages. For example, it has been shown that a higher proportion of Asian children are given bottles containing sweetened liquids than white children (Williams 1986). With the exception of the few who continue this habit after the age of about 6 years this would only affect the primary dentition. The sugar consumption in older Asian children may be more similar to that of white children. Alternatively it may be that different subgroups of Asians predominate in the younger and older samples, depending on the patterns of immigration over the past couple of decades. Gelbier and Taylor (1985) have pointed out that 'Asians' are not a homogeneous group. Like 'Europeans' the group comprises a number of subgroups. They may be broadly divided into those from India, Pakistan, and Bangladesh, although even these need to be subdivided into groups with different languages, religions and cultural patterns, some of which factors will affect behaviour related to dental health.

In the past, the caries prevalence in black children was found to be lower than that for white children in the United States. However, the racial differences seem to have disappeared (Bagramian and Russell 1973; Heifetz *et al.* 1976) or even reversed to a position where black children have more caries (Infante and Russell 1974). It is suggested that these changes have come about because the black children are adopting a similar diet to the white children.

The British studies show that in the primary dentition the Asian children have the lowest proportion of affected teeth which have received treatment but that in older children it is the Afro-Caribbean group which has least treatment relative to the need. In both age groups, the Afro-Caribbean sample exhibited the highest proportion of extracted teeth.

The dental attitudes and behaviour of the various ethnic groups have been studied by Beal and Dickson (1975*b*). It was found that, whilst the mothers of white children were best at visiting the dentist regularly themselves and favoured taking their children to the dentist before the age of five, they did not have as great a preference for the conservation of decayed teeth as the Asian mothers. Conversely, the Asian mothers who had the most favourable attitudes towards filling teeth, were least likely to make sure that their children visit the dentist early in life. The West Indian mothers, on the other hand, who had the children with the least decay, were the group most in favour of the extraction of decayed primary and permanent teeth, and these mothers themselves visited the dentist less frequently than the mothers from the other ethnic groups.

Other differences described recently relate to the standards of dental cleanliness. In 5-year-olds, Paul and Bradnock (1986) found white children to have cleaner teeth than Asians whilst Saxby and Anderson (1987) have found that dental cleanliness in teenagers was of a better standard in both Afro-Caribbean and Asian children than in white children of the same age.

There is also a difference in the service from which parents seek dental treatment for their children. The majority of white children are taken to a general dental practitioner whereas Asian children are more likely to go to a community dental service clinic, if they go anywhere (Paul and Bradnock 1986; J. F. Beal, unpublished data).

One factor which is bound to influence the availability of preventive dentistry, and thus how much is carried out, is the attitudes of the dental profession itself. Craft and Sheiham (1976) found that general dental practitioners in the north of England were more negative in their knowledge, attitudes, and behaviour towards prevention than their colleagues in the south. The northern dentists were also much less likely to employ dental hygienists, a finding confirmed by Rock and Bradnock (1976). If a patient's own dentist is not positively orientated towards prevention, not only will it reduce the amount of preventative therapy that is carried out, but it is less likely that the patient will be inspired to practise those aspects of self-care prevention which are necessary on a daily basis at home.

The results of the national study of children's dental health (Todd 1975) highlighted a difficult problem for dental policy makers and planners. Although treatment from the General Dental Services of the National Health Service is provided from an open-ended budget, in reality the total resources, including manpower, available for dental treatment are limited and are certainly insufficient to cope with the total need for treatment. Some form of rationing is therefore necessary. This has been done, not by restricting dental treatment to those who need it most, or to basic forms of treatment such as the relief of pain and simple operative procedures, but by providing comprehensive treatment to the self-selected group who demand it. In practice this has meant that restorative dentistry has been restricted to those with the most favourable attitudes and behaviour. The national dental health surveys have shown that the differences in dental health between regular and non-regular attenders is even more marked in young adults (Gray *et al.* 1970) than in children (Todd 1975). In other words, those children who are not being taken regularly to the dentist by their parents are being condemned to gradually deteriorating dental health and very low expectations of dentistry. This results in those persons then bringing up their children in the same pattern, hence continuing the cycle of deprivation (Todd and Dodd 1985).

However, in order to produce any major breakthrough, it will be necessary either to prevent a large proportion of dental disease, or to persuade those who do not at present demand dental treatment for themselves and their children to do so in future—or better still a combination of both. The recent reduction in the prevalence of dental caries in children (Anderson 1981*a,b*; Anderson *et al.* 1981), the increase in the number of dentists over the past couple of decades, and an increase in research into dental health education may all help to provide the conditions in which the required break in the cycle can be made (see Chapter 16, p. 480 *et seq.*).

Probably one of the most important factors will be to make sure that the maldistribution in dental manpower is reduced so that those who at present have less easy access to the dentist no longer suffer from living in dentally deprived areas. Whether this might best take place by market forces encouraging dentists to open new practices in areas where there are few if any dentists; by financial or other incentives to dentists to work in these areas; or by some other method should be considered by the profession and those responsible for the planning of dental services. The Dental Strategy Review Group (1981), set up to advise the British Government on future dental policy, were in no doubt that the minimizing of the social and geographical differences in dental health will require a co-ordinated manpower policy and cannot be left to chance. As Davis (1980) states: 'once people are actually in the dental system—in other words, once the hurdle of access has been surmounted—neither education nor income exert much influence on the volume of care received, a finding that suggests that ease of entry into the dental system is the crucial contingency'. This has been confirmed more recently by Eddie and Davies (1985).

However, in planning dental services it must be remembered that those living in deprived areas have greater needs. Carmichael (1985) has pointed out that 'equality means equal shares. Equity means fair shares. If two groups of dental patients have needs, a policy of equality will give each group half; but if one group has a large unmet need compared with the relatively smaller needs of the other group, a policy of equity would give the first group priority. Those living in inner city Britain deserve better than they get at present.'

Social factors and water fluoridation

The fluoridation of water differs from most other methods of preventive dentistry, in that it is neither a clinical technique carried out by the dentist nor a matter which is the individual responsibility of each member of the population. The decision on its implementation or otherwise is, therefore, neither a matter for the clinician exercizing the right of clinical freedom, nor one in which there is individual freedom for each person to decide for himself. It is a public health measure and the decision on whether to fluoridate or not is one which must be taken by the community. The method of making this decision differs from one community to another. It has been decided nationally in Eire; by local government in many parts of the United States; by health authorities in Britain; and by public referenda in other American communities.

In democratic communities, even if the decision is made without the direct involvement of the public by holding a referendum, it is usually necessary for there to be some indication of public support for such a measure before it is likely to be implemented. A number of surveys have been undertaken in order to ascertain the proportion of the population in favour of, or opposing fluoridation. The results of national polls in the United states have been summarized by Frazier (1980). All of the studies conducted since 1959 have shown that over 70 per cent of the adult population have heard about fluoridation. However, only a half know why it is added to the water supply although this proportion increases to three-quarters if respondents are asked to choose one reason from a list of possible replies. It is found that knowledge of the purpose of fluoridation is best in the high income groups and those with the highest levels of education (US General Accounting Office 1979). Between 1959 and 1972 when those who had heard of fluoridation were asked their opinion, between 65 and 77 per cent were found to be in favour and only 11 to 14 per cent against, the remainder not having an opinion one way or the other. Metz (1967) reported that support for fluoridation was related to income, age, and number of children. The most recent national study conducted in 1977 showed that 51 per cent of all respondents were in favour whilst 10 per cent opposed fluoridation.

In Britain many of the studies have been conducted in specific areas. However, several national samples have been asked about fluoridation. The earlier surveys showed that 46 per cent in 1968 (Jackson 1972); 48 per cent in 1971 (Jackson 1972); and 67 per cent in 1986 (West Midlands Regional Health Authority 1980) were in favour compared to 16, 14 and 16 per cent respectively who were opposed. The trend has been for an increasing level of support. Two studies for which the National Association of Health Authorities commissioned independent market research firms to conduct the investigation showed 71 per cent in favour in 1985 (British Fluoridation Society 1985) and 76 per cent in 1987 (British Fluoridation Society 1987) whilst opposition was 11 and 9 per cent. Other studies conducted between 1963 and 1973 showed between 26 and 70 per cent approve and 5 to 20 per cent disapprove (Beal and Dickson 1973). More recent local studies conducted in the North of England indicated support ranging from 54 to 92 per cent whilst opposition ranged from 5 to 23 per cent. Most of the British studies show a similar social gradient to that found in the United States. Those from the higher social classes were more knowledgeable and more likely to believe fluoridation to be desirable than those from the lower social classes.

Frazier (1980) notes that, although opinion polls consistantly show a large majority in favour of fluoridation, when it is voted upon in public referenda it is often defeated. It is, therefore, necessary to investigate why some people are opposed to fluoridation, what sort of people they are and what factors influence how an individual casts his or her vote in a referendum. There has been little research in this field in Britain and it is to the American literature that one must turn for much of the evidence. It is important to bear in mind, therefore, that some of the findings may not apply to Britain.

Although there are conflicting results from various studies, there is fairly general agreement about some of the factors associated with opposition to fluoride (Frazier 1980). Frequently anti-fluoridationists are found to be older, without young children, and with low levels of income, occupational status, and education. When their attitudes to fluoridation have been studied in relation to other beliefs, opponents have been described as anti-science, anti-authoritarian, politically conservative, and against government intervention. They have also been found to be those unable to cope with the world, poorly integrated into the social and organizational life of the community, and to have feelings of political powerlessness and deprivation, these factors producing the so-called 'alienation hypothesis' to explain anti-fluoridation stances. Negative attitudes to fluoridation are also associated with a lack of knowledge about fluoridation generally including whether the medical and dental professions support fluoridation (Simmel and Ast 1962). Favourable fluoridation attitudes are related to positive dental health practices (Mctz 1967) including regular visits to the dentist (Beal and Dickson 1973).

Sapolsky (1969) has described how a generally favourable public opinion can be converted into one of opposition during the arguments and debate associated with a referendum campaign. It is suggested that this change takes place because doubts and anxiety are introduced by the anti-fluoride lobby. Many people simply become confused by the conflicting evidence produced by two sets of so called 'experts'. This has given rise to the 'confusion hypothesis' of anti-fluoride attitudes. When leading anti-fluoridationists claim, for instance, that fluoride causes cancer, most members of the public are not equipped with the medical and scientific training necessary to interpret the data and form a reasoned opinion. Their subsequent confusion results in them voting against fluoridation, as they are unable to identify the scientific shortcomings in the anti-fluoridationists' argument. Often this decision is rationalized by suggesting that there are other less contentious and more effective methods of preventing dental decay which can be applied by each person individually. It is likely, therefore, that the alienation hypothesis fits more closely to the leaders of the anti-fluoride movement and the confusion hypothesis to the voters. It is certainly true that the anti-fluoridationists can form a small vociferous pressure group which can be very effective in generating conflict, doubt and subsequent rejection by the community.

Earlier in the fluoride controversy, those against fluoridation often suggested that it was not effective in reducing dental decay or that it only delayed the onset of caries (National Pure Water Association 1969). As there is abundant evidence that fluoridation is a true preventive measure this argument is heard less often now. Currently the two most common objections to fluoridation are that it is harmful to general health, for example, that it causes cancer, mongolism, or kidney disorders, and that it is mass medication or infringes personal liberty (Royal College of Physicians 1976; J. F. Beal, unpublished data). Those who are least knowledgeable tend to give the former of these two reasons for their opposition whilst those who are most knowledgeable give the latter (Arcus-Ting *et al.* 1977).

Frazier (1980) reviews a number of investigations into the most important factors in the acceptance and implementation of fluoridation. Crain *et al.* (1969) have shown that fluoridation is most likely to be adopted where there is a degree of centralization of decision-making authority; top level support from the mayor and other high-status, politically active leaders; and active support from health and non-health organizations. There is some disagreement about the importance of the level of active support from the dental profession. Sanders (1961) reported that in the 1950s, there was little correlation between activity of dentists and fluoridation outcome. More recently, however, others have found that the leadership roles of physicians and dentists are significantly related to outcome in smaller communities (Frazier 1980).

Frankel and Allukian (1973) stated that the most important factor is the level of pro-fluoride activity. Where the pro-fluoridationists out-campaigned opponents, the ballot was more likely to show a majority in favour of fluoridation. In Britain, the part of the country which has recently been most successful in implementing new fluoridation schemes is the West Midlands, where the Regional Health Authority has set up an action group which has initiated and co-ordinated activity amongst the dental and medical professions, members of health authorities, community health councils, and the water authority, teachers, the media, and key local politicians.

Adopters of an innovation have been categorized by Rogers and Shoemaker (1971) as innovators, early adopters, early majority, late majority, and laggards. Innovators do not seem to influence many community members and it may be counter-productive to involve them extensively in a pro-fluoridation campaign because they are seen as somewhat different from the rest of the community (Iverson 1980). The keys to success are the early adopters. They seem to exert the greatest degree of opinion leadership on most issues. Iverson recommends that dentists, physicians, and local political leaders should be counted as among the early adopters and subsequent opinion formers, but adds that this is not always the case. Frazier (1980) in her review of the role of the profession states that, 'under routine, non-campaign circumstances, the dental profession only infrequently communicates with patients or the public about fluoridation. Even under campaign conditions, approval of fluoridation by medical and dental organizations may not be widely known.' It is important, however, that the profession is not authoritarian, patronizing or arrogant in pressing for fluoridation as that too has been identified as a vote-loser (Gamson 1964).

If the profession does not provide the information about fluoridation, who does? The answer is the mass media. In 1966, O'Shea and Cohen reported that eight out of ten respondents identified the mass media (press, radio, or television) as the *one* source of information about fluoridation. Another group who might be expected to be providing information about fluoridation is school teachers. Much emphasis has been placed on the role of teachers in dental health education. A study carried out by Loupe and King (unpublished data), which is quoted by Frazier (1980), reveals in teachers a lack of knowledge about fluoridation, and little understanding of its importance.

As already indicated, many of the studies on the social/psychological aspects of fluoridation have been conducted in the United States. Those studies which have been carried out in Britain have tended to confirm their findings. It is an area in which more research is needed. This must not, however, stop the dental profession from actively propagating the information about fluoridation in order to counter the misleading and inaccurate claims of anti-fluoridationists. It must be remembered that the opponents of fluoride are constantly sending leaflets and other materials giving their point of views to members of parliament, local authorities and health authorities. The pro-fluoride case must not be allowed to go by default.

Social factors and dental health education

All too often in the past, dental health education programmes have been carried out without any evaluation into their effectiveness. Any measurement has usually consisted solely of the number of leaflets handed out, the number of posters displayed or the number of people contacted during the programme. Those projects in which a proper evaluation has been carried out have usually produced disappointing results (Davis *et al.* 1956; Parfitt *et al.* 1958; Goose 1960; Finlayson and Wilson 1962). Before focusing on some of the possible reasons for the comparative failure of much dental health education it is important to bear in mind some of its successes. One of the main messages of dental health educators has been concerned with the importance of regular tooth-brushing. In the national child dental health survey, Todd (1975) reported that 99 per cent of all mothers thought that children should be encouraged to brush their teeth. Traditionally the public has been told to brush their teeth because it will prevent dental decay, and this was given as the reason for brushing by 87 per cent of the mothers. In fact, the message communicated by the dental profession, even if not totally accurate, was known by the vast majority of those questioned. Other misguided but widely held beliefs, such as eating apples to clean the teeth, or massaging the gums to stimulate them and prevent gingivitis, are accepted by the public precisely because they have been part of the message communicated by the dental profession over a considerable period of time.

But what of the failures? What can be learnt from the mistakes of the past so that future programmes do not fall into the same errors?

Too often those responsible for carrying out dental health programmes do not start by setting out exactly what they are hoping to achieve. It is essential before any planning takes place that the objectives of the project are identified. One of the first tasks must then be to decide to which group or groups the message should be provided. Obviously a single campaign cannot hope to reach all sections of the community. It is important to bear in mind that the interests and problems, dental or otherwise, of one group will be quite different from another. Something suitable for one particular group, say those in an old persons' home, will be totally irrelevant to others, such as groups of expectant mothers. Clearly we must first decide to whom we are aiming our programme, that is we must define our *target group* or groups. Usually our resources, both manpower and finance, are limited so we must consider which of the potential target groups are most likely to benefit from our programme. With which section of the population do we stand most chance of success in improving dental health? Is it pre-school children, primary schoolchildren, secondary schoolchildren, young adults, expectant mothers, womens organizations, old people's clubs, or some other section of the community?

In order to make this assessment we need first to look at how everyday attitudes and behaviour in such matters as oral hygiene and diet, are formed. Most people do not consciously make a logical decision each day about whether they should clean their teeth or what sort of snacks they are going to eat. It is something that they have grown up with, a habit which they continue unless they are activated into changing their behaviour. The key to this is the process known as *socialization*. Little of man's behaviour is purely instinctive, rather it is learned behaviour. Each society, or group within society, has its own culture or set of shared values, norms, and beliefs. Socialization is the process by which culture is transmitted and a person learns the rules and practices of his or her social group. Just as we learn a game by playing it, so we learn life by engaging in it; we are socialized in the course of the activities themselves. For example, if we are untutored in manners, we learn the 'correct' manners for our society through the mistakes that we make and the disapproval that others display (Worsley *et al.* 1970). We receive reinforcement and support for appropriate behaviour whilst being subjected to sanctions for deviance.

In the early years of life socialization takes place mainly within the family. It is the mother particularly who is responsible for training the young child and teaching him or her the correct way to behave. This early learning is known as *primary socialization*, and it is during this early period that many of our attitudes and styles of behaviour are formed and much of this will remain with us all our life. However, the process of socialization is something which continues as we pass through successive stages of our life. When a child starts school, the teachers and other school children play an important role in the process. During adolescence, the young adult develops more and more as an independent person and begins to formulate his or her own beliefs, attitudes and behaviour. This continuing process of adaptation to different social expectations is known as *secondary socialization*.

How does this relate to dental health and the messages we wish to communicate? In childhood the main dental problem is that of dental caries. Apart from water fluoridation, the most effective way of preventing decay is by controlling sugar intake. In this respect of course, parents have a big influence. They provide most of the food that is eaten and also the pocket money which is often used for the purchase of sweets or snacks. Unfavourable habits, such as the craving for sugar (a condition known as 'having a sweet tooth'), are often established very early in life. It is known to be much harder, if not impossible, to change these habits later in life (Baric *et al.* 1974). It is, therefore, important to try to avoid their formation in the first place. As the mother is the main agent of primary socialization, an important target group for dental health education will be mothers during pregnancy and whilst they have a young pre-school child.

It should, however, be remembered that there are a number of sociological barriers to changing the pattern of sugar intake, even in persuading a mother to control the sugar she gives to her child. Sweet eating, for example, is accepted as the social norm within our society. It may be possible to convince a few mothers that they should be different from everyone else for the benefit of their children's dental health, but it is a much more difficult matter to try to change the accepted way of behaving so that it is the deviant mother who gives her child sweets between meals. One of the problems is that sweet eating is perceived by adults as differing from other sweet foods. Sweets are consequently used by them in a number of different ways (Baric *et al.* 1974). Sometimes they are indeed used as a foodstuff, either as part of a main meal or as a snack; at other times they are used as a gift, a treat, or a token of affection given by parents, grandparents, or other relatives or friends; in other circumstances they are used as a means of reinforcement, either as a reward for good behaviour or a bribe. In babies and

Table 11.10. The percentage of mothers of 5-year-old children giving eating/avoiding sweets and not brushing/brushing teeth as the cause/prevention of dental decay (Todd 1975)

	Sugar/sweets	Tooth-brushing
Cause	88	44
Prevention	47	73

young children, sweets and sugary drinks are also used as pacifiers. We thus find that when we suggest a modification of sweet-eating habits, we are in fact trying to change a practice which is deeply ingrained in our society. We are often seen as depriving children of something special or depriving adults of a method of showing affection or praise to their children. An indication of this problem can be found in the answers given by mothers to two questions in the national survey of child dental health (Todd 1975). The mothers were first asked 'What do you think causes teeth to decay—or go bad?' They were not prompted but their reply was written down verbatim. The next question asked 'What do you think can be done to help prevent decay?' Again their answer was recorded. The results are shown in Table 11.10. As more than one answer could be given the numbers total to more than 100 per cent. It can be seen that most mothers recognized that the eating of sweet things was the cause of dental caries. Only half as many mentioned lack of cleaning. However, the situation is reversed when the mothers were asked about preventing decay. Clearly, although they recognized the role of sugar in the cause of the disease, they did not perceive the control of sugar as a reasonable way of preventing decay. We are thus faced with the difficult problem of having to change the social norms in our community and this will involve an approach not just to individual mothers, perhaps in the dental surgery, but to all those in the group or subculture to which this target population belongs.

Perhaps we are also too negative in our message relating to sugar consumption. The dentist is frequently seen as someone who admonishes his patients and tells them *not* to have sweets, and *not* to have sugary snacks. Possibly a more positive attitude would be helpful. Advice should be given on controlling the frequency of sucrose consumption, suggesting that if sweets are to be eaten, then instead of eating them at intervals throughout the day, they should be eaten altogether, preferably at mealtimes when they will do least harm. Positive information should be given on less harmful and reasonably priced alternatives which can be eaten in place of a sweet snack. It is also sometimes possible to associate the behaviour we are recommending with other motivations which already exist in an individual. For example, the patient who is concerned about a weight problem can be advised about the link between sugar and obesity and advised to reduce sweet consumption in order to control his or her weight.

After the teenage years, dental caries frequently becomes less of a problem whilst periodontal disease increases in severity. The main factor in the prevention of periodontal disease is regular and thorough oral hygiene. From the dental health educator's point of view, this is fortunate because the recommendation that individuals should brush their teeth coincides with the social norm. This time the health educator is supported by social pressure rather than working against it. It is a matter of trying to refine a technique rather than introduce a new form of behaviour. As young adults are often more motivated to perform an action for social or cosmetic reasons than for health reasons the social benefits of tooth cleaning can be stressed. Indeed it has been shown (Hodge 1979) that tooth-brushing is not practised by adolescents as part of health behaviour but as an integral part of personal hygiene and grooming, and as such is influenced by their family and their peers. However, it is necessary to bear in mind that the purpose of brushing the teeth is to clean them. In the child dental health study, Todd (1975) showed that 99 per cent of mothers thought that children should be encouraged to brush their teeth, 92 per cent of mothers of 14-year-olds claimed that their child brushed at least once a day, but on clinical examination only 44 per cent of the children in that age group had clean teeth. The traditional message exhorting individuals to clean their teeth regularly is therefore not sufficient. Information on how to clean and, more important, how to check the efficiency of the cleaning must be provided. It is the thoroughness of cleaning which must be stressed.

Of course, providing information does not necessarily result in a change in behaviour or improvement in dental health. Nevertheless, if we wish people to use disclosing agents we must first make sure that they know about them and how to use them. However, even if a person believes that disclosing agents are a valuable aid in tooth cleaning it does not follow that he will use them. It is common for someone to believe in something which he or she does not practice, or to practice something they do not believe. Nurses who smoke are a good example. They know the evidence which shows that smoking is injurious to health. They believe that smoking is a major cause of ill health but they adopt a behaviour which seems to conflict with this belief. This separation of practice from belief has been called *cognitive dissonance* (Festinger 1957). When there is strong internal conflict between beliefs and attitudes, on the one hand, and behaviour on the other, then this may sometimes lead to a change taking place. This change can be either in the belief or the behaviour. We find, therefore, that behaviour may influence belief as well as beliefs influencing behaviour. In practice if a person does not use disclosing tablets for any of a variety of reasons, he or she may justify their behaviour by adopting an unfavourable attitude to the value of disclosing agents. Conversely, children who already use disclosing tablets because they are told to by parents, may well adopt a favourable attitude to their role in oral hygiene. Despite all these difficulties we do have the advantage, in the prevention of periodontal disease, that we are building on already established social norms rather than trying to modify them, and this social support should be our most vital asset.

Another reason for the lack of success in many campaigns is the complexity of the language used both in the spoken word and printed materials. Dentists are, by definition, 'middle class' and most others in the field of dental health education also have middle-class backgrounds. One of the attributes of the middle classes is their use of an *extended code* or wide vocabulary, often with the use of long words in lengthy complex sentences. Conversely, those from the working class use a *restricted code* composed of fewer and simpler words. Sentences are short. There are a number of methods of calculating reading age, one of which was devised by Gunning (1952). The Gunning index is based upon the number of difficult words (having three or more syllables) and the average length of the sentences. By using the prescribed formula, a number is calculated which represents the age at which a person could be expected to read and understand the passage concerned. Blinkhorn and Verity (1979) used this method to calculate the reading ages of both tabloid newspapers and the 'quality' papers and compared these with the reading age necessary for a variety of dental health leaflets. They found that the tabloids required a reading age of about 12 years compared with $16\frac{1}{2}$ years for the quality press. The reading age necessary for the dental health leaflets ranged from 13 to $17\frac{1}{2}$ years. Similar calculations performed on popular novels which 'the man in the street' might read indicated that they needed a reading age of 10–12 years (J. F. Beal, unpublished data). It can be seen, therefore, that the materials produced for dental health education are more difficult to read than the type of reading matter to which many people are accustomed. Indeed, some are more difficult than the quality newspapers. When leaflets are used it is, of course, essential that the recipient is able to read and understand them. In future it is most important that those responsible for the production of new leaflets take great care to make sure that they are understandable. One of the problems has been that most dental health leaflets are written by dentists who, naturally, use dental jargon. They use the word 'gingivitis' for 'gum disease'; 'dental caries' for 'tooth decay'; 'orthodontic appliance' for 'braces'. It must be remembered that materials produced for the layperson must be in lay language if they are to be understood. All too often we end up with dentists seeking to transmit middle-class behaviour in middle-class terminology to working-class people who speak another language. If the recipient of the message does not then adopt the behaviour recommended by the dentist, he or she is then criticized as being apathetic, not caring about their teeth, or just plain 'thick'. Dental health educators fail to understand that they do not pour their messages, exhortations, and appeals into a void, but rather into an existing culture in which, at minimum, some displacement must take place—what Polgar (1962) has termed the 'fallacy of the empty vessel'. Similarly five years at dental school have ensured that dentists can instantly recognize and comprehend a section through the jaw showing erupted and unerupted teeth, or a section through a tooth exposing its various components. Most members of the population have not had that advantage and are not able easily to understand the meaning of such diagrams.

Dentists and dental health educators earn their living from people's mouths. A major part of their lives is devoted to dental matters. Too often they forget that dental health is not of such vital importance to most other people. It is much lower down most people's order of priorities. It is, therefore, doubly essential that leaflets on dental health are attractive and easy to read. Otherwise most people will not bother to struggle through them. It is important also to recognize that, however well the materials are produced, they cannot take the place of personal contact and should be used as a back-up or *reinforcement* of a face-to-face communication.

Mention has already been made of incorrect or misleading information being included in dental health communication. Even when the message is scientifically accurate, it is important to make sure that it is not capable of misinterpretation by the reader. Not long ago, a very attractive poster was produced bearing the message that 'clean teeth don't decay'. Strictly speaking that is true. A tooth with no plaque present will not decay. Many readers, however, interpret this as 'if you brush your teeth they won't decay'. Of course, it is impossibly to totally remove all plaque from the tooth especially in pits and fissures, and also interdentally (except possibly with the use of floss). There is, therefore, the danger that many readers will so interpret that poster that they ignore the more important factor, namely the control of sucrose consumption. It is a wise measure to test draft materials with a selection of members from the target population in order to identify such potential problems and misunderstandings. This should be carried out before the materials are produced so that the necessary modifications can be made.

It is often claimed that the most effective dental health education is on a one-to-one basis in the dental surgery. There is no real evidence for this claim, and in fact, it ignores a number of factors which suggest that it may not be true. It must be remembered that most patients in the dental chair are not at ease; they are anxious and apprehensive and are thus not in the best frame of mind for understanding the new information they are being given, or learning the details of new techniques they are being taught. They are also receiving this information in isolation from their friends and those to whom they relate in their day-to-day life. They may not, therefore, be subject to the social support of others. Short visits to the dentist will do little by themselves to change a patient's ingrained habits (Blinkhorn 1981). In contrast, dental health education aimed at a group is able to utilize the peer group pressures which are exerted on members of that group. It therefore becomes possible for individuals within the group to influence each other and, it is to be hoped, help to resocialize deviant members of the group. This is not to argue, however, that the one-to-one relationship is of no value. Many people expect the dentist go give advice on how to care for their teeth. The dentist is able to adapt the message to the patient's individual needs and answer any questions which arise. It is also important for the dentist to be able to give his or her professional support and reinforcement to the advice which may have been given by others such as health visitors or teachers.

In every community there are certain key people who are opinion formers. It is to these persons that others turn for advice. In the field of dental health these include, besides dentists, the other members of the dental team, doctors, health educators, health visitors, midwives, teachers, and journalists. Such persons must, therefore, be kept informed of the correct messages to communicate, and encouraged to use their contacts with mothers, children and others to give dental advice whenever appropriate. The influence of these health and education personnel is not limited to those to whom they talk because the message becomes passed on to others in a *two-step* communication.

Lastly, it is unrealistic of the organizers to expect to achieve major changes in behaviour and health status by single, short-term campaigns. As already described, behaviour patterns are built up over a considerable period of time and handed down from one generation to another. Dental health educators must ensure that periodic *reinforcement* of the message is received by constant repetition. It is only in this way, like the wearing away of stone by constantly dripping water, that changes in a community level will be achieved.

The role of commerce and politics

In considering the promotion of oral hygiene, much support may be received from the manufacturers of products such as dentifrices and tooth-brushes. Commercial activity, including the use of the mass media for advertising campaigns, has undoubtedly contributed significantly to the increasing use of fluoride toothpastes and the more frequent replacement of tooth-brushes. In this respect, some of the interests of the manufacturers coincide with those of the dental profession. In addition to the advertising of their own branded products, the manufacturers of dental health aids have given financial and other support to a number of dental health education initiatives. The manufacturers of sugar products, however, may find that their commercial interests conflict rather more often with the message of the dental health educator. In the past, these companies have provided finance for the production of dental health materials, but this has provoked the accusation that the dental health message has been distorted and the role of sugar in the aetiology of dental caries not fully explained. Whilst any producer of dental health education materials should be free to accept help from any available source, it is essential for the credibility of the material that the message should be consistent with the scientific facts, and that the content of the materials must be decided by those involved in dental health education without interference from commercial sponsors.

The Black report (Report of a Research Working Group 1980) recommended a number of social and political policies which could be taken in order to benefit the general health of the population, especially those in the lower socio-economic groups. Similarly some have suggested, in relation to dental health, that political action should be taken in the control of sugar. Advocates of political action point to the commercial interests of the so-called 'sugar lobby' and the large sums of money spent annually on advertising in order to persuade the population to consume more sugar. This product they point out is responsible not only for dental caries, but is also associated with disorders such as obesity and heart disease. Various legal sanctions have been suggested including the taxation of sugar products, banning of advertising, and the printing of health warnings on wrappers and packets. Opponents of this point of view believe that these measures are either unworkable, ineffective, or infringe personal liberty in an unacceptable way. The dental profession has been reluctant to become involved in this type of political debate, but if all possible measures to reduce dental disease are to be considered then the merits and disadvantages of such political action will need to be discussed.

Conclusion

This chapter has attempted to identify some of the most important social factors which are relevant to the practice of dentistry and, in particular, preventive dentistry. It is hoped that by bearing these factors in mind, the dentist will be able to understand the attitudes and actions of his or her patients and others with whom he or she meets in a professional capacity. It is only upon this foundation that the dentist will be able to convert technical expertise in prevention into reality, and that an improvement in the dental health of the whole community becomes a possibility.

References

Anderson, R.J. (1981*a*). The changes in the dental health of 12-year-old school children in two Somerset schools: a review after an interval of 15 years. *Br. dent. J.* **150**, 218–21.

Anderson, R.J. (1981*b*). The changes in dental health of 12-year-old school children resident in a naturally fluoridated area of Gloucestershire: a review after an interval of 15 years. *Br. dent. J.* **150**, 354–5.

Anderson, R.J., Bradnock, G., and James, P.M.C. (1981). The changes in the dental health of 12-year-old school children in Shropshire: a review after an interval of 10 years. *Br. dent. J.* **150**, 278–81.

Arcus-Ting, R., Tessler, R., and Wright, J. (1977). Misinformation and opposition to fluoridation. *Polity* **10**, 281–9.

Bagramian, R.A. and Russell, A.L. (1973). Epidemiologic study of dental caries experience and between-meal eating patterns, *J. dent. Res.* **52**, 342–7.

Baric, L., Blinkhorn, A.S., and MacArthur, C. (1974). A health education approach to nutrition and dental health education. *Hlth Educ. J.* **33**, 79–90.

Beal, J.F. (1973). The dental health of five-year-old children of different ethnic origins resident in an inner Birmingham area and a nearby borough. *Archs. oral Biol.* **18**, 305–12.

Beal, J.F. and Dickson, S. (1973). The attitudes of West Midland mothers to water fluoridation. *Publ. Hlth.* **87**, 75–80.

Beal, J.F. and Dickson, S. (1974*a*). Diet and dental health. *Hlth Educ. J.* **33**, 8–12.

Beal, J.F. and Dickson, S. (1974*b*). Social differences in dental attitudes and behaviour in West Midland mothers. *Publ. Hlth* **89**, 19–30.

Beal, J.F. and Dickson, S. (1975*a*). Dental attitudes and behaviour related to vertical social mobility by marriage. *Commun. Dent. oral Epidem.* **3**, 174–8.

Beal, J.F. and Dickson, S. (1975*b*). Differences in dental attitudes and behaviour between West Midland mothers of various ethnic origins. *Pub. Hlth.* **89**, 65–70.

Beal, J.F. and James, P.M.C. (1970). Social differences in the dental conditions and dental needs of 5-year-old children in four areas of the West Midlands. *Br. dent. J.* **129**, 313–18.

Beal, J.F. and James, P.M.C. (1971). Dental caries prevalence in 5-year-old children following five and a half years of water fluoridation in Birmingham. *Br. dent. J.* **130**, 284–8.

Bergner, L. and Yerby, A.S. (1976). Low income and barriers to use of health services. In *The health gap. Medical services and the poor*, (ed. R.L. Kane, J.M. Jasteler and R.M. Gray). Springer, New York.

Bernstein, B. (1961). Social class and linguistic development: a theory of social learning. In *Education, economy and society*, (ed. A.H. Halsey, J. Floud and A.C. Anderson). Free Press, New York.

Bernstein, B. (1965). A socio-linguistic approach to social learning. In *Penguin survey of the social sciences*, (ed. J. Gould). Penguin Books, Harmondsworth.

Blau, P.M. (1956). Social mobility and interpersonal relations. *Am. Soc. Rev.* **21**, 291–5.

Blaxter, M. (1976). Social class and health inequalities. In *Equalities and Inequalities in health. Proceedings of the Twelfth Annual Symposium of the Eugenics Society*, London, 1975, (ed. C.O. Carter and J. Peel), pp. 111–25. Academic Press, London.

Blaxter, M. (1984). Equity and consultation rates in general practice. *Br. med. J.* **288**, 1963–7.

Blinkhorn, A.S. (1981). Dental health education. In *Dental public health*, (ed. G.L. Slack). Wright, Bristol.

Blinkhorn, A.S. and Verity, J.M. (1979). Assessment of the readability of dental health education literature. *Commun. Dent. oral Epidem.* **8**, 195–8.

Bradnock, G., Marchment, M.D. and Anderson, R.J. (1984). Social background, fluoridation and caries experience in a 5-year-old population in the West Midlands. *Br. dent. J.* **156**, 127–31.

British Fluoridation Society (1985). *Fluoridation. What the people say*. BFS, London.

British Fluoridation Society (1987). *Fluoridation Action Report 1987*. BFS, London.

Brotherston, J. (1976). The Galton Lecture: 1975. Inequality: is it inevitable? In *Equalities and inequalities in health. Proceedings of the Twelfth Annual Symposium of the Eugenics Society*, London, 1975, (ed. C.O. Carter and J. Peel), pp. 73–104. Academic Press, London.

Bulman, J.S., Richards, N.D., Slack, G.L., and Willcocks, A.J. (1968). *Demand and need for dental care*. Oxford University Press, London.

Carmichael, C.L. (1981). Social and geographical factors affecting the role and provisions of community dental services in Newcastle AHA(T). *Proc. Br. Ass. Study commun. Dent.* **3**, 38–44.

Carmichael, C.L. (1985). Inner city Britain: A challenge for the dental profession. A review of dental and related deprivation in inner city Newcastle-upon-Tyne. *Br. dent. J.* **159**, 24–7.

Cooper, M.H. (1975). *Rationing health care*. Croom Helm, London.

Corbett, E.M. and Moore, W.J. (1976). Distribution of dental caries in ancient British populations. 4. The 19th century. *Caries Res.* **10**, 401–14.

Craft, M. and Sheiham, A. (1976). Attitudes to prevention amongst dental practitioners: a comparison between the north and south of England. *Br. dent. J.* **141**, 371–6.

Crain, R.L., Katz, E., and Rosenthal, D.B. (1969). *The politics of community conflict: the fluoridation decision*. Bobbs-Merrill, New York.

Cushing, A.M. and Sheiham, A. (1985). Assessing periodontal treatment needs and periodontal status in a study of adults in north-west England. *Commun. dent. Hlth.* **2**, 187–94.

Davis, H.C., Parfitt, G.J., and James, P.M.C. (1956). A controlled study into the effect of dental health education on 1,539 school children in St. Albans. *Br. dent. J.* **100**, 354–6.

Davis, P. (1980). *The social context of dentistry*. Croom Helm, London.

Dental Strategy Review Group (1981). *Towards better dental health*. Department of Health and Social Security, London.

Downer, M.C. (1970). Dental caries and periodontal disease in girls of different ethnic groups: a comparison in a London secondary school. *Br. dent. J.* **128**, 379–85.

Eddie, S. and Davies, J.A. (1985). The effect of social class on attendance frequency and dental treatment received in the General Dental Service in Scotland. *Br. dent. J.* **159**, 370–2.

Festinger, L. (1957). *A theory of cognitive dissonance*. Row Peterson, Evanston.

Finlayson, D.A. and Wilson, W.A. (1982). Dundee's dental health education campaign: results of survey six months later. *Br. dent. J.* **112**, 88–9.

Frankel, J.M. and Allukian, M. (1973). Sixteen referenda on fluoridation in Massachusetts; an analysis. *J. publ. hlth. Dent.* **33**, 96–103.

Frazier, P.J. (1980). Fluoridation: a review of social research. *J. publ. hlth. Dent.* **40**, 214–33.

French, A.D., Carmichael, C.L., Furness, J.A., and Rugg-Gunn, A.J. (1984). The relationship between social class and dental health in 5-year-old children in the north and south of England. *Br. Dent. J.* **156**, 83–6.

Gamson, W.A. (1964). How to lose a referendum: the case of fluoridation. *Transaction* **2**, 9–11.

Gelbier, S. and Taylor, S.G.B.W.S. (1985). Some Asian communities in the UK and their culture. *Br. dent. J.* **158**, 416–18.

Goldthorpe, J.H., Lockwood, D., Bechhofer, F., and Platt, J. (1968). *The affluent worker; political attitudes and behaviour*. Cambridge University Press.

Goldthorpe, J.H., Lockwood, D., and Bechhofer, F. (1969). *The affluent worker in the class structure*. Cambridge University Press.

Goose, D.H. (1960). An oral hygiene campaign in Wellingborough. *Dent. Practit.* **10**, 258–62.

Gray, P.G., Todd, J.E., Slack, G.L., and Bulman, J.S. (1970). *Adult dental health in England and Wales in 1968*. HMSO, London.

Gunning, R. (1952). *The technique of clear writing*. McGraw-Hill, New York.

Heifetz, S.B., Horowitz, H.S., and Korts, D.C. (1976). Prevalence of dental caries in white and black children in Nelson County, Virginia, a rival southern community. *J. publ. hlth. Dent.* **36**, 79–87.

Hippocrates (c. 400 BC). On Airs, Waters and Places. Translated by F. Adams. In *Great books of the Western world. No. 10. Hippocrates and Galen*, (ed. R.M. Hutchins), pp. 9–19. Encyclopaedia Britannica, Chicago (1952).

Hodge, H. (1979). Factors associated with toothbrushing behaviour in adolescents. Ph.D. thesis, University of Manchester.

Infante, P.F. and Russell, A.L. (1974). An epidemiologic study of dental caries in pre-school children in the United States by race and socio-economic level. *J. dent. Res.* **53**, 393–6.

Iverson, D.C. (1980). Fluoride's role in health promotion: a national perspective. *J. Publ. hlth. Dent.* **40**, 276–83.

Jackson, D. (1972). Attitudes to fluoridation: a survey of British housewives. *Br. dent. J.* **132**, 219–22.

James, P.M.C. (1981). One hundred years of dental public health. *Br. dent. J.* **151**, 20–3.

Jenkins, P.M., Feldman, B.S., and Stirrups, D.R. (1984*a*). The effect of social factors on referrals for orthodontic advice and treatment. *Br. J. Orth.* **11**, 24–6.

Jenkins, P.M., Feldman, B.S., and Stirrups, D.R. (1984*b*). The effect of social class and dental features on referrals for orthodontic advice and treatment. *Br. J. Orth.* **11**, 185–8.

Lennon, M.A. (1976). An evaluation of the adequacy of the general dental service. *Br. dent. J.* **131**, 223–5.

Metz, A.S. (1967). The relationship of dental care practices to attitude toward fluoridation (1959 NORC data). *J. Hlth. socl. Behav.* **8**, 55–9.

National Pure Water Association (1969). *11 years of fluoridation: ineffective and unsafe: errors and omissions in government report.*

Newson, J. and Newson, E. (1976). Changes in the concept of parenthood. In *The sociology of modern Britain*, (revised edn.), (ed. E. Butterworth and D. Weir). Fontana/Collins, Glasgow.

Office of Population Censuses and Surveys (1980). *Classification of occupations.* HMSO, London.

Office of Population Censuses and Surveys (1986*a*). *Mortality statistics, perinatal and infant: social and biological factors for 1984*, Series DH3 No. 17. HMSO, London.

Office of Population Censuses and Surveys (1986*b*). *Registrar General's decennial supplement on occupational mortality 1979–83.* HMSO, London.

O'Mullane, D.M. and Robinson, M.E. (1977). The distribution of dentists and the uptake of dental treatment by school children in England. *Commun. Dent. oral Epidem.* **5**, 156–9.

O'Shea, R.M. and Cohen, L.K. (1966). The social sciences and dentistry, III Current opinion on fluoridation. *J. publ. hlth. Dent.* **26**, 331–3.

Parfitt, G.J., James, P.M.C., and Davis, H.C. (1958). A controlled study of the effect of dental health education on the gingival structures of school children. *Br. dent. J.* **104**, 21–4.

Paul, P.F. and Bradnock, G. (1986). The dental health of Asian and Caucasian four- and five-year-old children resident in Coventry. *Commun. dent. Hlth.* **3**, 275–85.

Perkins, P.C. and Sweetman, A.J.P. (1986). Ethnic differences in caries prevalence in 5-year-olds in north-west London. *Br. dent. J.* **161**, 215–16.

Polgar, S. (1962). Health and human behaviour: areas of interest common to the social and medical sciences. *Curr. Anthrop. J.* 159–79.

Report of a Research Working Group (1980). *Inequalities in health.* HMSO, London.

Rock, W.P. and Bradnock, G. (1976). The employment of dental hygienists within the General Dental Service in the United Kingdom. *Br. dent. J.* **140**, 351–2.

Rogers, E.M. and Shoemaker, F.F. (1971). *Communication of innovations: a cross-cultural approach* (2nd edn). Free Press, New York.

Rogers, J. Gelbier, S., Twidale, S., and Plamping, D. (1984). Barriers faced by parents in obtaining dental treatment for young children: a questionnaire evaluation. *Commun. dent. Hlth.* **1**, 207–12.

Rosser, C. and Harris, C. (1965). *The family and social change*. Routledge and Kegan Paul, London.

Royal College of Physicians (1976). *Fluoride, teeth and health*. Pitman Medical, Tunbridge Wells.

Sanders, J.T. (1961). The stages of a community controversy: the case of fluoridation. *J. soc. Issues* **17**, 55–65.

Sapolsky, H.M. (1969). The fluoridation controversy: an alternative explanation. *Pub. Opinion Q.* **33**, 240–8.

Saxby, M.S. and Anderson, R.J. (1987). Dental cleanliness in a West Midlands population aged 14–19 years according to sex, ethnic origin and the presence of 1 ppm fluoride in the drinking water. *Commun. dent. Hlth.* **4**, 107–15.

Sheiham, A. (1969). The prevalence and severity of periodontal disease in British populations: dental surveys of employed populations in Great Britain. *Br. dent. J.* 115–22.

Sheiham, A. and Hobdell, M.H. (1969). Decayed, missing and filled teeth in British adult populations. *Br. dent. J.* **126**, 401–4.

Simmel, A. and Ast, D.B. (1962). Some correlates of opinion on fluoridation. *Am. J. publ. Hlth.* **52**, 1269–73.

Susser, M.W. and Watson, W. (1971). *Sociology in medicine*, (2nd edn.). Oxford University Press, London.

Taylor, P.J. and Carmichael, C.L. (1980). Dental health and the application of geographical methodology. *Commun. Dent. oral Epidemiol.* **8**, 117–22.

Titmuss, R.M. (1969). *Commitment to welfare*. George Allen and Unwin, London.

Todd. J.E. (1975). *Children's dental health in England and Wales 1973*. HMSO, London.

Todd, J.E. and Dodd, T. (1985). *Children's dental health in the United Kingdom 1983*. HMSO, London.

Todd, J.E. and Walker, A.M. (1980). *Adult dental health*, Vol. 1. *England and Wales 1968–1978*. HMSO, London.

Townsend, P., Phillimore, P., and Beattie, A. (1987). *Health and deprivation*: inequality and the North. Croom Helm, London.

US General Accounting Office (1979). *Reducing tooth decay—more emphasis on fluoridation needed*. Publ. No. HRD-79-3. Government Printing Office, Washington.

Varley, T.F. and Goose, D.H. (1971). Dental caries in children of immigrants in Liverpool. *Br. dent. J.* **130**, 27–9.

West Midlands Regional Health Authority (1980). Summary of opinion survey on fluoridation. Mimeograph.

Whitehead, M. (1987). *The health divide: Inequalities in health in the 1980's*. Health Education Council, London.

Williams, S.A. (1986). Behaviour patterns affecting the dental health of infants. *Dent. Hlth.* (Lond.) **25**, 3–4, 6.

Worsley, P. *et al.* (1970). *Introducing sociology*. Penguin Books, Harmondsworth.

12

Role of dental health education in preventive dentistry

F. P. ASHLEY

Introduction

THE prevention of dental disease is considered by many to be the primary aim of dental health education. It could therefore be argued that this entire book is concerned with dental health education as it provides the scientific basis on which dental health education rests. In addition, the chapters on oral cleanliness and dental caries, prevention and control of periodontal disease, and social factors and preventive dentistry deal with specific aspects of dental health education. The aim of this section is to take a more general view of dental health education. Points which will be considered include the aims of dental health education, the selection of target groups, the importance of the correct message, as well as current messages and the effectiveness of dental health education.

There has been much discussion in recent years of whether we should be talking about health education or health promotion. Ian Sutherland's (1987) account of the rise and fall of the Health Education Council considers the use of these terms at some length. He suggests that health promotion expects to identify specific results in terms of reductions in the amount of disease and improvements in the quality of community and personal health. On the other hand, health education is an activity valuable in itself, enabling self-possession and self-determination. It is an important part of education in its entirety. Health promotion is the responsibility of all those who are concerned with bringing about the improvement of health, and is best seen as a banner under which a wide variety of people can gather to work for the enhancement of health. Health education is an aspect of health promotion and one of its roles is to provide people with information, skills, and experiences through which they can exercise a greater degree of control over their own health (French 1985).

Aims of dental health education

The general aim of dental health education is no different to the aim of dental treatment; that is to promote the life-long maintenance of a dentition which is comfortable, functional, socially acceptable, and promotes good general health. Comfort and function are largely determined by the individual and need no further comment. Social acceptability relates to factors such as appearance, ability to speak clearly, and the absence of halitosis associated with oral disease. The social acceptability of an individual's dentition is determined by the individual and the individual's peer group and not by the dentist or any other provider of dental health education. Promotion of good health through a healthy dentition is a more general concept and includes aspects such as reducing the risk of infective endocarditis from bacteriaemias of oral origin in susceptible individuals, through to ensuring that the individual can eat an adequate diet and has a good self-image.

However it should be emphasized that in order to promote the *life-long* maintenance of a dentition which will meet these requirements, changes in behaviour and provision of treatment are likely to be necessary at a time when no problems are apparent to the individual concerned.

It has to be recognized that some individuals with a high susceptibility to disease, perhaps combined with problems of compliance with appropriate preventive behaviour, may be incapable of maintaining a natural dentition over their lifetime. In view of this it may be worth considering the specific aims of dental health education under three headings:

(1) adoption of appropriate attitudes and life styles;
(2) making the best of conditions and disorders which cannot be prevented or treated adequately;
(3) encouraging better use of dental services.

The attitudes and life styles which are conducive to the prevention of dental disease would lead to effective, daily tooth cleaning with a fluoride toothpaste, and a reduction in the frequency of sugar intakes to three times a day or less. Adoption of appropriate attitudes might also help to bring about wider use of fluoridation and its attendant benefits.

The individual with a high susceptibility to disease has already been referred to. In addition there are dental conditions such as severe malocclusions, impacted teeth, and so on, which are not amenable to normal preventive procedures. Over-simplification of the dental health education message may result in unnecessary and incorrect feelings of guilt in the individual with the disease or condition. In the case of children the parents may feel that they are entirely responsible. In most cases such victim-blaming is entirely inappropriate.

Not only should individuals with established disease seek appropriate treatment but the providers of dental services should be encouraged to take a preventive approach.

Target groups

A phenomenon which is common to many of the chronic diseases afflicting mankind is the variation in individual susceptibility to the condition despite apparent similarities in their exposure to the recognized aetiological factors. This was illustrated in relation to periodontitis by the classic epidemiological study of Tamil tea-labourers by Loe *et al.* (1986). All subjects had consistently high levels of plaque and gingivitis but a tremendous variation in the severity of periodontitis was found. This ranged from the worst 10 per cent, who had lost most of their teeth with periodontal disease, to the best 10 per cent, who had virtually no bone loss. This latter group were presumably the dental equivalent of the 90-year-old who has smoked 40 cigarettes a day for all his adult life with no apparent adverse effects. It could be argued that the resistant group are not in any need of dental health education to prevent their periodontitis as their natural resistance will ensure that they retain sufficient periodontal support for their lifetime. A similar argument may be advanced in relation to dental caries. When 50 per cent of 5-year-olds are free from dental caries (Todd and Dodd, 1985), we should in theory be targeting our dental health education at the caries-prone group.

There are several objections to this approach. First, we are not yet in position where we can assess the susceptibility of an individual to disease with sufficient accuracy to have great confidence in our selection of targets. Second, many of the methods or predictive tests which are being developed are relatively expensive to administer on a population basis. The commercially available kits which estimate salivary buffering capacity and counts of lactobacilli and *Streptococcus mutans* are expensive in relation to the current expenditure on dental health education. Third, it is apparent that behaviour changes are far more likely to occur if the whole population is involved rather than just the highly susceptible group. Finally, if we go back to the example of 50 per cent of 5-year-olds in 1983 who were caries-free, it should be stressed that dental health education helped to achieve this improvement from the 25 per cent of 10 years before. We would not advocate abolishment of the legislation concerning the wearing of seat belts because the number of injuries to drivers and passengers has been reduced since seat-belt wearing was made compulsory.

This advocacy of a general population approach for dental health education rests on the continuing high prevalence of dental disease, and the need for changes in behaviour to achieve reductions in these diseases. It does not preclude some targeting of certain broad groups. Epidemiological data may be used to indicate which social, geographical, or age groups are most at risk to the various dental diseases. Other factors, such as the likely receptiveness of the target audience or their potential for influencing other people, may also be important.

The target groups identified by the Dental Health Programme Planning Group of the Health Education Council (1986) were:

1. The public—although all of the public were considered to be potentially in need of dental health education, the current and proposed target groups were:
   young children (3–5-years-old);
   adolescents;
   young adults (16–20-years-old);
   middle-aged adults;
   older people.
2. Professionals—all professionals, and in particular the members of the dental team.
3. Decision makers—ranging from those involved in decisions on such matters as fluoridation to food manufacturers, who may need encouragement to develop non-cariogenic, nutritionally acceptable snacks and drinks.

Even if the whole population is to be the target of dental health education, the message should be tailored to take account of the different needs of the individuals within the population. This is more easily achieved when the approach is on a one-to-one basis rather than to a group. Further discussion of this point has been presented in the chapter on the prevention and control of chronic periodontal disease. In theory, use of mass media, such as television, radio and newspapers, permits access to most of the population and is frequently advocated as the solution to all the problems of dental health education. There is very little evidence to support this opinion. Mass-media campaigns can raise public awareness but their effect on behaviour seems limited (Shou 1987; Rise and Sogaard 1988). The one-to-one approach is possible every time a patient attends a dental surgery, and this is one reason why the dental team is singled out as a target group and why the Health Education Council in its 1985–6 Dental Health Programme sought 'to foster a preventive approach by dental professionals'. Decision makers form another obvious target group—the most important decision made in recent years was probably that concerned with the marketing of fluoride toothpastes.

The importance of the correct message

In a review of dental health education in the previous 100 years Fox and Maddick (1980) noted that there had been three consistent messages during that time: regular dental visits; good oral hygiene; and a properly balanced diet. However they observed that there had been changes in the more specific recommendations and the reasons given for their justification. Some of the earlier messages, in particular concerning the relationship between diet and oral hygiene and caries, are now considered to be incorrect. The previous emphasis on diet was concerned with ensuring the correct development of the tooth structure rather than limiting the number of occasions on which acid was formed in the plaque in response to a sugar intake. Similarly, tooth-brushing was stressed as central to the prevention of caries, and apples were considered as nature's tooth-brush. It would be naive to suppose that changes in knowledge will not result in our successors in another hundred years finding some fault with our current messages.

The problems associated with changes in knowledge are compounded by the health educator's need for relatively simple messages. A message hedged around by too many 'ifs', 'buts', and 'howevers' ceases to be a message which can be easily understood and acted upon by the target audience. On the other hand, over-simplification of the facts may result in a message which will soon cease to be correct. This is particularly disturbing in view of the observation (I. Maddick and B. Fox, personal communication) that different generations retain the message which was in vogue during their school-days.

Cynics might argue that if there is any doubt at all about the message it is better to keep quiet. However, to do so may deprive people of knowledge which would enable them to improve their health. It should be emphasized that this problem is not unique to dental health education, indeed dental health education rests on a sounder scientific basis than most of health education. For instance, one of the current messages on prevention of heart disease concerns the beneficial effect of regular exercise yet, at the time of writing, the scientific evidence for this statement is minimal, in particular for women.

The Health Education Authority (formerly the Health Education Council) publish a policy document *The Scientific Basis of Dental Health Education* (Levine 1985), which has played a major role in ensuring that the providers of dental health education are aware of what is currently seen as the correct message. However as Towner (1987) points out: 'There is now a plethora of reports and studies available upon which dental health education can draw. Social science has revealed the complexity of developing, evaluating and disseminating effective materials and programmes. Perhaps paradoxically the self assurance demonstrated in the mass propaganda campaigns of the inter-war period is not so evident now and the way forward less certain.'

Current messages in dental health education

In *The Scientific Basis of Dental Health Education* (Levine 1985) the statement is made that in the past the information presented to the public by dental health educators has been unnecessarily complicated, frequently contradictory, and sometimes wrong. It is suggested that advice should be based on four simple statements:

1. **'Restriction of sugar-containing foods and drinks to meal times.**
   The number of times sugar enters the mouth is the most important factor in determining the rate of dental decay. If confined to meal times, the harmful effects of sugar will be reduced. Food and drinks not containing added sugar may be consumed between meals with little risk of causing decay.'

Examination of this first statement reveals that it is not as simple as suggested. The health educator might like to translate this into two simple messages, (i) 'sugar will not cause decay if it is only consumed at meals' and (ii) 'avoid decay by keeping to safe snacks and drinks between meals'. Although both messages would probably be a correct interpretation of the first statement for most of the population, exactly what constitutes a safe snack or drink is the subject of much discussion. Dried fruit has appeared on lists of safe snacks despite its high sugar content and Aristotle's reported observation in the fourth century BC of the relationship between eating figs and caries.

Another problem with suggesting 'safe snacks' is avoiding conflict with the general health education message. Cheese, crisps, and peanuts may be acceptable from a dental viewpoint but are open to criticism from a general health aspect because of their fat and salt content. It is important that we ensure that any dietary advice given as part of dental health education is consistent with the general health education guide-lines. At the same time the dental profession has to try and ensure that these guide-lines are consistent with good dental health. Current dietary trends encourage the consumption of fruit and fruit juices, which if excessive, may predispose to erosion. It is important to make the public aware of this.

2. **'Cleaning the teeth and gums thoroughly every day with a fluoride toothpaste**

   The removal of dental plaque is essential for the prevention of periodontal disease. The toothbrush is the only means of plaque removal that should be recommended to the public, other oral hygiene aids, apart from disclosing agents, being a matter for personal professional advice. Thorough brushing, every day, is of more value than more frequent cursory brushing, and a careful scrub technique should be advised. The toothbrush size and design should allow the user to reach all tooth surfaces and gum margins easily and comfortably. Regular toothbrushing by itself will not prevent dental decay, but a definite benefit will be gained by the use of a fluoride toothpaste or powder.'

This statement is clearly aimed at the prevention of both caries and periodontal disease, and by bringing the two aspects together it builds on the public perception that tooth-brushing is of positive benefit to dental health. This belief owes much to the success of previous dental health education activities. These were based on the concept that 'a clean tooth never decays'. Theilade and Theilade (1976) date this back to Greenwood (1760–1815). Towner's (1986) survey of 296 factory workers, aged 18–40 years indicated that brushing was directed at the prevention of tooth decay rather than gum disease. She also found that knowledge of gum disease was less than that of caries and the perceived susceptibility was also less. It would appear unwise to be over-critical of the value of tooth-brushing on its own in the prevention of caries as we wish people to continue to brush their teeth both to prevent periodontal disease and to deliver fluoride in toothpaste to reduce caries.

3. **'Water Fluoridation**

   Fluoridation of the water supply has a profound influence on the dental health of the community and should be implemented at the earliest possible time. Fluoride tablets or drops are an alternative for motivated parents.'

For many years health educators were cautious about promoting fluoride tablets or drops as it was considered that their use tended to undermine the case for water fluoridation. In addition, the relationship between caries and socio-economic status meant that the individuals most likely to benefit from their use would be least likely to take them on a regular basis unless they were administered at school. This latter comment is still true but the slow progress with water fluoridation, and cost considerations in those water authorities serving small populations, means that promotion of fluoride tablets or drops is appropriate.

4. **'Regular Dental Attendance**
   Studies on the control of periodontal disease have emphasised the importance of regular professional cleaning in addition to daily plaque removal. It is the dentist's responsibility to ensure that this is carried out effectively at intervals depending on the needs of individual patients, to monitor the health of the mouth and to provide dental health advice. Once decay is established and a definite cavity is present, it cannot be remineralized, but the tooth can be restored. Whilst many people may need fillings only infrequently, the importance of early detection and treatment makes regular attendance advisable.'

The vagueness of the term 'regular' as opposed to annual or 6-monthly reflects the state of the scientific literature in relation to attendance. In fact if the emphasis were to be placed on periodontal health, one study (Axelsson and Lindhe 1978) would lead us to believe that oral hygiene reinforcement, scaling, and necessary root planing, should be carried out every 2 to 3 months in adults.

These comments on the statements in *The Scientific Basis of Dental Health Education* are made to emphasize the point that they are open to debate and modification as the years pass. However the statements are an excellent summary of the consensus view of experts in the UK in 1985.

Effectiveness of Dental Health Education

One approach to the assessment of the effectiveness of dental health education would be to say that the programme concerned is not worth implementing unless it results in a significant reduction in dental disease. This is perhaps a reaction to well meaning but misguided efforts at dental health education, which in some cases were based on incorrect assumptions about methods of preventing dental disease. Such a hard-line approach underestimates the importance of achieving improvements in knowledge, attitudes, and behaviour. Indeed it could be argued that dental health education is justified if it results in a significant gain in knowledge and understanding of both the causes of dental disease and its prevention. In theory the individual is then able to make an informed choice but, in fact, the choices available may be restricted because of economic or other constraints. Even if the argument that everyone has the right to some dental health education is accepted, questions arise as to how effective the education is and how much of our resources should be devoted to health education. Inevitably we have to relate this to the overall cost of dental disease and the potential benefits of prevention. It is therefore customary to build evaluation into dental health education programmes.

Most programme initiatives have been related to children and the major effort in the UK has come from the Cambridge Dental Health Study of the Health Education Council. Between 1975 and 1986 the Dental Health Study Team, led by Michael Craft, carried out a range of studies into various aspects of dental health education. They developed, evaluated, and disseminated two programmes for children: '*Natural Nashers*' for adolescents and '*Good Teeth*' for pre-school children (Craft and Croucher 1979; Croucher *et al.* 1985). Coincident with the development of these programmes others were being developed and evaluated either in response to local needs (Hodge *et al.* 1985), or nationally, supported by toothpaste manufacturers (Maddick and Fox 1982; Towner 1984; Dowell 1983). Since then there has been a major cut-back in the activities of the toothpaste manufacturers but the programmes of the Health Education Council (now the Health Education Authority) continue to be available through commercial publishers and are backed up by a national network of co-ordinators. Almost all of the co-ordinators are drawn from the staff of the Community Dental Services and they provide an advisory and training service for users of the programmes.

Assessment of the contribution of dental health education to the improvement in dental health in the last 20 years is almost impossible. It may well be argued that the decision of the toothpaste manufacturers to promote fluoride toothpaste was the most important factor. However, dental health education may have contributed to this decision and its acceptability by the public as well as promoting the more widespread and frequent use of such toothpaste. When the reduction in rampant caries in very young children, associated with dietary changes such as the more limited use of sweetened comforters, is considered (Holt *et al.* 1982) then we are on firmer ground, as it is extremely doubtful that fluoride toothpaste would have affected this group, many of whom were not having their teeth cleaned on a regular basis.

It is unlikely that we will see such a rapid rate of improvement in the dental health of children in the future and we cannot be sure what level of dental health education is required even to maintain this improvement. In any event it will always be necessary to balance the cost of effective dental health programmes against the potential benefits. In this context we are not just talking about savings in treatment costs but other benefits, such as the reduction in experience of pain and general anaesthesia, as well as the contribution made to the general well-being of the individual. Currently, public awareness of health issues is increasing, creating fertile ground for dental health education, which should help to bring about further improvements in dental health.

References

Axelsson, P. and Lindhe, J. (1978). Effect of controlled oral hygiene procedures on caries and periodontal disease in adults. *J. clin. Perio.* **5**, 133–51.

Craft, M.H. and Croucher, R.E. (1979). Preventive dental health in adolescents. Results of a controlled field trial. *Roy. Soc. Hlth. J.* **2**, 48–56.

Crouchers, R.E., Rodgers, A.I., Franklin, A.J., and Craft, M.H. (1985). Results and issues arising from an evaluation of community dental health education: the case of the 'Good Teeth Programme'. *Commun. dent. Hlth.* **2**, 89–97.

Dowell, T.B. (1983). Dental health education. Yours for Life programme. *Dent. Advertiser Hygienists Forum* **No. 22** (Feb.), 16–18.

Fox, B. and Maddick, I. (1980). A hundred years of dental health education. *Br. dent. J.* **149**, 28–32.

French, J. (1985). To educate or promote health? *Hlth. Educ. J.* **44**, 115–16.

Health Education Council (1986). *Dental Health Programme Plan.* Health Education Council, London.

Hodge, H., Buchanan, M., Jones, J., and O'Donnell, P. (1985). The evaluation of the infant dental programme developed in Sefton. *Commun. dent. Hlth.* **2**, 175–85.

Holt, R.D., Joels, D., and Winter, G.B. (1982). Caries in pre-school children: the Camden study. *Br. dent. J.* **153**, 107–9

Levine, R.S. (1985). *The scientific basis of dental health education. A policy document.* Health Education Council, London.

Loe, H., Anerud, A., Boysen, H., and Morrison, E. (1986). Natural history of periodontal disease in man. *J. clin. Perio.* **13**, 431–40.

Maddick, I. and Fox, B. (1982). The assessment of a teacher-based programme of dental health education for 5–7 year olds. *J. dent. Res.* **61**, 540.

Rise, J. and Sogaard A.J. (1988). Effect of a mass media periodontal campaign upon preventive knowledge and behaviour in Norway. *Commun. Dent. oral Epidemiol.* **16**, 1–4.

Schou, L. (1987). Use of mass-media and active involvement in a national dental health campaign in Scotland. *Commun. Dent. oral Epidemiol.* **15**, 14–18.

Sutherland, I. (1987). *Health education—half a policy.* National Extension College, Cambridge.

Theilade, E. and Theilade, J. (1976). Role of plaque in the etiology of periodontal disease and caries. *Oral Sci. Rev.* **9**, 23–64.

Todd, J.E. and Dodd, T. (1985). *Children's dental health in the United Kingdom 1983.* HMSO, London.

Towner, E.M.L. (1984). The 'Gleam Team' programme: Development and evaluation of a dental health education package for infant schools. *Commun. dent. Hlth.* **1**, 181–91.

Towner, E.M.L. (1986). *The adult dental health education study.* Research Report No. 9. Health Education Council, London.

Towner, E.M.L. (1987). *History of dental health education.* Occasional Paper No. 5. Health Education Authority, London.

13

Handicap in perspective

JUNE H. NUNN

WITH few exceptions, handicap remains a 'Cinderella' area of medicine and dentistry. However, it would appear that handicapped children and adults are assuming such numbers that the problem of their care, including their dental care, can no longer be an issue to be side-stepped. Care of the chronically sick and of the handicapped in particular have always been neglected areas of the National Health Service, with dentistry the poor relation of medicine. Not unnaturally whilst numbers were small or demand non-existent, dentistry and the handicapped person were separate entities and only crossed paths on an emergency basis. Yet the need, if not the demand, is there. Dentistry in the past has relied too heavily on demand for its services so that the handicapped population have inevitably lost out. Much of what has been published in the way of provision of dental services to handicapped people has probably been dealing with the tip of the iceberg.

The increasing sophistication in medical care has meant that many more infants at risk now survive the neonatal period than would have done previously, so that the number of children handicapped by one or more conditions may therefore increase. These advances have also generated handicapping conditions. Those surviving may well do so with more severe or even multiple handicaps, often well into adulthood (Forrest *et al.* 1973; Morton 1977). One estimate now puts the survival rate of children with Down's syndrome at 80 per cent (Department of Health and Social Security 1976*a*).

Higher standards of paediatric care, whilst increasing the survival rate of already handicapped children (Henry and Sinkford 1972), are vital also in the primary prevention of disability, as is the increasing availability of genetic screening and counselling (Fitzimmons 1982). Regrettably, those most vulnerable are often the people to make least use of these services (Younghusband *et al.* 1970; Department of Health and Social Security 1976*a*; HMSO 1976; Department of Health and Social Security 1977*a*; Children's Committee 1980).

Terminology

It soon becomes apparent that there is a persistent dilemma in the terminology of handicap.

Assigning a 'label' to a child is not without its pitfalls: because of the complexity of some conditions, the way that they manifest in one child may be different from that in another, or the child may meet the criteria of assessment on one occasion and not on another (Morgan 1979). The condition may well regress or worsen, thus making a static definition inappropriate (Ewalt 1972).

Once the label has been placed, however, these changes may not readily bring about a recategorization. To a certain extent, the label assigned to a child with a handicap is dependent upon the agency through which the disabilities have first been diagnosed; this in turn may depend more on chance social class and presenting symptoms than on the child's actual needs (Younghusband *et al.* 1970). Categorization in this way of children and the schools which they attend is often convenient only for administrative purposes, for within each category of handicap there are many degrees of severity of condition, and indeed some children will have more than one handicap, e.g., the psychiatric disorders superimposed on physical handicap (Harding 1980). Further arguments against the use of such rigid categories have been put forward in the Report of the committee of enquiry into Education of Handicapped Children and Young People (HMSO 1978*b*); recommendations made in the report aim to abolish the statutory categorization of handicapped pupils, and to integrate such children more closely with the normal schoolchild.

A number of authors (Younghusband *et al.* 1970; Harris *et al.* 1971; Swallow 1972; HMSO 1976; Swerdloff 1980) have addressed themselves to the problem of definition of terms, and attempted to distinguish between defect, disability, and handicap. However, in the context of dentistry for handicapped people, the categories suggested by Soble (1974) have practical applications: 'dentally handicapped' refers to patients 'who have some gross condition or deficit in their oral cavities which necessitates special dental treatment considerations'; and, 'handicapped for dentistry' referring to patients 'whose oral health may be considered within the normal range, but who have some physical and/or mental or emotional condition which may prevent them from being treated routinely in the dental situation'. Neither of these two are mutually exclusive.

Classification

Classification of the different types of handicaps can be carried out either from an aetiological point of view (Morgan 1979) or from presenting symptoms (Kanar 1979). Even across the broad range of handicaps, classification is frequently carried out, for the purposes of education, on the basis of intelligence testing. The procedure of categorizing children so affected is complicated by those individuals who possess a number of handicaps (Younghusband *et al.* 1970; DHSS 1971; Capute 1974). This is almost inevitable because profoundly retarded people nearly always have significant neurological involvement and are more vulnerable to chronic diseases (Morgan 1979). In addition, handicap may be imposed on disability by psychological and social defects (Franks 1969).

In 1976, the Department of Education and Science subdivided handicap with reference to special educational needs as: physical handicap and delicate; educationally subnormal; deaf and hearing impaired; blind and visually handicapped; maladjusted; epileptic; speech defect; and autism (Harding 1980).

These have been superseded by the 1981 Education Act where all such children are designated as children with learning difficulties. Although a number of other classifications are still used in the dental literature, for the purposes of comparison of oral health, the format in common usage would appear to be mental, physical, medical, and sensory handicaps. Despite the inadequacies, already explored, of such a classification it is in this form that the dental health of the former three groups will now be presented.

Dental health of handicapped children

Difficulties also exist in defining oral health in special groups. This has led Beck and Hunt (1985) to conclude that categorization by the diagnostic label of developmental disability may be inappropriate, as it may not be the disability itself that influences dental disease rates, but how profound is the level of the disease. However, very few authors actually categorize their study groups in such a way, so that data presented give only mean values of dental disease prevalence for each type of disability.

The largest group of disabled children encountered are those with a mental handicap, and it is their dental disease experience which will be discussed first.

Mental handicap

This category as a whole constitutes the largest subgroup when considering the total number of children in receipt of special education, with 25 per thousand of the child population affected (HMSO 1976).

The causes of mental handicap are legion, but are arbitrarily divided into three groups of children: the mildly educationally subnormal (ESN(M)); the severely educationally subnormal (ESN(S)); and the child with Down's syndrome. Although the last group comes within the remit of one or other of the first two categories, the dental health of Down's syndrome children is sufficiently different for them to merit separate study. ESN(M) children are classified as those with an IQ between 50 and 70, whilst ESN(S) children have an IQ of less than 50 (Drillen *et al.* 1966; Morgan 1979).

There would, however, appear to be distinct sex and social class bias in the determination of the numbers of mentally handicapped, especially ESN(M) children (Kushlik 1964; Richardson *et al.* 1964; Stevens and Heber 1964; Pless and Douglas 1971; Broadhead 1972; Neer *et al.* 1973; HMSO 1978*b*; McCabe 1979). Indeed, of the prevalence figures quoted for ESN(M) per thousand of the child population by the Court Report (HMSO 1976) above, only one-third will have evidence of central nervous system pathology. The prevalence of ESN(S) handicap is of the order of four per thousand, occurs more uniformly across the social class spectrum (HMSO 1976), and with distinct pathological involvement in its aetiology rather than socio-cultural factors. Of the affected children, the majority are usually found to be male, as with most other types of handicap.

Dental health in mental handicap

Dental caries

Rhodes (1884) was one of the first people to examine and report on the dental health of the 'insane'; of the 350 inmates of a mental hospital in Cambridge, compared with 350 patients from Addenbrooke's Hospital in the same city, he commented that relative to other people of similar class, tooth quality was good. From the studies which have followed Rhodes', it would seem that overall the prevalence of dental caries in the mentally handicapped is similar to that found in normal populations and, in many cases, lower. A number of the studies encompassed the mentally handicapped in institutions where stricter dietary control may have encouraged a lower prevalence of caries attack (Brown 1980; Forsberg *et al.* 1985; Schwarz and Vigild 1987). However, there are exceptions to this general finding of lowered disease prevalence in institutions (MacEntee *et al.* 1985).

For some of the studies, the caries experience in 10- to 12-year-olds approaches, and in some cases is lower than the goal, adopted by the World Health Organization, of a global average DMF equal to 3 at 12 years of age by the year 2000 (World Health Organization 1982).

When the individual components of the mean DMF values are examined, whilst the previous findings are confirmed, disparities are apparent when comparing handicapped and normal children. Generally, the amount of decay may be similar or even greater for the normal group, but the handicapped group will have more missing and fewer filled teeth (Maclaurin *et al.* 1985*a*; Jones and Blinkhorn 1986; Nunn and Murray 1987).

Although lacking a formal control group, the study by Mellor and Doyle (1987) is most encouraging in that it demonstrates the reductions in caries prevalence to be gained by a very comprehensive system of dental prevention and treatment, undertaken by the community dental service. Forty-nine 13-year-olds showed a reduction in the mean number of decayed teeth from a value of 3.8 to 0.4 in 4-year period, with a concurrent increase in the restorative provision, an 'F' value of 0.7 in 1977 rising to 3.8 in 1982.

Periodontal disease

Periodontal disease was generally found to be prevalent, and oral hygiene poor, amongst the mentally handicapped, especially if they were institutionalized (Brown 1980; Tesini 1980; Maclaurin *et al.* 1985*a*; Jones and Blinkhorn 1986; Nunn and Murray 1987). Ferguson (1975) found that the age of onset for destructive periodontal disease in ESN(S) children in Newcastle was as low as 10 years for girls and 12 years for boys.

Malocclusion

Even the early study by Rhodes (1884) led to the conclusions that his group of patients had ill-formed maxillae and more than usual overcrowding. He gave detailed measurements for inter-canine widths, which he stated were much narrower than in a normal population.

Gullikson (1969) found that 67 per cent of his study group of 3- to 14-year-olds had a malocclusion, with a greater predominance of Angle's Class III malocclusions than expected in the normal population.

A more recent study, using criteria laid down by the World Health Organization (1971) on dentofacial anomalies, has found that nearly half of the mildly mentally handicapped and two-thirds of the severely mentally handicapped children had a handicapping malocclusion (Nunn and Murray 1987).

Dental health in Down's syndrome

Down's syndrome children

Down's syndrome is a chromosomal disorder with three distinct aberrations: trisomy, translocation, and mosaicism. There are marked physical features, and mental subnormality of varying degree is found in all patients. Approximately 1 in 600 newborns have Down's syndrome, although there is a marked variation with maternal age (Department of Health and Social Security 1976*a*).

Dental caries

From the epidemiological data available to date it would appear that, with few exceptions, dental caries is not as prevalent in children with Down's syndrome as compared with normal children (Brown and Schodel 1976; Nunn 1984), with as many as 50 per cent of Down's syndrome children caries free (Maclaurin *et al.* 1985*b*). The reasons given for this are various, ranging from alterations in tooth eruption and tooth form, to biochemical differences in the saliva of Down's syndrome children (Winer *et al.* 1965; Weyman 1971; Cutress 1971). The study by Orner (1975) of 212 Down's syndrome children and their siblings showed the reduced caries prevalence of Down's syndrome children. The Down's group had only one-third the caries experience of their siblings, although 100 of the Down's syndrome children were institutionalized. This study is particularly useful in that, unlike some others, the comparisons of caries prevalence were matched for stage of tooth eruption rather than just by the children's chronological ages. This meant that each group was at a comparable risk to disease.

Periodontal disease

Periodontal disease tends to be more prevalent in children with Down's syndrome. Much of the periodontal problem found in children with Down's syndrome is localized to the lower incisor region initially, and many studies report worse oral hygiene, bone loss, acute ulcerative gingivitis, gross calculus, and evidence of tooth loss confined to this segment, in young Down's syndrome populations (Cohen *et al.* 1960; Johnson *et al.* 1960; Brown and Cunningham 1961; Cohen *et al.* 1961; McMillan and Kashgarian 1961; Johnson and Young 1963; Harvey-Brown 1965).

Twelve- to 14-year-old children with mobile lower incisors, and 15- to 17-year-olds with missing lower incisors were not uncommon in the Johnson and Young (1963) study. In the Gullikson (1973) group of Down's syndrome children, twice as many had gingivitis compared with 'retarded' controls, and 50 per cent of the Down's syndrome children had missing teeth, compared with 9.8 per cent of the retarded group. In the study by Maclaurin *et al.* (1985*b*), double the proportion of Down's syndrome children required further assessment with a view to complex periodontal treatment than did other mentally handicapped children; a fraction which in turn was higher than for normal children. The authors felt that the increased prevalence of periodontal problems may be a function of immunodeficiency in Down's syndrome, and related to the congenital disorder rather than directly to the oral hygiene. This seems a likely explanation although Nunn (1984) found that poor gingival conditions were almost equally prevalent between Down's syndrome and other mentally handicapped children, 61 per cent and 53 per cent respectively.

Malocclusion

One of the more striking features of the facies of children with Down's syndrome is the relative under-development of the middle third of the face, and the consequent tendency to a Class III skeletal base relationship. A high vaulted palate is a common finding along with other intra-oral anomalies (Parkin *et al.* 1970; McIver and Machen 1979). Many researchers cite a tendency to an Angle's Class III malocclusion in Down's syndrome subjects, together with a posterior cross-bite (Brown and Cunningham 1961; Cohen and Winer 1965; Gullikson 1973).

Physical handicap

The main physical handicaps of particular concern to dentists are those of cerebral palsy, spina bifida, and muscular dystrophy, together with a range of other orthopaedic disabilities. However, not all these children will have so severe a defect that they merit special dental care.

Cerebral palsy

This is defined as a disorder of movement and posture resulting from a non-progressive lesion of the brain stem. There are five distinct types, with mental handicap superimposed on approximately three-quarters of the group (Capute 1974; Gurling *et al.* 1977; Rumble 1980). The prevalence of cerebral palsy is of the order of one to two per thousand children of school age. Manifestation of the disability varies enormously, from the quadraplegic child with sensory and intellectual impairments to the monoplegic with a barely discernible disability.

Dental health in cerebral palsy

Dental caries

Most researchers have found that, as with other groups, although the DMF values were not significantly different, the 'M' component was the highest and the 'F' the lowest (Kanar 1979).

A later study also found that restorative care was minimal for a group of 92 cerebral palsied children, and the amount of active deciduous decay was very high, a 'd' value of 4.1 or a 'df' value of 4.6 for 5-year-olds compared with 1.1 and 1.6 respectively for 5-year-olds a year later in the 1983 National Survey of Child Dental Health, using the same criteria (Nunn 1984; Todd and Dodd 1985).

Periodontal disease

Values for gingivitis and oral hygiene indices have been found to be similar for the cerebral palsied and normal controls in spite of the difficulties sometimes experienced by the palsied in performing the necessary oral hygiene measures (Fishman *et al.* 1967). Even without constant parental back-up, it has been shown (Melville *et al.* 1981) that, through weekly visits to special schools by dental therapists, improvements in poor oral hygiene and gingival conditions could be made, despite the difficulties some of the more severely handicapped children had in effectively cleaning their teeth. By contrast, other authors have found periodontal disease and oral hygiene to be worse in children with cerebral palsy largely, it is assumed, because of the difficulties imposed by the motor defects (Leonard 1950; Kanar 1979). Indeed it was found that in a group of 92 children with cerebral palsy (Nunn 1984), 50 per cent had poor oral hygiene and 53 per cent had poor gingival health, using the Good, Fair, Poor index of James *et al.* (1960).

Malocclusion

Given the varying abnormal degrees of muscle tonicity, and the involuntary movements of structures influencing the dental arches, not unexpectedly, cerebral palsied children are found to have a high prevalence of malocclusions (Leeds 1976; Kanar 1979; Strodel 1987). In the spastic cerebral palsied, hypertonic facial muscles and a tongue thrust predispose to a Class II division 2 type of malocclusion, often with a cross-bite and crowding, due to the constriction of the dental arches. The athetoid type suffer hypotonicity of the orbicularis oris muscle coupled again with tongue protrusion, tending therefore towards an Angle's Class II division 1 type of malocclusion in 90 per cent of cases, often with an anterior open bite. The ataxic type present with a variety of malocclusions (Koster 1956; Kastein 1957). No such data are available for the remaining two types of cerebral palsy.

Foster *et al.* (1974), also using cephalometry and matched controls, investigated the effects of cerebral palsy in 33 patients with varying severity of the defect; they concluded that the cerebral palsy did affect the size and form both of the jaws and skull, but that the severity of the defect and the age at which the lesion occurred were important variables in determining the effect. Stratifying groups according to these variables was vital if such differences were not to be masked in a large group.

Spina bifida

In spina bifida, there is a defective fusion of one or more posterior vertebral arches, with or without protrusion of some or all of the contents of the spinal canal. It is estimated that in 50–60 per cent of cases the condition is inherited, but that environmental agents may be responsible for the remainder. Unlike most other malformations, it is commoner in the female. Hydrocephalus may be present in 95 per cent of cases. One-quarter of patients with associated hydrocephalus suffer from epilepsy, and between 30–40 per cent may have impaired intelligence (Stark 1977). Spina bifida along with other CNS defects is the most frequent congenital malformation found in this country, with a prevalence of 2.5 per 1000 total births.

Dental caries

In a small subgroup of a larger sample of handicapped children (Nunn 1984), it was found that relative to the group as a whole, caries experience in the 53 children with spina bifida was lower, a dmf of 1.8 for the spina bifida group of 6–9-year-olds compared to 2.74 for a similar age range of handicapped children. In the permanent dentition, this picture was repeated with a DMF of 1.6 for 10–14-year-old spina bifida children, and 2.35 for other handicapped children of the same age. However, for children with spina bifida the ratios of decayed, missing and filled teeth were more unfavourable compared with the handicap group as a whole; 31, 25, and 43 per cent compared with 28, 20, and 52 per cent, respectively.

Periodontal disease

The oral hygiene status of children with spina bifida in one study of 53 children (Nunn 1984) was worse than that of other handicapped children, and more children with spina bifida had poor gingival health than did handicapped children generally; 59 per cent and 44 per cent, respectively. These figures highlight the danger of combining data for handicapped children as this practice often masks the range of disease values found in subgroups.

Malocclusion

No published studies are available on the occlusion of children with spina bifida.

Muscular dystrophy

This is a group of inherited diseases characterized by weakness and degeneration of affected muscles. Males are exclusively affected in the Duchenne type. Facial musculature is always affected in the fascio-scapulo-humeral type, rarely in other forms (Walton and Nattrass 1954). Walton and Nattrass (1954) quoted a prevalence of four per 100 000 children for two areas in the northern region of England. There is scant information on the dental health of these children; little difference from normal in the prevalence of caries experiences and periodontal disease has been found (White and Sackler 1954; Henderson 1968). Other authors have found an increased prevalence of malocclusions due to abnormalities of orofacial musculature (Cohen 1975; Cohen and Feldman 1978).

Medical handicap

Children with a medical handicap fall into two groups: first, those whose general health may be further jeopardized if they were to develop dental disease; and second, those in whom the need for dental care in itself constitutes a risk (Hobson 1980). The dental effects which have been found to be specific to particular medical conditions are summarized in Table 13.1. There is however, very little published information on the oral health in medically handicapped children and, for many of these conditions, it remains difficult to separate out the effects of treatment from those of the condition itself, leukaemia being a classic example.

The need for prevention of dental disease in special groups

Background

In spite of the accumulated evidence on the lack of treatment and consequent poor dental health of many handicapped children, which has been detailed in the preceding pages, little has been done through official channels actively to bring about a change in this state of affairs.

Early reports, both specific to handicap (Department of Health and Social Security 1971; HMSO 1978*a*; 1980) and general to dental health (Department of Health and Social Security 1976*a*,*b*; 1977*a*,*b*) make, if at all, only fleeting reference to preventive dentistry and handicapped groups in the population. The Royal Commission on the National Health Service (Department of Health and Social Security 1979*b*) reiterated much of what the Court Report (HMSO 1976) said with respect to dentistry in general, but neither the former Enquiry or the Government's immediate response to it, *Patients First* (Department of Health and Social Security 1979*a*), said anything about dentistry and the handicapped. A follow-up, Handbook on Policies and Priorities (Department of Health and Social Security 1981) merely states that services for the handicapped were poor, without being more specific.

Publication of the Dental Strategy Review Group's Report *Towards Better Dental Health* (HMSO 1981) saw not only the highlighting of the inadequate care for special and priority groups, but also suggestions, like discretionary payments

Table 13.1. Dental disease in medically handicapped children

Condition (authors)	Prevalence	No. and age (yrs.)	Caries	Periodontal disease	Orthodontics	Other
Asthma	22 in 1000					
(Wotman *et al.* 1973)		25, 10–15	—	100% with calculus	—	Clinical examination and saliva samples
		25 controls	—	43% with calculus	—	
(Hyppa and Paunio 1979)		15, 10–11 30 controls	DMFS 6.9 DMFS 8.6	53% with calculus 60% with calculus	— —	Increase in lactobacilli counts in asthmatics due to steroid inhalation
(Attrill and Hobson 1984)		30, 5 m–17	DMFT 3.3	Segments with plaque: 3.0	—	
		30 minor orthopaedic conditions (0)	DMFT 5.2	Segments with gingivitis: 1.2 plaque: 2.7 gingivitis: 0.9 (0)		
Cystic fibrosis (CF)	1 in 2000					
(Swallow *et al.* 1967)		63, 11	♂ DMFT 0 ♀ 1.8	3% with gingivitis 9.5% with calculus	—	Saliva samples. 1.5% with hypoplasia 36.5% with discoloured teeth
		1500 physically handicapped	♂ 3.5 ♀ 3.8	—	—	
(Brooks *et al.* 1970)		52, $2\frac{1}{2}$–$8\frac{1}{2}$	defs 2.9 DMFS 3.3	—	—	Clinical examination and full mouth x-rays
		sibling controls	defs 6.8 DMFS 6.4			
(Wotman *et al.* 1973)		25, 10–15	—	90% with calculus	—	Clinical examination and saliva samples
		25 control	—	43% with calculus	—	
(Jagels and Sweeney 1976)		21, 10–12	deft 2.57 DMFT 2.52	OH* score = 1.5; 10% cystic fibrosis	**Cl. I 82% CF 76% sibs Cl. II div. 1 15% CF 18% sibs	5% with hypoplasia
		19 siblings, 10–12	deft 2.42 DMFT 4.26	22% siblings	Cl. II div. 2. 4% CF 3% sibs Cl. III 0% CF 3% sibs	1% siblings with hypoplasia

(Blackharsh 1977)		42, 4–25	—	30 with mild gingivitis; 26 with mild plaque	—	30% with stains of clinical crown; no specific agent identified
		10 sibling controls	—	4 with mild gingivitis; 2 with mild plaque	—	
(Primosch 1980)		39, 16–19	DMFS 11.54	—	—	24% with discoloured teeth
		Controls	DMFS 15.92	—	—	42.7% with enamel defects
(Attrill and Hobson 1984)		30, 5 m–17	dmft/DMFT 3.5	Segments with plaque: 3.6 Segments with gingivitis: 1.8	—	—
		30 minor orthopaedic	dmft/DMFT 5.2	plaque: 2.7 gingivitis: 0.9		
(Kinirons 1985)		118 children				
		mean age 3.45 n = 42	dmf 0.5	21% with calculus	—	Salivary pH 6.89 (resting);
		mean age 8.15 n = 35	DMF 1.54	69 mild gingivitis	—	buffering capacity of
		mean age 12.22 n = 39	DMF 3.07	63 mild plaque	—	stimulated saliva, 1.5 ml
		85 siblings				
		mean age 3.02 n = 30	dmf 1.7	5% with calculus	—	Salivary pH 6.79
		mean age 8.38 n = 26	DMF 2.04	32 mild gingivitis	—	Buffering capacity of
		mean age 12.61 n = 26	DMF 5.38	26 mild plaque	—	stimulated saliva, 1.34 ml
(Mahaney 1986)		50 females mean age 12.38	—	—	—	Dental age 0.84 years behind chronological age
		50 control females	—	—	—	Dental age 0.04 years behind chronological age
Epilepsy (EP)	5–10 in 1000					
(Gingis *et al.* 1980)		46 (mean age 28) mentally retarded	—	Gingival overgrowth related to serum phenytoin levels	—	Abnormally short roots not related to high serum phenytoin
		45 mentally retarded	—	—	—	

Table 13.1. *continued*

Condition (authors)	Preval- ence	No. and age (yrs.)	Caries	Periodontal disease	Orthodontics	Other
(Lundstrom *et al.* 1982)				Plaque frequency per individual	Increase probing plaque depth (⩾0.75 mm) †GU	
		21, 9–17 (I) carbamalzepine	(I) DFS 5.7	60%	8.7	
		10, 8–17 (II) phenytoin	(II) DFS 8.0	41%	24.7	
		19, 7–22 (III) previous phenytoin	(III) DFS 13.2	58%	15.6	
		15, 8–14 (IV) epileptic, no medication	(IV) DFS 4.7	42%	7.8	
(Robinson *et al.* 1983)		229 medicated children 144 controls (c)	—	Gingival hyperplasia in 40% epileptics	—	Premolar volume 0.47 mm (Ep) 0.56 mm (c) Intercuspal width reduced in early-onset epileptics. Delayed shedding and eruption of teeth? due pseudohypopara-thyroidism effect of anti-convulsants
(Modeer *et al.* 1986)		30 phenytoin-treated	DFS 5.5	Visible plaque index (VPI): 42.8% Gingival bleeding index (GBI): 15.1% Increased probing depth (IPD) >4 mm: 8.9%	—	Lysozyme activity in saliva increased significantly in phenytoin group
		25 other anti-convulsants	DFS 6.3	VPI: 48.5% GBI: 10.6% IPD: 1.9%		
Cardiac disease (Kaner *et al.* 1946)	6–8 in 1000		Increase in carious lesions	Cyanotic soft tissues	Anterior open bite in some patients	Delayed eruption; dilation and engorgement of pulp vessels

(Gould and Picton 1960)		30 with cyanosis 30 without cyanosis	—	23% normal gums 43% overall redness 33% deep maroon 6% controls with overall redness Pocketing: 8% cyanotics >2 mm 3% controls >2 mm Oral hygiene: Good—14% cyanotics 24% controls Bad—5% cyanotics 3% controls	Cyanotics: Cl. III 5 Controls: Cl. III 2	
(Hakala 1967)		65 cyanotics, 6.1	dmf 2.7 (deciduous molars)	Marginal gingivitis (MG): 45.4% patients; calculus (Cal): 26.8%	Cl. I 92.4% II 1.8% III 1.8%	Enamel hypoplasia: 16.9%
		180 acyanotics, 6.9	dmf 3.1	MG 2.1% Cal 3.1%	Cl. I 90.1% II 6.2% III 1.0%	Enamel hypoplasia: 10.0%
		177 control hospital in-patients, 6.5	dmf 3.8	MG 2.5% Cal 4.0%	Cl. I 88.4% II 7.9% III 5.2%	Enamel hypoplasia: 5.2%
Diabetes (D)	1 in 1600					
(Sheppard 1936)		10, 10–19	—	80% minimal bone resorption 20% complete bone resorption	—	Full mouth radiographs. Disease controlled by insulin and diet
(Rutledge 1940)		20, 8–19	3 caries-free, 11 'lower than expected caries'	16, gums of normal colour 10, evidence of bony changes	—	Life caries index (Bodecker)
(Wegner 1971)		312, 10–18 388 matched controls	DMFT 12.6 DMFT 9.2	— —	— —	Included incipient lesions
(Matsson and Koch 1975)		33, 9–16	DFS 13.4	—	—	Children treated by diet and insulin
		Matched controls	DFS 20.5			

Table 13.1. *continued*

Condition (authors)	Prevalence	No. and age (yrs.)	Caries	Periodontal disease	Orthodontics	Other
(Wegner 1975)		13–15	DMFT 1.88	—	—	For diabetics diagnosed after 6 yrs of age
		Controls	DMFT 5.51			
(Faulconbridge *et al.* 1981)		94, 5–15	Males: 16% with caries Females: 19% with caries	Males PLQ†† = 0.57 Females PLQ = 0.55	—	Bay and Ainamo's Qualitative Index PLQ (1974)
		Matched controls (c)	Males: 16% with caries Females: 17% with caries	Males PLQ = 0.42 Females PLQ = 0.28	—	
(Goteiner *et al.* 1986)		169, mean 11.3 80 controls, mean 12.0	def/DMF 4.53 def/DMF 4.46	§GI: 1.39 (D) 1.34 (C) ‖PDI: 0.01 (D) 0.03 (C)	—	Children with family history of diabetes have lower caries prevalence
Blind/partial sighted	3 in 10 000					
(Greeley *et al.* 1976)		20, 11–16	DMFT 4.8	¶PHM–M 32.7	Cl. I 55% Cl. II 21% Cl. III 5%	23% with unrepaired fractured incisors
		44, 11–16 Partially sighted	DMFT 3.9	PHM–M 33.9	—	
(Anaise 1979)		434, 14–17	—	‡PI: 0.90 Debris: 1.86	—	
		460 sighted controls		PI: 0.23 Debris: 1.08		

* OH = Oral hygiene. ** Cl. = Class in Angle's classification. † GU = gingival units. †† PLQ = Stained plaque index. § GI = Gingival index. ‖ PDI = periodontal disease index.
¶ PHM–M = modified personal hygiene performance index. ‡ PI = periodontal index.

to general dental practitioners who treated handicapped individuals, for overcoming this problem. A few years later, a Scottish group (Scottish Home and Health Department 1984), addressing itself specifically to the subject of dentistry for the handicapped, came up with specific proposals for remedying the identified shortfall in care.

Reasons for inadequate dental care

There would appear therefore to be acknowledgement, recently at least, that dental care provision for special groups in the community is poor. Why this is so seems to arise from a number of factors, singly or in combination. Dentistry is largely a demand-led service relying on sufficient motivation on the part of potential recipients to seek out such care. Not surprisingly then, handicapped groups in many instances have lost out. Other factors have been, and to an extent still are, the attitudes of both provider and patient, as well as dental education, and finance.

Many dentists have unfounded fears about providing dental care for handicapped people, which culminate in negative attitudes in this sphere of their work (Gurney and Alcorn 1979). Many parents and guardians have low expectations of dentistry which, when coupled with the often overwhelming, competing needs of their handicapped child, result in only emergency attendances for dental treatment. In the past, very little attention, either didactic or practical, has been given to the topic of dentistry for handicapped people in undergraduate or even postgraduate education. This meant that dental practitioners with a plentiful supply of work on normal patients were able to ignore the special groups. In addition, many dentists feel that providing such care is inadequately reimbursed and that such patients should be treated under the auspices of the salaried services, either community or hospital. The advent of fees on the general dental services fee scale (with prior approval) for the application of topical fluorides and fissure sealants in those with special needs, may now go some way towards fostering a positive and preventive attitude on the part of practitioners to the care of these groups.

Whilst dental care is free for children and young adults in full-time education, as well as for those in receipt of certain state benefits, parents and guardians may incur other expenses, like loss of time from work and in travel, which make dentistry less accessible.

Need for special dental care

There is some evidence that provision of dental treatment may markedly alter the habits and appearance of handicapped children (Adelson, 1965; Ohmori *et al.* 1981), but there is general agreement that this on its own is not enough. The need for good quality dental services in such special groups is necessary for many reasons but two in particular are of prime importance. First, for a number of handicapped children, the need for dental treatment may impose a further handicap and secondly, the medical condition of some children is such that dental disease could be fatal (Hobson 1980; HMSO 1981).

Need for prevention

In a memorandum submitted to the Royal Commission on the National Health Service, the British Dental Association (1977) stated that *prevention* of dental disease for handicapped patients was of vital importance and should receive absolute priority. Following on this, others (Anderson 1978; Holloway and Downer 1979; Richardson *et al.* 1981) have made the point that such preventive measures are justified for special groups although they may not be cost-effective for the population as a whole. Yet others have emphasized this point by stating that there is a case for the dental care of handicapped children to be at least as good (HMSO 1981), if not better (Franks 1969), than that given to ordinary children.

This must be especially so in the light of such specific problem areas, common to many with disabilities, of, for example, the need to take medication long-term. Such therapy is often given in a syrup vehicle, with disastrous consequences for the dentition (Roberts and Roberts 1979; Hobson and Fuller 1987), although strenuous efforts are now being made by both the dental profession and the pharmaceutical industry to overcome this.

Preventive programmes

With this and other such difficulties in mind, a number of authors have stressed the importance of a vigorous approach to prevention, including fluoride supplements, dietary advice and oral hygiene instruction, and the importance of regular professional dental care (Franks and Winter 1974; Evans and Aledort 1978; Hall 1980; Goodman 1981; Pool 1981; Cooley and Sobel 1982; Pool 1982). However, Swallow and Swallow (1980) emphasize that prevention is not just up to the patient and/or parent but has to be the responsibility of the dentist.

Aside from the one-to-one relationship, other studies have documented the setting up and the success of programmes for groups of handicapped individuals, ranging from oral hygiene programmes (Bensberg *et al.* 1966; Melville *et al.* 1981; Fenton *et al.* 1982) to preventive programmes involving the application of agents topically (Nagel *et al.* 1971; Tarver 1976; Hobson and Slattery 1984). Others allude to the potential spin-offs, as, for example, in the prevalence study by Jones and Blinkhorn (1986) of children at special schools in Glasgow. This study highlighted again the lower prevalence of dental caries relative to a control group, attributing the difference to the publicity given to fluoride supplements for handicapped children. However, in that study, only eight out of 34 special schools distributed fluoride supplements and, of those 34 schools, only 10 had organized brushing programmes.

Fluoride supplements for handicapped children have been dealt with only briefly. Nowak (1976) suggested that for such groups a different dosage schedule should be adopted, higher than now generally accepted (Dowell and Joyston-Bechall, 1981), to compensate for the lack of fluoride intake from food and liquid sources by handicapped children. This is not dissimilar to the regimen described by Geddes *et al.* (1973). Dowell and Joyston-Bechall (1981) and Murray and Rugg-Gunn (1982), discussing fluoride supplement dosages, comment only that these may need to be altered for special groups.

A small number of texts, whilst supposedly addressing themselves to the topic of prevention for the handicapped, on the whole only discuss standard, accepted preventive techniques as used for non-handicapped groups in the population (Nowak 1976; Plotnick 1975; Hargreaves 1976). However, there are a number of locally based studies that give results, in terms of improvements in dental health, for special groups of children and young adults as a result of preventive dental programmes. Other studies, with more detailed results are given in Table 13.2. For some of the programmes (Brown 1975; Tarver 1976) it is difficult to separate out the benefits to be gained from treatment and preventive efforts in terms of improvements in dental health. An additional problem encountered with some preventive schemes for special groups is that of using retrospective controls in a time of changing caries prevalence (Stephen and MacFadyen 1977). In addition, there are many District Health Authorities who run intensive programmes for handicapped children but as yet details of their work remain unpublished.

Conclusions

Whatever the benefits to be gained from dental treatment *per se*, there will be a sizeable proportion of children with handicaps who, for example, will not or cannot tolerate dental treatment or for whom the provision of a prosthesis following the loss of the natural dentition is not feasible.

Svatun and Heloe (1975) found that 18 out of 29 handicapped patients in their study were unable to wear full dentures, emphasizing the importance of primary prevention. Allied to this, Mitchell *et al.* (1985) stressed the importance of preventive dentistry following conservation under general anaesthesia, so that the future approach might be a preventive rather than an invasive one.

Although it had no remit to address itself to the specific aspects of dental care for special groups, the UK Government's White Paper on *Primary Health Care* (HMSO 1987) inevitably encompasses this aspect, albeit indirectly. Its endorsement of a capitation system of payment in the general dental services for children, consequent on a successful outcome to the experimental period, should go some way towards enabling special groups of children to obtain the therapeutic and preventive services that they require.

The change of emphasis to a health promotional role for the community dental service should also foster a more preventive approach that would benefit these groups of children in particular.

Table 13.2. Preventive programmes for handicapped children

Study	Condition	Programme	Oral health: Dental caries	Periodontal disease	Other
Boyd (1943)	111 diabetic children, 14 m–14 yrs.	Controlled diet only	0.71 DMFS over 47 m	—	—
Ripa and Cole (1970)	91 severely mentally retarded, 5–10 yrs	Cyanoacrylate fissure sealant applied under rubber dam, with body restraints, to 278 Ds, Es, 6s	84.3% reduction in caries in permanent teeth (5 became carious, 32 in control teeth)	—	At 12 m one-third teeth sealed, one-third partly sealed, one-third lost all sealant; 63 teeth had some evidence of caries initially
Brown (1975)	53 children 7–18½ yrs, with variety of handicaps	Routine dental care plus home care to include fluoride supplements, diet control, oral hygiene measures, topical fluorides	DMFT increment over 18 m in 8–10-yr-olds = 0.6 (1.9 in normal controls)	Increments for 7–11-yr-olds over 18 m: debris: 12 → 6.5 calculus: 0.8 → 0.7 gingivitis: no change pocketing: 4 → 3 segments involved	Maintenance required less than half the time and one-third of the cost of the initial restorative programme
Richardson *et al.* (1977)	160 retarded children, 5–21-yrs-old; IQ 30–80	UV-polymerized fissure sealant, half-mouth controls, 812 1° + 2° molars		—	2-yr results: 40% retained on primary teeth; 61% retained on permanent teeth
Stephen and MacFadyen (1977)	57 cleft palate children, 3–5 yrs, 34 cleft palate children (retrospective control)	Dietary and oral hygiene advice, fluoride therapy and fissure sealing (Nuva-Seal)	defs after 3 yrs: 1.44 test 13.5 control Caries free: 74% test 0% control	—	Total costs: prevention for test group: £438; treatment for control group £426–£490. (Treatment 65%–90% more costly than prevention)
Dowell and Teasdale (1978)	Medical handicap 4 yrs 8 m	Health visitor and dental officer visits to home, fluoride tablets, OHI*. Surgery visits/4–6 m; topical fluorides and OHI.	80% caries-free; dmf 0.6	—	—
Loesche (1981)	Trisomy-21 and non-trisomy 21 children	Suspension of OH procedures and 5% Kanamycin (K) 3 × day or placebo (P) applied over 5 days at 5-wk intervals	—	Plaque weight (as % of initial value) K: 48% P: 114%, after 10 wks. Gingivitis (as % of initial value): K 87% P 106%, after 10 wks	Systemic metronidazole may also be useful for treatment of periodontitis

Richardson *et al.* (1981)	103 mentally retarded children (IQ 30–80); 5–21 yrs; 64% male	5-yr follow-up of UV polymerized fissure-sealant resin (half-mouth controls)	Less than 50% of the decay in test teeth compared with controls		
Atrill and Hobson (1984)	30 asthmatics (A), 30 cystic fibrosis (CF) 5–16 yrs 9 m 30 orthopaedic (O) controls	Dental treatment, OHI, fluoride tablets.	1st visit / 2nd visit d + D 1.5 (A) 0.4 1.7 (CF) 0.6 2.6 (O) — f + F 1.1 (A) 1.9 1.2 (CF) 2.4 1.5 (O) —	1st visit / 2nd visit plaque (segments) 3.0 1.3 3.6 1.3 2.7 — gingivitis (segments) 1.2 0.6 1.8 0.4 0.9 —	Fluoride tablet uptake continuing for 90.4% (28) children at 2nd visit. Uptake of care: 77% asthmatics; 87% cystic fibrosis by 2nd visit
Mellor and Doyle (1987)	Special schools children (1977) n = 106, 14 yrs (1982) n = 49, 14.3 yrs	Home visits, fluoride tablets, school brushing, comprehensive dental treatment	1977 1982 D 3.8 0.4 M 1.4 0.8 F 0.7 3.8 similar in 1982 to other Rochdale children	—	Uptake of treatment in community dental service: 1978 80% 1982 79% **GA requirements for ESN(S) children: 1977 34.8% 1982 7.0%
Schwarz and Vigild (1987)	329 mentally retarded, 6–9-yr-olds (resident and non-residents)	Community and personal preventive measures quarterly, bimonthly or not available, plus comprehensive dental care	40% caries-free (i) Non-residents had 25% more caries than normal individuals of same age (ii) 40% 13–19-yr-olds DMFS > 8 with preventive programme; 60% DMFS > 8 without preventive programme	(Non-residents) severe gingivitis: Supervised tooth-brushing 12% Unsupervised tooth-brushing 28%	

* OHI = oral hygiene instruction.
** GA = general anaesthesia.

References

Adelson, J.J. (1965). The effects of dental treatment on the behaviour of handicapped patients. *J. Am. dent. Ass.* **71**, 1411–15.

Anaise, J.Z. (1979). Periodontal disease and oral hygiene in a group of blind and sighted Israeli teenagers (14–17 years). *Commun. Dent. oral Epidemiol.* **7**, 353–6.

Anderson, R.J. (1978). Preventive dental care—do we need it and can we afford it? *Br. Ass. Study commun. Dent. Newsletter*. No. 18, 6–16.

Attrill, M. and Hobson, P. (1984). The organisation of dental care for groups of medically handicapped children. *Commun. dent. Hlth.* **1**, 21–7.

Beck, J.D. and Hunt, R.J. (1985). Oral health status in the United States: problems of special patients. *J. dent. Educ.* **49**, 407–26.

Bensberg, G.J., Barnett, D.D., and Menius, J.A. (1966). A survey: dental services in state residential facilities. *Ment. Retard.* **4**, 8–13.

Blackharsh, C. (1977). Dental aspects of patients with cystic fibrosis: A preliminary clinical study. *J. Am. dent. Ass.* **95**, 106–10.

Boyd, J.D. (1943). Long term prevention of tooth decay among diabetic children. *Am. J. Dis. Child.* **66**, 349–61.

British Dental Association. (1977). Editorial—Memorandum to the Royal Commission on the National Health Service. *Br. dent. J.* **142**, 53–63.

Broadhead, G.D. (1972) Social class factors in special education. *J. biosoc. Sci.* **4**, 315–24.

Brooks, H.T., Zacherl, W.A., and Rule, T.T. (1970). Caries prevalence in children with cystic fibrosis. IADR. Abstr. No. 338 North American Division.

Brown, J.P. (1975). Dental treatment for handicapped patients. (1) The efficacy of a preventive programme for children. (2) The economics of dental treatment—a cost benefit analysis. *Australia dent. J.* **20**, 316–25.

Brown, J.P. and Schodel, D.R. (1976). A review of controlled surveys of dental disease in handicapped persons. *J. Dent. Child.* **43**, 313–20.

Brown, J.P. (1980). The efficacy and economy of comprehensive dental care for handicapped children. *Int. dent. J.* **30**, 14–27.

Brown, R.H. and Cunningham, W.M. (1961). Dental manifestations of mongolism. Oral Surg. **14**, 664–76.

Capute, A.J. (1974). Developmental disabilities: an overview. In: Symposium on Dentistry for the Handicapped. *Dent. Clin. Am.* **18**, 557–77.

The Children's Committee (1980). *Second Annual Report, 1979–1980*. Mary Ward House, London.

Cohen, M.M., Winer, R.A., and Shklar, G. (1960). Periodontal disease in a group of mentally subnormal children. *J. dent. Res.* **39**, 745.

Cohen, M.M., Winer, R.A., Schwartz, S., and Shklar, G (1961). Oral aspects of mongolism. Oral Surg. **14**, 92–107.

Cohen, M.M. and Winer, R.A. (1965). Dental and facial characteristics in Down's syndrome (mongolism). *J. dent. Res.* **44** (supp.), 197–208.

Cohen, M.M. (1975). Congenital, genetic and endocrinologic influences on dental occlusion. *Dent. Clin. N.Am.* **18**, 499–574.

Cohen, M.M. and Feldman, B.S. (1978). *Oral aspects of muscular dystrophy*. Proceedings of the fourth International Association of Dentistry for the Handicapped. London.

Cooley, R.O. and Sobel, R.S. (1982). Dental treatment considerations for the medically compromised child. *Pediatr. Clin. N.Am.* **29**, 613–29.

Cutress, T.W. (1971). Dental caries in trisomy 21. *Archs. oral Biol.* **16**, 1329–44.

Department of Health and Social Security (1971). *Better Services for the Mentally Handicapped*, Cmnd. 4683. HMSO, London.

Department of Health and Social Security (1976*a*). *Prevention and health: everybody's business. A reassessment of public and personal health.* HMSO, London.

Department of Health and Social Security (1976*b*). *Priorities for health and personal social services in England. A consultative document.* HMSO, London.

Department of Health and Social Security (1977*a*). *Prevention and Health*, Cmnd. 7047. HMSO, London.

Department of Health and Social Security (1977*b*). *The Way forward. Priorities in the health and social services.* HMSO, London.

Department of Health and Social Security (1979*a*). *Patients first.* HMSO, London.

Department of Health and Social Security (1979*b*). *Royal Commision of Enquiry into the National Health Service*, Cmnd 7615. HMSO, London.

Department of Health and Social Security (1981) *Care in action. A handbook of policies and priorities for the health and personal social services in England.* HMSO, London.

Dowell, T.B. and Joyston Bechall, S. (1981). Fluoride supplements—age related dosages. *Br. dent. J.* **150**, 273–5.

Dowell. T.B. and Teasdale, J. (1978). A preventive scheme for infants. *Br. dent. J.* **144**, 117–18.

Drillen, C.M., Jameson, S., and Wilkinson, E.M. (1966). Studies in mental handicap. Part 1—prevalence and distribution by clinical type and severity of defect. *Archs. Dis. Child.* **41**, 528–38.

Evans, B.E. and Aledort, L.M. (1978). Haemophilia and dental treatment. *J. Am. dent. Ass.* **96**, 827–32.

Ewalt, J.R. (1972). Classification of mental retardation. *Am. J. Psychiatr.* 128 (supp.), 18–20.

Faulconbridge, A.R., Bradshaw, W.C.L., Jenkins, P.A., and Baum, J.D. (1981). Dental status of a group of diabetic children. *Br. dent. J.* **151**, 253–5.

Fenton, S.J., DeBiase, C., and Portugal, B.V. (1982). A strategy for implementing a dental health education program for state facilities with limited resources. *Rehab. Lit.* **43**, 290–3.

Ferguson, M. (1975). Dental condition of handicapped children. A thesis submitted for the Diploma in Dental Public Health. Royal College of Surgeons of England.

Fishman, S.R., Young, W.O., Haley, J.B., and Sword, C. (1967). The status of oral health in cerebral palsied children and their siblings. *J. Dent. Child.* **34**, 219–27.

Fitzimmons, J.S. (1982). *The provision of regional genetic services in the United Kingdom.* 19 March. Times Health Supp, London.

Forrest, A., Ritson, B., and Zealley, A. (1973). *New Perspectives in Mental Handicap.* Churchill Livingstone, Edinburgh.

Forsberg, H., Quick-Nilsson, I., Gustavson, K.H., and Jagell, S. (1985). Dental health and dental care in severely mentally retarded children (SMR). *Swed. dent. J.* **9**, 15–28.

Foster, T.D., Griffiths, M.I., and Gordon, P.H. (1974). The effect of cerebral palsy on the size of the skull. *Am. J. Orthodont.* **66**, 40–9.

Franks, A.S.T. (1969). Dental care for patients with chronic disease and disability. *Br. dent. J.* **126**, 189.

Franks, A.S.T. and Winter, G.B. (1974). Management of the handicapped and chronic sick in the dental practice (2). *Br. dent. J.* **136**, 62–7.

Geddes, D.A.M., Jenkins, G.N., and Stephen, K.W. (1973). The use of fluoride in caries prevention. *Br. dent. J.* **134**, 426–9.

Gingis, S.S., Staple, P.H., Miller, W.A., Sedransk, N., and Thompson, T. (1980). Dental root abnormalities and gingival overgrowth in epileptic patients receiving anti-convulsant therapy. *J. Perio.* **51**, 474–82.

Goodman, J.R. (1981). Dental treatment of children with congenital heart disease. *Proc. Br. paedodont. Soc.* **11**, 15–17.

Goteiner D., Vogel, R., Deasy, M., and Goteiner, C. (1986). Periodontal and caries experience in children with insulin-dependant diabetes mellitus. *J. Am. dent. Assoc.* **113**, 277–9.

Gould, M.S.E. and Picton, D.C.A. (1960). The gingival condition of congenitally cyanotic individuals. *Br. dent. J.* **109**, 96–100.

Greeley, C.B., Goldstein, P.A., and Forrester, D.J. (1976). Oral manifestations in a group of blind students. *J. Dent. Child.* **43**, 39–41.

Gullikson, J.S. (1969). Oral findings of mentally retarded children. *J. Dent. Child.* **34**, 59–64.

Gullikson, J.S. (1973). Oral findings in children with Down's syndrome. *J. Dent. Child.* **40**, 293–5.

Gurling, F.G., Fanning E.A., and Leppard, P.I. (1977). The handicapped child population in South Australia in 1975. *Australia dent. J.* **22**, 107–12.

Gurney, N.L. and Alcorn, B.C. (1979). The concept of attitudes. In *Dentistry for the Handicapped Patient*, Postgraduate dental handbook series. 5 (ed. K.E. Wessels), pp. 1–19. John Wright PSG Inc., Boston.

Hakala, P.E. (1967). Dental and oral changes in congenital heart disease. *Suom. Hammaslaak. Toim.* **63**, 284–324.

Hall, R.K. (1980). Oral and dental changes and management of children with cardiac disease. *J. int. Ass. Dent. Child.* **11**, 19–29.

Harding, T.W. (1980). *The role of a constructional furniture system in special schools.* Handicapped Persons Research Unit, Newcastle-upon-Tyne Polytechnic.

Hargreaves, J.A. (1976). Preventive dentistry for handicapped children. *J. Dent.* **42**, 352–3.

Harris, A.I., Cox, E., and Smith, C.R.W. (1971). *Handicapped and impaired in Great Britain.* HMSO, London.

Harvey-Brown, R. (1965). Dental treatment of the mongoloid child. *J. Dent. Child.* **32**, 73–81.

Henderson, P. (1968). Changing patterns of disease and disability in school children in England and Wales. *Br. med. J.* **2**, 259–63.

Henry, J.L. and Sinkford, J.C. (1972). Community dental care for developmentally disabled children. *J. Am. Coll. Dent.* **39**, 184–7.

HMSO (1976). *Fit for the future.* The Report of the Committee on Child Health Services, Vol. 1., Cmnd. 6684. London.

HMSO (1978*a*). *Development team for the mentally handicapped, first report, 1976–1977.* London.

HMSO (1978*b*). *Special educational Needs*, Report of the Committee of Enquiry into Education of Handicapped Children and Young People. London.

HMSO (1980). *Development team for the mentally handicapped, second report, 1978–1979.* London.

HMSO (1981). *Towards better dental health*, Report of the Dental Strategy Review Group. London.

HMSO (1987). *The promotion of health*, White paper on Primary Health Care. London.
Hobson, P. (1980). The treatment of medically handicapped children. *Int. dent. J.* **30**, 6–13.
Hobson, P. and Slattery, G.R. (1984). Treatment needs of medically handicapped children in the North District of Manchester. *Commun. dent. Hlth.* **1**, 173–80.
Hobson, P. and Fuller, S. (1987). Sugar based medicines and dental disease—progress report. *Commun. dent. Hlth.* **4**, 169–76.
Holloway, P.J. and Downer, M.C. (1979). The benefit of preventive procedures for high risk groups. *Int. dent. J.* **29**, 118–24.
Hyppa, J. and Paunio, K. (1979). Oral health and salivary factors in children with asthma. *Proc. Finn. dent. Soc.* **75**, 7–10.
Jagels, A.E. and Sweeney, E.A. (1976). Oral health of patients with cystic fibrosis and their siblings. *J. dent. Res.* **55**, 991–6.
James, P.M.C., Jackson, D., Slack, G.L., and Lawton, F.E. (1960). Gingival health and dental cleanliness in English school children. *Archs. oral Biol.* **3**, 57–66.
Johnson, N.P., Young, M.A., and Gallios, J.A. (1960). Dental caries experience of mongoloid children. *J. Dent. Child.* **27**, 292–4.
Johnson, N.P. and Young, M.A. (1963). Periodontal disease in mongols. *J. Perio.* **34**, 41–7.
Jones, M.G. and Blinkhorn, A.S. (1986) The dental health of children attending special schools in Glasgow. *J. pediatr. Dent.* **2**, 61–6.
Kaner, A., Losch, P.K., and Green, H. (1946). Oral manifestations of congenital heart disease. *J. Pediatr.* **29**, 269–76.
Kanar, H.L. (1979). Cerebral palsy and other gross motor and skeletal problems. In *Dentistry for the handicapped patient*. Postgraduate dental handbook series. 5 (ed. K.E. Wessels), pp. 33–9. John Wright PSG Inc., Boston.
Kastein, S. (1957). Oral, dental and orthodontic problems of speech in cerebral palsy. *J. Dent. Child.* **24**, 243–6.
Kinirons, M.J. (1985). Dental health of children with cystic fibrosis: an interim report. *J. paediatr. Dent.* **1**, 3–8.
Koster, S. (1956). The diagnosis of disorders of occlusion in children with cerebral palsy. *J. Dent. Child.* **23**, 81–3.
Kushlik, A. (1964). The social distribution of mental retardation. *Develop. Med. Child. Neurol.* **15**, 748–59.
Leeds, J.J. (1976). Clinical modifications for the treatment of handicapped children. *J. Dent. Child.* **43**, 43–5.
Leonard, R.C. (1950). Dentistry for the cerebral palsied. *J. Am. dent. Ass.* **41**, 152–7.
Loesche, W.J. (1981). Plaque control in the handicapped. The treatment of specific infections. *Can. dent. Assoc. J.* **47**, 649–86.
Lundstrom, A., Eeg-Olofsson, O., and Hamp, S.E. (1982). Effect of anti-epileptic drug treatment with carbamazepine or phenytoin on the oral state of children and adolescents. *J. clin. Perio.* **9**, 482–8.
McCabe, M. (1979). Handicap in Newcastle-upon-Tyne. Thesis submitted for the degree of B.Ed (Hons). University of Newcastle-upon-Tyne.
McIver, F.T. and Machen, J.B. (1979). Prevention of dental disease in handicapped people. In *Dentistry for the handicapped patient*, Postgraduate dental handbook series, 5. (ed. K.E. Wessels), pp. 77–93. John Wright PSG Inc., Boston.
McMillan, R.S. and Kashgarian, M. (1961). Relation of human abnormalities of structure and function to abnormalities of the dentition II. Mongolism. *J. Am. dent.* **63**, 368–73.
MacEntee, M.I., Silver, J.G., Gibson, G., and Weiss, R. (1985). Oral health in a long term care institution equipped with a dental service. *Commun. dent. oral Epidemiol.* **13**, 260–3.

Maclaurin, E.T., Shaw, L., and Foster, T.D. (1985*a*). Dental study of handicapped children attending special schools in Birmingham. Parts 1 and 2. *Commun. dent. Hlth.* **2**, 249–58; 259–66.

Maclaurin, E.T., Shaw, L., and Foster, T.D. (1985*b*). Dental caries and periodontal disease in children with Down's syndrome and other mentally handicapping conditions. *J. paediatr. dent.* **1**, 15–20.

Mahaney, M.C. (1986). Delayed dental development and pulmonary disease severity in children with cystic fibrosis. *Archs. oral. Biol.* **31**, 363–7.

Matsson, L. and Koch, G. (1975). Caries frequency in children with controlled diabetes. *Scand. J. dent. Res.* **83**, 327–32.

Mellor, J. and Doyle, A.J. (1987). The evaluation of a dental treatment service for children attending special schools. *Commun. dent. Hlth.* **4**, 43–8.

Melville, M.R.B., Pool, D.M., Jaffe, E.C., Gelbier, S., and Tulley, W.J. (1981). A dental service for handicapped children. *Br. dent. J.* **151**, 259–61.

Mitchell, L., Murray, J.J., and Ryder, W. (1985). Management of the handicapped and the anxious child: a retrospective study of dental treatment carried out under general anaesthesia. *J. pediatr. Dent.* **1**, 9–14.

Modeer, T., Dahllof, G., and Theorell, K. (1986). Oral health in non-institutionalized epileptic children with special reference to phenytoin medication. *Commun. Dent. oral Epidemiol.* **14**, 165–8.

Morgan, S.B. (1979). Mental Retardation. In *Dentistry for the Handicapped Patient*, Postgraduate dental handbook series. 5, (ed. K.E. Wessels), pp. 21–28. John Wright PSG Inc., Boston.

Morton, M.E. (1977). Dental disease in a group of adult mentally handicapped patients. *Publ. Hlth.* **91**, 23–32.

Murray, J.J. and Rugg-Gunn, A.J. (1982). Fluoride tablets and drops. In *Fluorides in caries prevention*, Dental Practitioner Handbook, p. 95. Wright, Bristol.

Nagel, J., Pearson, P., Pool, D., and Tulley, W.J. (1971). Dental care of the handicapped child in the community. *Guy's Hosp. Gazette.* **85**, 339–45.

Neer, W.L., Foster, D.A., Jones, J.G., and Reynolds, D.A. (1973). Socioeconomic bias in the diagnosis of mental retardation. *Except. Child.* **40**, 38–9.

Nowak, A.J. (1974). Dental health for the mentally retarded citizen—our shared concern. *J. Acad. dent. Handicap.* **1**, 3–12.

Nowak, A.J. (1976). *Dentistry for the handicapped patient*. Mosby, St. Louis.

Nunn, J.H. (1984). The dental health of handicapped children in the Northern Region and the resources available to them for dental care. A thesis submitted for the degree of Ph.D. University of Newcastle-upon-Tyne.

Nunn, J.H. and Murray, J.J. (1987). The dental health of handicapped children in Newcastle and Northumberland. *Br. dent. J.* **162**, 9–14.

Ohmori, I., Awaya, S., and Ishikawa, F. (1981). Dental care for severely handicapped children. *Int. dent. J.* **31**, 177–84.

Orner, G. (1975). Dental caries experience among children with Down's syndrome and their siblings. *Archs. oral Biol.* **20**, 627–34.

Parkin, S.F., Hargreaves, J.A., and Weyman, J. (1970). Children's dentistry in general practice: dental care of physically and mentally handicapped children. *Br. dent. J.* **129**, 575–8.

Pless, I.B. and Douglas, J.W.B. (1971). Chronic illness in childhood: Part 1. Epidemiology and clinical characteristics. *Paediatrics.* **47**, 405–14.

Plotnick, S. (1975). A survey of preventive dentistry programmes for the handicapped child. NY *J. Dent.* **45**, 160–3.

Pool, D. (1981). Dental care of the handicapped. *Br. dent. J.* **151**, 267–70.

Pool, D. (1982). Dental care for the handicapped adolescent. *Int. dent. J.* **32**, 194–202.

Primosch, R.E. (1980). Tetracycline discoloration, enamel defects and dental caries in patients with cystic fibrosis. *Oral. Surg.* **50**, 301–8.

Rhodes, W.A. (1884). The mouths of the insane. *J. Br. dent. Assoc.* **5**, 413–15.

Richardson, W.P., Higgins, A.C., and Ames, R.G. (1964). Rates of attendance and reasons for non-attendance at a clinic of handicapping conditions. *Am. J. publ. Hlth.* **54**, 1177–83.

Richardson, B.A., Smith, D.C. and Hargreaves, J.A. (1977). Study of fissure sealants in mentally retarded Canadian children. *Commun. Dent. oral Epidemiol.* **5**, 220–6.

Richardson, B.A., Smith, D.C., and Hargreaves, J.A. (1981). A 5-year clinical evaluation of the effectiveness of a fissure sealant in mentally retarded Canadian children. *Commun. Dent. oral Epidemiol.* **9**, 170–4.

Ripa, L.W. and Cole, W.W. (1970). Occlusal sealing and caries prevention: results after 12 months, after a single application of adhesive resin. *J. dent. Res.* **49**, 171–3.

Roberts, I.F. and Roberts, G.J. (1979). Relation between medicines sweetened with sucrose and dental disease. *Br. med. J.* **2**, 14–16.

Robinson, P.B., Harris, H., and Harvey. W. (1983). Abnormal skeletal and dental growth in epileptic children. *Br. dent. J.* **154**, 9–13.

Rumble, J.D. (1980). Dentistry for handicapped children. Can we do more? *Dent. Pract.* **18**, 23–5.

Rutledge, L.E. (1940). Oral and roentgenographic aspects of the teeth and jaws of juvenile diabetes. *J. Am. dent. Ass.* **27**, 1740–50.

Schwarz, E. and Vigild, M. (1987). Provision of dental services for handicapped children in Denmark. *Commun. dent. Hlth.* **4**, 35–42.

Scottish Home and Health Department (1984). Dental Services for the Handicapped. London, HMSO.

Sheppard, I.M. (1936). Alveolar resorption in diabetes mellitus. *Dent. Cosmos* **78**, 1075–9.

Soble, R.K. (1974). Sociological and psychological considerations in special patient care: the dentist, the patient and the family. *Dent. Clin. N.Am.* **18**, 554–6.

Stark, G.G, (1977). *Spina bifida. Problems and management.* Blackwell, Oxford.

Stephen, K.W. and MacFadyen, E.E. (1977). Three years of clinical caries prevention for cleft palate patients. *Br. dent. J.* **143**, 111–16.

Stevens, H.A. and Heber, R. (1964). *Mental retardation—a review of research.* University of Chicago Press.

Strodel, B.J. (1987). The effects of cerebral palsy on occlusion. *J. Dent. Child.* **54**, 255–60.

Svatun, B. and Heloe, L.A. (1975). Dental status and treatment needs among institutionalized mentally subnormal persons in Norway. *Commun. Dent. oral. Epidemiol.* **3**, 208–13.

Swallow, J.N., Dehallis, J., and Young, W.F. (1967). Side effects to antibiotics in cystic fibrosis: dental changes in relation to antibiotic administration. *Archs. Dis. Child.* **42**, 311–18.

Swallow, J.N. (1972). Dental disease in handicapped children—an epidemiological study. *Israeli J. dent. Med.* **21**, 41–51.

Swallow, J.N. and Swallow, B.G. (1980). Dentistry for the physically handicapped in the International Year of the Child. *Int. dent. J.* **30**, 1–5.

Swerdloff, M. (1980). The problems and Concerns of the handicapped. *J. dent. Educ.* **44**, 131–5.

Tarver, R.D. (1976). Preventive dentistry program for mentally retarded and handicapped children. *Alaska Med.* **18**, 81–7.

Tesini, D.A. (1980). Age, degree of mental retardation, institutionalisation and socioeconomic status as determinants in the oral hygiene status of mentally retarded individuals. *Commun. Dent. oral Epidemiol.* **8**, 355–9.

Todd, J.E. and Dodd, T. (1985). *Children's dental health in the United Kingdom in 1983*. HMSO, London.

Walton, J.M. and Nattrass, F.J. (1954). On the classification, natural history and treatment of the myopathies. *Brain* **88**, 169–231.

Wegner, H. (1971). Dental caries in young diabetics. *Caries Res.* **5**, 188–92.

Wegner, H. (1975). Increment of caries in young diabetics. *Caries Res.* **9**, 91–6.

Weyman, J. (1971). *The dental care of handicapped children*, (1st edn). Longman, London.

White, R.A. and Sackler, A.M. (1954). Effect of progressive muscular dystrophy on occlusion. *J. Am. dent. Ass.* **49**, 449–54.

Winer, R.A., Cohen, M.M., Feller, R.P., and Chauncy, H.H. (1965). Composition of human saliva, parotid gland secretory rate, and electrolyte concentration on mentally subnormal patients. *J. dent. Res.* **44**, 632–4.

World Health Organisation (1971). Oral health Surveys. Basic Methods. Geneva, WHO.

World Health Organization (1982). Goal for oral health in the year 2000. *Br. dent. J.* **152**, 21–2.

Wotman, S., Mercadente, J., Mandel, D.L., Goldman, S.R., and Denning, C. (1973). The occurrence of calculus in normal children, children with cystic fibrosis and children with asthma. *J. Perio.* **44**, 278–80.

Younghusband, E., Birchall, D., Davie, R., and Kellmer Pringle, M.L. (1970). *Living with handicap*. National Bureau for Co-operation in Child Care, London.

14

Preventive orthodontics

J. R. E. MILLS

THE human face is almost infinitely variable and the human eye has the gift of distinguishing quite minor variations so that we recognize our friends and acquaintances, even if they are encountered in unexpected circumstances. The exception to this is the case of identical twins, whose appearance is so similar as to deceive all but their closest friends. Similar, although less marked, is the facial resemblance of close relatives. Facial appearance reflects the underlying bony skeleton, together with the covering of soft tissues, and these are the factors which most influence the occlusion of the teeth. Identical twins share the same chromosomes and a study of twin pairs by Lundstrom (1949) has used this fact to show that the arrangement, and especially the inter-arch occlusion of the teeth, is to a large extent genetically determined, and this has been confirmed by Saunders *et al.* (1980) in a study of 147 families, and by Lobb (1987), although there are differences even in monozygotic twins. These are presumably the result of environmental factors. Eugenics has never become popular, nor indeed, has it ever been suggested in the case of dental occlusion, so there is comparatively little that can be done to intercept the development of a malocclusion. In this chapter therefore, certain suggestions will be put forward concerning interceptive mechanisms and while these are necessary and desirable, they will play only a limited part in controlling malocclusion.

Development of the deciduous dentition

The most important role which the general dental practitioner or paedodontist can supply is in monitoring the development of the deciduous and later the permanent dentitions, to ensure that all teeth develop normally, in their correct position and in their correct number. The order of eruption of the deciduous teeth is well known to every dental student, and yet Leighton (1968) has shown that there are many variations and in fact only a minority of children follow the textbook plan. It is not uncommon, for example, to find upper deciduous lateral incisors erupting before the centrals. In general this does little harm and the full deciduous dentition is eventually developed but in the rare case of crowding of the deciduous anterior teeth, a late-erupting incisor could be displaced, or presumably even impacted. The deciduous incisors are normally spaced when they erupt and remain so until they are replaced by permanent incisors. If the deciduous incisors are in contact it is probable that the permanent incisors will be crowded; if the deciduous incisors are themselves crowded, then crowding of the permanent successors is almost invariable. Contrary to popular belief, malocclusion of the dental arches, giving an Angle Class II or Class III relationship, is quite frequently seen in the deciduous dentition, but there is no justification for intervening at this stage. Supplemental incisors may be seen in the deciduous dentition and are almost always followed by a supplemental permanent incisor in the same location. This is a useful pointer so that appropriate action can be taken when the permanent incisors erupt.

Early loss of deciduous teeth

Deciduous incisors are occasionally lost early as the result of trauma, and generally this calls for little action except for radiographic examination to ensure that the root is not retained and to see whether the developing permanent tooth has been misplaced. If this has occurred, it is likely to be dilacerated.

Problems are more likely to arise where deciduous molars are lost, and this is a traditional cause of crowding of the permanent teeth. In fact this does not cause any decrease in the size of the dental bases, so that the effect is essentially a localization of pre-existing crowding and if the patient is not inherently crowded, then it is unlikely that the space will close to any appreciable extent. The effect of the loss of deciduous molars has been thoroughly investigated by Richardson (1966), who followed 74 children for several years after the loss of deciduous molars, and by Ronnerman (1965), who followed the fate of 187 patients. Their findings generally agree and may be summarized as follows:

1. Following extraction of deciduous molars, the space may close to a variable extent, may remain of its original width, or occasionally, may partly close and then re-open.

2. This would seem to be dictated by the degree of inherent crowding. Spaces will not close in an uncrowded mouth. Ronnerman implies that crowding anterior to the first molar only occurs in 10 per cent of those who lose deciduous molars, and in whom it would not have occurred had the molars been retained.

3. The greatest space loss occurs after extraction of the upper second deciduous molar, followed by the lower second deciduous molar, the upper first deciduous molar and least of all following the loss of the lower first deciduous molar. The last has little effect on later crowding but a unilateral loss may cause the lower centre line to displace towards that side. Clinch (1959), in a serial study, indicated that even this effect may have been exaggerated.

4. The greatest space loss would seem to occur where the deciduous molars are lost early and, in particular, extraction of the second molar before the first

permanent molar erupts almost always causes some loss of space. It would seem desirable therefore, to retain the deciduous molars until the first permanent molars are in occlusion, even if they have to be lost shortly thereafter.

It has been suggested that where a deciduous molar is unavoidably extracted, this should be 'balanced' by extracting its antagonist and even the corresponding teeth on the opposite side of the mouth. There would seem to be little justification for such a procedure and indeed, the remaining deciduous molar will tend to prevent forward movement of the first molar and the occlusion may well assist in maintaining a space in the opposing arch.

The fitting of space maintainers is happily less fashionable than was the case some years ago. In the majority of cases they would be unnecessary and serve no useful purpose, and they may even have an adverse effect by promoting caries and periodontal disease. If a removable space maintainer, or a fixed lingual arch, is used for this purpose, it may interfere with slight natural increase in intermolar width which occurs with growth.

In general, the loss of space following the extraction of deciduous molars could be corrected by the extraction of a premolar in the appropriate quadrant and this would probably have been necessary for the relief of general crowding in any case. The effect of the loss of the deciduous tooth is to localize the crowding in the permanent canine and premolar areas. Perhaps the one case where a space maintainer might be indicated is where the first permanent molars are in Angle Class II relationship before the upper second deciduous molar is lost. If, in a crowded mouth, the upper first permanent molar migrates even further mesially, it will not be possible to correct the malocclusion by the loss of a single premolar in this quadrant, and the orthodontist will be committed to the more difficult procedure of moving the permanent molar distally.

Retention of deciduous teeth

Deciduous teeth may be retained beyond their normal time of shedding, either locally or generally. Individual teeth may be retained as a result of infection, either following a blow, usually in the incisor region, or from caries, more often posteriorly. Occasionally, a deciduous molar may be retained over-long because the premolar is somewhat misplaced and consequently one root of the deciduous molar does not resorb normally, as shown in Fig. 14.1(a). In any case the retained deciduous tooth will frequently have the effect of displacing the erupting permanent tooth, as shown in Figs. 14.1(a) and (b). If the deciduous remnant is removed, the permanent tooth will have a strong tendency to move to its correct position, provided this is not prevented by the occlusion of the teeth. In the case shown in Fig. 14.1(b), the deciduous incisor was removed and the permanent incisor came forward into a normal occlusion. Had the deciduous incisor not been removed, the permanent successor would have erupted inside the bite and been held by the occlusion as shown in Figs. 14.16(c) and (d). If left uncorrected, the adjacent teeth may crowd together, so that later treatment

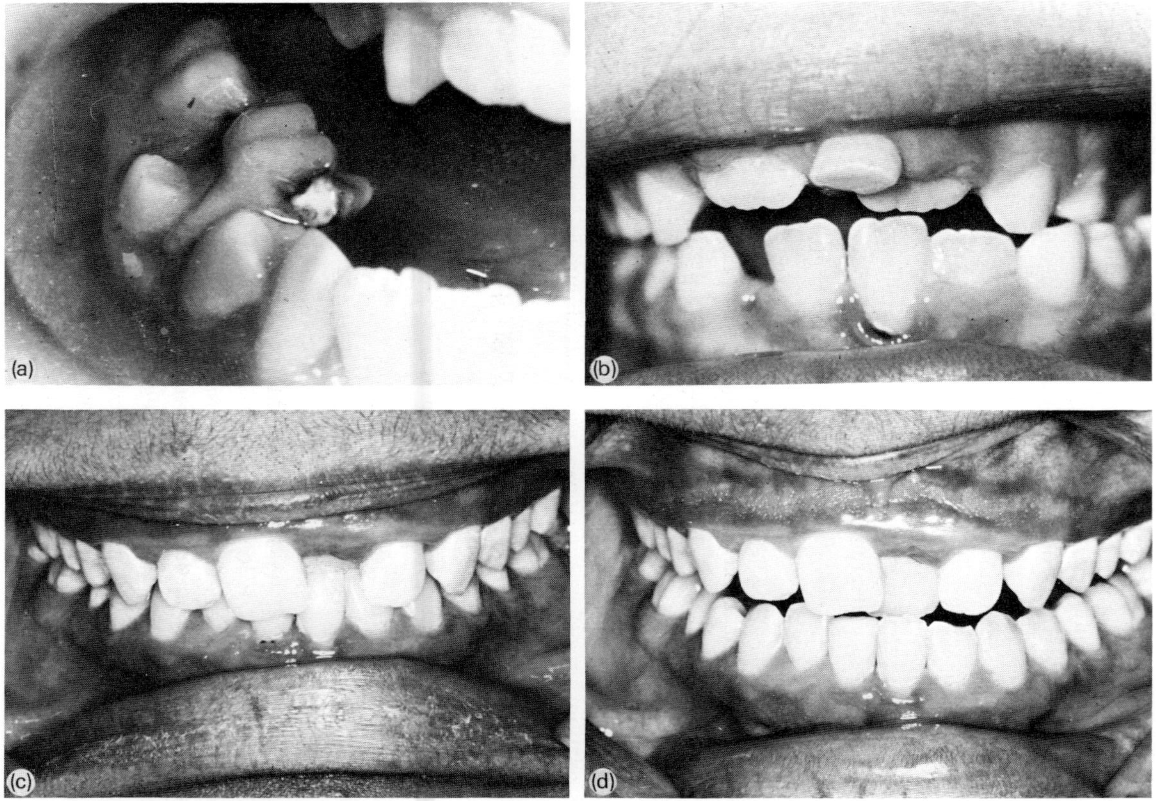

Fig. 14.1. (a) Retention of $\overline{E}|$ due to failure of mesial root to resorb, causing buccal deplacement of $\overline{5}|$. (b) Retention of non-vital $|\underline{A}$ causing lingual displacement of $|\underline{1}$. Note unilateral cross-bite on patient's left side. (c) Adult patient with lingually displaced $|\underline{1}$. (d) Note that the patient can achieve edge-to-edge occlusion on this tooth.

becomes difficult. Similarly, the premolar in Fig. 14.1(a) could be locked in cross-bite if the deciduous molar had not been removed.

Occasionally a patient is seen in whom the deciduous molars and canines fail to shed in a normal fashion. Quite often the roots have resorbed but the teeth remain firm well beyond the normal age for shedding. If the deciduous molars are present after the fourteenth birthday, serious thought should be given to their extraction. If the premolars are present, close beneath the crowns of the deciduous molars, and at least one-quarter of their roots has formed, then the deciduous molars should be extracted and the premolars will usually erupt within a matter of a few months.

At this point, one might mention the submerged deciduous molar. It is not uncommon to find that, as the dento-alveolar structures develop vertically, one or more deciduous molars will fail to keep pace and thus appear to be submerged relative to their neighbours. These teeth are usually ankylosed and the corresponding permanent tooth may be absent. In most cases the deciduous molar will free itself and shed normally, and routine extraction is not indicated. Very occasionally the submergence will continue and the tooth may even disappear into the bone. Such teeth should, therefore, be kept under observation. They should be extracted if they are not shedding at the same time as other deciduous molars and in any case if the permanent tooth is missing.

Development of the permanent dentition

Here again a close watch should be kept and, in examining a child's dentition, it is not sufficient merely to diagnose caries and gingivitis. At the age of 9 years, the presence and position of all developing permanent teeth should be checked radiographically. Absence of the third molar at this age is no indication that it will not eventually calcify and this tooth may not put in its first appearance until 14 or 15 years in exceptional circumstances. The need to check for the presence of all teeth should be self-evident but presumably the dentist who extracted the lower left first molar shown in Fig. 14.2(a) was unaware of the congenital absence of the lower second premolar and third molar. The teeth most usually missing are upper lateral incisors, second premolars, and lower central incisors, although any tooth may be congenitally absent, alone or in combination with others. Even upper permanent canines occasionally fail to form. In the case of congenitally absent premolars, some thought may be given to early extraction of the deciduous molars in the hope that the space will close naturally by mesial drift of the first permanent molars. If the deciduous molar is extracted in such cases, it may be advisable to extract also the opposing permanent premolar. Lindqvist (1980) has suggested that deciduous molars should not be extracted in these cases before 8 years in girls and 6 months later in boys, as the first radiographic evidence of the premolar may sometimes be as late as this. They should ideally be extracted as soon as possible after these ages to minimize tilting of the adjacent teeth. Where upper lateral incisors are congenitally absent, orthodontic

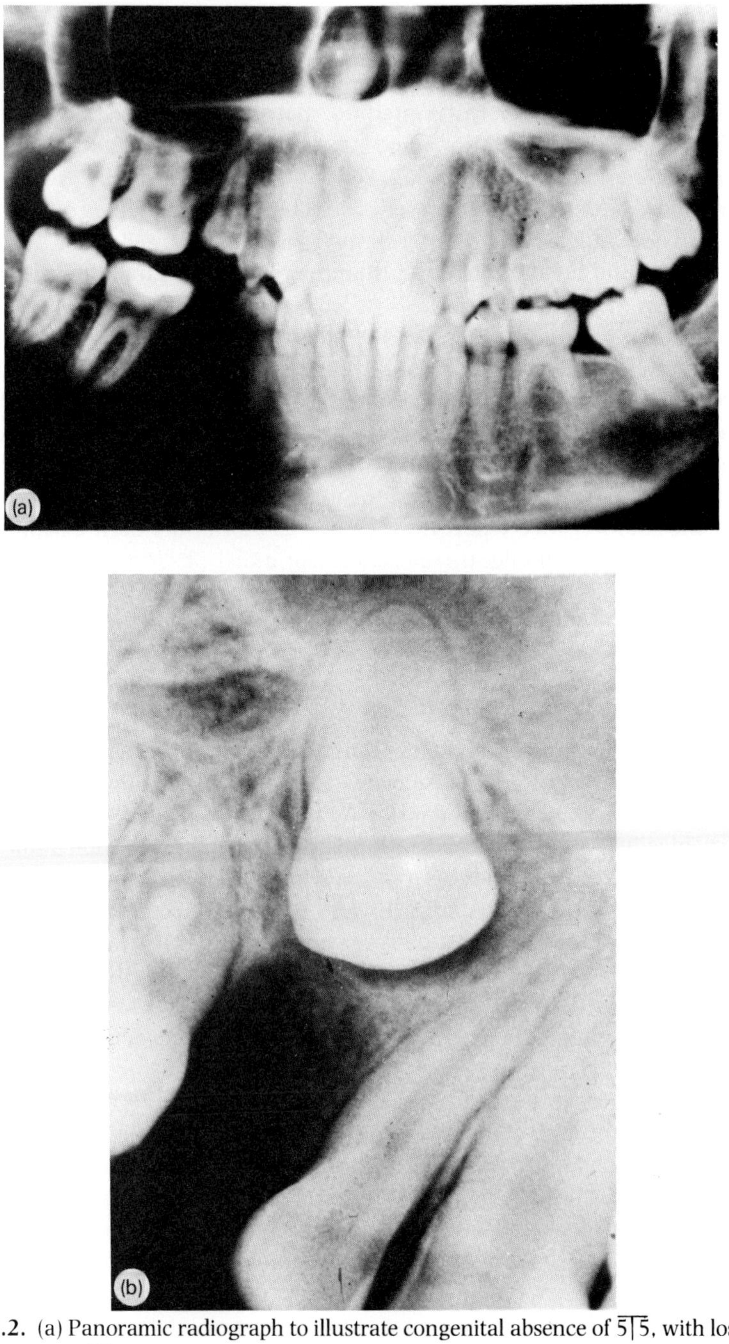

Fig. 14.2. (a) Panoramic radiograph to illustrate congenital absence of $\overline{5|5}$, with loss of $\overline{|6}$ and absence of $\overline{|8}$. (b) Radiograph of $\underline{4321|}$ region. Note foreshortening of $\underline{3|}$ which indicates probable displacement from the line of the arch.

advice should be sought at an early stage. In some cases the space may be closed by bringing forward the upper permanent canines, whereas in a less crowded mouth, it is desirable to maintain the space for an ultimate prosthesis. The absence of a lower incisor can easily be overlooked if the remaining teeth are well aligned and in contact. Congenital absence of third milars is seldom a disadvantage.

It is equally important to check at this stage that the developing permanent teeth are in their normal position. Any tooth may develop in a misplaced position but the most frequent offender is the upper permanent canine, probably because of its late eruption compared with its neighbours. While a single radiograph will not position the tooth accurately, the picture seen in Fig. 14.2(b), with the grossly foreshortened permanent canine, was a hint that this tooth was not in its normal position. It may be misplaced either palatally or in the labial sulcus. If it is found to be misplaced, then orthodontic opinion should be sought. The teeth will generally erupt along their long axes, and also have a strong tendency to progress towards the surface. If these factors would tend to bring the crown of the unerupted canine into contact with the roots of the anterior teeth, then action should be taken as soon as possible. In the majority of cases, the crown of the permanent canine is well removed from the roots of the anterior teeth and can safely be left and monitored to see if it will correct itself. If it fails to do so, or show signs of growing in an abnormal direction, then orthodontic treatment is probably called for without delay.

Crossbites

Figure 14.1 shows examples of cases where retained deciduous teeth may cause permanent teeth to fall into a local crossbite. This is not the only cause of such a localized condition but in almost any case where a single tooth erupts into crossbite, it should be corrected as soon as possible. This applies particularly to upper incisor teeth. Where an upper central incisor is lingually displaced quite frequently a single lower incisor will be displaced labially through the outer plate of bone and unless it is corrected fairly quickly a dehiscence will develop. Another effect of delay is seen in Figs. 14.1(c) and (d). The upper left central incisor in this East African patient erupted inside the bite and this was accompanied, as it frequently is, by a forward displacement of the mandible in occlusion, so as to avoid the premature contact of this upper incisor. The remainder of the dentition developed in this displaced position, while the teeth on either side of the displaced incisor crowded mesially so that there was no longer sufficient space to correct the tooth. Such a condition, if seen after development of the entire permanent dentition, is quite difficult to correct, and the problem could have been prevented had the tooth been moved over the bite as soon as it was noted. This situation is very common in the case of instanding lateral incisors and to correct such teeth it is frequently necessary to extract the deciduous canine so as to give the necessary space.

Occasionally, where the upper dental arch is narrower relative to the lower, the buccal cusps of the upper teeth will erupt in a cusp-to-cusp relationship, bucco-lingually, with the lower posterior teeth. This is uncomfortable and the patient therefore displaces the mandible to the appropriate side thus producing what appears to be a unilateral posterior crossbite. An example of this is seen in Fig. 14.1(b). Opinions differ as to whether this should be treated as soon as it is seen or whether it is better left to the very early permanent dentition. The case shown in Fig. 14.1(b) in fact corrected itself as the permanent premolars erupted, but nevertheless orthodontic advice should be sought in such a case.

Other factors

Edward Angle, who practised around the turn of the century, has been called the father of orthodontics. It has also been said of him 'American orthodontics would be forever indebted to and hampered by the Angle tradition'. One of his principal precepts was that every individual is born with the potential for ideal occlusion, from which it followed that all malocclusion, were due to environmental factors. Although this belief is thoroughly discredited, it gave rise to certain aetiological beliefs which die hard.

Digit sucking

Basic to the practice of orthodontics is the belief that the teeth are normally in a position of balance between the activity of the lips and cheeks on the one hand and the tongue on the other. If a force is applied which disturbs this balance, then the teeth will move until a new position of balance is achieved. If this is the result of an orthodontic appliance, and that appliance is then withdrawn, the teeth are once again in a position of imbalance and will revert to their original position. In this context a thumb, finger, or other part of the human hand can be used as an orthodontic appliance. About half of all children suck a digit or digits. This usually commences in the first year of life and seldom ceases much before the age of four. It varies considerably in intensity and frequency but if the habit continues for several hours a day, it will have the effect of moving the appropriate teeth. The traditional picture is seen in an exaggerated form in Fig. 14.3, which shows the teeth of a 14-year-old boy who was in the habit of sucking the knuckle of his right index finger. Typically, the upper incisors are proclined, while the corresponding lower incisors may be slightly retroclined. There is an anterior open bite. The deformity is usually asymmetrical and in a child who sucks a digit of the right hand it is normally displaced to that side. It will vary considerably in extent, and that shown in Fig. 14.3 is an extreme case. In some cases, although not here, digit sucking is associated with a tendency to crossbite of the posterior teeth.

Most children cease this habit before the permanent incisors erupt. Bowden (1966), followed a group of thumb-suckers up to the age of 8 years and he found

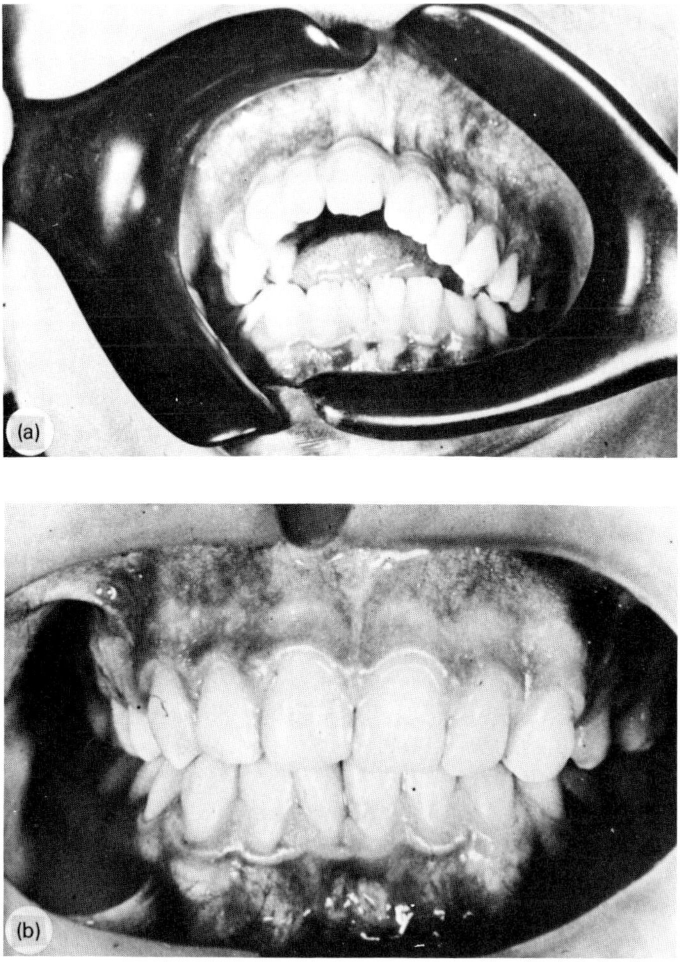

Fig. 14.3. (a) The result of persistent sucking of knuckle of right hand in 15-year-old boy. (b) The result following simple orthodontic treatment.

that after withdrawal of the habit the overjet corrected itself in about 12 months, although the overbite took up to 3 years to re-establish itself to normal levels. Attempts to break the habit are usually unproductive. A child will even develop a taste for bitter aloes, as his elders develop a taste for bitter beer. Appliances attached to the hand or the teeth do not usually have the required effect and there is certainly no cause to attempt to break the habit before the eruption of the permanent incisors. The effect is a purely local one on the labial segment of teeth and can easily be corrected by orthodontic treatment. I am very doubtful whether preventive measures are ever justified. When the time comes for mechanical correction, the placing of an orthodontic appliance, which the child accepts as clearly doing something useful, also provides a deterrent and the habit normally disappears without difficulty.

Mouth breathing

Very many children have their lips apart at rest. The overwhelming majority of these produce a seal anteriorly between the tongue and lower lip and, posteriorly, between the soft palate and dorsum of the tongue. Humphreys and Leighton (1950) showed many years ago that the true mouth breather is rare. The traditional but erroneous picture of a mouth breather is of a child with prominent upper anterior teeth, a narrow upper arch, a high vault to the palate and a 'pinched' appearance of the external nose. The place of mouth breathing as an aetiological factor therefore fell into disfavour until the work of Linder-Aronson (1979). This worker approached the problem from the opposite end. He visited an ear, nose, and throat hospital and examined 81 children who were unable to breath through their noses to an adequate extent due to pathological conditions, normally adenoid tissue. He found a reasonably constant clinical picture of a patient with a steep lower border of the mandible, an increased lower facial height, a narrow upper dental arch with a tendency to crossbite, and, surprisingly, retroclined upper and lower incisor teeth. Although the children differed from a control group to a statistically significant extent, the average effect was nevertheless comparatively mild. After removal of the offending obstruction, Linder-Aronson followed the children for some years and found a tendency to self-correction which again was statistically significant, although in the case of inter-molar width the increase was only 0.6 mm greater than his control group. He explained the situation as follows:

Being unable to breathe through the nose, the child had to lower the mandible so as to be able to breathe through the mouth. Consequently, the tongue was removed from the vault of the palate and failed to oppose the action of the cheeks and lips. The former caused the posterior teeth and their alveoli to grow downwards rather than downwards and buccally, giving a narrow upper arch but increasing the maxillary alveolar height and therefore rotating the mandible in a downward and backward direction. Similarly, the absence of the tongue caused retroclination of the anterior teeth under lip activity, other things being equal. It would seem that mouth breathing only occurs in children who are, either permanently or temporarily, unable to breathe normally through their noses. Clearly if this is the case, the obstruction should be removed on the grounds of general health, but while this may cause some slight improvement in the occlusion and facial appearance, the improvement is likely to be small although further deterioration may be avoided.

Interceptive orthodontics

This is closely allied to the subject of preventive orthodontics and a number of procedures, some of which have already been described, are used in the hope of preventing or reducing the need for subsequent orthodontic treatment.

Serial extractions

This procedure was popularized shortly after the last war by Kjellgren (1948) and its advantages and pitfalls are well described by Dewel (1969). It is intended for use in patients with crowding of the anterior teeth, and briefly the procedure is to extract the deciduous canines to allow a natural alignment of the anteriors. This is followed by extraction of the first deciduous molars to encourage the eruption of the first premolars, which are then extracted in their turn. In my opinion it is seldom or never indicated in its complete form and in considering its use, certain points should be carefully observed.

Firstly, it should be remembered that when the incisor teeth erupt, they are normally somewhat crowded and may align themselves during their eruption. Even if they are fully erupted, they may occasionally align spontaneously. Secondly, if the deciduous canine is extracted too early, the socket will heal and bone will be laid down so that eruption of the permanent canine will be impeded; this tooth may then well erupt through the labial plate of bone and difficulty may be encountered in bringing it down to its correct position. Moorrees *et al.* (1963) have suggested that the deciduous canine should not be extracted until half the root of the permanent canine has formed. The purpose of extracting the first deciduous molar is to encourage the eruption of the first premolars well ahead of the canines but in my opinion this is a barbarous procedure which is unnecessary. If it is practised then the deciduous molars should not be extracted, again according to Moorrees, until at least one-quarter of the root of the permanent premolar has formed and the crown thereof is close beneath the crown of the resorbed deciduous molar. Finally, the first premolar should be extracted when it has erupted. In the upper arch the space will show a great tendency to close spontaneously by mesial movement of the posterior teeth and an upper space maintainer is essential in the vast majority of cases. The extraction of the first premolar may allow the canine to align itself but will usually have comparatively little effect on the incisor teeth. In the lower arch some judgement is necessary but, unless space is very critical, a space maintainer need not be fitted, provided a constant monitoring of the arch is undertaken. In this arch, the canines show some tendency to drift distally and incisor teeth may be well aligned, provided none of them is rotated. Rotations are not usually self-correcting. The procedure should only be used in carefully selected cases, which should be of Class I malocclusions on a Class I or preferably mild Class III skeletal base. It is necessary to see the patient at least every 4 months, and it is unlikely that an ideal occlusion will be achieved although later mechanical orthodontic treatment may be somewhat shortened and simplified.

Modifications of this practice are possible. It is quite often useful to extract the first premolars before the canines have erupted and to allow the canines therefore to drift distally into the space, preventing their labial exclusion. Once again, an upper space maintainer and possibly a lower space maintainer are indicated. Some authors advocate the extraction of the first deciduous molar and the surgical removal of the developing first premolar at the same visit. This practise cannot be too strongly deprecated. It involves the unnecessary admission of the child to hospital, it almost always involves the destruction of considerable alveolar bone, including the outer plate thereof and, because this does not reform, a good contact between the canine and second premolar is seldom achieved. Finally, it usually fails in its purpose of aligning the anterior teeth, at least so far as the upper arch is concerned.

Extraction of first permanent molars

Wilkinson (1944) must bear much of the responsibility for the popularization of this practice as an aid to a good occlusion. The claims which he made were, to say the least, extravagant, involving as they did the complete elimination of both caries and periodontal disease. Unfortunately, the first permanent molar is singularly caries prone and its extraction is sometimes unavoidable. This almost always has the effect of relieving any possibility of impaction of the third molars but, apart from this, its effect on the occlusion is likely to be for the worse. Salzmann (1938) showed that in the upper arch the space will usually close completely but this occurs almost entirely by mesial drift with mesio-lingual rotation of the upper second molar. The premolars will drift distally, usually only one or at the most two millimetres, and this will provide little relief of anterior crowding. In the lower arch the effect is more equally divided between the second molar and the second premolar, with the former tilting mesially and the latter drifting distally, often with a space developing between the two lower premolars. Frequently, residual space is left while the occlusion between the lower second molar and the upper teeth leaves much to be desired, and may occasionally give rise to temporomandibular joint problems. On the other hand, the lower extraction may relieve lower anterior crowding at least to some extent. If the extraction of a first permanent molar becomes necessary, Thilander *et al.* (1963) have indicated that the best time is around the age of 10 or 11 years; specifically after eruption of the lateral incisor and first premolar, but before the eruption of the canine or second permanent molar. If extraction is delayed until the second permanent molars are in occlusion the space will virtually never close naturally.

Wilkinson in fact advocated the extraction of all four first permanent molars as a 'balanced' procedure. When the loss of a permanent molar is unavoidable the condition should be considered on its merits with attention given to the occlusal relations of the teeth in working out the final likely effect of extractions. In general, if it is necessary to extract a lower first molar and orthodontic treatment is not intended, it is usually advisable to balance this by extracting the corresponding upper molar, although the latter extraction may be delayed for some months after the lower tooth is lost to allow some mesial movement of the lower second molar. If it is the upper molar which is unsaveable, then providing the lower first molar is quite sound, or can be saved in the long term, its extraction is usually contraindicated, as the upper second molar will erupt to occlude with the lower first molar and the upper third with the lower second molar. Caries is often symmetrical and it may be that the first molars on the opposite side of the mouth are also in a desperate condition, but unless this is the case, I can see no good reason for extracting the contralateral first molars. Happily, the problem of carious first molars is less common than was the case a few years ago.

Enucleation of third molars

Some years ago the practice became popular of removing the developing tooth germs of the third permanent molars in children as soon as these were visible radiographically. The third permanent molars are seldom useful teeth, frequently become impacted, and very occasionally give rise to problems which necessitate their extraction. This is the only possible justification for enucleating these teeth in a young child and therefore necessitating an unpleasant operative procedure in hospital. Their loss at this stage will not give space for the relief of crowding and it would seem that third molars have little or no effect in causing later crowding of the anterior teeth.

It would seem probable that modern and future preventive treatment can do much to decrease substantially the incidence of dental caries and periodontal disease. Unfortunately, the same is not true of malocclusion; indeed such measures may increase its incidence. Nevertheless, the dentist should be constantly aware of the developing occlusion and be ready to intervene where this is indicated. It has been said: the dentist says 'open wide' and misses the malocclusion, the orthodontist says 'close together' and misses the caries. Both should mend their ways.

References

Bowden, B.D. (1966). A longitudinal study of the effects of digit and dummy sucking. *Am. J. Orthodont.* **52**, 887–901.

Clinch, L.M. (1959). A longitudinal study of the results of premature extraction of deciduous teeth between 3–4 and 13–14 years of age. *Dental Pract.* **9**, 109–26.

Dewel, B.F. (1969). Prerequisites in serial extraction. *Am. J. Orthodont.* **55**, 633–9.

Humphreys, H.F. and Leighton, B.C. (1950). A survey of antero-posterior abnormalities of the jaws in children between the ages of two and five and a half years of age. *Br. dent. J.* **88**, 3–15.

Kjellgren, B. (1948). Serial extractions as a corrective procedure in dental orthopedic therapy. *Trans. Eur. Orthodont. Soc.* 134–60.

Leighton, B.C. (1968). Eruption of deciduous teeth. *Practitioner* **200**, 836–46.

Linder-Aronson, S. (1979). Respiratory function in relation to facial morphology and the dentition. *Br. J. Orthodont.* **6**, 59–71.

Lindqvist, B. (1980). Extraction of the deciduous second molar in hypodontia. *Eur. J. Orthodont.* **2**, 173–82.

Lobb, W.K. (1987). Cranio facial morphology and occlusal variation in monozygous and dizygous twins. *Angle Orthodont.* **57**, 219–33.

Lundstrom, A. (1949). An investigation of 202 pairs of twins regarding fundamental factors in the aetiology of malocclusion. *Dental Rec.* **69**, 251–64.

Moorrees, C.F.A., Fanning, E.A., and Grøn, A.M. (1963). The consideration of dental development in serial extraction. *Angle Orthodont.* **33**, 44–59.

Richardson, M.E. (1966). The relationship between the relative amount of space present in the deciduous dental arch and the rate and degree of space closure subsequent to the extraction of a deciduous molar. *Dental Pract.* **16**, 111–18.

Ronnerman, A. (1965). Early extraction of deciduous molars and canines. *Trans. Eur. Orthodont. Soc.* 153–67.

Salzmann, J.A. (1938). Study of orthodontic and facial changes and effects on dentition attending loss of first molars in five hundred adolescents. *J. Am. dent. Ass.* **15**, 892–905.

Saunders, S.R., Popovich, F., and Thompson, G.W. (1980). A family study of craniofacial dimensions in the Burlington Growth Centre sample. *Am. J. Orthodont.* **78**, 394–403.

Thilander, B., Jakobsson, S.O., and Skagius, S. (1963). Orthodontic sequelae of extraction of permanent first molars. *Odontologisk Tidskrift* **7**, 381–412.

Wilkinson, A.A. (1944). The early extraction of the first permanent molar as the best method of preserving the dentition as a whole. *Dental Rec.* **64**, 2–8.

15

The changing pattern of dental disease

J. J. MURRAY

Introduction

DENTAL disease very rarely causes death and is widely accepted by the public at large as something they all get and have to live with. However, dental disease is not static and the dental health of the population depends on the amount of disease, on the attitude of the patient, and on the type of treatment offered by the dental profession. Important changes have been noted in the caries experience of children, particularly over the last 10 or 15 years in many developed countries, and this reduction in disease should eventually result in a changing type of dental treatment in adulthood.

The changing pattern of caries experience in children

Jackson (1974) summarized the results of over 70 published and unpublished surveys of caries experience in English children and young adults during the period 1947 to 1972. With regard to 5-year-old children (Table 15.1), he concluded that there had been little change in the mean dmf between 1947–1960 and 1960–1972. In the permanent dentition an apparent *increase* in mean DMF values for 12-year-old children was reported according to the Ministry of Education quinquennial surveys (HMSO 1958–68; Table 15.2) between 1948–1968, and this trend was supported by results from other studies (Jackson 1974). However the available evidence with regard to 15-year-old English schoolchildren between 1950–1977 (Table 15.3) suggested that little or no *increase* in caries had occurred. In contrast, one year later, an opposing view, that the dental health of children was improving, was cautiously put forward by Palmer (1980), who suggested that the dental health of children in Somerset had improved in recent years. His view was based on personal observations and the comments of practitioners in both the general and community dental service. Data for both 5- and 14-year-old children showed a downward trend between 1975 and 1979 (Table 15.4).

The weakness in the type of analysis put forward by Jackson (1974) is that the

Table 15.1. Caries experience of 5-year-old English children during the years 1947–1972. (References in Jackson 1974)

Year of survey	Author	Area	No. of children	Mean dmf
1947	Miller (1950)	Manchester	128	4.80
1947	Mellanby and Mellanby (1948)	London	1590	4.06
1948	*HSC (1958–59)	7 areas, England	15158	4.29
1948	Miller (1950)	Manchester	42	6.07
1949	Miller (1950)	Manchester	109	5.39
1949	Weaver (1950)	North Shields	500	4.45
1949	Mellanby and Mellanby (1950)	London	692	5.34
1950	Miller (1950)	Manchester	74	5.50
1950	Jackson (1952)	Accrington	142	4.16
1960	Sanderson (1960)	West Riding	521	4.60
1961	Sanderson (1961)	West Riding	534	4.19
1962	Bulman *et al.* (1968)	Darlington	66	4.80
1962	Bulman *et al.* (1968)	Salisbury	101	4.90
1962	Dodd (1965)	Cheshire	300	5.74
1963	HSC (1962–63)	7 regions, England	16390	5.10
1964	Smyth *et al.* (1964)	Gloucestershire	90	2.98
1966	Millward (1967)	Maidstone	45	4.29
1967	Murray (1969a)	York	527	4.09
1967	Beal and James (1970)	Balsall Heath	257	5.24
1967	UKF Studies (1969)	Sutton	119	2.80
1967	Beal and James (1971)	Dudley	329	5.24
1967	Beal and James (1970)	Sutton Coldfield	304	3.27
1967	Beal and James (1971)	Northfield	335	5.02
1968	BES (1972)	Leicestershire	1757	4.07
1968	BES (1972)	Lincolnshire	409	4.06
1968	Beal and James (1971)	Dudley	274	4.80
1968	HSC (1966–68)	7 regions, England	15781	4.50
1969	Clayton (1969)	West Riding	403	5.10
1969	Timmis (1971)	Essex	959	4.19
1969	**BES (1972)	Scunthorpe	196	4.28
1969	BES (1972)	Corby	205	4.28
1969	Beal and James (1971)	Dudley	255	5.04
1969	Hesterman (1969)	Shropshire	542	5.09
1969	Bride (1969)	Manchester	390	3.89
1970	Beal and James (1971)	Dudley	229	5.09
1970	BES (1972)	Devon	1150	4.70
1970	Teasdale (1972)	Huddersfield	224	4.17
1970	Awath-Behari (1970)	Wolverhampton	100	4.47
1970	Whitehouse (1970)	Nottinghamshire	193	3.82
1970	Gordon (1973)	6 areas, England	1909	4.26
1972	Lowery (1972)	West Riding	257	4.48
		Total	63586	4.59

* HSC = Health of the School Child.
** BES = Birmingham Epidemiological Studies.

studies are not strictly comparable, having been carried out by different investigators, all with different standards of diagnosis. Palmer recognized the problem, even from his own area, because he acknowledged that his records did not satisfy strict epidemiological requirements in that the methods were not calibrated nor standardized. Nevertheless, his samples were large and included vir-

Table 15.2. Caries experience of 12-year-old children—Source: *Health of the School Child*. Quinquennial Surveys (HMSO 1954—68)

Area	1948	1953	1958	1963	1968
Manchester	3.7	3.5	4.1	4.4	4.5
Middlesex	—	4.6	5.1	5.8	5.4
Northumberland	2.5	3.6	5.6	5.6	5.3
Nottinghamshire	4.2	3.0	3.8	4.1	4.9
Somerset	2.7	4.3	5.6	5.4	5.0
West Riding	2.9	4.2	6.1	6.1	6.3
West Sussex	2.7	3.2	—	—	—
East Sussex	—	—	4.5	5.3	5.1
All areas	2.9	3.8	5.5	5.3	5.5

Table 15.3. Caries experience in 15-year-old English children 1950–1977 (Jackson 1974)

Year of survey	Author	Area	No. of children	Mean DMF
1950	Jackson (1952)	Accrington	148	7.9
1957–59	Starkey (1966)	Naval recruits	4795	10.8
1958–59	Jackson (1961)	Leeds	94	9.5
1963–65	Starkey (1966)	Naval recruits	5156	11.2
1964	Bulman *et al.* (1968)	Salisbury	22	9.8
1964	Bulman *et al.* (1968)	Darlington	58	8.5
1965	*HSC (1969–71)	England	14 025	9.8
1967	Murray (1969)	York	381	8.9
1968	Bristow (1975)	Portsmouth	437	9.5
1973	Todd (1975)	England	576	8.0
1974	Papyanni (1974)	Halifax	300	8.0
1977	Crossland (1977)	Bury	309	9.6
1977	Jackson (1978)	Yorkshire	2827	9.7
1977	Fairpo (1978)	Harrogate	208	7.5
1977	Williams (1978)	York	174	9.1

* HSC = Health of the School Child.

Table 15.4. Somerset Area Health Authority statistics (Palmer 1980)

Year	5-year-olds		14-year-olds	
	No. of children	Mean def	No. of children	Mean DMF
1975	3022	2.6	2294	7.2
1976	3369	2.5	2259	6.4
1977	3426	2.1	3402	6.3
1978	3279	1.8	2612	5.8
1979	3528	1.7	3149	5.3

Table 15.5. Changes in caries experience in England

Author	Date	Age of children (yrs.)	Place	Year of examination	Mean DMF
Anderson	1981*a*	12	Somerset	1963	5.4
		12	Somerset	1978	3.4
Anderson	1981*b*	12	Shropshire	1970	4.5
		12	Shropshire	1980	3.1
Anderson	1981*c*	12	Gloucestershire	1964	4.5
		12	Gloucestershire	1979	2.2
Andlaw *et al.*	1982	11	Bristol	1970	4.6
		11	Bristol	1979	2.9
		14	Bristol	1973	9.5
		14	Bristol	1979	6.7

Table 15.6. Changes in caries experience of pre-school children

Author	Date	Age of children (yrs.)	Place	Year of examination	Mean def
Winter *et al.*	1971	3	London	1967	1.4
Holt *et al.*	1982	3	London	1981	0.7
Silver	1982	3	Hertfordshire	1973	1.5
Silver	1982	3	Hertfordshire	1981	0.6

Table 15.7. Declining dental caries in various countries (references in, Glass 1982)

Author	Country	Age of subjects (yrs.)	Year of examination	Mean DMFT
Fejerskov *et al.*	Denmark	20	1972	16.6
Fejerskov *et al.*	Denmark	20	1982	11.8
O'Mullane	Eire	8–9	1961	2.8
O'Mullane	Eire	8–9	1979	1.3
O'Mullane	Eire	13–14	1961	8.0
O'Mullane	Eire	13–14	1979	4.4
Brown	New Zealand	12–13	1950	7.9
Brown	New Zealand	12–13	1982	4.1
Von der Fehr	Norway	15	1970	*32.0
Von der Fehr	Norway	15	1979	*15.0
Downer	Scotland	10	1970	5.0
Downer	Scotland	10	1980	3.6
Carlos	USA	6–11	1971–74	1.7
Carlos	USA	6–11	1979–80	1.1
Carlos	USA	12–17	1971–74	6.2
Carlos	USA	12–17	1979–80	4.6

* DMFS values.

tually all children attending state-maintained schools in Somerset, in particular age bands. Shortly afterwards there followed a steady stream of papers, by research workers using strict epidemiological techniques, confirming Palmer's assertion that caries experience in English children was declining (Table 15.5). Similar findings were reported in pre-school children (Table 15.6).

The theme of a decline in dental caries took on an international flavour when the first international conference devoted to this topic was held in Boston in June 1982. Speakers from Denmark, Eire, the Netherlands, New Zealand, Norway, Scotland, Sweden, and the United States all confirmed that a downward trend in dental caries in children and young adults had occurred in the 1970s (Glass 1982; Table 15.7).

Data from various surveys in the Netherlands was given in the form of a diagram for 6-year-old and 12-year-old children (Figs. 15.1; 15.2); Kalsbeek 1982). These data suggested a gradual decline in caries in the 1970s. A report from Australia (Burton *et al.* 1984) suggested that caries experience of 12-year-old children had declined by 84 per cent from 1963 to 1982 (Table 15.8).

This downward trend was confirmed by a Working Group of the FDI (1985) and WHO who had access to figures from the WHO Global Oral Data Bank (Fig. 15.3). They concluded that the most probable reasons for the decrease in dental caries in children in the developed countries were considered to be associated with:

(1) the widespread exposure to fluoridated water and/or fluoride supplements, especially the regular use of fluoride toothpaste;

(2) the provision of preventive oral health services;

(3) the increased 'dental awareness' through organized oral health education programmes;

(4) the ready availability of dental resources.

The factor common to all countries with a substantial reduction in caries was fluoride, either as fluoridated water or toothpaste.

National Dental Health Surveys of Child Dental Health in England and Wales 1973–1983

The first national survey of children's dental health in England and Wales was carried out in 1973. The Office of Population Censuses and Surveys was responsible for drawing up a stratified random sample of over 12 000 children, aged 5–15 years, attending over 500 schools in the two countries. Dental examinations were undertaken at the schools by 70 dentists who had been specially trained and calibrated for the study. In addition, parents of children aged 5, 8, 12 and 14 years were visited in their homes by Social Survey Interviewers, to obtain information on social class, patterns of dental attendance, and other issues.

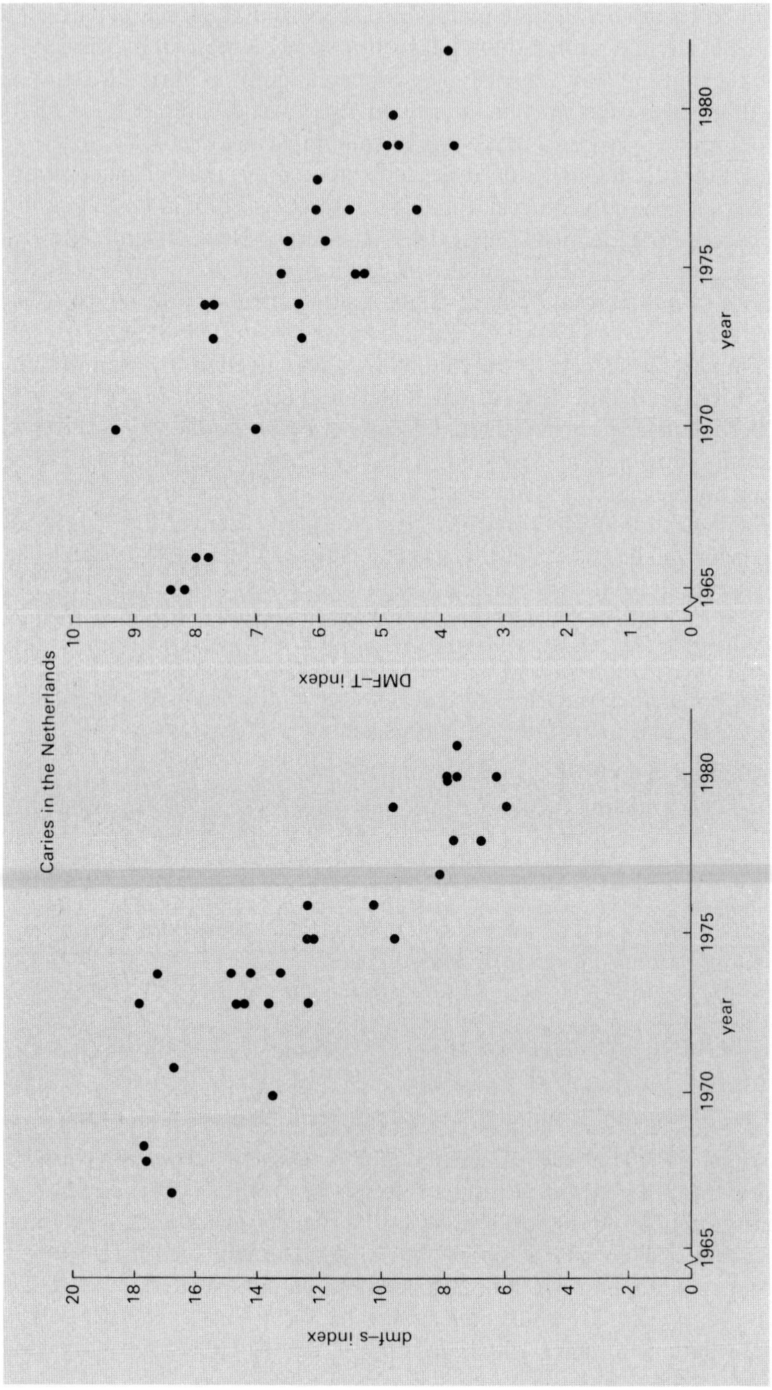

Fig. 15.1. dmfs values for 6-year-old children from the Netherlands (Kalsbeek 1982).

Fig. 15.2. DMFT values for 12-year-old children from the Netherlands (Kalsbeek 1982).

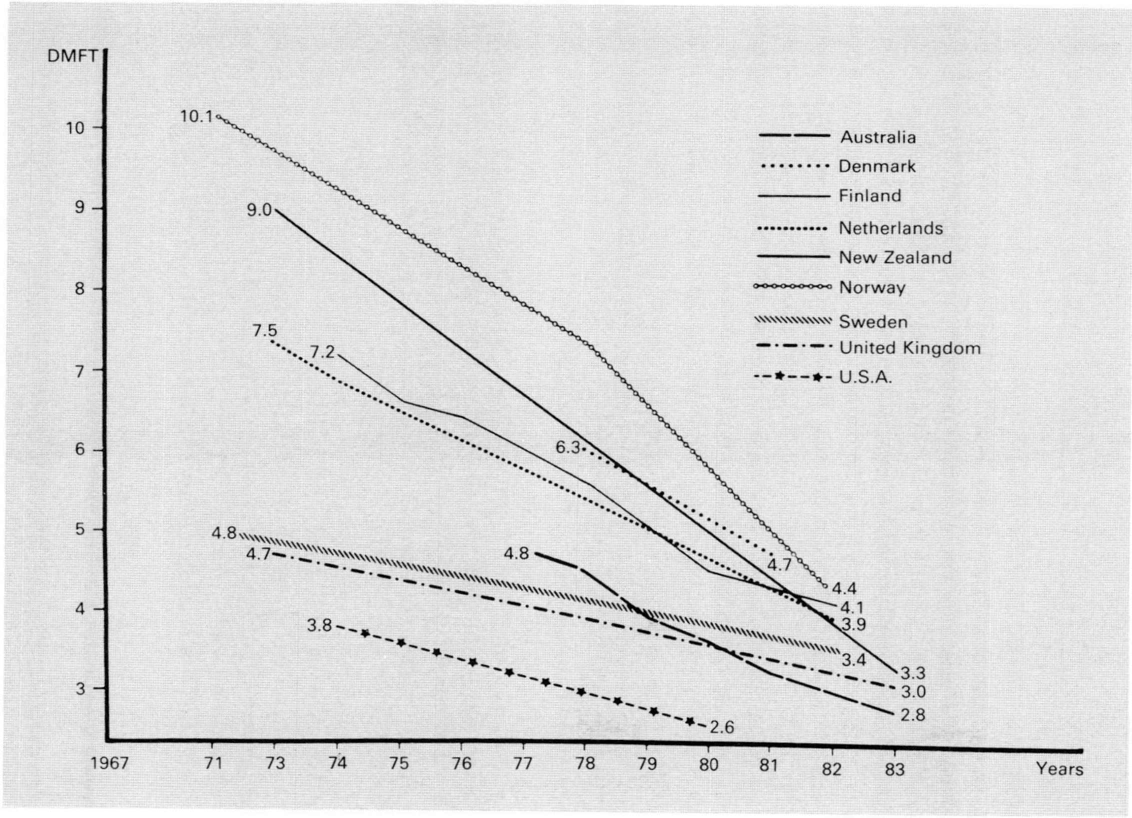

Fig. 15.3. Trends in dental caries 1967–1983 DMFT as 12 years. (Source WHO Global Oral Data Bank (Renson *et al.* 1986).)

Table 15.8. Changes in caries experience of 12-year-old Sydney children (Burton *et al.* 1984)

1963		**1982**	
No. of children	**Mean DMFT**	**No. of children**	**Mean DMFT**
426	8.5	736	1.4

The second national survey was held ten years later, in 1983; this time Scotland and Northern Ireland were included, and the sample size was increased to over 20 000 to enable data from the four countries in the United Kingdom to be presented separately. Seventy-six dentists, many of whom had been involved in the previous survey, carried out the examinations at school, after participating in a training and calibration exercise. In order to reduce costs, information from parents was obtained mainly from a postal questionnaire. In both surveys the level of co-operation was very high—between 88–95 per cent of selected children were examined successfully. For the purposes of this review the state of children's dental health for England and Wales between 1973 and 1983 will be compared.

(i) Dental caries in deciduous teeth

Dramatic reductions in caries in 5-year-old children were observed (Table 15.9) over the 10-year period. The proportion of children with untreated decay in deciduous teeth was much less in 1983 compared with 1973 (Fig. 15.4), and more importance was being placed on the preservation of deciduous teeth through restorative treatment among the older children than was the case in 1973 (Fig. 15.5). There was therefore a considerable reduction in the number of untreated carious deciduous teeth over the 10-year period.

(ii) Dental caries in permanent teeth

A similar general trend was observed in the permanent dentition. The proportion of children with decay was lower for every age group. In 1973, 50 per cent of 7-year-olds had some decay in their permanent teeth, but in 1983 this point was not reached until children were 9 years of age (Fig. 15.6). The mean DMFT had fallen from 8.4 to 5.6 for 15-year-old children, a reduction of approximately 33 per cent (Fig. 15.7).

The DMFT values for England and Wales in 1983 are compared with those re-

Table 15.9. Caries experience in 5-year-old children in England and Wales 1973–1983

	1973	**1983**
Per cent caries-free	28	51
Mean dmft	4.0	1.8

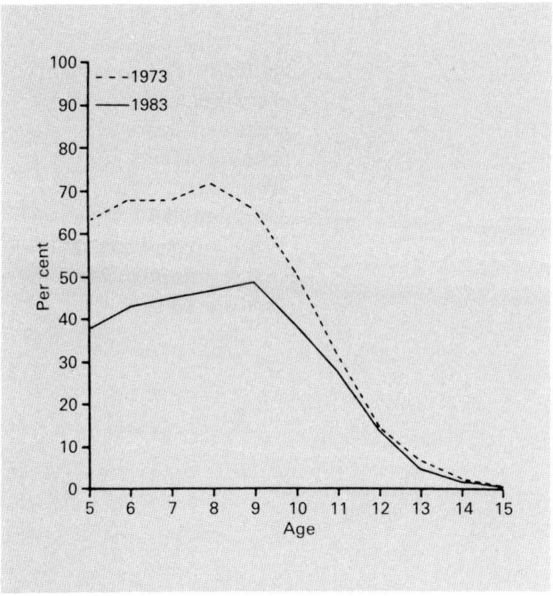

Fig. 15.4. The proportion of children with some decayed deciduous teeth in England and Wales in 1973 and 1983 (Todd 1985). (Reproduced by kind permission of Miss Todd and OPCS.)

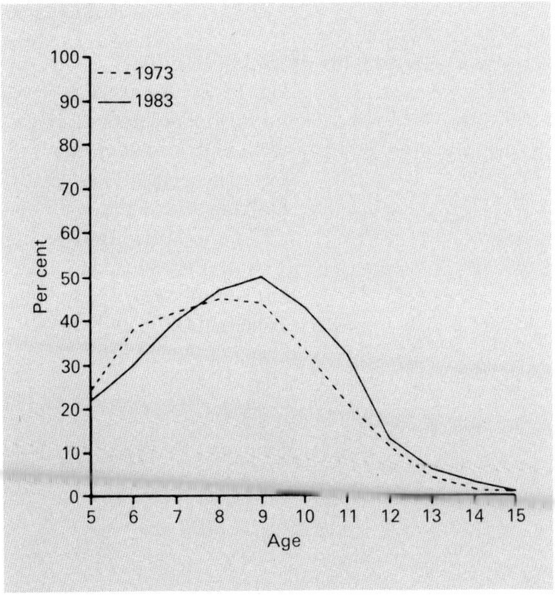

Fig. 15.5. The proportion of children with some filled deciduous teeth in England and Wales in 1973 and 1983 (Todd 1985). (Reproduced by kind permission of Miss Todd and OPCS.)

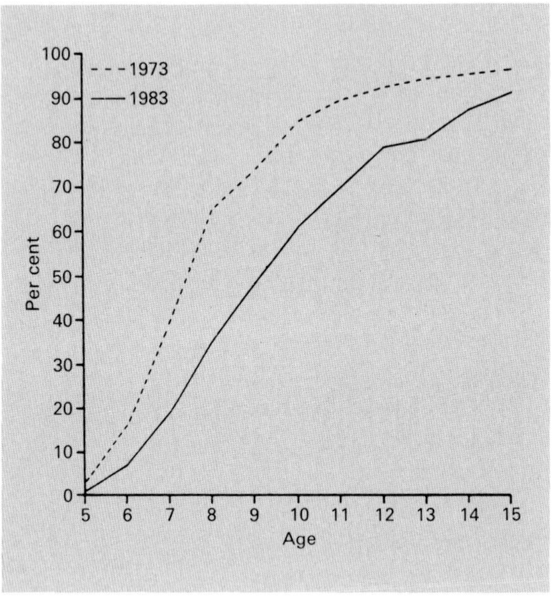

Fig. 15.6. The proportion of children with known decay experience of permanent teeth in England and Wales in 1973 and 1983 (Todd 1985). (Reproduced by kind permission of Miss Todd and OPCS.)

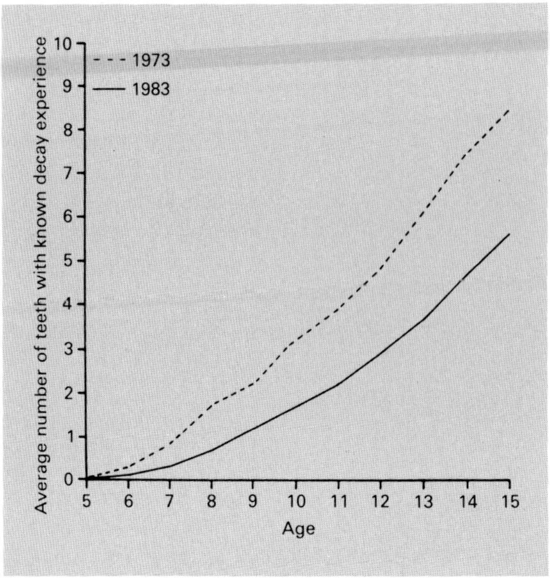

Fig. 15.7. The average number of permanent teeth with known decay experience (DMFT) in England and Wales in 1973 and 1983 (Todd 1985). (Reproduced by kind permission of Miss Todd and OPCS.)

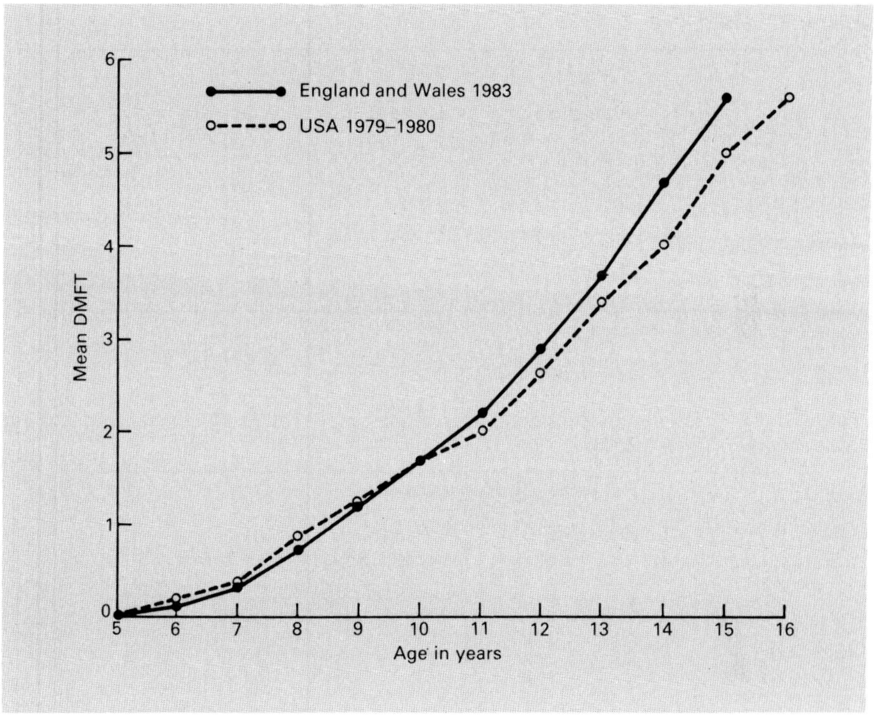

Fig. 15.8. Mean DMFT values in permanent teeth of 5–16-year-old children from USA (1979–80) and England and Wales (1983).

Table 15.10. Proportions of children with gum inflammation, calculus, and debris in England and Wales, 1973–1983

Age (yrs.)	Gum inflammation		Calculus		Debris	
	1973	**1983**	**1973**	**1983**	**1973**	**1983**
5	20	18	5	3	39	29
8	56	47	15	13	67	55
12	57	50	28	21	64	49
15	51	49	34	33	51	47

Table 15.11. The prevalence of specific occlusal problems in England and Wales children 1973–1983

	Proportion (per cent) of children with					
	Instanding or edge-to-edge incisors		Overjet 5–6 mm		Overjet 7 mm or more	
Age (yrs.)	1973	1983	1973	1983	1973	1983
8	12	9	11	16	7	8
12	9	10	11	13	7	8
15	9	13	11	12	3	4

Table 15.12. Crowding, orthodontic extractions and decay extractions in England and Wales children 1973–1983

	Per cent children with					
	crowding		orthodontic extractions		decay extractions	
Age (yrs.)	1973	1983	1973	1983	1973	1983
8	65	70	—	—	4	2
12	55	65	13	15	23	13
15	53	66	21	29	33	22

Table 15.13. Proportions of children who had had appliance therapy and who were in need of orthodontic treatment

	Per cent who					
	had a brace at the examination		had had a brace		were in need of orthodontic treatment	
Age (yrs.)	1973	1983	1973	1983	1973	1983
8	—	—	1	1	57	56
12	5	7	7	7	37	41
15	1	3	16	20	27	31

ported in the survey of United States children in 1979–80 in Fig. 15.8 (Miller *et al.* 1981).

(iii) Periodontal disease in children

In contrast to the good news on dental caries, there was virtually no change in gum inflammation and calculus between 1973 and 1983 (Table 15.10). There was a slight trend towards less debris in 1983, although this still meant that half

Table 15.14. Prevalence (per cent) of accidental dental damage among children in the United Kingdom 1983

Age (yrs.)	Males	Females	Both sexes
8	12	7	10
12	29	16	23
15	33	19	26

Table 15.15. Proportion (per cent) of children in the United Kingdom with damaged incisors that have not been treated in 1983

Age (yrs.)	Males	Females	Both sexes
8	89	84	88
12	89	93	90
15	85	81	84

the children from the age of 7 years had debris present on the day of the examination.

(iv) Orthodontic condition of children

The orthodontic assessment in 1983 was not identical to that carried out 10 years earlier, but incisor problems, crowding and orthodontic treatment and need could be compared. Very little change in 'incisor problems' was observed (Table 15.11). In contrast the prevalence of crowding had increased substantially between 1973 and 1983. This may be related at least in part to a sharp decrease in proportion of children who had teeth extracted for decay reasons (Table 15.12). During the dental examination in both 1973 and 1983 the dentist asked the children whether they had ever worn a brace and also recorded whether each child was wearing a brace at the time of the examination. In addition, an assessment was made by the dentist as to whether orthodontic treatment was needed (Table 15.13). Despite the differences between the orthodontic examinations of 1973 and 1983, it is clear that orthodontic extractions increased, appliance therapy increased (although not apparently statistically significantly) but there was still almost one-third of 15-year-old children who were regarded by the survey dentists as in need of orthodontic treatment. Parents were asked some questions about what they thought about the appearance of their child's teeth, especially whether they thought the teeth were crooked or protruding, and they were asked whether they would like their child to have their teeth straightened. Among children whom the dentist assessed as not needing any orthodontic treatment for crowding about four out of five parents said their child's teeth were not crooked. However, among those for whom the dentist said there was an orthodontic treatment need for reasons for crowding, fewer than half the parents said their child's teeth were crooked. The results

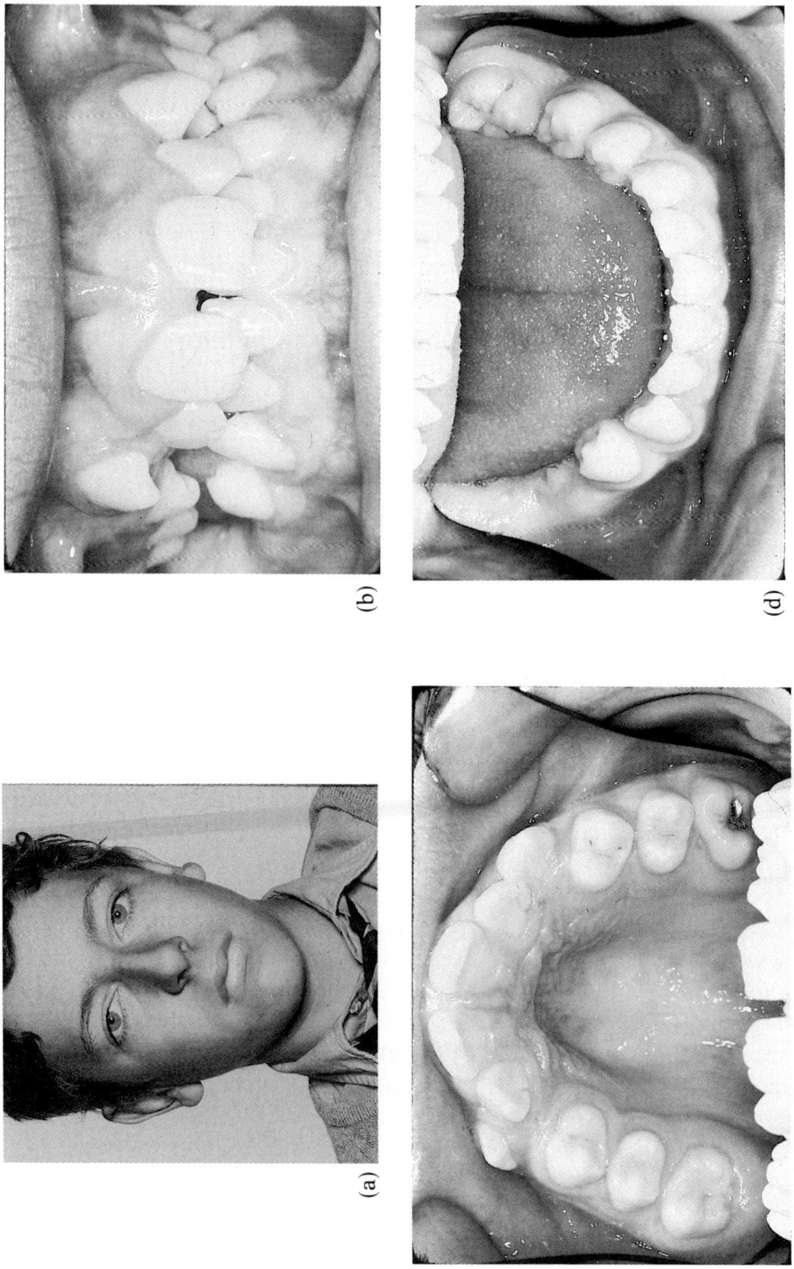

(a) (b) (c) (d)

showed that crowding that was of dental significance to the examiner was not recognized as being a problem by over half of the parents.

These findings raise an interesting point with regard to aesthetics and the need for treatment, which was referred to in the Schanschieff Report into Unnecessary Dental Treatment (Department of Health and Social Security 1986). Are dentists over-emphasizing the problem and advocating treatment when parents do not perceive an aesthetic problem? The alternative explanation is that the general public are not aware of crowding, especially in the premolar and canine regions, and that dentists are using their professional judgement to score crowding which parents had not appreciated.

(v) Trauma to anterior teeth

By the age of 15 years over a quarter of children in England and Wales had suffered accidental damage to their front teeth. The prevalence was much higher in boys than in girls (Table 15.14) These findings were much higher than in 1973, probably because there had been a very large reported increase in the number of incisors with fracture of the enamel only (the least serious traumatic injury). In the vast majority of cases the damaged incisors received no treatment (Table 15.15). Among 12-year-olds for example, only 10 per cent of incisors with traumatic injury had been treated. When the information from the questionnaire to the parents relating to damage to the incisors was correlated with the clinical findings, it was obvious that parents were not as aware of accidental damage to the teeth as were the dental examiners. For example, among 15-years-olds, the dentist recorded 26 per cent with traumatic injury whilst the parents felt only 16 per cent had damaged a permanent incisor.

The need for treatment in children and its effect on treatment needs in later life

The results of these surveys show clearly the direction in which the dental services should move in order to provide a better standard of dental health for children. Although great emphasis has been placed on the welcome reduction in caries in many western countries, there has not been the same reduction in the prevalence of periodontal disease. As parental awareness increases there will be an increasing demand for orthodontic treatment, and for the treatment and prevention of trauma to anterior teeth. Experience in the United States has shown that, in spite of the substantial decrease in the prevalence of dental caries, the de-

---

Fig. 15.9. (a) Facial appearance of a 13-year-old patient. (b) View of anterior teeth showing upper canines crowded out of the arch. (c) Occlusal view of upper arch showing lack of space in the upper canine region. First permanent molars had been extracted and second permanent molars had moved forward closing the space. (d) Occlusal view of the lower arch showing the poor alignment of second permanent molars, following the extraction of first permanent molars.

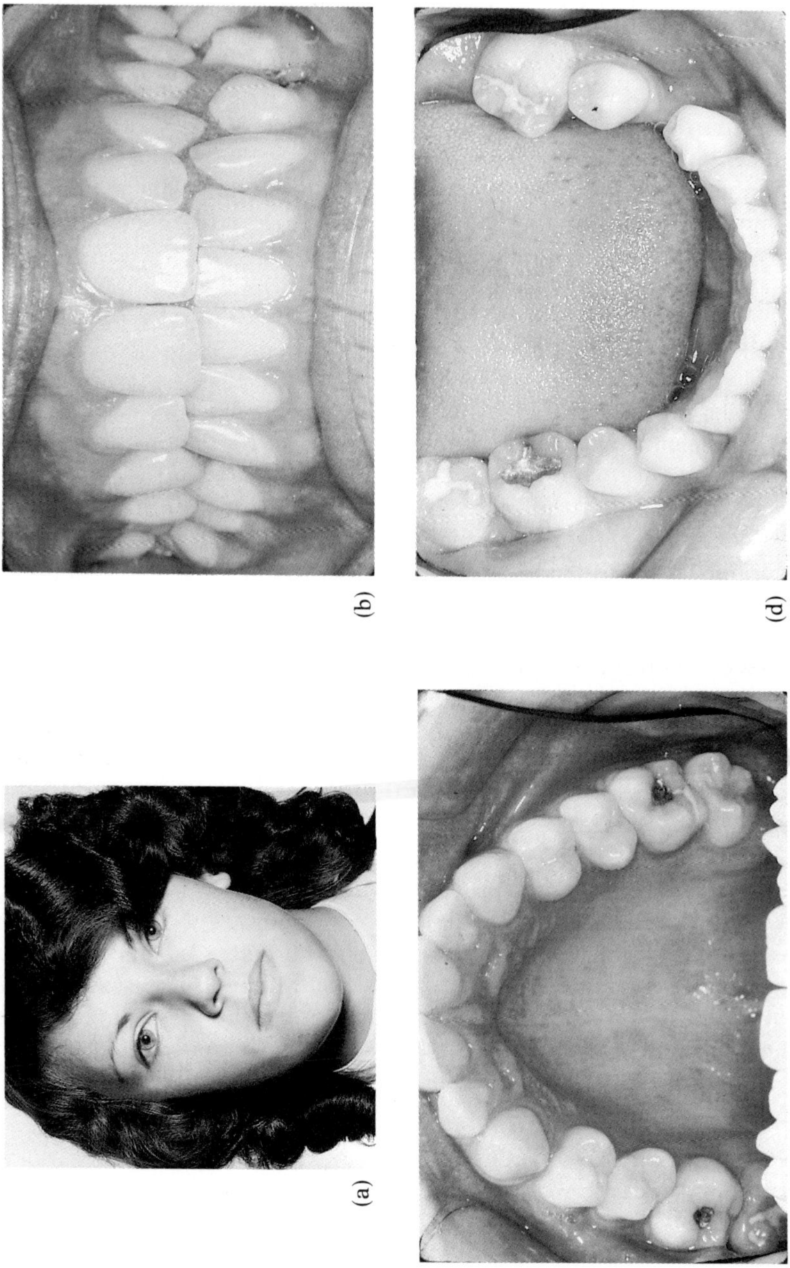

(a) (b) (c) (d)

mand for dental services by children aged between 5 and 17 years did not decline. There was an increase in the ratio of filled teeth to total caries experience, and an extension of dental care to a large proportion of the population, together with more complete maintenance care and a growing awareness of the need for programmes for prevention of all dental diseases (Waldman 1987).

The prevention of dental caries by a combination of public health and individual preventive measures gives us the opportunity to ensure that the whole dental environment for children is improved so that their future dental needs are reduced and simplified. It may be a gross simplification and generalization to say that by the age range 12–14 years the future dental needs of a patient are largely determined, but consider the following examples.

The first, a 13-year-old boy, had his first permanent molars extracted some years ago (Fig. 15.9). He was referred for orthodontic treatment of misplaced maxillary canines. The failure to manage the space created by extraction of first molars some years previously means that complex orthodontic treatment will be necessary and more teeth may have to be extracted in the upper arch in order to provide him with a reasonable occlusion. The next patient has fared so much better (Fig. 15.10). She has very good oral hygiene, well-aligned incisor and canine teeth, and an excellent upper arch. All second permanent molars have been fissure sealed, three first permanent molars have been restored but, for some reason, the lower left first permanent molar was extracted shortly after eruption. The resulting occlusion in that quadrant is poor, the contact points non-existent, and she will have to concentrate more effort in that quadrant to ensure that periodontal disease is kept to a minimum in later life.

The next patient (Fig. 15.11) also has a beautiful smile and good oral hygiene. Her upper arch shows true prevention, with all four permanent molars fissure sealed. The lower arch has been preserved by amalgam restorations in the occlusal and buccal surfaces. Which arch will require further dental attention in future years? How often will those amalgams be replaced and extended in the next 50 years? Why were we able to prevent caries in the upper arch but only 'manage' caries in the lower arch? The bitewing radiographs (Fig. 15.11(e), (f)) certainly suggest that some of the occlusal amalgams are minimal and might have been obviated by a more preventive approach.

This preventive philosophy can be illustrated by the next case (Fig. 15.12). If one sees a small brown line or the earliest signs of decalcification in first perman-

---

Fig. 15.10. (a) Facial appearance of a 14-year-old patient. (b) View of anterior teeth showing incisor and canine teeth well aligned. (c) Occlusal view of upper arch: teeth are well aligned; the upper first permanent molars have been restored with amalgam and the upper second molars have been fissure sealed. (d) Occlusal view of the lower arch showing fissure sealants on both lower second molars, and occlusal restoration in the lower right first permanent molar, but a poor occlusion on the left side because the lower left first permanent molar has been extracted some years ago.

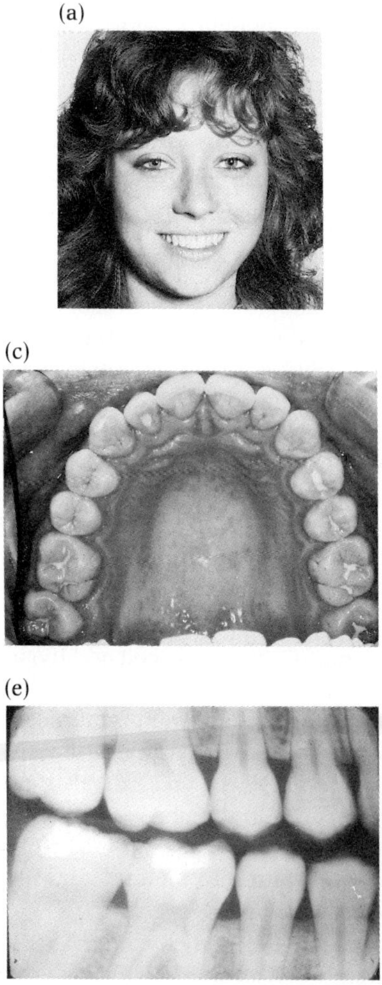

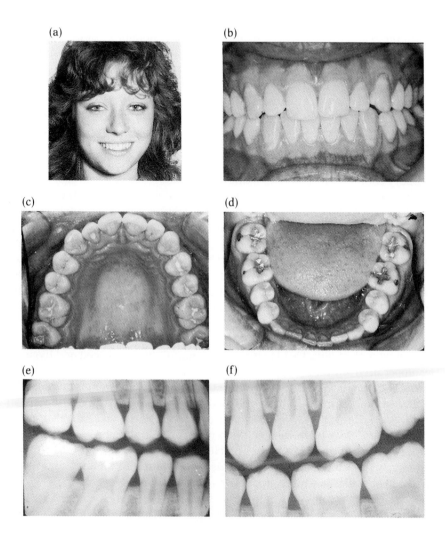

Fig. 15.11. Facial appearance of a 17-year-old patient. (b) View of anterior teeth showing good alignment of incisor and canine teeth. (c) Occlusal view of upper arch showing a caries-free arch with all molars fissure sealed. (d) Occlusal view of lower arch showing amalgam restoration in all four permanent molar teeth. (e, f) Bitewing radiographs of this patient showing shallow amalgam restorations.

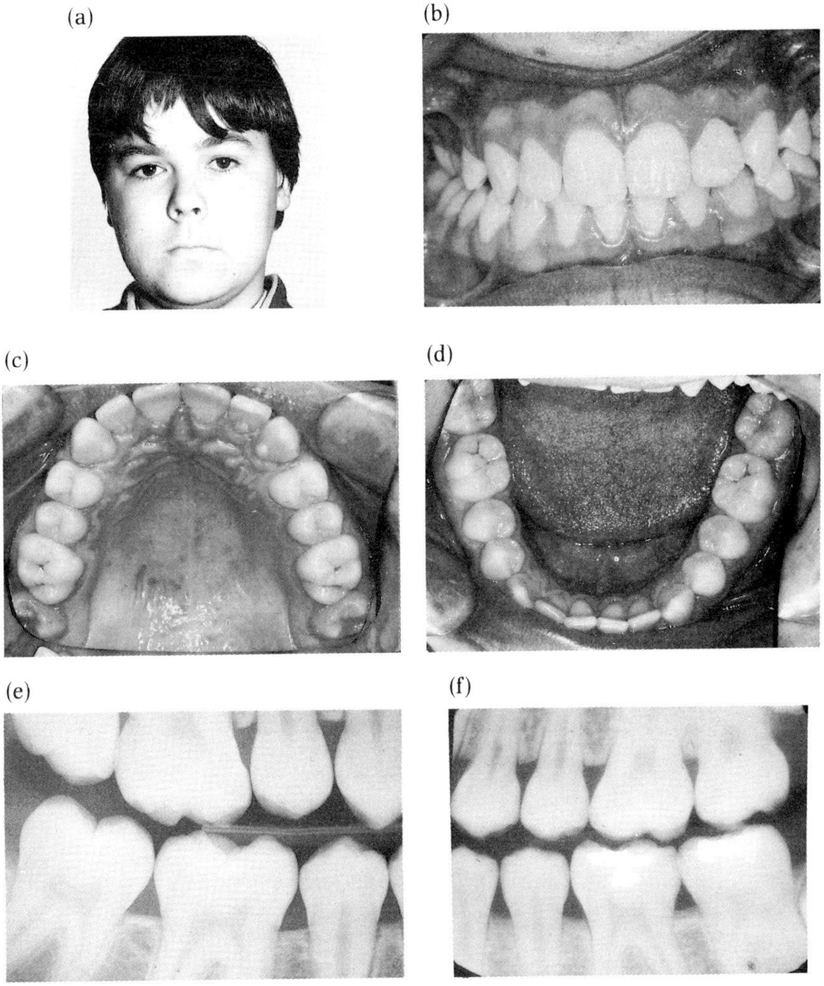

Fig. 15.12. (a) facial appearance of a 13-year-old patient. (c) View of anterior teeth showing anterior teeth well aligned. (c) Occlusal view of upper arch: a small amount of staining is evident in the fissures of the upper first permanent molars, but these teeth have been fissure-sealed. (d) Occlusal view of lower arch: the lower first permanent molars have been fissure-sealed with a clear sealant. (e) Bitewing radiographs of this patient showing a caries-free dentition.

Table 15.16. Prevalence of edentulousness in various European countries (WHO 1986)

	Per cent edentulous	
Country	**35–44 yrs.**	**65+ yrs.**
Austria	—	30
Denmark	8.0	60
Finland	15.0	65
GDR	0.5	58
Hungary	—	18
Ireland	12.0	72
Malta	—	50
Morocco	2.8	—
Netherlands	18.0	70
Poland	13.5	—
Portugal	2.0	—
Sweden	1.0	20
Switzerland	—	25
United Kingdom	13.0	79

Table 15.17. Mean number of sound, decayed and treated teeth among adults with some natural teeth in England and Wales (Todd and Walker 1980)

Tooth condition	1968	1978
Sound and untreated	12.8	13.2
Crowned or bridged	0.1	0.3
Filled (otherwise sound)	6.8	7.8
Filled, and decayed, or not restorable	2.2	1.9
Missing	10.1	8.8

Table 15.18. Missing teeth per person, age 35–44 years (WHO 1986)

Czechoslovakia	8.0
Denmark	4.5
Finland	15.0
GDR	5.0
Hungary	13.0
Ireland	10.6
Malta	6.5
Morocco	7.3
Netherlands	9.9
Portugal	6.7
Spain	5.6
Sweden	5.0
Switzerland	5.0
United Kingdom	9.2

ent molars in a 7-year-old child, it is very easy to feel that caries will inevitably occur in all first permanent molars, and that the patient is caries-susceptible. However, if by fissure sealing and oral hygiene instruction those same surfaces can be kept free from amalgams, the same child when 13 years of age, with all premolar and second molar teeth in occlusion, is labelled caries-immune. The bitewings show a caries-free dentition (Fig 15.12(e), (f)) and with reasonable oral hygiene it can be predicted that this patient will keep his teeth for life with the minimum of restorative treatment being required.

National Surveys of Adult Dental Health

(i) Prevalence of edentulousness

The standard of dental health in a country depends in part on the attitude of the population to dental care, and the resources available for dental treatment. There is also a historical perspective in that treatment available to a population in the past often makes itself felt in the statistics of the present. For example, the 'management' of periodontal disease in the 1930s–1950s in the United Kingdom by the extraction of teeth and the provision of dentures has resulted in a high prevalence of edentulousness. The finding in the first national survey in England and Wales carried out in 1968 (Gray *et al.* 1970), that 37 per cent of adults over the age of 16 years had no natural teeth, certainly focused attention on the dental needs of adults. Even if the pattern of dental treatment changed immediately from extraction towards restoration and prevention, those already rendered edentulous will feature in the statistics until they die. A summary of edentulousness in various European countries (WHO 1986) shows the United Kingdom almost at the bottom of the list in terms of edentulousness at two age groups (Table 15.16).

(ii) The dentate population

Two factors, regional variations and dental attendance, were found to affect the dental health of dentate adults in the 1968 survey in England and Wales (Gray *et al.* 1970). Considering the 16–34-year-olds with some natural teeth, the best group, in terms of the number of standing teeth, was from London and the South-East, who attended regularly at the dentist. The worst group were those from the North, who attended only when having trouble. However, there was a higher proportion of people in the North with sound and untreated teeth, compared with those in London and the South East, who had many more restored teeth, particularly in the premolar region (Fig. 15.13). The report found no evidence to suggest that there were major differences in the occurrence of tooth decay among the regions of England and felt that the reasons for the variations found between London and the North, regular and irregular attenders, was due partly to a difference in the attitudes of patients to dental health and treatment, and partly to a difference in the treatment given by dentists.

Ten years later, the 1978 survey (Todd and Walker 1980) again enabled a

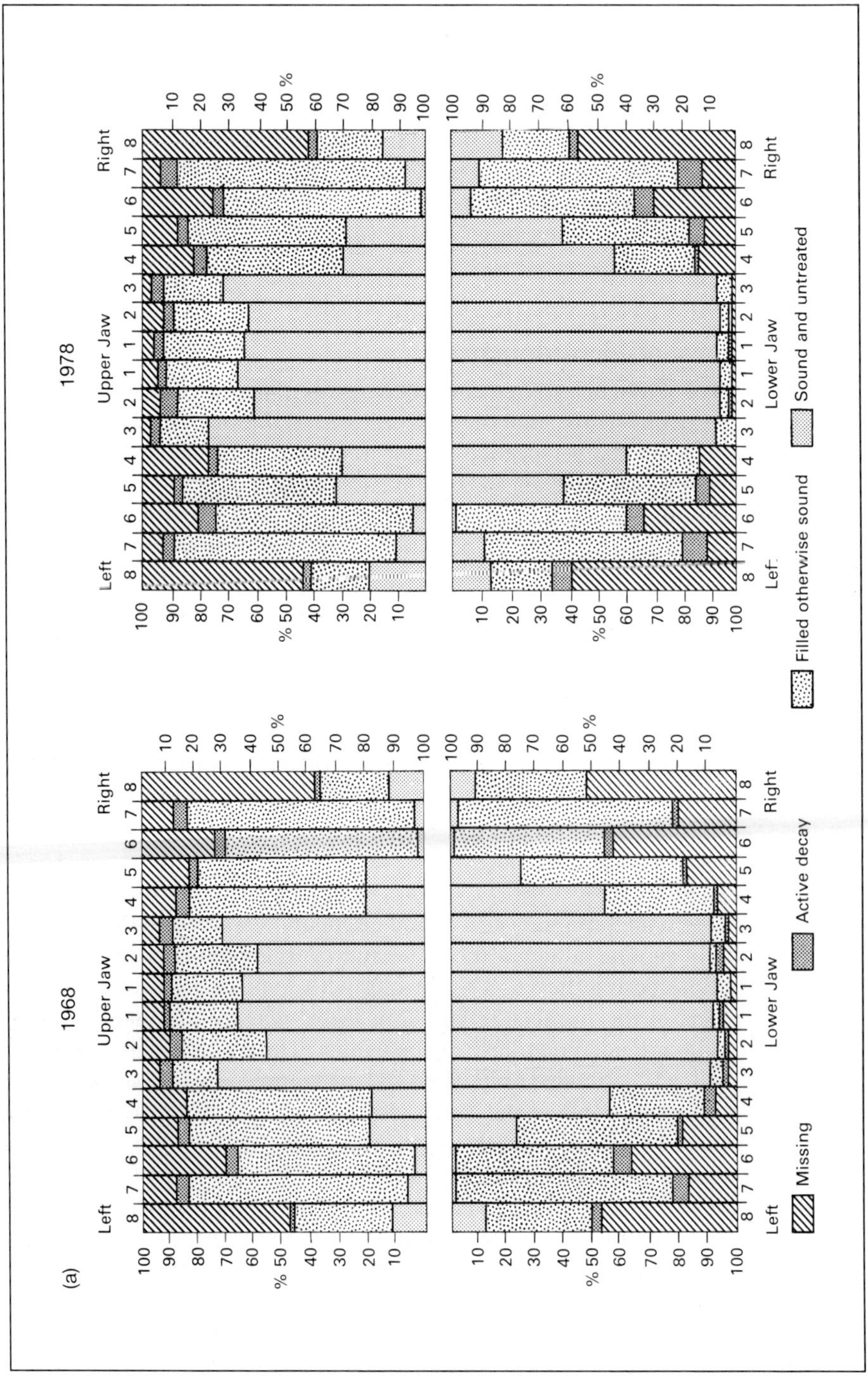
(a)
1968
1978
Upper Jaw
Lower Jaw
Left
Right
Missing
Active decay
Filled otherwise sound
Sound and untreated

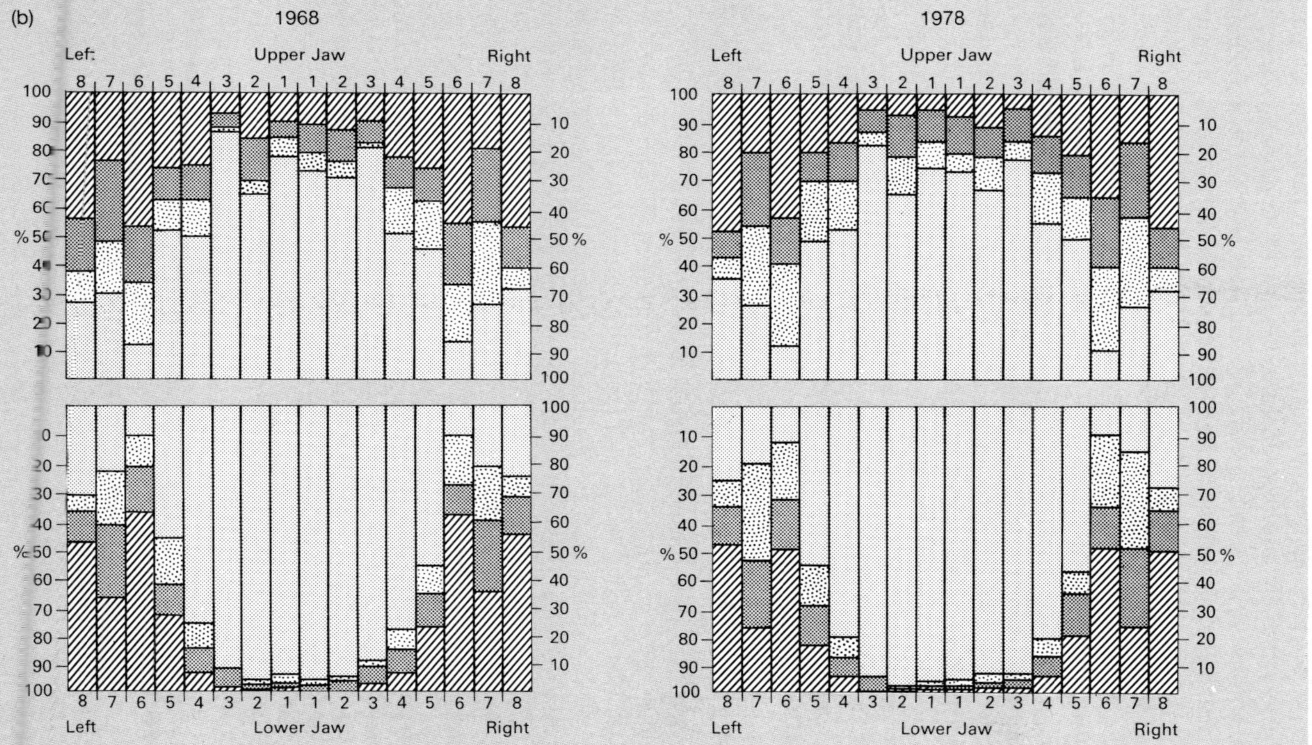

Fig. 15.13. The distribution of tooth conditions (missing, active decay, filled otherwise sound, sound, and untreated) around the mouth for adults, aged 16–34 years, with some natural teeth. A comparison of two subgroups, those from (a) London and South-East, who attend for a regular check up and (b) those from the North, who attend only when having trouble, for 1968 and 1978. (Reproduced by kind permission of Miss Todd and OPCS.)

comparison to be made between the same groups of regular and irregular attenders. These data are also reproduced in Fig. 15.13. Comparing these two subgroups, 10 years apart, it can be seen that relatively little has changed in the pattern of dental care for dentate adults. In the London and South-East regular attenders there is a slightly higher proportion of sound, untreated teeth and a small decrease in the proportion of filled teeth among premolars and wisdom teeth. In the 'worst group'—young dentate adults in the North who only go to the dentist when they are having trouble, the level of untreated decay was still very high, but there was a slight increase in the number of molar teeth that had been filled rather than extracted. Overall, very little change had occurred in the mean number of sound, decayed and treated teeth among adults with some natural teeth in England and Wales between 1968 and 1978 (Table 15.17).

The position of the United Kingdom in comparison to the rest of Europe in terms of missing teeth in dentate adults, aged 35–44 years, is shown in Table 15.18. The worst figure (15.0) was found in Finland and the best figure (4.5) in Denmark. On the basis of this table the UK is in the middle band with respect to missing teeth in dentate adults.

Conclusion

The important reduction in caries observed in children should now begin to be seen in statistics for young adults. This will only occur if both dentists' and patients' attitudes to dental health and treatment change. If caries is declining, real improvements in the number of sound teeth should be seen. This change will be accelerated if emphasis can be directed onwards from restoration to prevention.

References

Anderson, R.J. (1981*a*). The changes in dental health of 12-year-old school children in two Somerset schools. A review after an interval of 15 years. *Br. dent. J.* **150**, 354–6.

Anderson, R.J., Bradnock, G., and James, P.M.C. (1981*b*). The change in dental health of 12-year-old school children in Shropshire. A review after an interval of 15 years. *Br. dent. J.* **150**, 278–81.

Anderson, R.J. (1981*c*). The changes in the dental health of 12-year-old school children resident in a naturally fluoridated area of Gloucestershire. A review after an interval of 15 years. *Br. dent. J.* **150**, 354–6.

Andlaw, R.J., Burchell, C.K., and Tucker, G.J. (1982). Comparison of dental health of 11-year-old children in 1970 and 1979 and of 14-year-old children in 1973 and 1979: studies in Bristol, England. *Caries Res.* **16**, 257–64.

Burton, V.J., Rob, M.I., Craig, G.G., and Lawson, J.S. (1984). Changes in the caries experience of 12-year-old Sydney school children between 1963 and 1982. *Med. J. Australia* **140**, 405–7.

FDI (1985). *Changing patterns of oral health*, Commission on Oral Health, Research and Epidemiology, Joint FDI/WHO Working Group 5, 72nd Annual World Dental Congress, Helsinki, Finland (August 1984).

Glass, R.L. (ed). (1982). *The first international conference on the declining prevalence of dental caries. J. dent. Res.* **61** (spec. iss.), 1301–83.

Gray, P.G., Todd, J.E., Slack, G.L., and Bulman, J.S. (1970). *Adult dental health in England and Wales in 1968*. HMSO, London.

HMSO (1954). *Health of the school child*, Report of the Chief Medical Officer of the Ministry of Education for the years 1952 and 1953. London.

HMSO (1958). Health of the school child, Report of the Chief Medical Officer of the Ministry of Education for the years 1956 and 1957. London.

HMSO (1960). Health of the school child, Report of the Chief Medical Officer of the Ministry of Education for the years 1958 and 1958. London.

HMSO (1962). Health of the school child, Report of the Chief Medical Officer of the Ministry of Education for the years 1960 and 1961. London.

HMSO (1964). Health of the school child, Report of the Chief Medical Officer of the Department of Education and Science for the years 1962 and 1963. London.

Holt, R.D., Joels, D., and Winter, G.B. (1982). Caries in pre-school children. *Br. dent. J.* **153**, 107–9.

Jackson, D. (1974). Caries experience in English children and young adults during the years 1947–1972. *Br. dent. J.* **137**, 91–8.

Kalsbeek, H. (1982). Evidence of decrease in prevalence of dental caries in the Netherlands: an evaluation of epidemiological caries survey on 4–6 and 11–15-year old children between 1965 and 1980. *J. dent. Res.* **61** (spec. iss.), 1321–6.

Miller, A.J., Brunelle, J.A., Carlos, J.P., and Scott, D.B. (1981). *The prevalence of dental caries in United States children 1979–80*. National Institute of Dental Research, U.S. Department of Health and Human Services, Public Health Service, National Institutes of Health.

Palmer, J.D. (1980). Dental health in children—an improving picture? *Br. dent. J.* **149**, 48–50.

Renson, C.E. (1986). Changing patterns of dental caries: a survey of 20 countries. *Ann. Acad. Med. Singapore*. **15**, 284–98.

Schanschieff Report (1986). *Report of the Committee of Enquiry into Unnecessary Dental Treatment*. HMSO, London.

Silver, D.H. (1982). Improvements in the dental health of 3-year-old Hertfordshire children after 8 years. *Br. dent. J.* **153**, 179–82.

Todd, J.E. (1975). *Children's dental health in England and Wales 1973*. HMSO, London.

Todd, J.E. and Walker, A.M. (1980). *Adult dental health, Vol. 1, England and Wales 1968–1978*. HMSO, London.

Todd, J.E. and Dodd, T. (1985). *Children's dental health in the United Kingdom in 1988*. HMSO, London.

Waldman, B.H. (1987). Increasing use of dental services by very young children. *J. dent. Child.* **54**, 248–50.

Winter, G.B., Rule, D.C., Marker, G.P., James, P.M.C., and Gordon, P.H. (1971). The prevalence of dental caries in pre-school children aged 1 to 4 years. *Br. dent. J.* **130**, 271–7; 434–6.

World Health Organization (1986). *Country profiles on oral health in Europe 1986*. WHO, Geneva.

16

Resources, treatment, and prevention

J. J. Murray

THERE is a dynamic relationship between the natural history of any disease and the response by society in trying to combat the problem. As far as dental disease is concerned, in Britain and in many other countries, the original response to a carious tooth was to extract it. Historically this was usually a painful and hazardous procedure performed by poorly trained operators. Society's response was to encourage the development of professional skills and to allow the practice of dentistry to be limited to those who had received appropriate professional training. As knowledge and skill increased, attention turned to the preservation of teeth and the treatment of caries by restoration rather than extraction. This trend from extraction to restoration depended not only on the skill of the dental profession but also on the reaction of society with respect to the economic resources that individuals and government were prepared to commit to dental treatment, and the attitude of individuals to the advice proffered by professionals. Real improvements in health can only occur when both the community at large and the health professionals share the same objectives, which surely should be the primary prevention of disease.

Simplistically, the progress of dentistry can be represented as one in which there is movement from extraction to restoration and onwards to prevention (Fig. 16.1). The main thrust of this book has been to gather together information on diet, fluoridation, preventive measures for the individual, and oral hygiene, all of which would have an effect on the prevention of the two main dental diseases, caries and periodontal disease. But it would be facile to assume that these measures alone can exert a beneficial effect without appreciating that they can only work within a favourable framework agreed by society. Patients' attitude, dentist's attitude, remuneration and manpower all have a crucial role to play in the prevention of dental disease.

In the 1940s the major dental treatment option in the United Kingdom was extraction, but in the 1950s and 1960s there was a definite shift towards restoration. A number of factors were responsible for this change in direction. The introduction of high-speed rotor cutting instruments revolutionized restorative dentistry and, in particular, enabled more complex restorative procedures,

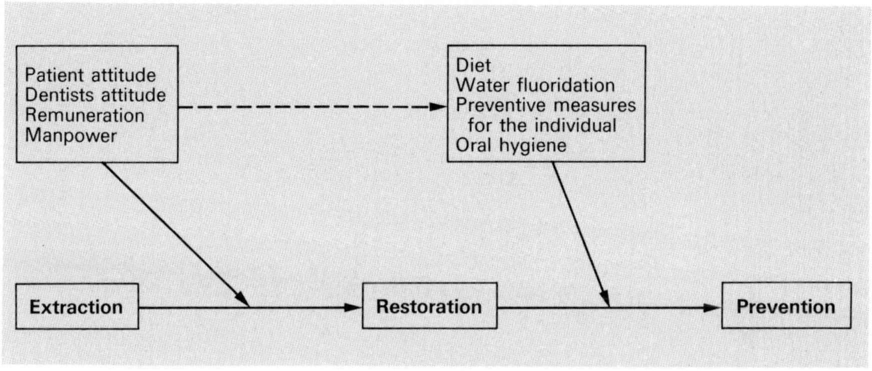

Fig. 16.1. Factors affecting changes in dental treatment and prevention.

crowns, and bridgework to be completed more quickly, and with less discomfort to the patient. The attitude of the patient has certainly changed—to give just one example, in 1968 27 per cent of adults with some teeth found the thought of full dentures very upsetting, (Gray *et al.* 1970) whereas in 1978 the figure had almost doubled to 48 per cent (Todd and Walker 1980).

The interaction between dentists' attitude and remuneration can be seen by examining the changes in the pattern of dental treatment carried out in the general dental services in England and Wales over the last 35 years. The uptake of more complex restorative procedures—crowns, bridges, endodontic treatment—has occurred partly because of the increasing technical skills acquired by the dental profession and partly because the regulations of the Dental Estimates Board (DEB) have expanded so that more complex restorative procedures have been allowed within the National Health Service (Fig. 16.2).

The number of permanent teeth extracted in the general dental services has fallen from nearly 18 million in 1950 to 3.7 million in 1985. The number of general anaesthetics has fallen at a similar rate, from 1.5 million in 1955 to 433 000 in 1986. The provision of dentures (and this includes remaking dentures for those rendered edentulous many years ago) has fallen from its high point of almost 3 million in 1950 to a plateau of approximately 1.25 million in the 1980s (Fig. 16.2).

The habit of regular attendance at the dentist was one of the factors reported by the Adult Dental Health Surveys to be of significance to the dental conditions of adults. Since the inception of the NHS the number of dental exminations (Fig. 16.2) has increased steadily each year and, in 1985, reached 30 million (this examination, until changes in regulations by the Government in 1988, was free as far as the patient was concerned). The number of amalgam and synthetic restorations increased extremely rapidly in the 1950s and 60s, reaching a peak of 32 million in 1975. Over the last 10 years this particular aspect of treatment has reduced. What are the reasons for this? Could it be that the fall in caries noticed in children is coming through with young adults and so fewer teeth need to be

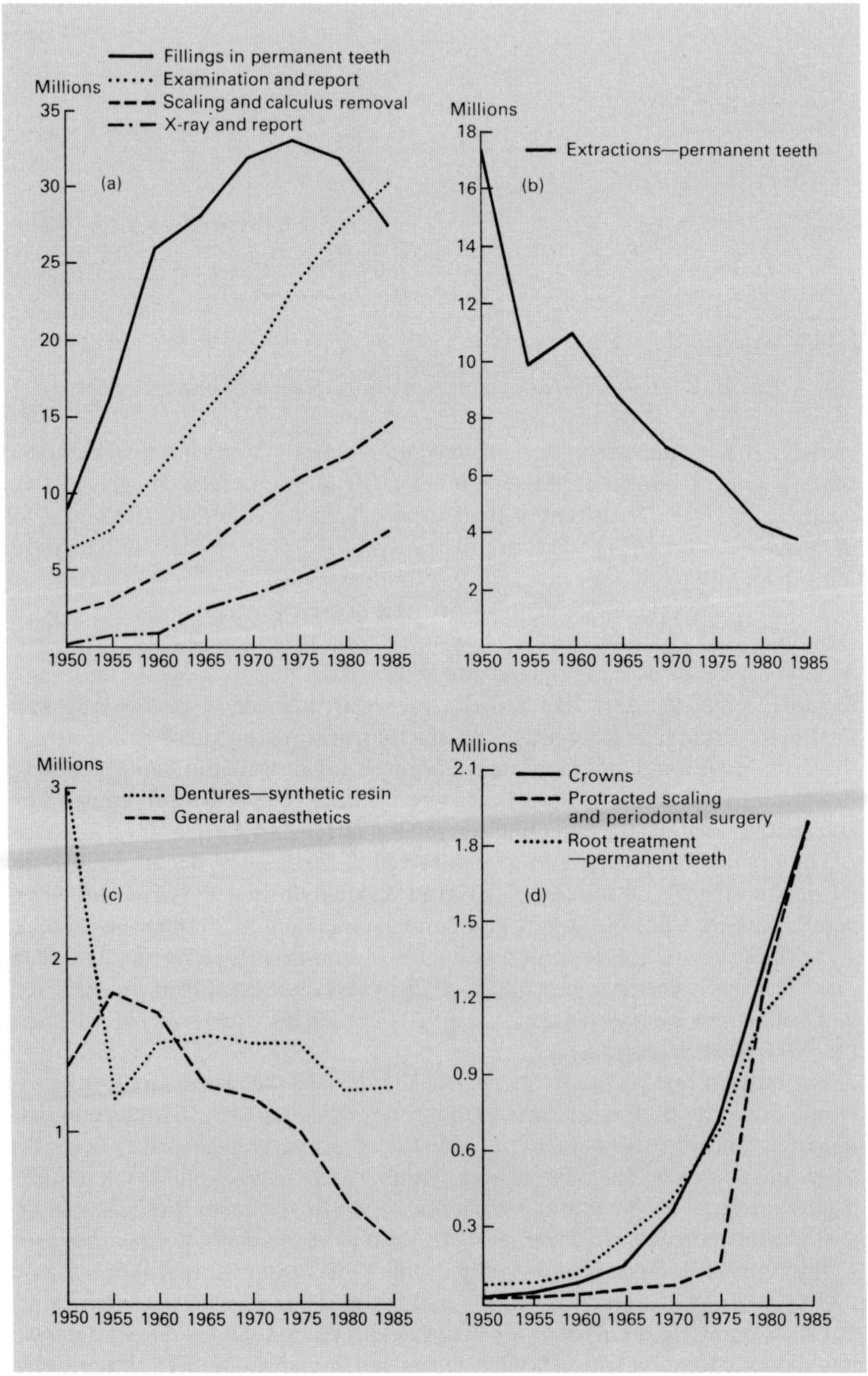

Fillings in permanent teeth
Examination and report
Scaling and calculus removal
X-ray and report
Millions
35
30
25
20
15
10
5
(a)
1950 1955 1960 1965 1970 1975 1980 1985
Millions
18
16
14
12
10
8
6
4
2
Extractions—permanent teeth
(b)
1950 1955 1960 1965 1970 1975 1980 1985
Millions
3
2
1
Dentures—synthetic resin
General anaesthetics
(c)
1950 1955 1960 1965 1970 1975 1980 1985
Millions
2.1
1.8
1.5
1.2
0.9
0.6
0.3
Crowns
Protracted scaling and periodontal surgery
Root treatment —permanent teeth
(d)
1950 1955 1960 1965 1970 1975 1980 1985

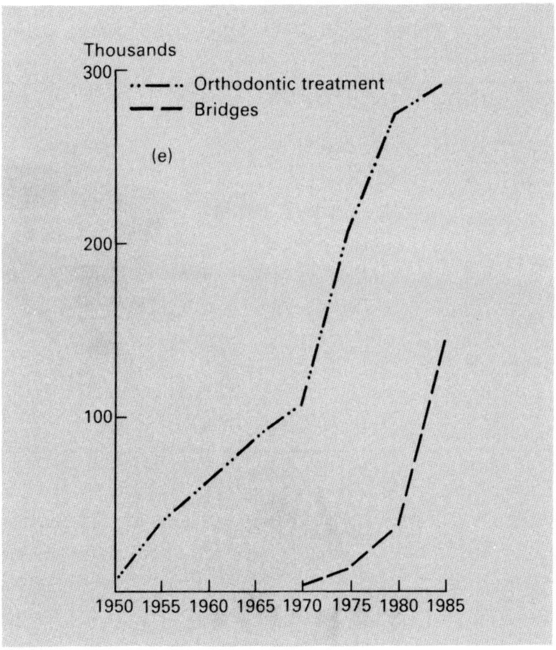

Fig. 16.2. The changing pattern of dental treatment in the general dental services of the National Health Service in England and Wales, 1950–1985. (By kind permission of the Chairman of the Dental Estimates Board.)

restored? Is there a change of attitude on the part of the dentist, who is becoming more aware that the 'repair of repair'—replacing fillings with new fillings—is not as vitally important as it may have been thought in the past? Are patient charges having an effect in that as patients have to pay an increasing amount for NHS dental treatment, they are beginning to resist simple restorative treatment?

Elderton and Davies (1984), in their follow-up study of dental treatment provided in the General Dental Service for 720 randomly selected dentate adults in Scotland, showed that overall 66 per cent of the surfaces restored over a 5-year period were replacement restorations. They also reported that 12 per cent of the sample were recipients of half of all the restorative treatment and commented: 'It seems that once a person has a number of teeth filled, he tends to have an ever increasing commitment to receiving further restorative treatment. It would seem that the 12 per cent are a high risk group—at high risk of having their teeth re-filled'. They concluded that owing to the general decline in caries prevalence it may well be that many morphologically imperfect restorations do not now warrant replacement. If dentists and the dental service understood the characteristics of restorative care provided, it might be possible to slow down the cycle of replacement restorations by employing a more selective approach when deciding which restorations should be placed.

More complex restorative treatment in the general dental services increased very slowly in the 1950s and 60s, but the rate of change increased dramatically

Table 16.1. Cost of various items of dental treatment in the general dental services of the National Health Service in England and Wales for children aged 0–15 years (Dental Estimates Board Annual Report 1980/1986)

	1980		1986	
	£m	per cent	£m	per cent
Examination and X-rays	19.4	31.0	34.1	33.9
Restoration of teeth				
(i) deciduous	6.0	10.0	9.0	8.9
(ii) permanent	16.0	26.0	16.8	16.7
Dentures	0.3	0.5	0.3	0.3
Periodontal treatment	4.6	7.5	11.6	11.5
Extractions, other surgical treatment (except periodontal), and general anaesthetics	3.8	6.0	7.5	7.5
Orthodontics	12.0	19.0	21.3	21.2
Total	62.1	100.0	100.6	100.0

in the 1970s and 80s (Fig. 16.2). Over 2 million teeth were crowned, 1.4 million teeth were root-treated, and 156 000 bridges were placed in 1986. How much are these increases due to changing patient attitudes so that they are now demanding a more sophisticated service, or to dentists realizing that it is more profitable and satisfying to provide more complex restorative treatment?

The emphasis on restoration of teeth has, in a sense, overshadowed the need for the treatment of malocclusion, especially in children. It has been suggested that about 50 per cent of British children have malocclusions sufficiently severe as to warrant orthodontic treatment, but only about half of these children receive treatment (Todd 1975; Todd and Dodd 1985). Although the total cost of orthodontic treatment in the General Dental Services was £23 million in 1986 or 3 per cent of the total (see Chapter 1), the vast majority of this treatment is completed by the time children have reached 15 years of age. A summary of the cost of the service to children, aged 0–15 years, in the General Dental Services only, (Table 16.1) shows that, in 1980, 35 per cent of the fees were for the treatment of caries, compared with 19 per cent for the treatment of malocclusion, whereas in 1986, the restoration of teeth accounted for 25.6 per cent of the cost and orthodontic treatment had increased slightly to 21.2 per cent of the total cost in this age group.

Government financial policy may also have an impact on dental treatment. The number of dental examinations in the general dental services in England and Wales has risen steadily every year since the inception of the National Health Service. In 1986 dentists were paid for 30.6 million 'examinations and report' by the DEB. This part of dental treatment was free as far as the patient was concerned. In 1987 the Government announced in its White Paper *Promoting Better Health* (HMSO 1987) that the dental examination was now to be included in fees paid for by the patient, although children, expectant nursing mothers, and those receiving social security payments, would still receive all

Table 16.2. Studies concerning the general dental services in England and Wales (from D. Scarrott, personal Communication 1988)

Year	Number of dentists	Total treatment cost £m	Patients' contributions £m	Treatment cost for exchequer £m	1987 (4) £m	Average cost per GDP at 1987 prices £m
1950	9657 (1)	40.6 (2)	— (3)	40.6	492.5	51 000
1955	9788	33.3	7.1	26.1	241.8	24 700
1960	10 254	50.6	9.2	41.4	337.5	32 900
1965	10 405	59.0	11.2	47.8	329.1	31 600
1970	10 843	90.3	16.5	73.8	406.5	37 500
1975	11 737	191.4	32.2	159.2	474.3	40 400
1980	13 039	410.2	93.9	316.3	481.8	37 000
1985	15 076	667.6	198.1	469.5	505.7	33 500
1987	15 545	811.7	244.2	567.5	567.5	36 500

(1) At end of year, to 1960; at September 30 from 1965.
(2) Treatment fees only—that is, the total cost of the general dental services apart from employers' superannuation contributions and (from 1970) seniority payments.
(3) Contributions actually paid, net of remitted charges for low-income patients.
(4) Exchequer cost at 1987 prices inflating by the retail prices index (all items).

their dental treatment free. The patient will now pay a proportion of the total cost of dental examination and treatment. It will be interesting to see whether this policy change will influence the number of dental examinations in the general dental services in the coming years, and whether the change affects the quality of adult dental health in the long term.

Much more emphasis is now placed on the management of periodontal disease. Scaling and calculus removal approached the 15 million mark in 1985, and protracted scaling and periodontal surgery has rocketed from 1975 (100 000) to almost 2 million courses of treatment 10 years later, helped by changes in the narrative of the DEB (Table 16.2).

The changes in the DEB regulations, which gave dental practitioners greater opportunity to engage in more complex restorative and periodontal procedures, certainly helped to emphasize the importance of preservation as against extraction. The statistics reflect a situation where the dentist's attitude and remuneration, and the patient's attitude or acceptance of the treatment suggested, react together to produce change. In addition, manpower and the availability of dental services also play an important part in helping to promote the trend from extraction to restoration. The number of dental practitioners in the general dental services in England and Wales has grown from 9359 in 1955 to 15 076 in 1985. More dentists serving a community should allow more time to be spent on the preservation of the dentition rather than extracting teeth.

The cost of treatment in the general dental services in 1987 was £753 million (Table 1.1), of which almost 50 per cent was paid for fillings, crowns, bridges, and root canal therapy. This is apparently a very significant increase on the sum of £420.2 million for 1980. Four points should, however, be borne in mind: first, the rate of inflation; second, the fact that increasingly sophisticated treatment

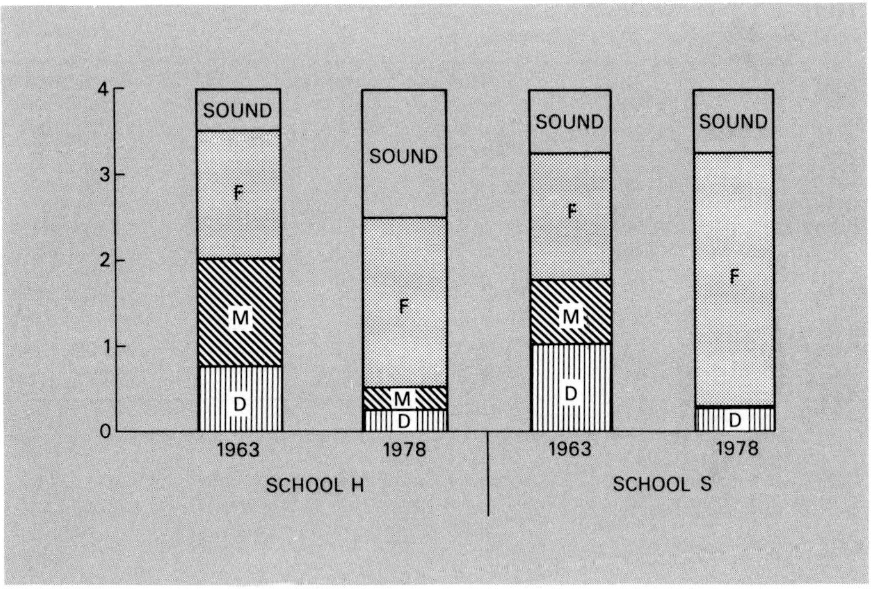

Fig. 16.3. The average number of decayed, missing, filled, and sound first permanent molars of 12-year-old children from two schools examined in 1963 and 1978. (With permision of the Editor, *British Dental Journal*.)

means higher laboratory costs; third, the number of dentists had increased by more than 2000 (from 13 039 to 15 256) between 1980 and 1986; fourth, patient charges contribute substantially to the total sum.

The number of dentists in the general dental services, total treatment cost, patient contributions, and the net amount received by GDPs, having been standardized for inflation, from 1950 to 1987, are given in Table 16.2. These data show that although the total treatment cost has increased from £40.6 million in 1950 to over £800 million in 1987, the real cost per GDP, that is, the mean annual sum each dental practitioner receives from the DEB, has not changed a great deal in real terms over the last 27 years. Constraints on public expenditure mean that any new initiative in health has to be looked at carefully, but how will the next movement, from restoration onwards to prevention, be achieved?

First, dental attitudes to the management of the dentition need to change. Anderson (1981) reported the changes in dental health of 12-year-old children from two Somerset schools over a 15-year period. Dental caries prevalence had fallen by 35 per cent. One interesting finding from the survey of the two schools was that the DMF had fallen much more in one school than the other; the difference was most marked in the DMF values for first permanent molars (Figure 16.3) In both schools the amount of untreated decay had fallen dramatically and the need for extracting first permanent molars had been reduced almost to zero, but the number of fillings had increased slightly in one school and virtually doubled in the other school. In the first school, dental treatment was provided by the same practitioners as 15 years ago, but there had been a marked change in the provision of general dental services in the catchment area of the second school, with the opening of new multi-practitioner surgeries. Anderson (1981) pointed out that if carious lesions have been prevented, the dental profession must not spoil the situation by continuing to fill occlusal surfaces in teeth which may not become carious. He suggested that dentists' attitudes should change and that the maxim 'If in doubt fill' should be changed to 'If in doubt, wait', especially for occlusal fissures of the permanent dentition of younger children. It is now known that dental caries is not simply a process of demineralization but an alternating process of destruction and repair. Once a cavity has formed, repair will not 'fill up the hole', but if caries can be detected in its earliest stage, clinician and educated patient can then combine their efforts to ensure that operative intervention is not required. Unless practitioner and informed patient have the courage to 'watch the early lesion' they will never know whether prevention would have been preferable to restoration (see Chapter 6, p. 239).

Second, just as restorative dentistry gained an increasing share of the general dental services' cake in the 1970s and 80s, so measures aimed to prevent disease need to be given more resources in the next phase of the development of dental services. Until 1986 GDPs received no payment for applying topical fluorides or fissure sealants. Now a fee is allowed for topical fluoride therapy and fissure sealants may be applied, having received prior approval, for children with special needs. The introduction of a capitation scheme will give practitioners the opportunity to practise preventive measures and so help to tip the balance from restoration to prevention. The provision of resources are essential if the goal to reduce dental caries still further is to be realized.

What is a realistic objective to aim for with respect to the prevention of dental disease? The World Health Organization and the International Dental Federation have proposed that the following indicators of improved oral health should be adopted, covering the young, the mature, and the elderly (WHO 1982):

The following global goals for the year 2000 are proposed:

Goal 1. 50 per cent of 5–6-year olds will be caries free.

Goal 2. The global average will be no more than 3 DMF teeth at 12 years of age.

Goal 3. 85 per cent of the population should retain all their teeth at age 18.

Goal 4. A 50 per cent reduction in present levels of edentulousness at age 35 to 44 will be achieved.

Goal 5. A 25 per cent reduction in present levels of edentulousness at age 65 and over will be achieved.

Goal 6. A data-based system for monitoring changes in oral health will be established.

According to the Child Dental Health Survey figures for England (Todd 1985), about 51 per cent of 5-year-olds are caries-free, and the mean DMF for 12-year-olds is 2.9 teeth. This means that the first two goals suggested by the FDI for the year 2000 have already been reached in England. However, there is still no room for complacency. Even with the reduction in caries noted in the 1983 survey, the impact of dental caries on British children is still unacceptable. By the age of 8 years, 27 per cent of children were reported to have had teeth extracted under a general anaesthetic, and by the age of 15 the figure had risen to 49 per cent. Even accepting that some of these in the 8–15-year age group were orthodontic extractions, the stigma of caries is still casting far too long a shadow over a large proportion of our children. By the year 2000 90 per cent of our 5-year-old children should be caries-free, and the mean DMF rate for 12-year-old children should be no higher than 1.0 DMFT. These objectives would be better than the first two global goals suggested by FDI and would enable more resources to be allocated to the treatment of traumatized anterior teeth, the management of malocclusion, and the prevention of periodontal disease in children. However, if the decline in the prevalence of dental caries is to continue, more emphasis on the prevention of dental disease will be required. Two recent studies (Holt *et al.* 1988; Rugg-Gunn *et al.* 1988) have reported little change in caries levels in young English children between 1980 and 1986.

The next three goals suggested by the FDI depend very heavily on the successful prevention of periodontal breakdown. The prospect of absolute periodontal health on a large scale is remote as it requires the widespread adoption of meticulous plaque control. A more realistic objective is the reduction in the rate of progress of periodontal disease to a level compatible with tooth survival for life. The success of standardized programmes of professional tooth cleaning and oral hygiene education, such as that described by Suomi *et al.* (1971), show that this may be achieved when resources are made available to interested patients. The benefits of this approach, however, can only apply to individuals who present themselves to a dentist who recognizes the value of a plaque-control programme. A further drawback to the dentist-based approach to periodontal care is the excessive consumption of time and resources involved. These factors, therefore, suggest that a satisfactory community-based strategy of periodontal care must be developed before the benefits will be enjoyed by the population as a whole.

In the United Kingdom there has been a welcome reduction in the percentage of the adult population who are edentulous. In the 15-year period between 1968 and 1983 the proportion of the population in England and Wales age 16 years and over who had no natural teeth fell from 37 per cent to 25 per cent. This was in part due to changing attitudes on the part of the public and the dental profession, and the increased opportunity to carry out restorative and periodontal treatment in the general dental service. Nevertheless, there is still a long way to go before the prevalence of edentulousness in the United Kingdom falls to the levels enjoyed by other countries, for example, Scandinavia, Japan, and America.

Although some aspects of this book have discussed pevention mainly in the United Kingdom context, most of the information in this book applies to dental disease world-wide. The reports of a fall in caries and improvement in the level of gingivitis in North America, the United Kingdom, and much of northern Europe and in Australasia indicates that dental disease is preventable on a country-wide scale. More disturbing are the reports of the increase in dental caries prevalence in the developing countries of the world, and it is obligatory that information on prevention of dental disease is available to those in charge of their dental services. The delivery of dental care to the community was considered by a WHO expert committee in 1985 (WHO 1987). In their document they pointed out that all the member states of WHO have adopted the goal of health for all by the year 2000, and all national oral-health care systems must take their share of responsibility in efforts to meet this goal. In their view most oral health services, while providing acceptable treatment-orientated care financed by various direct or third-party payment systems, are now faced with difficulties when a change is needed in order to provide a preventive-orientated service and different restorative care to deal with rapidly changing levels of oral disease, social patterns, and priorities. 'Profound changes are needed not only in the type of care offered and in the way it is provided, but also in the way providers are trained, employed, supervised and supported. Yet in all the major industrialized countries, as well as a number of developing countries, there now exist deeply entrenched systems which have evolved over many decades and which represent security and continuity to those working within them. There is therefore an understandable reluctance to change even when the need for change is overwhelmingly evident.' They concluded that there is a need to revise financing systems so as to improve rewards for effective prevention and care, and to facilitate access and coverage.

The aim of this book has been to draw together the available evidence concerning the prevention of dental caries and periodontal disease. There is no doubt that, even on the basis of our present knowledge concerning the pathogenesis of dental diseases, if this information were put into practice, a vast amount of dental disease afflicting the Western World in particular could be eliminated, and much unnecessary suffering could be prevented. If this is to be achieved, the dental profession must extend its horizons beyond the traditional role of clinical, diagnostic, and technical expertise for individual patients in the surgery, and become more aware of the psychological and social factors relevant to the prevention of dental disease.

References

Anderson, R.J. (1981). The changes in the dental health of 12-year-old school children in two Somerset schools. *Br. dent. J.* **150**, 218–21.

Annual Reports, Dental Estimates Board 1950–1986.

Elderton, R.J. and Davies, J.A. (1984). Restorative dental treatment in the general dental service in Scotland. *Br. dent. J.* **157**, 196–200.

Gray, P.G., Todd, J.E., Slack, G.L., and Bulman, J.S. (1970). *Adult dental health in England and Wales 1968*. HMSO, London.

HMSO (1987). *Promoting better health*. White Paper. The Governments programme for improving primary health care. HMSO, London.

Holt, R.D., Joels, D., Bulman, J., and Maddick, I.H. (1988). A third study of caries in pre-school aged children in Camden. *Br. dent. J.* **165**, 87–91.

Rugg-Gunn, A.J., Carmichael, C.L., and Ferrell, R.S. (1988). Effect of fluoridation and secular trend in caries in 5-year-old children living in Newcastle and Northumberland. *Br. dent. J.* **165**, 359–64.

Suomi, J.D., Greene, J.C., Vermillion, J.R., Doyle, J., Chang, J.J., and Leatherwood, E.C. (1971). The effect of controlled oral hygiene procedures on the progression of periodontal disease in adults: results after third and final year. *J. Perio.* **42**, 152.

Todd, J.E. (1975). *Children's dental health in England and Wales 1973*. HMSO, London.

Todd, J.E. and Dodd, T. (1985). *Children's dental health in England and Wales 1983*. HMSO, London.

Walker, A.M. and Dodd, P. (1980). *Adult dental health United Kingdom 1978*, Vol. 2. HMSO, London.

World Health Organization (1982). Goal for oral health in the year 2000. *Br. dent. J.* **152**, 21–2.

World Health Organization (1987). *Alternative systems of oral care delivery*. Technical Report Series 750. Geneva.

INDEX

Abbreviatons: APF = acidulated phosphofluoride; DMF = decayed, missing, filled; GMA = bis-glycidyl-methacrylate; GTF = glucosyltransferase.